Rehabilitation
Nursing Practice

D1128783

NOTICE

Medicine is an ever-changing science. As new research and clinical experience broaden our knowledge, changes in treatment and drug therapy are required. The editors and the publisher of this work have checked with sources believed to be reliable in their efforts to provide information that is complete and generally in accord with the standards accepted at the time of publication. However, in view of the possibility of human error or changes in medical sciences, neither the editors nor the publisher nor any other party who has been involved in the preparation or publication of this work warrants that the information contained herein is in every respect accurate or complete, and they are not responsible for any errors or omissions or for the results obtained from use of such information. Readers are encouraged to confirm the information contained herein with other sources. For example and in particular, readers are advised to check the product information sheet included in the package of each drug they plan to administer to be certain that the information contained in this book is accurate and that changes have not been made in the recommended dose or in the contraindications for administration. This recommendation is of particular importance in connection with new or infrequently used drugs.

Rehabilitation Nursing Practice

Edited by

Patricia A. Chin, RN, DNSc
Associate Professor
School of Nursing
Azusa Pacific University
Azusa, California

Darlene N. Finocchiaro, RN, MS, CRRN
Lecturer and Clinical Instructor
Nursing Department
California State University, Los Angeles
Los Angeles, California

Anita Rosebrough, RN, MS, MSN, CRRN
Associate Professor
School of Nursing
Azusa Pacific University
Azusa, California

McGRAW-HILL
Health Professions Division

New York   St. Louis   San Francisco   Auckland   Bogotá
Caracas   Lisbon   London   Madrid   Mexico City   Milan   Montreal
New Delhi   San Juan   Singapore   Sydney   Tokyo   Toronto

McGraw-Hill

A Division of The McGraw·Hill Companies

Rehabilitation Nursing Practice

Copyright © 1998 by The McGraw-Hill Companies, Inc. All rights reserved. Printed in the United States of America. Except as permitted under the United States Copyright Act of 1976, no part of this publication may be reproduced or distributed in any form or by any means, or stored in a data base or retrieval system, without the prior written permission of the publisher.

1 2 3 4 5 6 7 8 9 0 DOC DOC 9 9 8 7

ISBN 0-07-105482-0

This book was set in Adobe Garamond by BiComp, Inc. The editor was John Dolan; the production supervisor was Rick Ruzycka; project management was by Spectrum Publisher Services; the cover designer and text illustrator was Acclaimed Media & Graphics. R. R. Donnelley and Sons was printer and binder.

This book is printed on acid-free paper.

Cataloging-in-publication data is on file for this title at the Library of Congress.

Contents

Section V   Generational Issues

Section VI   Transition to the Community

Contributors

Susan Arakaki, BS, OTR
Occupational Therapist II
Rancho Los Amigos Medical Center
Downey, California

Patricia A. Chin, RN, DNSc
Associate Professor
School of Nursing
Azusa Pacific University
Azusa, California

Darlene N. Finocchiaro, MS, RN, CRRN
Lecturer and Clinical Instructor
Nursing Department
California State University,
    Los Angeles
Los Angeles, California

Michael V. Finocchiaro, MD
Urologist
Rancho Los Amigos Medical Center
Downey, California

Honor Duderstadt Galloway, BS, OTR
Occupational Therapist II
Rancho Los Amigos Medical Center
Downey, California

Aloma R. Gender, MSN, RN, CRRN
Chief Operating Officer
Chief Nursing Officer
Columbia Mission Bay Hospital
San Diego, California

Shari Herzfeld, RN, MN, CRRN
Nursing Instructor
Rio Hondo College
Whittier, California

Lynda Jones, RN, BSN
Orthopedic Clinical Nurse Specialist

Riverside Community Hospital
Riverside, California

Kathryn A. S. Kumagai, PT, NCS
Physical Therapist
Western Physical Therapy
Downey, California
Neurological Clinical Specialist
Casa Colina Hospital for
    Rehabilitation
Granada Hills, California

Mary Lee Lacy, MSN, RN, CRRN
Clinical Nurse Specialist
Rehabilitation Services
Children's Hospital of Orange County
Whittier, California

Carol Lea Melvin, MSN, RN, CRRN
Spina Bifida Coordinator
Shriners' Hospital for Children,
    Los Angeles
Rancho Cucamonga, California

Kimberly D. Mory, MA, CCC-SP
Director, Adult Day Health Care
Casa Colina Centers for Rehabilitation
Pomona, California

Wendy E. B. Perez, MA, CCC-S
Associate Professor
Communication Department
Biola University
La Mirada, California

Barbara Kammerer Quayle, MA
Image & Social Skills Training
    Consultant and Seminar Leader
Seal Beach, California

Lorise Rodriguez, MSN, RN
Cardiac Educator/Disease Manager

HealthCare Partners Medical Group
Los Angeles, California

Anita Rosebrough, RN, MS, MSN, CRRN
Associate Professor
School of Nursing
Azusa Pacific University
Azusa, California

Susan McKeever Smith, RNC, MN
Associate Professor
School of Nursing
Azusa Pacific University
Azusa, California

Linda E. Swofford-Ten Eyck, RN, BSN, CRRN
Ten Eyck and Associates
San Diego, California

Shila Wiebe, RN, MSN
Assistant Professor
School of Nursing
Azusa Pacific University
Azusa, California

Elizabeth A. Yetzer, MA, MSN, CRRN
Rehabilitation Nursing Educator
(PACT) Program
Long Beach Department of Veterans
Affairs Medical Center
Long Beach, California

Robin Johnson Zableckis, BS, OTR
Occupational Therapist II
Rancho Los Amigos Medical Center
Downey, California

Preface

Rehabilitation nursing is a specialty practice area that is gaining importance in today's dynamic and ever-changing health care environment. Nurses in a variety of practice settings are required to incorporate rehabilitation concepts into everyday clinical practice. *Rehabilitation Nursing Practice* is written to acquaint the undergraduate nursing student and practicing health care professional with the basic concepts of rehabilitation nursing. It is intended to serve as an introduction to the practice of rehabilitation nursing.

This book contains six sections and 34 chapters. Each chapter begins with a list of key terms and objectives for the reader. Most chapters contain nursing interventions for specific neurological deficits, client/family teaching/learning needs, and common nursing diagnoses. Section I introduces the theoretical foundations of rehabilitation nursing, including a chapter that discusses the interdisciplinary rehabilitation team process. Section II focuses on psychological and psychosocial concepts as they relate to the client and family experiencing rehabilitative nursing care. Major neurological deficits and common rehabilitation disorders are addressed in Section III. In Section IV, the emphasis is on the self-care skills necessary to promote optimal functional living in a variety of settings. Section V discusses the developmental issues related to the concepts of pediatric rehabilitation. The final section addresses issues related to transitioning to the community and to successful community reintegration.

Acknowledgments

We the co-authors thank our clients, families, colleagues, and students for all that we have learned from them. The encouragement, support, and hard work of many people made this book possible.

As always I thank my husband, William; my daughter, Pamela; and my son, Will, for their continued love and support. I would also like to offer a special thank you to my parents, Harry and Mollie Naymick, for providing me with the foundation on which I built my life and mission of teaching and caring.

—Patricia A. Chin

I give special thanks to Pat and Anita, you were wonderful to work with; to my mom, who always encouraged me to go further in my profession; to my loving husband, Mike, who told me I could even though I didn't believe I could, to his constant love and support; to my friends, especially Mary, Yvette, and Ed, who gave me constant support; to Cheryll, who did *all* my typing; to the nursing department of California State University, Los Angeles, especially Judy, Diane, Marlene, and Marilyn, for their guidance, support, and time off when needed; and to my Lord Jesus Christ.

—Darlene N. Finocchiaro

My special gratitude goes to my husband, Radford, for his constant support and tolerance of my preoccupation with the book; and to my sons, Christopher and Mark, and their families for their support. A special thank you to Christopher for his computer graphic talents and contribution.

—Anita Rosebrough

Rehabilitation
Nursing Practice

THEORETICAL FOUNDATIONS OF PRACTICE

CHAPTER 1
Scope of Rehabilitation and Rehabilitation Nursing

Aloma R. Gender

Key Terms

Advanced Practice Rehabilitation Nurse
American Academy of Physical Medicine and Rehabilitation
Americans with Disabilities Act (ADA)
Association of Rehabilitation Nurses
Caregiver
Certified Rehabilitation Registered Nurse (CRRN)
Certified Rehabilitation Registered Nurse–Advanced (CRRN-A)
Client Advocate
Coordinator of Care
Counselor
Educator
Expert Witness
Goal
International Classification of Impairments, Disabilities, and Handicaps
Legal Consultant
Length of Stay
Philosophy
Practice Settings
Process
Rehabilitation
Rehabilitation Nursing
Rehabilitation Nursing Generalist
Researcher
Howard A. Rusk
Standards of Care
Standards of Professional Performance

Objectives

1. Describe the history of rehabilitation nursing.

2. Define the goals and philosophy of rehabilitation nursing.

3. Describe the characteristics of rehabilitation nursing and the roles of a rehabilitation nurse.

4. Identify target populations for rehabilitation nursing practice.

5. Identify various practice settings for rehabilitation nurses.

6. Describe the standards of care and practice for basic and advanced practice.

7. Identify important health care policy for persons with disabilities.

8. Describe the development of the Association of Rehabilitation Nurses.

Introduction   One nurse, in describing why she chose rehabilitation as a specialty area, stated that rehabilitation nursing is like being a "bridge over troubled waters." Another nurse said, in a lighter vein, "I don't look good in white. Rehabilitation allows me to wear street clothes or colored tops." Yet another said,

> What I like about rehabilitation nursing is the chance to interact with both the client and the family. The length of stay is longer so you really get to know them and to develop a relationship. As a rehabilitation nurse, I am a caregiver, educator, confidante, advocate and friend to both the patient and their family. Each adapts and adjusts to the disability at a different rate. I must treat the entire family unit and help each with the physical changes and psychosocial adjustment that is necessary.

Rehabilitation nurses help clients and their significant others through a very difficult health care crisis. A client newly injured from a stroke, brain injury, or spinal cord injury, unlike a person having a cholecystectomy, will not leave the hospital in the same condition in which they entered. The rehabilitation nurse, along with members of an entire interdisciplinary team, helps clients with physical disabilities to reach the highest level of independent functioning possible within the limits of their disability. The nurse and the interdisciplinary team enable the client to cross that bridge from hospital to home and back into the community.

In the 1960s, the development of specialties within nursing began to occur. Rehabilitation nursing was one of those specialties. This chapter explores the history of rehabilitation nursing and its early origins, goals, and philosophy. It also covers the roles of a rehabilitation nurse, the standards of care, the different practice settings, the target populations, and the development of the Association of Rehabilitation Nurses and important health care policy for persons with disabilities.

Definition of Rehabilitation   The word **rehabilitation** originates from the Latin word *habilitas* or *habilitare,* which means "to render fit." The Latin word *rehabilitare* means "to render fit again" (Partridge, 1963, p. 273). Rehabilitation was used as a term in the sixteenth century when restoring someone to a former rank or privilege. In the late nineteenth century, it came to be used as an architectural expression, meaning to repair or to restore buildings (Young, 1989).

Today, in addition to these two definitions, Webster (Neufeldt, 1994, p. 1131) described rehabilitation as "to put back in good condition . . . to bring or restore to a normal or optimal state of health, constructive activity, etc. by medical treatment and physical or psychological therapy . . . to prepare (a disabled or disadvantaged person) for employment, as by vocational counseling or training."

In the medical literature, the word *rehabilitation* first appeared in 1918 in an article in the *Journal of the American Medical Association.* It described the Red Cross Experimental School for re-educating the persons disabled in World War I. Written by Douglas C. McMurtrie, the article was entitled "Human Factors in the Reconstruction of Disabled Soldiers and Sailors."

The Roots of Rehabilitation and Rehabilitation Nursing
Early Societies through the Nineteenth Century

Stryker (1977, p. 5) stated that the "history of rehabilitation reflects mankind's persistent discomfort, apathy and insensitivity toward disadvantaged persons, whether they be old, poor, mentally impaired or physically disabled." Primitive people believed that only the fit should survive; therefore, ancient societies did not treat the disabled or elderly with any degree of caring or respect (Stryker, 1977). The Eskimos left the disabled and elderly on free-floating pieces of ice and sent them off to sea. The Native Americans placed poisonous snakes in tents and hoped for a swift death. In U.S. society, people with disabilities were kept in basements or in the back rooms of hospitals (Martin, Holt, & Hicks, 1981). The initial change in attitude toward persons with disabilities came with an interest in crippled children around the turn of the nineteenth century, particularly with the outbreak of poliomyelitis. Religious organizations, in particular, accepted this cause. The first U.S. schools for crippled children were developed in 1893, and the first clinic was developed in 1904 (Mumma, 1987).

As a philosophy in nursing, the roots of rehabilitation can be traced to Florence Nightingale. In her *Notes on Nursing* (1992, p. 22), concerning the Crimean War in 1854, she stated, "Whatever a patient *can* do for himself, it is better, *i.e.* less anxiety, for him to do for himself. . . ." When Nightingale returned from the war, she established nursing schools in London. The first U.S. nursing schools were organized after the American Civil War (Young, 1989).

As a practice in nursing, rehabilitation began in convalescent and sanatorium units, which developed before the turn of the nineteenth century (Stryker, 1977). Literature on convalescent nursing describes patients eating in a small dining room, decorating their rooms similar to a home, and bringing their personal belongings (Fowler, 1928). Education for the nurses focused on anatomy and physiology of bones and muscles, massage, range of motion, and applying electrical stimulation to weakened muscles (Weeks, 1882). Massage was believed to prevent wasting and deformity (Stanton, 1900).

There was a great deal of idle time when people were convalescing. In 1907, a nursing teacher, Susan Tracy, began working on ways to "occupy" patients' time. The foundation of occupational therapy for people who were infirm and disabled was then established (McCourt, 1993).

World War I to World War II

World War I (1914–1918) had a tremendous impact on the field of physical medicine. There was a need not only to treat the wounded and disabled soldiers, many of whom were amputees or had spinal cord injuries, but to bring educational and vocational resources together to restore a sense of purpose to their lives (McCourt, 1993). In 1926, the first physical therapy school opened at Northwestern University Medical School in Chicago. Nurses were recruited to enter the physical therapy programs (Young, 1989). The **American Academy of Physical Medicine and Rehabilitation** was founded in 1938 to set standards and requirements for the practice of rehabilitation medicine.

World War II

World War II (1939–1945) brought about an increased interest in rehabilitation, again to respond to the needs of disabled soldiers. The continued epidemic of poliomyelitis also contributed to the expanding need for rehabilitation services. In 1941, an Australian nurse, Sister Elizabeth Kenny, changed the method of treatment for polio in America. She demonstrated her method of using muscle manipulation and hot fomentations instead of rigid orthoses at the Mayo Clinic in Rochester, Minnesota (Young, 1989). The Sister Kenny Institute, bearing her name, was founded in Minneapolis in 1942 (Mumma, 1987).

Post–World War II to Present

After World War II, **Howard A. Rusk,** head of the Air Force Convalescent Training Program, recommended the establishment of separate convalescent centers for disabled veterans (Rusk, 1948). Having experienced the benefit of these centers, he advocated the same care for the civilian disabled population. In an article he wrote in 1948, he stated that there were 19,000 amputees in the military as a result of the war but that, during that same period, 120,000 civilians suffered major amputations from disease and accidents. He established the first rehabilitation program in a community hospital at Bellevue, New York.

The ward for rehabilitation at Bellevue was designed to emphasize a homelike atmosphere. Clients were to eat in the dining room instead of in their rooms, the design of larger rooms allowed more space for wheelchairs, and laundry facilities were built as clients were encouraged to wear their own clothes. Recreation rooms also were created and home passes promoted to practice learned skills (Jones, 1948). In describing rehabilitation care, Rusk (1948, p. 76) stated, "Properly nurtured and developed, its contribution will mean the difference between independence and hopelessness for millions of America's disabled. As with all medical care, however, much of its success will be dependent upon good nursing."

Early rehabilitation nursing duties, as described by Jones (1948), included encouraging correct bed posture to prevent deformities, avoiding tight top sheets over client's feet, and using foot boards to prevent foot drop. Extra pillows were encouraged for good positioning, rocker knives to aid independence in feeding, and the use of ropes at the foot of the bed to help clients lift themselves. Every 2-hour voiding schedules and reducing fluids after 6:00 P.M. to prevent incontinence characterized early bladder programs. Well-trained attendants were used to provide care in addition to the professional nurse.

In 1949, Morrissey wrote about the importance of nutrition and the need for the rehabilitation client to consume more calories and protein. She stated that there are an estimated 99 daily activities that a person must perform to meet the demands of daily living. She emphasized that "each sick person is regarded not as a patient with a disease but as a person with a future" (Morrissey, 1949a, p. 453). This was a new concept for nursing care at that time.

After World War II, society moved from an agrarian to an industrial way of life. This led to an increase in industrial injuries requiring rehabilitation care. The advent of the automobile also resulted in a rise in accidents and permanent injuries (Stryker, 1977). The shortening of the work week to 5 days permitted more leisure time and, therefore, more recreational activities, some of which involved physical injuries (McCourt, 1993). With the cure of polio in the late 1950s, rehabilitation medicine and nursing expanded to include strokes, cardiac conditions, arthritis, orthopedic injuries, brain injury, and so on. Centers for rehabilitation care began to form both as free-standing hospitals and as units in existing acute care hospitals. An accrediting body specific for setting rehabilitation standards, the Commission on Accreditation of Rehabilitation Facilities, was established in 1966. In 1974, a group of rehabilitation nurses in Illinois, spearheaded by Sue Novak, established the **Association of Rehabilitation Nurses.**

The Specialty Practice of Rehabilitation Nursing Philosophical Overview

See Table 1 for a summary of rehabilitation philosophy, goal, and process.

Philosophy. The basic **philosophy** at the core of rehabilitation is that the disabled individual has the right to become expert in his or her own health care management (McCourt, 1993). Rehabilitation nurses believe that a person with a disability has intrinsic worth that transcends the disability, and that each person is a unique, holistic being who has both the right and the responsibility to make informed personal choices regarding health and lifestyle (American Nurses' Association & the Association of Rehabilitation Nurses, 1988).

Table 1
Rehabilitation Philosophy, Goal, and Process

Rehabilitation philosophy: individual has the right to be an expert

1. Goal: transfer of accountability to the client
2. Process used to achieve goal:
   a. Education
   b. Development of self-care skills

Goal. Given this philosophy, the **goal** of rehabilitation then becomes the transfer of accountability for self-care from the health care professional to the client (McCourt, 1993). The major goal of rehabilitation nursing is to assist persons with disability and chronic illness in attaining maximum functional ability, maintaining optimal health, and adapting to an altered lifestyle (American Nurses' Association & the Association of Rehabilitation Nurses, 1988).

In *Rehabilitation Nursing: Concepts and Practice—A Core Curriculum,* Mumma (1987) listed six specific goals of rehabilitation:

1. To achieve maximal functional potential and self-sufficiency
2. To achieve and maintain an acceptable quality of life
3. To ensure that the client's specific needs are addressed
4. To promote adaptation and adjustment of the client and family to a changed life
5. To prevent complications and promote optimal wellness
6. To return to successful function within the community

Patients are assisted to formulate goals that are realistic and attainable and that consider their continuing accountability for optimal wellness (American Nurses' Association & the Association of Rehabilitation Nurses, 1988).

Process. Education of the client and the development of self-care skills are the operations, or the **process,** carried out by the rehabilitation team to support the person with a disability in achieving this goal (McCourt, 1993). The process of rehabilitation nursing involves a problem-solving approach that is based on the nursing process of assessment, planning, interventions, and evaluation (American Nurses' Association & the Association of Rehabilitation Nurses, 1988).

International Classification of Impairments, Disabilities, and Handicaps.
The World Health Organization (WHO) developed an **international classification** for the words *impairment, disability,* and *handicap* that provides a conceptual framework for working with the rehabilitation client. According to the WHO

model, an impairment occurs at the organ level and does not in itself result in a disability. A disability occurs when there is restriction or lack of ability to perform an activity in a manner considered normal for a human being. A handicap is present when the impairment or disability limits or prevents the fulfillment of roles that the person was able to do in the past (Storck & Thompson-Hoffman, 1991). In rehabilitation, the goals need to be aimed at preventing handicaps, not just disability. The rehabilitation nurse and the interdisciplinary team members must address the roles the client participated in before impairment and disability, and prepare interventions that will enable the person to perform those roles again.

An example of the preceding concepts put into action might be that of Mr. S., a 60-year-old gentleman with a newly diagnosed stroke (impairment). He has weakness on the left side of his body and is unable to walk, dress himself, or perform grooming and hygiene activities independently (disability). One of the roles Mr. S. performs that he takes great pleasure in doing is the grocery shopping for his family. He has been doing this since the 1970s. He is currently unable to perform this role (handicap). The rehabilitation team could address his disability (the weakness of his left arm and leg) by performing range-of-motion exercises, strengthening and coordination activities, and gait exercises that would help him walk and dress and feed himself. But will these techniques alone help him to drive to the grocery store, manipulate a shopping cart, choose the correct food items, pay for the food, and unload and store the items once he is home? The rehabilitation team must look at the roles Mr. S. performs, identify the barriers to performing those roles (given the impairment and disability), and set up interventions to deal with those barriers so that the roles can again be achieved.

Definition of Rehabilitation Nursing

The definition of **rehabilitation nursing** is "the diagnosis and treatment of human responses of individuals and groups to actual or potential health problems stemming from altered functional ability and altered lifestyle" (American Nurses' Association & the Association of Rehabilitation Nurses, 1988, p. 4).

Characteristics of Rehabilitation Nursing

The characteristics of rehabilitation nursing are described by Mumma (1987, p. 13) as follows:

1. Practiced within a dynamic, therapeutic, and supportive relationship that is constantly changing, progressing, or regressing as nurse and client influence one another.
2. Practiced within a wide variety of health care and community settings.
3. Necessitates an expanded knowledge base.
4. Utilizes the nursing process to achieve individualized quality outcomes for the client as defined in the *Standards of Rehabilitation Nursing Practice* (Arn, 1994).

5. Is practiced in collaboration with the other members of the interdisciplinary rehabilitation team to facilitate overall achievement of goals of rehabilitation.

Major Roles of Rehabilitation Nurses

The roles of a rehabilitation nurse relate back to the philosophical belief that the disabled client has the right to become an expert in his or her care. The primary role, therefore, is that of teacher or client **educator** (McCourt, 1993). Information is provided to the client and his or her significant others, to help them become thoroughly knowledgeable about their injury or illness and to teach them how to prevent complications in the future. The focus is to move from illness to wellness and to learn how to maintain a well state for the rest of the client's life, not just for the duration of the hospital stay. When teaching, skills progress from the simple to the complex.

The second role is that of **caregiver.** The nurse is the major caregiver on the rehabilitation team. The nurse provides hands-on care until the client or family member develops the skills. Activities are aimed at restoration of function, maintenance of function, and prevention of complications and further functional loss (Mumma, 1987). The knowledge needed to provide this care is extensive. The rehabilitation nurse must not only be an expert in rehabilitation nursing concepts, but must also be a generalist and have knowledge of medical, surgical, pediatric, obstetric, psychiatric, and critical care procedures and techniques. Depending on the client population at a given time, a rehabilitation nurse will have the opportunity to use all of the knowledge gained in his or her undergraduate education program. The nurse must also understand the knowledge used by the other interdisciplinary team members, because part of the caregiver role is to help clients transfer and apply skills learned in therapy into their activities throughout the day (Stryker, 1977).

To provide this care, Stryker (1977, p. 20) stated that a rehabilitation nurse needs to be slightly "slow-geared." The nurse must have patience and understanding while allowing the client to struggle with dressing or turning or performing a catheterization. Time must be allowed for the patient to practice and learn the new skills. The nurse must know what makes the difference between dependence and independence (Stryker, 1977) and when to do "for" the patient and when to insist that the patient do the task alone.

Counselor is the third role. The rehabilitation nurse helps the client and client's family see strengths of which they may not yet be aware. They assist the client toward self-actualization. Expert communication and listening skills are needed for this role to be effective. The nurse must practice viewing the world around each patient with new eyes; to view them from an ability-oriented perspective. The rehabilitation nurse helps both the patient and family visualize a new life (Stryker, 1977).

The fourth rehabilitation nursing role is that of **coordinator of care.** The nurse is the only member of the rehabilitation team whose work influences the patient 7 days a week, 24 hours a day. A knowledge and understanding of group dynamics is critical as the rehabilitation nurse interfaces and coordinates care with professional and lay members of the team (Dittmar, 1989). Clients are aided in acquiring effective problem-solving skills and eventually to become their own health care expert (McCourt, 1993).

In the role of **client advocate** the nurse conveys the patient's needs and insights to others and is a collaborative partner with the patient. The nurse bridges the gap between the medical profession and nonmedical professionals that are working on behalf of the patient (McCourt, 1993; Mumma, 1987).

The sixth role of the rehabilitation nurse is that of **researcher.** Research findings, pertinent to rehabilitation, must be put into practice. The rehabilitation nurse must also participate in research studies or design studies as appropriate (McCourt, 1993).

Finally, as rehabilitation nurses gain experience and expertise in the field, they may be called on to be a **legal consultant** or **expert witness.** In this role, the nurse provides the knowledge and skills essential in litigation proceedings or may be asked to do life care planning as a service to clients, families, and the medical and legal professionals. Life care plans project current and future health care needs and costs (McCourt, 1993).

Family Involvement

The need to view the family or significant other, as well as the client, as an integral part of the rehabilitation team has been previously mentioned. The family must be included in the rehabilitation process from the onset (Dittmar, 1989; Watson, 1987). They, as well as the client, are going to have to deal with the disability and live with its consequences long after the inpatient stay or home health service is over. For the rehabilitation treatment and teaching to be incorporated into daily life, full cooperation and commitment from the family are crucial (Mumma & Nelson, 1996).

Rehabilitation nurses need to assess the family members' emotional states; their physical ability to care for the client, if this will be required; and their current knowledge base and educational needs. Cultural and religious barriers must also be identified. Potential problems with caregiver role strain, ability to cope, and so on, can be identified early in the rehabilitation process. The emotional changes that caregivers will go through must be addressed. The nurse needs to be aware that social isolation and role fatigue can result if a particular family member is the only one caring for a relative. An assessment of whether other family members or friends are available to help should be made and information on support groups, respite care, and other community resources given (Muslof, 1991).

Agreement from the family, as well as the client, on the plan of care is obtained on the day of admission or soon thereafter. The rehabilitation nurse must be able to allow family members to ask questions and to receive emotional support and understanding (Watson, 1987). Their opinions and concerns must be listened to and any conflicts resolved.

Generalist and Advanced Practice Rehabilitation Nursing Roles

Rehabilitation nurses may practice in generalist or advanced practice roles. At the level of **rehabilitation nursing generalist** a nurse's educational background is a diploma, associate's degree, or bachelor's degree (McCourt, 1993). The Association of Rehabilitation Nurses developed a certification examination in 1984 "to validate the basic knowledge and skill level of rehabilitation nurse generalists" (McCourt, 1993, p. 18). Those who pass the examination receive a **Certified Rehabilitation Registered Nurse (CCRN)** credential. Areas of practice in which rehabilitation nurses at this level may be involved include clinical nursing, management, pre-admission evaluation, education, case management, outpatient nursing, home health nursing, and so on. Knowledge and skills are usually acquired through a "combination of on-the-job training and both formal and informal continuing education" (McCourt, 1993, p. 18).

An **advanced practice rehabilitation nurse** has a master's or doctorate degree. Practice roles may include functioning as a clinical nurse specialist, nurse practitioner, researcher, administrator, educator, case manager, or consultant (McCourt, 1993). The Association of Rehabilitation Nurses developed and administered the first advanced practice certification examination in 1997. The credential is as a **Certified Rehabilitation Registered Nurse–Advanced (CRRN-A).**

Standards of Care and Standards of Professional Performance

The Association of Rehabilitation Nurses revised their standards of rehabilitation nursing practice in 1994. The new document is entitled *Standards and Scope of Rehabilitation Nursing Practice* (3rd edition). The document follows the American Nurses' Association standards and covers both standards of care and standards of professional performance. There are six **standards of care** and eight **standards of professional performance** (see Table 2).

The *Scope and Standards of Advanced Clinical Practice in Rehabilitation Nursing* was published in 1996 by the Association of Rehabilitation Nurses. Six standards of care and seven standards of professional performance are identified (see Table 3).

Practice Settings

Rehabilitation nursing occurs in a variety of **practice settings.** Even though the majority of rehabilitation nurses can be found in rehabilitation units or free-standing rehabilitation hospitals, the subacute or skilled rehabilitation arenas are expanding as are the outpatient, home health, and insurance company areas. Private practice, educational institutions, general hospitals, and hospices are other practice settings. All ages of clients are treated, from pediatrics to adolescents to adults and geriatrics, depending on the clinical site.

Table 2
Rehabilitation Nursing Standards of Care and Standards of Professional Performance

Standards of Care

Standard I.   Assessment
  The rehabilitation nurse collects client health data

Standard II.   Diagnosis
  The rehabilitation nurse analyzes the assessment data when determining diagnoses

Standard III.   Outcome Identification
  The rehabilitation nurse identifies expected outcomes individualized to the client

Standard IV.   Planning
  The rehabilitation nurse develops a plan of care that prescribes interventions to attain expected outcomes

Standard V.   Implementation
  The rehabilitation nurse implements the interventions identified in the plan of care

Standard VI.   Evaluation
  The rehabilitation nurse evaluates the client's progress toward attainment of outcomes

Standards of Professional Performance

Standard I.   Quality of Care
  The rehabilitation nurse systematically evaluates the quality and effectiveness of rehabilitation nursing practice

Standard II.   Performance Appraisal
  The rehabilitation nurse evaluates his or her own nursing practice in relation to professional practice standards and relevant statutes and regulations

Standard III.   Education
  The rehabilitation nurse acquires and maintains current knowledge in nursing practice

Standard IV.   Collegiality
  The rehabilitation nurse contributes to the professional development of peers, colleagues, and others

Standard V.   Ethics
  The rehabilitation nurse's decisions and actions on behalf of clients are determined in an ethical manner

Standard VI.   Collaboration
  The rehabilitation nurse collaborates with the client, significant others, and health care providers in providing client care

Standard VII.   Research
  The rehabilitation nurse uses research findings in practice

Standard VIII.   Utilization
  The rehabilitation nurse considers factors related to safety, effectiveness, and cost in planning and delivering client care

Table 3
Scope and Standards of Advanced Clinical Practice in Rehabilitation Nursing

Standards of Care

Standard I.   Assessment
The advanced practice nurse in rehabilitation collects comprehensive client health data

Standard II.   Diagnosis
The advanced practice nurse in rehabilitation critically analyzes the assessment data in determining diagnoses for clients with chronic illness or disability

Standard III.   Outcome Identification
The advanced practice nurse in rehabilitation identifies expected outcomes derived from the assessment data and diagnoses and individualizes expected outcomes with clients who have chronic illness or disability and with the health care team when appropriate

Standard IV.   Planning
The advanced practice nurse in rehabilitation participates in the development of a comprehensive plan of care with the client and significant others that includes interventions and treatments to attain expected outcomes

Standard V.   Implementation
The advanced practice nurse in rehabilitation prescribes, orders, and implements interventions and treatments for the plan of care
   a. Case Management/Coordination of Care
   b. Consultation
   c. Health Promotion, Health Maintenance, and Health Teaching
   d. Prescriptive Authority and Treatment
   e. Referral

Standard VI.   Evaluation
The advanced practice nurse in rehabilitation evaluates the client's progress in attaining expected outcomes

Standards of Professional Performance

Standard I.   Quality of Care
The advanced practice nurse in rehabilitation develops criteria for and evaluates the quality of care and effectiveness of advanced practice nursing

Standard II.   Self-Evaluation
The advanced practice nurse in rehabilitation continuously evaluates his or her own nursing practice in relation to professional practice standards and relevant statutes and regulations and is accountable to the public and to the profession for providing competent clinical care

Table 3
Scope and Standards of Advanced Clinical Practice in Rehabilitation Nursing (*Continued*)

Standard III.   Education
  The advanced practice nurse in rehabilitation acquires and maintains current knowledge and skills in the specialty practice area of rehabilitation nursing

Standard IV.   Leadership
  The advanced practice nurse in rehabilitation serves as a leader, effective team member, and role model in the professional development of peers, colleagues, and others

Standard V.   Ethics
  The advanced practice nurse in rehabilitation integrates ethical principles and norms in all areas of practice

Standard VI.   Interdisciplinary Process
  The advanced practice nurse in rehabilitation promotes an interdisciplinary process in providing care for the client

Standard VII.   Research
  The advanced practice nurse in rehabilitation uses research to discover, examine, and evaluate knowledge, theories, and creative approaches to health care for persons with chronic illness and disability

Stryker (1977) emphasized that rehabilitation is a part of health care, not a phase of it. She wrote that for a patient to receive the greatest benefit from rehabilitation, it is imperative that it be seen as a process that begins when the patient first encounters the acute disease or trauma. Rehabilitation, Stryker says, has often been referred to as the third phase of medical care, which implies that it is separate from acute and convalescent care. "This kind of thinking deprives a patient of several vital aspects of rehabilitation," Stryker observed (1977, p. 12), such as learning how to prevent pressure sores and contractures, or how to maintain existing abilities. It prevents the client from being able to visualize a satisfying future and it does not help families to prepare themselves or their environment for the necessary changes. The same interventions taught in rehabilitation should begin at the onset of the illness or disease. Stryker (1977) wrote that measures taken during acute care can shorten and enhance the rehabilitation process. Rehabilitation must begin when the client first experiences the onset of an acute disease or trauma or the early symptoms of a progressively disabling condition (Stryker, 1977).

Third-party payers today are shaping and influencing the type of setting in which rehabilitative care will be provided, once the client is medically stable. Owing to rising health care costs, insurance companies, as well as Medicare and Medicaid programs, are pushing for the lowest level of rehabilitation care that is appropriate. Therefore many clients (such as those with orthopedic injuries, e.g., fractured hips and knee surgeries), who once would have been placed in an acute rehabilitation setting after their surgery, are now being transferred to a skilled unit or discharged home with home health services. The push for all medical procedures and care to be provided in less costly settings is redefining how rehabilitation care is delivered.

The average inpatient **length of stay** for acute rehabilitation has dramatically decreased over the years, from 52.2 days in 1978 (S. Sonic, personal communication, March 23, 1993) to 18 days in 1994 (Fiedler, Granger, & Ottenbacher, 1996). This presents a challenge for the rehabilitation nurse and rehabilitation team to educate and enable a client to be as independent as possible in a shorter time frame. Outpatient and home health follow-up services become crucial.

Changing Demographics and the Future Need for Rehabilitation Services

In the early 1900s, life expectancy in the United States was only 47 years (Kluger, 1996; Watson, 1987). People did not live long enough to develop a chronic disease. Medical technology was limited, at best, and antibiotics had not been invented. If a major accident occurred, survival rates were extremely low.

In 1987, the average life expectancy had increased to 71 years (Watson, 1987). Today, it is about 76 years (Kluger, 1996). By the year 2000, it is predicted that there will be 118,000 people who are more than 100 years old (Celtron, 1992). As people live longer, there is an 80 percent probability of acquiring one or more chronic disabling conditions. Currently three-fourths of people older than 75 years have at least one limitation in their ability to perform activities of daily living.

In addition to longer life spans, members of the largest segment of the American population, the baby boomers, are growing older. Today, one in eight Americans is 65 years of age or older. "By 2050, the elderly population is expected to be 80.1 million or one in five people" (Estill, 1996, p. A-1). With the increase in life expectancy and the baby boomer population, there will be large numbers of people who can expect to have at least one disabling condition over the course of an extended life span (McCourt, 1993).

Medical advances have also now made it possible for people with disabilities, such as spinal cord injury and brain injury, to live normal life spans. As these people grow into adulthood and old age, health problems will arise that did not previously need to be addressed. An increase in dual disabilities will occur as people age. A client with a spinal cord injury may now have arthritis, or a person with Parkinson's disease may fracture a hip or incur a stroke.

Experience in trauma care from the two world wars and the Korean and Vietnam wars has improved the survival rates for traumatically injured persons (Mc-

Court, 1993). Many who live have functional impairments not experienced before. Medical technology is also enabling premature infants to survive birth weights not previously encountered. Many of these children have physical disabilities that need rehabilitative care. As medical advances in the past saved lives that created opportunities for rehabilitation services, so new diagnoses will be seen in the future, thus creating new challenges.

Target Populations

Target populations for rehabilitation services continue to expand. Two to 3 percent of the U.S. population, or 5 million, have chronic diseases and disabilities, the treatment of which requires rehabilitation services (Kottke & Lehman, 1990). "Stroke is the third leading cause of death in the United States and the leading cause of disability among adults" (Gresham et al., 1995, p. 1), with 550,000 cases occurring each year (Gresham et al., 1995). As such, it is the leading diagnosis seen in most rehabilitation settings. In addition to stroke, orthopedic injuries, musculoskeletal diseases, spinal cord injuries, brain injury, multiple sclerosis, Guillain-Barré syndrome, clients with pulmonary and cardiac conditions, oncology, pain, burns, acquired immunodeficiency syndrome (AIDS), chemical dependency, general deconditioning, postpolio syndrome, and so on, are diagnoses being treated.

National Health Policy for the Disabled

Craven and Gleason (1996, p. 62) state that a chronologic review of legislation important to rehabilitation "quickly illuminates how changes in the social construction of disability [have] influenced healthcare delivery for persons with disabilities." Just as World War I had an impact on physical rehabilitation care, it also had an impact on legislation to provide vocational training for the war disabled. The War Risk Act of 1914 specified vocational rehabilitation training for those who incurred a disability while in the service. The National Defense Act of 1916 gave men who served in the armed services vocational adjustments, which included educational benefits (Craven & Gleason, 1996).

World War II also had an impact on legislation. In 1943 The Vocational Rehabilitation Act was passed, making funds available for professional training and research for the disabled (Mumma, 1987).

In 1954, the Hill-Burton Act provided amendments to the 1943 Vocational Rehabilitation Act. Training grants became available for the education of rehabilitation professional staff, such as nurses, physicians, rehabilitation counselors, social workers, physical therapists, and occupational therapists. This bill also gave grants to states to use for the establishment, alteration, or expansion of rehabilitation facilities and workshops (Mumma, 1987).

Accessibility standards for buildings being constructed, altered, or leased by the federal government or financed by federal grants were set in place by the Architectural Barriers Act in 1968.

In 1973, an important piece of legislation for the disabled, the Rehabilitation Act, was passed. A Rehabilitation Service Administration was established within the Department of Health, Education, and Welfare (HEW). State rehabilitation agencies were required to develop individualized written rehabilitation program plans for each client served. An Architectural and Transportation Barriers Compliance Board was organized to ensure compliance with the Architectural Barriers Act of 1968. All new facilities constructed with federal funds had to be barrier-free. Discrimination in recruitment, advertising, hiring, rates of pay, and benefits was prohibited toward persons employed by programs receiving federal money. Disabled children were entitled to a free, appropriate public education in a setting as close to normal as possible (Mumma, 1987).

In 1990, another landmark bill for the disabled was passed with the **Americans with Disabilities Act (ADA).** This act extended the civil rights laws to the physically disabled, mentally disabled, and the chronically ill. According to Chai Feldblum (1992), who helped draft the bill, it achieves what would have been in place all along for the disabled had those with disabilities been in the mainstream of society. Instead, the disabled were kept hidden behind walls while airplanes, restaurants, streets, automobiles, housing, and so on, were built without them in mind. With the ADA, access is guaranteed to employment, transportation, communication, and recreation (Craven & Gleason, 1996). Reasonable work site accommodations for disabled workers must be made at the company's expense. This can be accomplished by altering work stations, such as raising a desk or purchasing a tabletop copier for someone in a wheelchair, or by restructuring the job through revised schedules. Other aspects of the act include modification of public services to be accessible, such as bathrooms, telephones, and commuter rail services. All common telecommunication carriers must provide relay services for the hearing and/or speech impaired. Physician offices must be accessible and the same level of care must be provided by physicians to all of their patients, regardless of their disabilities (Craven & Gleason, 1996).

Conclusion

Rehabilitation is a life-long process carried out by the client, family, and interdisciplinary team working together (Dittmar, 1989). The rehabilitation nurse is a critical member of this team. Without the coordination, education, and carry-through of rehabilitation principles provided by the nurse, the rehabilitation process cannot occur. Morrissey (1949b) stated that the nurse must use his or her skills much as a musician does. The fabric of life is woven together much like a theme of music. A skillful nurse uses "her knowledge and her experience to create harmony within the whole structure" (Morrissey, 1949a, p. 454). The rehabilitation nurse helps clients and their families weave their lives back together and return to the community and to their roles as productive members of society.

References

American Nurses' Association & the Association of Rehabilitation Nurses. (1988). *Rehabilitation nursing: Scope of practice: Process and outcome criteria for selected diagnoses.* Kansas City, MO: Author.

Association of Rehabilitation Nurses. (1994). *Standards and scope of rehabilitation nursing practice* (3rd ed.). Skokie, IL: Author.

Association of Rehabilitation Nurses. (1996). *Scope and standards of advanced clinical practice in rehabilitation nursing.* Glenview, IL: Author.

Celtron, M. (1992, August). *Future issues.* Paper presented at the 25th anniversary celebration of the Commission on Accreditation of Rehabilitation Facilities, Washington, DC.

Craven, G. T., & Gleason, C. A. (1996). In S. P. Hoeman (Ed.), *Rehabilitation nursing: Process and application* (2nd ed., pp. 61–69). St. Louis: Mosby.

Dittmar, S. (1989). *Rehabilitation nursing: Process and application.* St. Louis: Mosby.

Estill, B. (1996, May 21). "Human tidal wave" of the old approaching. *The San Diego Union,* pp. A1, A13.

Feldblum, C. (1992, August). People issues. In A. Toppel (Chair), *A nation united: 25th anniversary celebration.* Symposium conducted at the meeting of the Commission on Accreditation of Rehabilitation Facilities, Washington, DC.

Fiedler, R. C., Granger, C. V., & Ottenbacher, K. J. (1996). The uniform data system for medical rehabilitation. Report of first admissions for 1994. *American Journal of Physical Medicine and Rehabilitation 75*(2), 125–129.

Fowler, H. A. (1928). Convalescent care as one nurse sees it. *American Journal of Nursing, 28*(12), 1205–1208.

Gresham, G. E., Duncan, P. W., Stason, W. B., et al. (1995). *Post-stroke rehabilitation. Clinical practice guideline, no. 16.* Rockville, MD: U.S. Department of Health and Human Services, Public Health Service, Agency for Health Care Policy and Research. AHCPR Publication No. 95-0662.

Jones, F. T. (1948). The nurse's responsibility in rehabilitation. *American Journal of Nursing, 48*(2), 76–79.

Kluger, J. (1996). Can we stay young? *Time, 148,* 89–98.

Kottke F. J., & Lehmann, J. F. (1990). Preface. In F. J. Kottke & J. F. Lehmann (Eds.), *Kruesen's handbook of physical medicine and rehabilitation* (4th ed., p. xvii). Philadelphia: W. B. Saunders.

Martin, N., Holt, N. B., & Hicks, D. (1981). *Comprehensive rehabilitation nursing.* New York: McGraw-Hill.

McCourt, A. E. (Ed.). (1993). *The specialty practice of rehabilitation nursing: A core curriculum* (3rd ed.). Skokie, IL: Rehabilitation Nursing Foundation.

McMurtrie, D. C. (1918). Human factors in the reconstruction of disabled soldiers and sailors. *Journal of the American Medical Association, 70,* 2013.

Morrissey, A. B. (1949a). Rehabilitation care for patients. *American Journal of Nursing, 49*(7), 453–454.

Morrissey, A. B. (1949b). The nursing technics in rehabilitation. *American Journal of Nursing, 49*(9), 545–551.

Mumma, C. M. (Ed.). (1987). *Rehabilitation nursing: Concepts and practice—A core curriculum* (2nd ed.). Evanston, IL: Rehabilitation Nursing Foundation.

Mumma, C. M., & Nelson, A. (1996). Models for theory-based practice of rehabilitation nursing. In S. P. Hoeman (Ed.), *Rehabilitation nursing: Process and application* (2nd ed., pp. 21–33). St. Louis: Mosby.

Musolf, J. M. (1991). Easing the impact of the family caregiver's role. *Rehabilitation Nursing, 16*(2), 82–84.

Neufeldt, V. (Ed.). (1994). *Webster's new world dictionary* (3rd college ed.). New York: Prentice-Hall.

Nightingale, F. (1859). *Notes on nursing: What it is, and what it is not.* London: Harrison & Sons.

Partridge, E. (1963). *Origins: A short etymological dictionary of modern English.* London: Routledge & Kegan Paul.

Rusk, H. A. (1948). Implications for nursing in rehabilitation. *American Journal of Nursing, 48*(2), 74–76.

Stanton, A. (1900). Massage in the treatment of infantile paralysis. *American Journal of Nursing, 4*(3), 211–212.

Storck, I. F., & Thompson-Hoffman, S. (1991). Demographic characteristics of the disabled population. In J. S. Thompson-Hoffman & I. F. Storck (Eds.), *Disability in the United States: A portrait from national data* (pp. 1–12). New York: Springer-Verlag.

Stryker, R. (1977). *Rehabilitative aspects of acute and chronic nursing care.* Philadelphia: W. B. Saunders.

Watson, P. G. (1987). Family participation in the rehabilitation process: The rehabilitator's perspective. *Rehabilitation Nursing, 12*(2), 70–73.

Weeks, C. (1882). *Textbook of nursing.* New York: D. Appleton & Co.

Young, M. A. (1989). A history of rehabilitation nursing. *Fifteen years of making the difference.* Skokie, IL: Association of Rehabilitation Nurses.

CHAPTER 2
Theoretical Bases for Rehabilitation

Patricia A. Chin

Key Terms *Family Interaction Theory*
Methods of Assisting
Role Theory
Self-Care Actions
Self-Care Limitations
Self-Care Theory
Social Learning Theory
Stress Theory
Systems Theory

Objectives 1. Discuss the purpose of a theory-based approach to rehabilitative nursing practice.

2. Discuss the concept of self-care and the assessment and development of self-care abilities and capabilities in rehabilitation nursing.

3. Discuss the usefulness of systems theory to rehabilitative nursing.

4. Discuss the usefulness of stress theory to rehabilitative nursing.

5. Discuss the usefulness of family interaction theory, role theory, and social learning theory to rehabilitative nursing.

Introduction This chapter presents concepts and principles important for understanding the content of this book. The concepts in this chapter should be used to comprehend and clarify the philosophy of rehabilitative nursing presented throughout this text. These concepts and principles form the bases

- For defining rehabilitative nursing practice, and the role of the nurse and other various team members
- For using the nursing process to design, implement, and evaluate a holistic plan of care for the client and caregivers
- For promoting mastery and independence
- For preventing complications and further disability
- For developing a view of rehabilitation as a process of health care and education, involving the client and caregivers across the life span

The rehabilitation team strives to develop the abilities and capabilities of the client regardless of any physical, cognitive, or psychological impairment experienced. The team also strives to develop the greatest level of independence and self-sufficiency possible for the client. Theoretical perspectives from various disciplines and specialty areas are used to achieve these goals. Those theories range from the very abstract family theories to the more focused mid-range theories of stress and loss. No one theory adequately addresses the issues, behaviors, or problems of rehabilitation nursing. Any theory used will depend on the client's situation; the nurse's skills and knowledge; the goals of the client, family, and nurse; and the philosophies of the agency and treatment teams.

A nursing model provides a way to conceptualize the domain of nursing. Adherence to a specific model of nursing will provide the practitioner with the parameters for data collection (assessment); identify the nature and source of patient problems (nursing diagnosis), direct patient goals, nursing goals, and nursing actions (planning/implementation/modification); and delineate mechanisms for the evaluation of nursing interventions.

Self-Care Theory

The concepts that compose **self-care theory** have great relevance and suitability to the rehabilitative process. The self-care approach is extremely pragmatic and seems most logical for working with clients in rehabilitation settings. In philosophical terms, providing personal self-care is essential for developing or maintaining a sense of self-worth and independence. The relationship between the client and the health care provider, in terms of the self-care approach, is a mutual and contractual partnership.

Many of the concepts presented in the following discussion are grounded in Orem's theory of self-care. Although the theory's conceptualization of the person and health is individualistic in nature, the family is an important factor. When the client is unable to engage in self-care actions the role of the family member is to assist with the meeting of the care demand.

Self-care actions are activities that individuals perform to maintain health, life, and well-being (Orem, 1985), and are very personal in nature. They include rituals, habits, timing, and practices learned in childhood (Hoeman, 1996). Three categories of self-care activities have been identified and include those actions taken to meet requisites (needs) for

1. Physical life and well-being (i.e., air, food, water, rest, interactions with others)
2. Development and maturity
3. Needs that arise following a change or deviation in health state (Orem, 1985)

Self-care practices are not random acts. They are deliberate, purposeful, and goal-directed actions taken to accomplish some goal or to meet a need. Deliberate action proceeds step by step to achieve a state different from the one that was present when the action began (for example, oral care). Deliberate action is driven by three sequences: (1) planning, (2) doing, and (3) checking. To engage in deliberative self-care the client will have to possess the abilities to carry out this sequence of action. The goal of self-care–oriented nursing is to empower the client and family with the knowledge and skills necessary to reach optimal safe performance of self-care and maximum independence. In the context of rehabilitation, self-care is the process that offers the client and family an opportunity to acquire the ability to function effectively following injury or disease and to assume responsibility for personal care (Hoeman, 1996).

A variety of conditions and impairments can affect the client's ability to perform self-care. In some cases a single disease process can interfere with the client's self-care capabilities and in other cases multiple processes combine to limit the client's capabilities. These processes can involve functional limitations; cognitive impairments; impaired reasoning; problems with decision making, problem solving, and judgment; and communication disorders.

The client may have sensory alteration, restriction in mobility, or decreased energy levels. Examples of common conditions that may affect the client's ability to engage in self-care include paralysis or paresis, decreased sensation in the extremities, disturbances in spatial orientation, agnosia, apraxia, hemianopsia, limitations in range of motion, extremity amputation, spasticity, ataxia, and tremors. Cognitive impairments may include decreased attention, lack of orientation, problems in sequencing of actions, and limitations in generalizing from one situation to other situations.

A number of factors influence the client's ability to engage in self-care with any level of proficiency. These factors are easy to assess and should be taken into consideration when building a database on the client and before the planning of care. The information on these basic self-care–condoning factors can be organized as follows:

1. Age, sex, developmental stage, and conditions of living
2. Family system, sociocultural orientation, and lifestyle
3. Health state of the client, and health care system and services available to the client

The nurse can facilitate the client's ability to engage in self-care activities. Orem (1985) identified three types of nursing systems. In the wholly compensatory system the nurse provides all the care necessary to meet self-care needs. The client or family lacks the skills or knowledge to provide the care needed to maintain physical well-being. An example would be a client in a coma following a traumatic head injury. In a partly compensatory system the nurse and the patient both participate in the actions necessary to meet the client's self-care needs. An example might be a client who, while in an inpatient rehabilitation unit, develops the skills to care for a stump following amputation. The degree of nursing involvement in performing or assisting in self-care activities is dependent on the client's self-care limitation, readiness, and capability to perform self-care activities.

In a supportive-educative system, the nurse provides the support and education necessary for the client to be independent in meeting self-care needs. The role of the nurse in this type of nursing is to assist the client or family to develop the skills and knowledge to be independent in self-care and to support the client and family in their efforts to be independent. An example would be that of a nurse assisting a discharged client to modify self-catheterization techniques.

Using the self-care model, nursing assesses each category of self-care needs, identifies deficits in meeting self-care needs, and designs and implements a plan of care for assisting clients to develop those self-care skills necessary for independent living, personal growth, and optimal health. When working with children or dependent adults the nurse assists caregivers to maintain therapeutic care supporting life processes and facilitating personal development and maturation.

The client will have the demand to meet a variety of needs to maintain physical integrity and functioning, to grow and mature, and to adjust to changes in health state. There is a set of needs common to all human beings. The actions to meet these needs bring about the internal and external conditions that maintain human structure and functioning. That set of needs includes

- The ability to obtain and use sufficient air, food, and water
- The ability to provide care associated with eliminative processes and excrements
- An adequacy and balance of rest, sleep, and activity
- The ability to interact with others; socialization to obtain resources essential to life, growth, and development
- The ability to make needs known to others; communication processes
- The ability to protect the self and others from hazards
- The promotion of human functioning and normalcy

Also common to all humans is the need to maintain physiological well-being. When the developmental needs are met it contributes to the prevention of developmental disorders and promotes development according to the client's potential. Two types of conditions influence client development: (1) conditions that support and promote the processes of development and maturation (e.g., going to school, marriage, and vocational preparation) and (2) conditions that prevent the processes of normal development and maturation (e.g., educational deprivation, failures of healthy individuation, loss of occupational security, and oppressive living conditions). Nurses will assist clients to learn and develop personally no matter what types of barriers exist to that development.

Another set of needs exists for clients who are ill, injured, or have a specific form of pathology including defects, deficits, or disabilities (Orem, 1985). Disease or injury not only affects specific structures and physiological or psychological mechanisms but also integrated client functioning. The needs that clients develop because of a change in health state or injury include

- Seeking and securing appropriate assistance in the event of a change in health state
- Being aware of and attending to the effects of a change in health state, or effects of injury
- Effectively carrying out prescribed diagnostic, therapeutic, and rehabilitative measures
- Detecting, attending to, and regulating the discomfort or deleterious effects of treatment and rehabilitation
- Modifying the self-concept and body image in accepting oneself as being in a particular state of health
- Learning to live with the effects of a change in health state in a lifestyle that promotes continued personal development (Orem, 1985)

Nursing intervention can be directed toward accomplishing patient's self-care actions, compensating for the patient's inability to engage in self-care activities, or supporting and protecting the patient (Orem, 1985). To accomplish this, there are at least five general **methods of assisting** that nurses can use to help clients meet their self-care needs. These methods can be applied in a variety of care situations and settings. They are as follows:

1. Doing for, acting for—acting in place of the client (e.g., positioning a paralyzed client)
2. Teaching—providing factual, technical information
3. Supporting physically and emotionally—sustaining the client in efforts made to gain self-care abilities or in coping and adapting
4. Providing an educational environment—creating an environment that motivates the client to establish appropriate goals and adjust behavior to achieve specific results
5. Guiding and directing—assisting the client to make choices or pursue a course of action

The nurse may assist the client by using any or all of these methods.

Self-care limitations are expressions of that which restricts the client in providing the amount and kind of self-care needed under existent and changing conditions and circumstances (Orem, 1985, p. 125). The rehabilitation client can experience limitations in knowledge, restrictions in judgment and decision making, and restrictions in result-achieving actions. The entire range of **self-care limitations** can be seen in rehabilitation clients. Some of the ways in which these limitations can be operationalized are

- Limitations in knowledge
- Limitations in developed skills
- Lack of resources for self-care
- Lack of sufficient energy for sustained action
- Inability or limited ability to control body movements
- Inability or limited ability to attend to self or exercise vigilance

- Changed modes of functioning that are new or not understood
- Unrecognized new needs associated with injury or change in health state
- Impaired sensory functioning, or perception, and/or impaired memory that interferes with ability to engage in self-care
- Lack of interest in meeting self-care needs
- Goal orientation and value placed on self-care inadequate to sustain actions for meeting needs
- Lack of support systems needed to sustain self-care

The rehabilitation client's potential for self-care is dependent on the client's overall capability to care for the self. Rehabilitation requires deliberate action by the client and health care provider to adapt or adjust functioning to compensate for disorders that restrict human functioning (Orem, 1985). Self-care theory provides an appropriate framework for the practice of rehabilitative nursing because of its focus on client and family autonomy for self-care and the inclusion of the client's participation in all aspects of the rehabilitation process. The clients engaged in the rehabilitation process require nursing when their own self-care abilities and capabilities are not adequate to meet their health care needs.

These areas should be assessed by the nurse to identify the types of limitations clients or families might have in meeting self-care needs. Problems clients experience in developing self-care after the onset of an illness, disease, injury, or disability will be related to one of these limitations. If that information is available the treatment team can identify appropriate interventions to overcome or mitigate the effects of the client's or family's problems by reducing the self-care limitation.

Systems Theory

A basic understanding of **systems theory** is also essential for rehabilitation nursing. General systems theory was first delineated by Von Bertalanffy (1950), a biologist. Systems theory was also described by sociologists around the same time (Parsons, 1951). Systems theory is an organized way of looking at and explaining a *unit.* The unit can be a group, a family, a community, or a society. It relates to the relationships and interactions within the unit as well as between a unit and other units. It is used to explain how forces or events affect the whole and how the whole influences each part (Friedman, 1992).

A *system* is a goal-directed unit characterized by its wholeness. This system is made up of interdependent, interacting parts that endure over time. A system has *structure,* which refers to the arrangement and organization of the system's parts. It also has *function,* which refers to the purposes or goals of the system that make possible the system's survival, continuity, and growth (Von Bertalanffy, 1950).

Systems are open or closed in interactions with the surrounding environment. An *open system* interacts with the environment to derive its input (resources) and output (products). All living systems are open systems. A *closed sys-*

tem does not interact with its environment. No totally closed system has been identified in reality (Parsons & Bales, 1955). Each system has *boundaries,* which act as filters that control the degree of exchange of input, output, and feedback with the external environment. Systems with porous boundaries receive a free exchange from the environment. Systems with less porous boundaries are more isolated from the environment. The system relies on feedback to maintain equilibrium or *homeostasis.*

Social systems are models of social organization (Parsons, 1951). The family is a dynamic social system composed of family members (Friedman, 1992). The family members represent the internal units of the system. The family functions interdependently with extrafamilial systems (e.g., school, church, rehabilitation team). When the family is unable to meet its functions because of a deficiency in resources it must turn to outside systems to achieve homeostasis.

The need for rehabilitation services can affect the entire family system. Many challenges experienced throughout the rehabilitation process can disrupt its structure and function. This disruption in equilibrium will drive the family to cope and adjust in order to reorganize and conserve its resources. If the family system is to survive the rehabilitation nurse must be able to determine the degree of disruption experienced by the family members. Internal and external factors must be considered as well as the nature of the family's interactions with the external environment.

Working with the families of rehabilitation clients can be stressful for the nurse. The family is a system with boundaries. The nurse and the rehabilitation team form a new subsystem for the family. The nurse will be influenced as much by the family as the family is by the nurse. The nurse will enter into a long-term relationship with the family. While the relationship can be very rewarding the nurse must be alert for signs of attachment and dependency. The nurse can become caught in a nurse-client-family triangle. The nurse may experience depression when the family fails to make progress or change.

Family Interaction Theory

Family interaction theory is used to explain the nature of the relationships between and among various members of the family. Using this approach, the nurse considers the personalities of the family members, and the dynamics arising from the interactions among the family members. The issues to be assessed and interpreted in family processes are role assignments, status, communication patterns, decision-making styles, problem-solving techniques, coping strategies, and socialization (Friedman, 1992).

The interaction approach attempts to interpret the interactions of family members in terms of the family's internal functioning (Friedman, 1992). When viewing the family as an interacting unity the nurse's perspective for working with the family shifts from seeing it as a social institution to seeing it as an internal network of family relationships. The nurse can then center attention on how family members function together to accomplish the tasks of the family as a whole as well as meeting the developmental tasks of each member. This approach makes it easier for the nurse to assess and specify potential sources of difficulty the family might encounter during rehabilitation to illness, injury, disease, or disability. Its major contribution is in explaining family communications, roles, decision-making, and problem-solving. These are critical areas of concern for effective treatment of the multiple needs of the client in rehabilitation who is working toward reentry into the community and toward optimum levels of self-management and independent living.

This theoretical approach does present the family as a self-contained system; but because the family does actively interact with the external environment, these exchanges must also be considered. The family cannot exist in a vacuum. The nurse must consider the nature of the exchanges between the family and the external environment and determine how the exchange might be affected by the rehabilitation process. The knowledge obtained about the client and family from this perspective helps to create a comprehensive picture of the client and family and is essential to providing effective care.

Role Theory

Role theory is used to analyze and explain the interactions and roles that family members assume during various situations. *Roles* are patterns or sets of expected behaviors. Status and power are conferred to the individual through acquired or assumed roles. The rehabilitation nurse can use role theory to identify the effects of illness, injury, disease, or disability on both the client and the family (Johnson, 1986). The rehabilitation nurse needs to be alert for family role strain and role conflicts arising from shifting family organization. Changing role responsibilities and transfer of role status involving the rehabilitation client can have a demoralizing effect on the client and may interfere with the accomplishment of rehabilitation goals or client adherence to the suggestions and recommendations of the treatment team.

Alteration in the client's ability to fulfill role expectation and responsibilities can result in feelings of inadequacy and insecurity for the client. Both the client and family members may be required to learn, voluntarily or involuntarily, new skills and role behaviors, resolve role conflicts, and relinquish roles. Family members who are required to take on new roles and responsibilities may feel angry or resentful. The rehabilitation nurse should be alert for signs that the client or family members are experiencing difficulty in adjusting to changing roles and the conflicts that can arise from the necessity to transfer roles from one member to another.

Stress Theory

An understanding of stress and coping, as encompassed in **stress theory,** is essential for rehabilitative nursing. The concept of stress was initially introduced by

Selye (1978) to health sciences as a physiological response: general adaptation syndrome (GAS). Selye's model is classified as a nonspecific systemic response model. Stress arising within a person, Selye proposed, is experienced in three general adaptation stages: an alarm reaction phase, a shock phase (when resistance is lowered), and a counterattack phase (activation of defenses—physiological fight or flight). During the phase of resistance maximum adaptation occurs. The adaptive response to a stressor during the stage of resistance involves the use of coping strategies. If the resistance phase is prolonged the individual can experience a loss of control or helplessness. If the individual's exposure to the stressor persists over time, or if coping strategies are inadequate, the individual can become exhausted, adaptation mechanisms can fail, and disease or even death can occur (Selye, 1978).

When a family member requires rehabilitative services the family is confronted with multiple stressors and challenges. Each member of the family will feel the need to accommodate to the client's changed circumstances (Freidman, 1992). This accommodation can be accomplished by supporting the client (functional) or by attacking the client (nonfunctional). The family will be bombarded with transitional stresses as well as situational stressors. By assessing the balance between the stressors and the strengths of supportive or protective elements the nurse and rehabilitation team can attempt to eliminate or reduce the strength of the stressors or supplement and enhance the family's resources and ability to cope with stress.

An assessment of the family's stressors and other risk factors and its psychosocial, physical, and environmental assets provides the nurse with the information necessary to anticipate family risk factors and then reduce or eliminate certain stressors. Some stressful life events cannot be avoided. Their effect on the family can be lessened by preparing the family for the event (stress inoculation) or by providing reality, present-oriented, short-term counseling before the time that the family becomes overwhelmed by the stressor(s) (Friedman, 1992). Stress theory is discussed in more detail in Chapter 10.

Social Learning Theory

Social learning theory stems from behavioral psychology. Bandura (1977) first described social learning theory. He broadened the learning models by placing a greater emphasis on the social aspect of learning and the mutual interactive effects of personal behavior and environment on learning. This theory stresses the cognitive aspects of learning and points out the importance of role modeling to facilitate skill development and behavioral change. The concept of *perceived self-efficacy* is a subset of social learning theory (Bandura, 1977; 1986). Social learning theory proposes that people make choices about behaviors on the basis of their ability to predict consequences of the actions. Social learning theory stresses reinforcement as a key to learning.

The nurse in the rehabilitation setting can apply the principles of this theory when considering how clients are socialized, how they communicate and function in family roles, and the strategies the client can develop and use to cope and adjust to change and stress. The principles of social learning theory are important for learning and teaching processes in the rehabilitation setting. Cognitive retraining often uses techniques grounded in social learning theory. The theory also has implications for the development of self-care and self-management mastery.

Conclusion

Basic concepts from several theories relevant to comprehending and clarifying the philosophy of rehabilitative nursing have been presented. The theories discussed provide a foundation for using the nursing process to design, implement, and evaluate a holistic plan of care for the client and caretakers, to promote mastery and independence, to prevent complications and further disability, and to develop a view of rehabilitation as a process of health care and education. Several additional theories (presented in subsequent chapters) include change theory, adaptation theory, the social construction of disability, and theories of loss necessary for effective client care in the rehabilitation setting.

References

Bandura, A. (1977). *Social learning theory.* Englewood Cliffs, NJ: Prentice-Hall.

Bandura, A. (1986). *Social foundations of thought and action.* Englewood Cliffs, NJ: Prentice-Hall.

Friedman, M. M. (1992). *Family nursing theory and practice* (3rd ed.). Norwalk, CT: Appleton & Lange.

Hoeman, S. P. (1996). *Rehabilitation nursing: Process and application* (2nd ed.). St. Louis: Mosby.

Johnson, S. L. (1986). Role theory strategies. In P. L. Johnson (Ed.), *High risk parenting: Nursing assessment and strategies for the family at risk.* (pp. 388–401). Philadelphia: J. B. Lippincott.

Orem, D. E. (1985). *Nursing concepts of practice.* New York: McGraw-Hill.

Parsons, T. (1951). *The social system.* Glencoe, IL: Free Press.

Parsons, T., & Bales, R. F. (1955). *Family socialization and interactions process.* New York: Free Press.

Selye, H. (1978). *The stress of life.* New York: McGraw-Hill.

Von Bertalanffy, L. (1950). The theory of open systems in physics and biology. *Science, 111,* 23–29.

CHAPTER 3
Ethical Issues in Rehabilitation

Darlene N. Finocchiaro and *Michael V. Finocchiaro*

Key Terms   *Advance Directives*
Blue Form
Capacity
Competency
Confidentiality
Conservator
Decision-Making Process
Declaration to Physicians (DP)
"Do Not Resuscitate" (DNR) Order
Deontology
Durable Power of Attorney for Health Care (DPAHC)
Egoism
Ethical Decision-Making Principles
Ethics
Fidelity
Informed Consent
Legal Decision
Living Will
Moral Issues
Morality
Physical Restraints
Placebo
Religious Perspective
Utilitarianism
Veracity

Objectives   1. Describe the purpose of an advance directive and what this document consists of.

2. Compare and contrast the three types of advance directives: durable power of attorney for health care, declaration to physicians, and a living will.

3. Discuss the nurse's role in the signing and implementation of a client's advance directive.

4. Determine when a "do not resuscitate" order might be ordered, and the nurse's responsibility.

5. Discuss the concept of veracity/truth telling in the administration of placebos.

6. State what the nurse is witnessing in the signing of a client's "informed consent."

7. Discuss seven or eight rehabilitation ethical issues and explain their significance to nursing practice.

8. Describe the three steps of the decision-making process.

9. Discuss the purpose and membership of the bioethics committee.

Introduction

The scope of nursing practice requires ethical decision making on a daily basis. A nurse must evaluate his or her own value system so as to implement it in the decision-making process. This value system is formed from several aspects including culture; religious background; family values; societal values; nursing theories; and law, both state and federal; these are influenced by ethical principles. Ethical issues specific to the field of rehabilitation nursing are addressed in this chapter, as they require further explanation to be applied in practice.

Definitions

Ethics: Ethics is the study of rightness of conduct, the processes used to judge moral behavior, and the problems encountered when applying principles of morally correct behavior. It involves studying values held by individuals and groups in the perspective of society. In nursing, the values developed by nursing professionals and educators are applied to the practice of nursing in its social role (Wywialowski, 1997).

Morality: Morality is one's values, choices, and actions resulting in living a good, upright life (Sparks, 1996).

Moral issues: Moral issues differ from ethical issues in that the decisions made will depend on loyalty to the employer or loyalty to the client.

Ethical decision-making principles: Within the study of ethics, several principles are involved. Foundation for ethical concepts, standards, codes, and ethical nursing practice.

Utilitarianism: Utilitarianism relates to doing the greatest good for the greatest number of individuals; that which is good for all.

Deontology: The principle of deontology has to do with rights, duties, and obligations. Therefore, it includes (1) preventing harm (nonmaleficence), (2) promoting good (beneficence), (3) being fair (justice), and (4) encouraging autonomy (the client's independence).

Egoism: Egoism describes the driving force behind actions taken for the good of the person who is acting.

Veracity: Communications must be truthful and accurate (Wywialowski, 1997).

Confidentiality: Principle guarding the right to privacy of clients and hospital committee meetings.

Fidelity: Being careful to follow up on one's own word to make sure you are following the details of a client's care (Wywialowsky, 1997).

Religious perspective: Decision making influenced by one's religious belief system (especially in life-and-death decision making).

Legal decision: When there are legal conflicts or the need for a legal decision, the input from a lawyer may be required.

Advance directive: A legally binding document that is signed in front of and sealed by a notary public. The document names a person or persons the client has appointed to make health care decisions in case of client incapacitation. On issuing such a document, it is presumed that the client and his or her appointed decision maker have discussed the issues thoroughly. One type of advance directive is also known as *durable power of attorney for health care.*

A *living will* is a document, legally executed by a lawyer, in which various medical situations are described and the decision the client wants is explicitly indicated. This document becomes effective when the client is incapable of making his or her own medical decisions.

Advance Directives

To preserve the right of all clients to make their own health care decisions, Congress enacted the Patient Self-Determination Act in October 1990, which became effective in December 1991. With the federal law in place, any hospital, nursing home, or hospice center that receives federal funds must ask on admission if a client has an advance directive. Also, if the client does not know what this is, the hospital must inform the client about his/her right to refuse treatment or to make other health care decisions. Therefore, the hospital must inform the client that he/she may execute an advance directive. The law also requires documentation on the client's chart of the existence of an advance directive for the client, with placement of a copy on the chart. This insinuates the formulation of hospital policies and procedures for advance directives. As an outcome of the law, staff and community education is a must. Home health care agencies and managed care organizations must provide their members with this information on enrollment (Berrio & Levesque, 1996).

An advance directive is a legally binding document that is formulated before an incapacitating illness or injury occurs. It allows a client to provide for decision making about his or her medical treatment if the client becomes unable to make those decisions. The advance directive can be of two types: (1) one that appoints a decision-making agent, or (2) a document that states a client's wishes about medical treatment in case the client becomes incapacitated. As a variant, both functions can be stated in a single document. Each state has its own laws, but in California there are three documents that serve as advance directives: (1) **durable power of attorney for health care,** (2) **declaration to physicians,** and (3) a **living will** (Rancho Los Amigos Medical Center, 1994).

1. A *durable power of attorney for health care* (DPAHC) is the preferred document, as it is considered a "legal document," that is, appoints an agent who makes decisions for the client who is incapacitated. The document can also specify which medical treatment a client does or does not want under certain circumstances. The DPAHC is signed, dated, witnessed or notarized, and is valid indefinitely until changed or canceled by the client.

2. A *declaration to physicians* (DP; California Natural Death Act) is a document specific to the state of California, as enacted by law. This is a legal document that is signed, dated, witnessed, and can be valid indefinitely. It directs physicians either to withhold or withdraw life-sustaining treatment from a client who is irreversibly unconscious as a result of a terminal illness. This action requires adequate documentation by a physician or, preferably, two physicians. A DP is very limited, as it refers to terminal illness only and no assigned decision maker is required (Rancho Los Amigos Medical Center, 1994).

3. A *living will* is considered a legal document in some states (not California). It consists of a written statement wherein the client relates his or her personal wishes concerning what care is wanted or not wanted. The declaration to physicians and the DPAHC are types of living wills in that they state the options given by clients for their treatment. The living will gives information to the health care deliverer in the client's terms to inform them what the client wants and does not want. Again, no surrogate decision maker is named (Rancho Los Amigos Medical Center, 1994).

The preceding are important documents that are intended to help in a client's care. Some authorities say it is even better to have a living will and DPAHC to attain maximum benefits. It is important that the document be executed correctly. The following are reasons clients do not initiate advance directive documents: (1) procrastination, (2) lack of knowledge about advance directives, (3) a desire not to face the issue, (4) dependency on other family members to make decisions, (5) passivity (e.g., "let the doctor inform me about it"; an attitude sometimes mirrored by physician passivity, e.g., "let the client ask me"), (6) misinformation, i.e., the perception that a lawyer is needed, (7) a "will of God" attitude, or (8) fear of not receiving treatment or of signing their life away (Berrio and Levesque, 1996). The rehabilitation nurse, in the role of client advocate, can make the difference by educating the client.

The rehabilitation nurse must know what an advance directive is and the state laws that regulate it. The nurse must be familiar with the hospital's policy and procedure on advance directives. As part of the nurse admission database, the question of whether the client has an advance directive or similar document needs to be addressed. If it is determined that a document is not present or completed, the nurse should explain the purpose of the advance directive in simple, nonmedical terminology. A member of the hospital ethics committee or a social worker might be helpful in obtaining necessary information to complete the document. A witness is necessary, when the client is ready to sign. This is usually done by a notary public assigned to the hospital. The nurse does not witness the client's signature. Once signed, a copy of the document is placed where easily visible in the medical record. The original copy should be kept by the client in a safe place. Once the document is signed, the nurse needs to be familiar with the client's decisions for health care, and also must know who will be responsible for health care decisions. The nurse should be certain that the client's physician is also aware of the client's wishes and that the physician has discussed these decisions with the client. The nurse needs to inform all members of the team caring for the client of the existence of the directive and any important issues contained therein. Depending on hospital policy, the nurse may or may not be responsible for advising clients as to why the advance directive is necessary. If it is the nurse's responsibility, the nurse may seek assistance from the hospital ethics committee as needed.

Follow-up of a client's care must be performed as instructed by the advance directive, if the client becomes incapacitated. If the client's wishes are not followed, the nurse and the health care team could be liable for assault and battery of the client. If the nurse's personal religious or ethical viewpoint precludes following the client's requests as laid out in the directive, the nurse should notify his or her superior for assistance. (See Figure 1 for a standard form of an advance directive.)

More research needs to be done by academics or research-oriented nurses as related to outcomes and the effectiveness of advance directives (Johns, 1996).

"Do Not Resuscitate" Order

The **"do not resuscitate" (DNR) order,** although a separate document, is an outgrowth of advance directives. DNR orders are addressed in every hospital's policy and procedures documents. The DNR order is written by a physician, after discussion between the physician and client or between the physician and client's decision maker. This is usually done for a client who has end-stage cancer or other devastating illness, if resuscitating the client would lead to a further life of misery. An example would be a client who decides that if he or she were to become totally paralyzed by a neurological disease, on an endotrachial tube, and that the only way he or she will live is in bed and on a ventilator; the client may tell the physician that if a cardiopulmonary arrest occurs he or she does not want to be resuscitated.

The thorough discussion must be documented in the medical record, and then the physician must write the order. These medical records are usually marked in some way so that all hospital personnel know not to resuscitate the client.

In some cases a physician's personal beliefs or religion will not permit the writing of this type of order. If, after personal reflection, the physician feels hesitant about implementing these orders, the physician must discuss it with a supervisor.

- Warnings to person executing the document:
  - a) Creation of durable power of attorney
  - b) Health Care Agent

I, _____ (client's name), do hereby designate and appoint:

Name: _____

Address: _____

Telephone number: _____

as my agent to make health care decisions for me.

- One may state here if client wants to donate body parts.
- Desires about life-prolonging care procedures, etc., may be listed here, along with *limitations* of power.

Alternate agent (if desired)

Name: _____

Address: _____

Telephone number: _____

- The power of attorney will exist indefinitely. It may revoke previous durable power of attorney.
- Signed and dated in front of notary public or two witnesses (nonmembers of the health care team or hospital staff, unless so designated by the hospital). One witness must *not* be a blood relative.

Fig 1. *A sample form for durable power of attorney for health care (California Health Care Association, 1997).*

Some states and counties have developed a bracelet or tag that is given to specific clients who have discussed these issues with their private doctor and requested a DNR order. These orders are housed in a special computer database. Therefore, if the client wearing such a bracelet or tag is rushed to an emergency room, the ER staff can proceed to take all measures to save the client, short of complete cardiopulmonary resuscitation.

Veracity   *Veracity,* known as truth, is absolutely necessary in all aspects of nursing. This is especially so in the administration of **placebos.** The truth must be told to the client. It is known that placebos can stimulate the release of endorphins under some clinical conditions and help relieve pain in and of themselves. The way this is told to the client is as follows: "This is a sugar substance that has been shown to relieve pain in some clients. Therefore, it is being given to you on a trial basis." The client should be informed by the physician.

Informed Consent

The purpose of **informed consent** is to ensure that a client who has the capacity to make decisions (or if not, the client's conservator) is informed of the benefits expected from the procedure in question. At the same time, possible complications that can occur need to be explained so that a balanced decision can be made.

The *expected benefits* are the end results hoped for following the procedure. *Possible risks* are the complications that could occur if the procedure is done. In the discussion with the client a relative rate of occurrence of the different complications should be discussed. What will happen if the procedure is not done (or what is the usual chain of events expected if no action is taken) needs to be addressed. This includes potential positive as well as negative effects.

The consent form can list all of the preceding items, including the chance of death as a complication. Before any invasive procedure can be performed there must be a signed consent.

The client's signature must be on the consent, with a date and time of signature. Also, a witness's signature must be present with date and time. Often, the nurse is the person who witnesses the consent. What does that mean? The nurse is witnessing only that the client is the one signing the consent. The nurse is witnessing that the client signed freely. If the nurse suspects that someone is pressuring the client into signing the consent, the nurse must notify the physician and his or her supervisor. The explanation of the procedure along with risks, benefits, complications, or side effects is the physician's responsibility. The nurse is not witnessing that the physician explained the procedure, or that he or she was present for that discussion.

When witnessing the signing of the consent, ethically the nurse must be sure that the client understands or can relate what the operation or procedure is in "lay terms." It needs to be verified that the physician did explain the procedure. If the nurse feels that the client needs further information, he or she should inform the physician. It is obligatory that the nurse affirm that the client has not received any narcotic or sedative medications that may alter the client's ability to think clearly when signing the consent.

In an emergency, a physician may elect to sign a form some facilities call a **"blue" form.** In some county facilities, this is present in the operating room. It is used for a transient or other client for whom no relative or legally appointed decision maker is available. The client is in imminent danger of bleeding to death, or of some other catastrophe, if action is not taken immediately. The blue form requires the signature of two licensed physicians. It presumes that there is not enough time to contact or find a legal guardian and the operation needs to be done immediately. In most cases, the client is unconscious or lacks the ability to understand or comprehend information. This form may also be used if after explaining the information the client still does not understand the imminent danger. This form must never be used to force a client to have an operation he or she does not want. Once the client has been operated on, the courts must be petitioned for legal guardianship by the social worker.

In such situations the **capacity** of the client becomes important. A client's capacity may be judged by whether the client can explain in lay terms what the operation is, the significance of having (or not having) the operation, and whether he or she appears to understand that it could lead to death—and the significance of that. If capacity to make decisions with regard to health care or even financial matters does not exist, then, with the assistance of a lawyer, the client needs to be presented to a judge. In the courtroom, the competency of the client will be determined.

The **competency** of a client must be determined by a judge. Competency is documented and declared in a court document sealed by the court judge.

A **conservator** is an agent appointed for a client to make financial and/or health care decisions. This is usually a consequence of a client being declared incompetent by a judge. Therefore, to protect the client, a judge appoints a conservator, who is usually someone the client knows or requests. However, any inconsistencies are subject to review by the court in case of dispute.

Rehabilitation Issues

The rehabilitation client, whether he or she has a spinal cord injury, multiple sclerosis, Guillain Barré syndrome, brain injury, cardiovascular accident (CVA), or chronic pulmonary obstructive disease, has special needs. These are not always addressed in acute nursing care. Ethical issues in all phases of nursing practice incite many questions, but few answers. Rehabilitation nursing has as one of its tenets that clients need to be part of the decision-making process, because the client is the one that is going to benefit from rehabilitative care. Many facilities have bioethics or ethics committees (to be discussed subsequently in this chapter) that help form policies and procedures. They can also act as an aid in the decision-making process.

There are limited funds available to rehabilitation clients with certain permanent disabilities. This may limit the extent of rehabilitation, or may incite family conflicts or legal questions. This places additional burdens on the rehabilitation nurse who is in charge of the client's rehabilitation. The nurse may need to ask for legal assistance, or the courts for a resolution.

Specific ethical issues include the following (Patterson, 1993):

• Does a client have the right to receive funds for his/her choice of treatment after he/she has refused the recommended treatment?

- Does there exist a right for all clients, to receive rehabilitation? Does this right extend to illegal aliens or to those who commit violent acts and are injured as a result?
- Who on the rehabilitation team makes the decision about discontinuing services owing to lack of progress toward specified goals?
- If a client for rehabilitation makes the statement that he/she wants to die, and therefore does not wish to be rehabilitated, should the team follow the request and stop treatment?
- What should the members of a rehabilitation team do if they have a homeless individual who is ready for discharge, but there is no adequate place to which the client can go?
- With a comatose client, when should staff discontinue gastrostomy or nasogastric tube feedings?
- When should restraints (either chemical or physical) be initiated?
- Do clients in a persisting vegetative state have the right to receive publicly funded organ transplants?
- Is parental consent needed to discuss sex education with a disabled adolescent?

Physical Restraints

Physical restraints can be initiated if the physician's order is clearly written on the chart. Such an order needs to be renewed every day, depending on the client's progress. These orders are usually written when there exists a high level of risk that the client will hurt him- or herself. Parameters need to be explicitly stated on the chart as to what behavior pattern needs restraining, and how long restraints need to be in place. It is necessary to review the hospital policy and procedure along with state regulations. A PRN (*pro re nata,* as circumstances may require) order cannot be written, as per regulations (state). If an emergency order is obtained over the phone, the physician must sign it within 24 hours of the order. The same should apply to chemical restraints, but there may be other parameters that need to be followed.

Candidate for Rehabilitation

The issue of certain clients receiving or not receiving rehabilitation needs to be evaluated in terms of *equity,* a principle about the "same" cases needing to be treated alike. In reference to health care, it refers to a system that provides similar services to people who have similar health problems or needs (Association of Rehabilitation Nurses, 1994).

Decision-Making Process

Clients that have a devastating illness or injury such as spinal cord injury may say "I want to die." This situation needs a complete evaluation to ensure that the client is not in a severe state of depression. Depression needs treatment before any decision can be made about not resuscitating the client. It may also be necessary to discuss the situation thoroughly with the client, and come to a compromise.

Case Study

A client sustained a CVA that was so severe that the client was unable to swallow, and a feeding gastrostomy tube needed to be inserted. The client wanted it removed and to be left to die. However, this client had not yet experienced the benefits of the complete rehabilitation program. The physician discussed the client's desires with the client and his family.

The client and physician were able to come to the following decision: The client would keep the gastrostomy tube for 3 months; during this time he would receive rehabilitation to strengthen him and to be able to see how much function would return. After 3 months the client, physician, and family would re-evaluate the situation. If the client, after this initial therapy trial, still wanted to die, the gastrostomy tube would be removed and nature left to take its course. The client would still be kept as comfortable as possible. Ultimately, the client elected to keep the gastrostomy tube in place.

The **decision-making process,** as summarized in Figure 2, can be used to approach all ethical situations. The "packaging" of these situations (see Figure 2) simplifies the approach. Ethical situations must be reviewed in their entirety before a decision can be correctly made.

Bioethics Committee

The bioethics committee should be available to assist the staff of a hospital on how to make an ethical decision. It should not be a "watch dog"–type committee, looking over everybody's shoulder. It should be a group educated in basic ethics and multidisciplined. There should be representatives from nursing, especially if the "shared governance" approach to hospital management is being used. In that situation, one of the members of the nursing practice council should be on the bioethics committee as a nursing representative. As a separate member of the committee, nursing administration may desire to have their own representative if

---

A. What are the benefits (beneficence) of making the calculated decision? What good will come out of it?

B. What are the possible negative returns (maleficence) from making that decision?

C. In a similar fashion, if I make the opposite decision, what are the good points or benefits of doing it this way?

D. Conversely, what are the negative points of making the opposite decision?

Fig 2. *A summary decision-making process to be used in approaching ethical situations. (Adapted from Brummel-Smith, 1990.)*

a position is available. The membership should include a physician, administrator, nursing personnel, recording secretary, psychiatrist, legal council, and a chaplain.

If it is protected under the auspices of a medical staff meeting, there may be an element of confidentiality to it, to protect what is discussed and its members. The committee should report to the medical director, and the nursing representative usually reports to either the practice council chair or director of nursing.

In some facilities, the committee has members who go out and evaluate clients in regard to certain ethical decision-making issues. They may also make suggestions to the treating primary physician. It is necessary to evaluate each particular facility, its policy and procedures and evaluate how the committee functions. In some instances it may have an obscure reputation, as staff may not understand how it functions. Nurses should become familiar with the hospital's bioethics committee, so they can make better ethical decisions regarding requests from clients.

Case Study

One bioethics committee became involved with a client who had end-stage pulmonary disease, who was intubated and put on a ventilator. The client wanted to be taken off the ventilator. The committee and its members started their decision-making process with the point that the client was making the decision. Through a long and careful thought process with a psychologist, psychiatrist, administrator, legal council, and clergy, the client decided he wished to be disconnected from the ventilator. This was carefully planned, accomplished, and the client expired. Staff was shocked by this end result, but the decision was made by means of a thorough process of ethical decision making as noted previously.

Case Study

A 60-year-old male developed Wegener's granulomatosis that required the client to have a tracheostomy and ventilator. Before the client ever came to the hospital he had executed an advance directive and, in the process, named a daughter as his agent. When the client became incapacitated, the agent requested that the tracheostomy be removed. This decision was made on the basis of the father's discussion with the daughter about these very issues. When the decision was made, some family members disagreed. The bioethics committee had to convene and make recommendations based on the facts. Ultimately, the tracheostomy was removed and the father expired very peacefully in no pain. The ethics committee had to advocate for the client's stated desires. The family also needed emotional support, which was provided.

Bioethics committees are involved in the decision-making process regarding removal of feeding tubes, removal of fluids, clients who are unable to swallow, and so on. These committees are being evaluated academically to determine where they fit in the comprehensive scope of health care. Also being questioned is what role the committee should serve so as to act in the most beneficial way. Many bioethics centers have opened across the country. Nurses should know about any bioethics centers available in their community as resources.

Conclusion

Ethics is a large field that is just beginning to come alive on its own. Many issues are being brought up, owing to the expansion of medical knowledge and technology. Many unheard-of questions have risen and will continue to be explored. The role of bioethics committees, centers, and ethicists is taking shape. The role of the bioethics committee is very important for the protection of clients, staff, and the whole decision-making process. The case studies presented suggest the immensity and scope of practice. More nursing research needs to be done in the field, under adequate research guidelines. This will clarify the role of nursing in these issues and decisions.

Bioethics is an expanding field and will establish its place in the nursing and medical arenas. Its role will expand to meet increasingly visible and ever-growing needs. The legal implications are also expanding and opening more doors to unthought-of issues, such as the rights of surrogate mothers.

The field of bioethics has been explained and its principles discussed; it is hoped that this discussion initiates a desire for further study and research.

References

Association of Rehabilitation Nurses. (December 1994–January 1995). ARN position statement: Ethical issues. *ARN News, 10*(10), 10–11.

Berrio, M. W., & Levesque, M. E. (1996). Advance directives: Most patients don't have one. Do yours? *American Journal of Nursing 96*(8), 25–29.

Brummel-Smith, K. (1990, Summer). *Bioethics.* Presentation given to medical staff at Rancho Los Amigos Medical Center, Downey, CA.

California Health Care Association. (1997). *Consent manual: A reference for consent and related health care law.* Sacramento, CA: Author.

Johns, J. L. (1996). Advance directives and opportunities for nurses. *Image, 28*(2), 149–153.

Patterson, T. (1993). Ethics in rehabilitation nursing. In A. E. McCourt (Ed.), *The specialty practice of rehabilitation nursing: A core curriculum* (3rd ed.). Skokie, IL: Rehabilitation Nursing Foundation.

Rancho Los Amigos Medical Center. (1994, March 1). *Advance directives (administrative policy and procedure).* Downey, CA: Author.

Sparks, R. C. (1996). *Contemporary Christian morality: Real questions, candid responses.* New York: Crossroad Publishing Co.

Wywialowski, E. F. (1997). *Managing client care* (2nd ed.). St. Louis: Mosby–Year Book.

CHAPTER 4
Interdisciplinary Rehabilitation Team: Composition, Models, Functions

Patricia A. Chin

Key Terms *Collaboration*
Communication
Conflict Resolution
Interdisciplinary Team
Multidisciplinary Team
Team Building
Team-Managed Care
Transdisciplinary Team

Objectives 1. Describe the characteristics, benefits, and limitation of various practice models used in rehabilitation settings.

2. Describe how the interdisciplinary rehabilitation team differs from the traditional medical model of health care delivery.

3. Identify the mission and goals of the interdisciplinary rehabilitation team.

4. Identify the strengths of the interdisciplinary rehabilitation team approach in the rehabilitation setting.

5. Discuss the composition of the rehabilitation interdisciplinary team and identify each professional team member's role and functions.

6. Identify the characteristics of a successful rehabilitation interdisciplinary team and team leader.

7. Discuss how collaboration, communication, and conflict resolution facilitate the effectiveness of the rehabilitation interdisciplinary team.

The Team Approach Rehabilitation is actually a philosophy of care. When attempting to meet the multiple physical, psychological, emotional, social, spiritual, and economic needs of the rehabilitation client, and the client's family, it is foolish to believe that one professional from any one discipline can be effective in accomplishing the task. A compromise between the specialization of disciplines and a comprehensive approach to client care is the team approach (Rothberg, 1981). Multidisciplinary care assumes that many qualified health care professionals contribute to comprehensive care. Nurses, physicians, public health workers, therapists, and social workers all have something of value to offer the client.

Multidisciplinary care shifts the focus from an episodic patient–health care provider relationship to a relationship between the client and a variety of different health care professionals. These professionals work as a coordinated system centered around client care. The focus shifts from the traditional illness-based approach to a community-based health approach. Instead of seeing the client apart from the environment the client is instead identified within the context of the community to ensure holistic care. The multidisciplinary team attempts to blend individual professions and their roles and responsibilities into a system focused on client needs and care (Henry, 1996).

The team approach for the delivery of care and services to clients with rehabilitative needs has been the foundation of rehabilitation care. The rehabilitation client is the most significant member of the rehabilitation team. Each client possesses unique and complex physical, psychosocial, and spiritual attributes and characteristics contributing to overall sense of self and identity. The common goals of the therapeutic rehabilitation team are to maintain client individuality; promote client autonomy within the parameters of the disability or chronic illness; and facilitate continued client maturity, growth, and development as a human person.

The strengths of the team approach to rehabilitation include promotion of communication, collaboration among health care providers, and the holistic view of the client and family. There is some evidence that the team approach energizes the staff and team members (O'Toole, 1992). Diller (1990) and Rothberg (1981) identified team member problems with role diffusion, care provider ambiguity, status concerns, interpersonal conflicts, lack of commitment of some team members, and staff competency as limitations of the team approach. Weaknesses of the team approach that might negatively influence its future role in rehabilitation practice include cost, inefficiency, reduced time for direct patient care, and the psychological strain on staff (Rothberg, 1981).

The mission of the rehabilitation team is to treat the multiple needs of the whole person. This requires the coordinated efforts of various specialists to enable the client to reach maximum potential (Keith, 1991). The core members of the rehabilitative team, as identified by the Joint Commission for Accreditation of Healthcare Organization (JCAHO, 1993) include the rehabilitation nurse, physician, physical therapist, occupational therapist, speech-language therapist, and social worker (see Table 1). The Commission for Accreditation of Rehabilitation Facilities (CARF, 1993) has extended that core list to include the psychologist and therapeutic recreational therapist. Additional rehabilitative team members are

Table 1
Core Members of the Rehabilitative Team and Their Roles

Member	Roles
Rehabilitation nurse	1. Provides direct care 2. Maintains and restores functions and prevents complications and further impairment 3. Reinforces the use of skills taught and practiced in therapy sessions 4. Coordinates daily schedule and team activities 5. Creates a therapeutic environment 6. Acts as client and family educator 7. Acts as client and family advocate
Physician	1. Establishes a medical diagnosis and prognosis 2. Provides medical management 3. Interprets radiologic and laboratory findings 4. Requests and interprets special testing procedures 5. Prescribes treatments, medications, and therapeutic aids 6. Directs the progress of the treatment plan
Physical therapist	1. Assists client in functional restoration of mobility 2. Deals with issues of range of motion, strength, reflexes, tone, posture, gait, orthotic or prosthetic fit and function, and sensorimotor function 3. Engages in treatment modalities: of heat/cold, hydrotherapy, electrical stimulation, massage, joint mobilization, and exercise 4. Provides training in locomotion using orthoses, prostheses, crutches, canes, walkers, and wheelchairs
Occupational therapist	1. Assists client in restoration of function for optimal participation in activities of daily living (work, school, community, recreation) 2. Assists with activities of daily living (ADL) and with independent living skills 3. Deals with issues of joint function and protection, coordination, endurance, body mechanics and positioning 4. Deals with issues of adapting and adopting assistive equipment and prosthetic devices 5. Evaluates home environment, home management, prevocational activities, and social skills
Speech-language therapist	1. Provides therapy for verbal and written language, articulation, speech fluency, and interactive communication 2. Provides therapy for cognitive deficits, memory, and comprehension 3. Coordinates use of verbal and nonverbal communication augmentation 4. Directs treatment plan for dysphagic clients
Social worker	1. Assists with personal issues 2. Assesses coping history and current adaptation to disability 3. Assesses availability of family members and support networks 4. Provides counseling and support 5. Deals with issues of housing, living arrangements, employment, and education 6. Deals with issues of financial resources 7. Deals with transportation issues 8. Expedites discharge issues 9. Acts as liaison between client and the family and community resources
Psychologist	1. Evaluates and treats client's psychological and neurospsychological impairments associated with disability 2. Assesses emotional and cognitive status 3. Provides counseling to client and family members
Recreational therapist	1. Assists clients with individual and group recreational and leisure activities 2. Assists with the promotion of social skills and resocialization

Sources: Diller (1990); Dittmar (1989); Hoeman (1992); Rothberg (1992).

added to the team depending on individual client needs, the care setting, and specific needs of client populations. Other professional members of the team may include audiologist, chaplain, driving evaluator/instructor, nutritionist, orthotic/prosthetic specialist, pharmacist, rehabilitation engineer, respiratory therapist, image consultant, and vocational counselor.

The team approach has been the model for providing care and services to individuals with rehabilitation needs and disabilities. However, the current health care crises, and flux in health care delivery models and health coverage plans, in the United States are shifting the structure of health care delivery models. Some rehabilitation authors have noted that the current health crisis, attempts at reform, and the economic flux challenge the team approach as currently conceived (Diller, 1990; Keith, 1991; Melvin, 1989). Alternative treatment models may need to be developed as government and third-party payers demand tighter cost containment, expenditure controls, and resource utilization. It is important for those professionals involved in rehabilitative nursing, and other team members, to demonstrate and support the effectiveness of team functioning in order to ensure quality care to individuals with disabilities and chronic illnesses.

Characteristics, Benefits, and Limitations of Rehabilitation Team Models

A variety of models exist for directing practice in rehabilitation settings. Not all of the models currently in use are effective for providing comprehensive care or for achieving the desired client rehabilitation outcomes. The choice of a rehabilitation practice model can be determined by the types of delivery setting available, types of service providers available, and types of services offered to clients. Other factors driving rehabilitation practice model selection are as follows: cost, the market for rehabilitation services, client care demands, consumer expectation, reimbursement issues, and existing practice regulations.

Existing rehabilitation practice models can be classified by focusing on the client, the setting, the provider, or the form of collaborative practice (see Table 2).

Collaborative Practice Models
Interdisciplinary Team

An **interdisciplinary team** is a group of professionals from a variety of disciplines whose activities are directed toward the accomplishment of a common goal. An interdisciplinary team approach is the practice model required by both the Joint Commission on Accreditation of Healthcare Organization (JCAHO, 1993) and the Commission on Accreditation of Rehabilitation Facilities (CARF, 1993). When this practice model is used members are engaged in problem solving beyond the confines and domain of their own disciplines (Diller, 1990). The members of the treatment team meet regularly to share information about the client and the client's needs and to discuss progress toward commonly agreed-on goals. The scheduling and timing of these meetings will depend on the client's stage of the rehabilitation process. During the stabilization period and early in the rehabilitation process team meetings will be more frequent than toward the termination and community reintegration stages of the rehabilitation experience.

Table 2
Current Classification of Rehabilitation Practice Models

Model	Characteristics	Specialization based on
Client focused	Consumer driven Recognizes the role of client needs, values, expectations Culturally sensitive Family oriented Specialization of care	• Type of disability (i.e., cancer rehabilitation, burn rehabilitation, cardiac rehabilitation) • Client developmental levels (i.e., pediatric rehabilitation, geriatric rehabilitation, adult rehabilitation)
Setting focused	Differentiated by the type of setting in which rehabilitation is provided	• Acute care rehabilitation settings (i.e., free-standing rehabilitation hospital, rehabilitation units in acute care hospitals) • Long-term care settings (i.e., long-term care facility, subacute hospital settings), community-based settings, home settings, religious-based settings
Provider focused	Considers cost and effectiveness of care outcomes Concerned with staffing levels, supply of health care providers, and patient demand for service Model differentiated by role of care provider	• Primary care provider model • Case management model • Nurse-managed care model • Independent practice/consultation model
Collaborative practice	Coordinated, concurrent care by multiple health care providers Team made up of professionals from variety of disciplines united in goal to effect positive rehabilitation outcomes for the patient Core members of the team determined by the needs of the client Client and family are considered critical team members Concerned with holistic care	• Interdisciplinary team • Transdisciplinary team • Multidisciplinary team

Sources: O'Toole (1992); Melvin (1989); Diller (1990); Hoeman (1992); Howard (1991).

Interdisciplinary team meetings are a priority activity for rehabilitation nursing. The rehabilitation nurse is a major asset to the treatment team. Rehabilitation nursing staff often have the opportunity to spend more time with the client while they are engaged in a variety of activities. Nursing personnel can be privy to vital information regarding client needs and problems because of the intimate nature of the nurse-client relationship. The effectiveness of the treatment team depends on the accuracy of nursing's assessment of the client's progress and the on-going input from nurses who coordinate client activities (O'Toole, 1992).

The interdisciplinary team approach to rehabilitation offers identified benefits to the client, the client's caregivers, and the treatment team. This approach provides the team members with a holistic view of client needs. This comprehensive, consistent, nonsegmented approach fosters optimal client outcomes. When the interdisciplinary team is productive there can be a reduction in health care cost, efficient use of health care resources, and appropriate use of health care personnel (O'Toole, 1992). Limitations to the interdisciplinary model have been identified. This model is more complex and time-consuming than the multidisciplinary model. There is a greater need for coordination and collaboration, and there can also be more incidents of conflict and disagreement regarding the treatment plan. One of the most often encountered issues experienced when using this approach is the controversy over who is designated as the interdisciplinary team leader (Diller, 1990).

Transdisciplinary Team

The **transdisciplinary team** is similar to the interdisciplinary team. In the transdisciplinary team approach one or two health care providers are responsible for the implementation of the treatment plan instead of professionals from all of the involved disciplines who might provide service to meet the client's needs. The use of this practice approach requires the primary health care provider to be able to provide a wide spectrum of care and to possess a broad scope of knowledge and skills. Members from the other disciplines are available for use by the primary care providers as consultants regarding client care. The focus of this approach is reinforcement and teaching across all disciplines (Diller, 1990). This approach to care requires a high degree of communication, interaction among health professionals, staff development, and flexible thinking (Hoeman, 1992).

One of the benefits associated with the transdisciplinary team approach is a reduction in the amount of stimulation and stress the client experiences in working with a limited number of individuals. The approach is beneficial for clients with cognitive disorders or developmental disabilities, who may have greater difficulty tolerating multiple and frequent changes of health care providers. The transdisciplinary practice conserves staff resources. Melvin (1989) emphasized that this practice approach could pose problems in meeting client needs because the primary health care provider may not possess the required expertise in all aspects of the treatment plan to produce established client outcomes. This practice approach has demonstrated neither effectiveness in the accomplishment of treatment team goals nor reductions in health care cost.

Multidisciplinary Team

The **multidisciplinary team** approach uses the skills and knowledge of a wide variety of disciplines. The practitioners are required to possess only the knowledge and skills of their own discipline. Each discipline assumes responsibility for its specific aspects of the treatment plan. The members of the multidisciplinary team do not participate in the collaborative planning of care, treatment implementation, or evaluation of treatment outcomes that occurs among the members of the interdisciplinary team. There is minimal coordination of client care in this practice approach. The client and family members are not encouraged to participate in the rehabilitation process in this approach. The benefit for team members is that less time is spent in team meetings. However, the trade-off for time savings is fragmented treatment, duplication of services, limitations in creative planning and problem-solving, and compromised client care (Howard, 1991).

An evolving form of the multidisciplinary practice model is **team-managed care.** This approach combines case management and the multidisciplianry treatment team. A case manager is designated to oversee treatment team activities. The case manager is the overall coordinator, provides supervision, and determines the selection of client services (Rothberg, 1992). The priorities of the treatment plan are determined by the entire treatment team. The benefits and limitations of the team-managed approach have yet to be established.

Core Membership and Functions of the Rehabilitative Team

The Joint Commission on Accreditation of Healthcare Organization (JCAHO) and the Commission on Accreditation of Rehabilitation Facilities (CARF) have established the membership of the treatment team as well as the core functions of the rehabilitative team members. The core functions of the team are consistent with the components of the nursing process and include assessment, designing of a plan of care, implementation of the treatment plan, evaluation and modification of the treatment plan, and discharge planning (Table 3). Each member of the rehabilitation team is responsible for the contribution of his or her specific discipline to the treatment team.

Understanding and Building the Effective Rehabilitation Team

Program Manager

The Commission on Accreditation of Rehabilitation Facilities (CARF, 1993) requires that one individual be designated as the program manager for the interdisciplinary team. The functions of this manager are to coordinate team activities, monitor appropriate use of resources, and facilitate the timely discharge of the client. The team leader often assumes a leadership role among the rehabilitation team members. It should be noted that team leadership is not vested in one person but really is the responsibility of the entire team (Campbell, 1992).

Leadership is defined as a set of behaviors and skills (Campbell, 1992) that can be taught and learned. Francis and Young (1979) identified leadership style as the single most important element in determining the quality of teamwork. The effectiveness of the rehabilitation team is enhanced when leadership activities are based on competence, expertise, and information rather than on the formal

Table 3
Core Functions of the Rehabilitation Team

Function	Specifics of Function
Assessment of functional needs and functional ability	Initial assessment of client's functional abilities and capabilities (baseline assessment) Initial assessment of the client's biological, psychological, social, and spiritual needs Assessment of the client's disabilities Continual monitoring of intervention results and treatment outcomes Assessment of client's and family's skills and capabilities necessary for discharge
Development and documentation of an interdisciplinary treatment plan	Developing and defining the treatment team's purpose Developing treatment strategies that are meaningful to client and family Developing clear, specific, measurable, and verifiable client goals and objectives Developing realistic and attainable goals that are congruent with available personnel, resources, and funding Developing interventions among disciplines Establishing client-centered outcome evaluation criteria Continuous documentation of treatment interventions and client's responses to interventions
Interdisciplinary team implementation of the treatment plan	Planning interventions aimed at achievement of rehabilitation goals based on client health care problems, etiology, and overall team goals Coordinating treatment team interventions focusing on attainment of independent living goals Providing opportunities for the client and family members to provide care and demonstrate that they have learned the skills and techniques needed for effective care
Evaluating the rehabilitation treatment plan for the degree of goals achievement	Evaluating summative and formative indicators of client's progress toward achievement of treatment goals Developing new goals as original treatment goals are achieved Modifying treatment goals as necessary to achieve goal completion Monitoring quality of care in conjunction with cost containment
Preparing for client discharge	Designating a discharge coordinator Setting discharge goal at onset of rehabilitation process Coordinating treatment team planning to meet discharge date successfully Discussing the client's discharge needs among treatment team members Communicating discharge needs to the care coordinator Determining what equipment and supplies will be necessary for continued care after client discharge Making appropriate referrals to available and accessible resources Insuring continuity of care through verbal and written communication with referral agencies and programs Facilitating client transitions to the discharge setting Initiating disengagement from client-rehabilitation team relationship to promote independence after discharge

Sources: Joint Commission on Accreditation of Healthcare Organizations (JCAHO, 1993); Commission on Accreditation of Rehabilitation Facilities (CARF, 1993).

status of an individual within the team. Leadership is most effective when it is balanced and shared among the members of the treatment team (Garner, 1988).

Team Building

A primary leadership activity is team building. **Team building** (Farley & Stoner, 1989) is a process of deliberately creating and unifying a group of people into an effective and efficiently functioning work unit. This occurs in order to accomplish specific goals established by the team. Team building must occur if the team is to become more adept in pursuing its objectives and in identifying and resolving work-related problems.

The effective rehabilitative team works in a cohesive manner to achieve a common purpose and mutually determined treatment goals. Each member of the team will bring to the team experience different training and skills, unique personalities, individualism, and unique discipline-specific expertise. Numerous factors can be barriers to team work that will ultimately decrease the effectiveness of the team and the achievement of client goals. Competition may exist among professionals from different disciplines. Role ambiguity, overlapping role functions, and conflicting expectations can also be barriers to the effective functioning of the team. If there is to be commonality among health care providers engaged in the rehabilitation process there must be a sense of trust and confidence among the team members. A sense of interdependence is essential.

Effective team work involves developing creative solutions to problems, creative constructive opinions, open communication of varied ideas, and consensus. The effective team leader is a skillful communicator and leader. The productive team is led by someone who is knowledgeable regarding group process, role relations, facilitation of collaboration, and conflict resolution.

Weekly meetings of the health care providers and the client do not make an effective working team. Team members may assume too much about other team members' knowledge, skills, or capabilities or they may know too little or have erroneous information about the role and functions of other team members. Team member interactions can be more effective if the team can establish

- The specific goal or target of the team
- The required tasks of the team and each team member
- The nature of team member and staff input and feedback and communication channels for disseminating that information
- The way team members can best work together to achieve team goals
- The guidelines and procedures necessary to facilitate team member task achievement
- The potential areas of conflict among the team members (Hoeman, 1993)

Effective teams are nurtured and developed through the efforts of team members who consciously work at the process of team building. The productivity of the therapeutic rehabilitative team is enhanced by fostering and supporting creativity, by risk taking, and by dealing with controversy and avoiding stagnation (Campbell, 1992). Three key elements that will promote effective group functioning are collaboration, communication, and conflict resolution.

Collaboration

Collaboration is a complex phenomenon. In the context of the provision of health care, "collaboration" refers to an interpersonal process occurring among two or more individuals who have made a commitment to function constructively to solve problems and accomplish identified goals, purposes, or outcomes (Hanson & Spross, 1996, p. 232). This definition implies shared values, commitments, and goals. Individuals may come to the rehabilitative team with expert skills and different strengths. By working side by side with a shared purpose, team members can combine energies and produce a synergistic effect. It is the shared vision and commonality of purpose that produce success and improves outcomes (Senge, 1990).

Prerequisite characteristics for collaboration are common purpose, clinical competency, interpersonal skills, trust, and a sense of humor (Hanson & Spross, 1996). Spross (1989) described three essential elements of collaboration: a common purpose, diverse and complementary professional knowledge, and an effective communication process. In nursing literature collaboration has also been described as a force for achieving desired outcomes (Evans, 1994). Clinicians engaged in collaboration use a communal, intellectual effort, sharing problem-solving, goal setting, and decision-making approaches (Evans, 1994).

Failure to collaborate affects care providers and the client. Job satisfaction and attitude were negatively affected and territoriality and competitiveness increased when there was a lack of collaborative effort (Alpert, Goldman, Kilroy, & Pike, 1992). A negative effect on client care is the most significant result of treatment team failure to collaborate (Baggs, 1989; Hanson & Spross, 1996).

Collaboration is achieved through open communication and harmony among team members. A collaborative team possesses a strong philosophy of acknowledging human dignity and respect (Roseman, 1985). The collaborative team uses negotiation to seek creative, integrated solutions to clinical problems. Boundaries and roles are well defined in a collaborative team (Cohen, Rubin, & Gombash, 1992). Information is communicated clearly and decision-making responsibilities are clearly outlined and supported by group consensus.

There are several processes that drive effective collaboration. Team members require recurring interactions. Through these interactions the members acquire understanding of role requirements and functions. They also learn to develop constructive, productive, and supportive patterns of interaction (Hilderley, 1991; Dickinson, Mateo, Jackson, & Swartz, 1995). Recurring interactions help clinicians to understand other team members' scope of practice and responsibilities

(Hanson & Spross, 1996). A skill identified by Krumm (1992) as a component of collaboration is bridging. She describes bridging as the ability to recognize and rearrange practice boundaries. Bridging occurs when tasks are redistributed among team members. Consultation also drives collaboration. Consultation is a process of communication through which those who are caring for a client seek advice regarding client concerns from other professionals. The primary care giver retains responsibility for care during the consultation process.

Constraints to an effective collaborative process can be tradition ((Hanson & Spross, 1996 ; Safriet, 1992) sexism and stereotypical images (Siegler & Whitney, 1994). Turf issues also interfered with both formal and informal collaborative efforts, especially between nurses and physicians.

Communication

Effective **communication** is an extremely important factor in the success of an interdisciplinary team (Moulder, Staal, & Grant, 1988). The rehabilitation nurse communicates with the client, family, and other health care providers regarding the provision of care. The rehabilitation nurse also communicates client data so that information is integrated into the interdisciplinary treatment plan. It is also important for the rehabilitation nurse to provide peers with constructive feedback regarding their practice. Ineffective communication can result in frustration and stress for team members, inappropriate actions and interventions based on incomplete or inaccurate information, and client and family receiving conflicting messages and instructions (Garner, 1988). Dysfunctional communication patterns include a self-perpetuating syndrome, inability to focus on one issue, and closed areas of communication.

Attributes of an Effective Communicator. Effective communicators accept differences in perspectives of others, and can tolerate constant review and challenge of their own ideas, thought, and beliefs. They possess personal identity and integrity. They can function independently and are willing to take risks. They are good at negotiating roles with other team members and accept the team philosophy of care (Givens & Simmons, 1977). Effective communicators are functional senders of messages as well as receivers of messages.

Functional senders firmly state their case. Their messages are highly congruent, intense, and explicit. They use communication techniques to increase clarification and qualification of statements. Functional senders send direct statements and ask direct questions. They elicit feedback to validate that their messages are being correctly received. They are open and receptive to feedback.

Functional receivers use attentive listening skills. They provide and elicit feedback to ensure that they are correctly receiving messages. They seek validation, clarification, and clarity by asking questions, making associations, and checking perceptions.

Dysfunctional senders make many assumptions. They often speak for others. Their perceptions or evaluations cannot be altered. They send incomplete messages. They assume that the perceptions, thoughts, and feelings of others are the same as their own. They generalize; one instance exemplifies all instances. They are unclear in their expression of feelings. There is an inability to express needs. They make covert requests of others instead of direct requests. Their messages are filled with complaints, sarcasm, superreasonableness, silent resentment, expression of hurt as anger, judgmental expressions, and put-down statements. There is a silent need for nurturance.

Dysfunctional receivers fail to listen. In their messages they use disqualifying "yes-but" statements. They are evasive, tangential, and distracted in their communications. Their statements are often offensive. Their messages are filled with negativity, there is a lack of exploration, and they do not seek validation from others.

Formal and Informal Communication Channels. Communications between and among team members will be either formal or informal. Formal communication channels include regular team meetings required by accrediting agencies for the discussion of client progress and goal achievement. Periodically, family conferences will be held to promote open communication among the client, the family, caregivers, significant support systems, and the health care providers. Administrative meetings provide another formal channel for the evaluation of team process, program goals, financial resources, and future team directions. Newsletters highlighting program activities and current practices are also formalized communication channels, as are computerized schedule sheets or scheduling boards. Administrative reports provide formal documentation of the team's contributions to client outcomes.

Informal communication channels that often provide team members with current information are impromptu confidential conversations in hallways, at lunch, and at the bedside. Information is often circulated more quickly through informal communication channels than through the formal channels.

Conflict Resolution

Conflict is inevitable (Weeks, 1992). Conflict is common and necessary for team development. Conflict can be relational, situational, and moral. Professionals can become angry or frustrated when others disagree with them, especially regarding client issues. Most professionals expect others to agree with them and may interpret disagreement as confrontation. Conflict always has consequences. Conflict can serve as a catalyst for needed change. Unresolved conflict can undermine the effectiveness of a treatment team (Frank & Elliot, 1992).

Conflict is an outgrowth of diversity. This diversity need not be a destructive force in relationships. It can result in mutual growth and improved relationships. Conflict does involve incompatible self-interest or desires but it also involves values, needs, perceptions, power, and feelings. Conflict may be interpreted as absolutes between right and wrong or between good and bad. However, conflict can be constructive when the possibility is explored that a particular conflict may arise because of subjective preferences rather than professional values. Conflicts between or among members of the interdisciplinary team are issue specific and should not be allowed to disrupt the interpersonal relationships of team members.

See Table 4 for a summary of several areas that may be the cause of conflicts among the members of the rehabilitation team.

How we understand conflict will influence how we approach **conflict resolution** (Weeks, 1992, p. 61). Four principles should be applied in conflict resolution situations:

1. Those involved need to be able to separate the people from the problem.
2. The focus should be on the interests of those involved, not on the positions they have taken.
3. Those involved should invent options for mutual gain.
4. Those involved should insist on using objective criteria—agreed-on independent standards (Fisher & Ury, 1981).

Cornett-Cooke and Dias (1984) identified strategies that would be useful for preventing conflicts among rehabilitation team members. Those involved in the team should clearly identify roles and reach consensus on the role functions of each team member. The team should identify areas of potential role overlap and negotiate role boundaries. The treatment team's purpose should be clearly articulated and treatment goals and outcomes negotiated. Communication can be improved by encouraging constructive criticism regarding the team's process. New members to the team should be oriented to the team's structure, function, process, objectives, and goals. Support should be provided for new team members and those experiencing staffing shortages or involved in treating a complex and challenging client. The team's process can be facilitated by identifying the role of the group, the informal and formal groups leaders, and the team's responsibilities.

Conflicts should be resolved in an effective and sustainable manner. Those determining how the conflict is perceived and resolved must take into consideration the future of the team members' working relationship. This is possible through a conflict partnership approach (Weeks, 1992).

Table 4
Rehabilitation Team Conflict

A. Possible Sources of Rehabilitation Team Conflict*

Source	Examples
Status issues	• Controversy over leadership of the team • Equality among team members • Professional rivalries • Power conflicts
Communication obstacles	• Using discipline-specific professional jargon • Inattentive listening skills and habits • Blockers to channels of communication • Time limitations
Practice issues	• Role ambiguity • Overlapping of professional roles • Unclear role boundaries • Role incongruity • Questions related to professional competency of team members • Too little understanding about the roles of various team members • Discrepancies in goals and outcome expectations
Decision-making issues	• Professional and personal value differences • Uncertainty regarding the decision-making process
Organization issues	• Differences among institutional policies and priorities • Competing goals • Constraints on time and resources • Large client case loads
Personal issues	• Feelings of burnout among team members • Ignoring the needs of other team members • Self-perception conflicts • Conflicts involving perceptions of situations • Unclear personal values and internal conflicts • Responding to personal emotional and feeling states
Ineffective conflict resolution skills	• Avoiding conflicts, believing that they will go away on their own • Using forceful confrontation or the conquest approach to resolving the conflict • Using bargaining skills as though conflict were a competition • Using a Band-Aid approach to conflict resolution

Table 4
Rehabilitation Team Conflict (*Continued*)

B. Stages of Conflict[†]

Latent conflict	Conflict is anticipated on the basis of certain conditions such as scarcity of resources, changing environment, or unclear role boundaries
Perceived conflict	Cognitive awareness occurs that a stressful situation is present
Felt conflict	Affective states (presence of stress, tension, anxiety, anger, hostility) are stimulated
Manifest conflict	Overt behavior results from perceived or felt conflict and can be constructive or destructive
Conflict aftermath	The conflict is resolved or avoided

* *Sources:* Roseman (1980); Weeks (1992).
[†] *Sources:* Marriner (1980).

1. Create an effective atmosphere.
   a. Personal preparation:
      (1) Remember that conflict can be positive.
      (2) Remember that an I-versus-you atmosphere is an obstructive approach.
      (3) Avoid getting locked into rigid demands of what the conflict solution should be.
   b. Timing:
      (1) Don't jump into an intense conflict resolution process prematurely; do some ground work.
      (2) Choose an appropriate time, free from distractions, that maximizes concentration and communication.
   c. Place:
      (1) Choose a place that promotes a sense of being connected.
      (2) In conflicts involving differing cultural or socioeconomic groups, choose a place that does not offend cultural mores or favor one group over another.
2. Clarify perceptions of the conflict, of the self, of the other parties involved.
3. Focus on individual and shared needs. Needs are the building blocks for effective conflict resolution.
4. Build shared positive power that actually constructs the process and moves it toward conflict resolution. Positive power energizes a "power with" process rather than a "power over" pattern (Weeks, 1992, p. 151).
5. Look to the future, learn from the past.
6. Generate options. Be open to all possibilities.
7. Develop "do-able" stepping stones to action—things that have a chance of being accomplished and meet one or more shared needs. Be sure each do-able is not a temporary quick-fix or a delaying tactic.

8. Make mutual benefit agreements that replace demands.

Additional strategies for resolving conflict have been identified by Levenstein (1984):

1. Clarify the common purpose of the treatment team.
2. Keep discussions relevant to and focused on client's needs, problems, and issues.
3. Agree on the terminology that the team members will use in communication and documentation.
4. Concentrate on the facts during team meetings.
5. Look for potential trade-offs when negotiating.
6. Listen to each other and avoid using debating tactics.
7. Recognize the uniqueness of each individual in the group—their values, emotions, feelings, and perceptions.
8. Be logical in discussions and arguments.
9. Pursue multidimensional solutions to problems.

Conclusion

An effective, productive, interdisciplinary team demands a strong commitment to the team by its members. A productive team is cohesive. There is mutual support and trust among team members and there is concession for differences in values, personalities, and skills. Members of a productive team have a high expectation of accomplishing their established goals and tasks. A strong team possesses a common language and a process for decision-making. Members of an effective team possess effective communication skills, are assertive, have clear role definitions, and deal with conflicts in a constructive manner. The goal of team building should be to increase team cohesiveness through improving interpersonal relationships, problem-solving, communication, and team member support. Effective team building requires work, education, and role clarification. Effective team membership must be learned and experienced.

References

Alpert, H., Goldman, L., Kilroy, C., & Pike, A. (1992). 7 Gryzmish: Toward an understanding of collaboration. *Nursing Clinics of North America, 27*, 47–59.

Baggs, I. (1989). Intensive care unit use and collaboration between nurses and physicians. *Heart and Lung, 18*, 332–338.

Campbell, L. J. (1992). Team maintenance and enhancement. In: *American Congress of Rehabilitation Medicine guide to interdisciplinary practice in rehabilitation settings* (pp. 173–187). Skokie, IL: American Congress of Rehabilitation Medicine.

Cohen, H., Rubin, A. M., & Gombash, L. (1992). The team approach to treatment of the dizzy patient. *Archives of Physical Medicine and Rehabilitation, 73*, 703–708.

Commission on Accreditation of Rehabilitation Facilities. (1993). *Standard manual for facilities serving people with disabilities.* Tucson, AZ: Author.

Cornett-Cooke, P., & Dias, K. K. (1984). Team-building: Getting it all together. *Nursing Management, 15*(5), 16–17.

Dickinson, C. P., Mateo, M., Jackson, D., & Swartz, W. (1995). BO-GYN consultants and Sharp, the birthplace: An exemplar of nurse-midwife and obstetrician independence and integration. *Advanced Practice Nursing Quarterly, 1*(2), 40–48.

Diller, L. (1990). Fostering the interdisciplinary team, fostering research in a society of transition. *Archives of Physical Medicine and Rehabilitation, 71,* 275–278.

Dittmar, S. S. (1989). *Rehabilitation nursing.* St. Louis: Mosby.

Evans, J. A. (1994). The role of the nurse manager in creating an environment for collaborative practice. *Holistic Nursing Practice, 8*(3), 23–31.

Farley, M. J., & Stoner, M. H. (1989). The nurse executive and the interdisciplinary team. *Nursing Administration Quarterly, 13*(2), 24–30.

Fisher, R., & Ury, W. (1981). *Getting to yes.* New York: Viking Penguin.

Francis, D., & Young, D. (1979). *Improving work groups: A practical manual for team building.* San Diego, CA: University Press.

Frank, R. G., & Elliot, T. R. (1992). Conflict resolution and feedback. In: *American Congress of Rehabilitation Medicine guide to interdisciplinary practice in rehabilitation settings* (pp. 143–157). Skokie, IL: American Congress of Rehabilitation Medicine.

Garner, H. G. (1988). *Helping others through teamwork.* Washington, DC: Child Welfare League of America.

Givens, D., & Simmons, S. (1977). The interdisciplinary health care team. *Nursing Forum, 16*(2), 165–184.

Hanson, C. M., & Spross, J. A. (1996). Collaboration. In A. B. Hamric, J. A. Spross, & C. M. Hanson (Eds.), *Advanced nursing practice: An integrative approach.* (pp. 229–248). Philadelphia: W. B. Saunders.

Henry, R. C. (1996). An update on the community partnerships. In R. W. Richards (Ed.), *Building partnerships educating health professionals for the communities they serve* (pp. 33–50). San Francisco: Jossey-Bass.

Hilderley, L. (1991). Nurse-physician collaborative practice: The clinical nurse specialist in a radiation oncology private practice. *Oncology Nursing Forum, 18,* 585–591.

Hoeman, S. P. (1992). Community-based rehabilitation. *Holistic Nursing Practice, 6*(2), 32–41.

Hoeman, S. P. (1993). A research-based transdisciplinary team model for infants with special needs and their families. *Holistic Nursing Practice, 7,* 63–72.

Joint Commission on Accreditation of Healthcare Organization. (1993). *Rehabilitation services: Accreditation manual for hospitals.* Oakbrook Terrace, IL: Author.

Howard, M. E. (1991). Interdisciplinary team treatment in acute care. In P. M. Deutsch & K. B. Fralish (Eds.), *Innovation in head injury rehabilitation* (pp. 3–26). New York: Mathew Bender Company.

Keith, R. A. (1991). The comprehensive treatment team in rehabilitation. *Archives of Physical Medicine and Rehabilitation, 72,* 269–274.

Levenstein, A. (1984). Negotiating vs. confrontation. *Nursing Management, 15*(1), 25–28.

Melvin, J. L. (1989). Status report on interdisciplinary medical rehabilitation in the twenty-first century. *Nursing Economics, 11,* 163–169.

Moulder, T. A., Staal, A. M., & Grant, M. (1988). Making the interdisciplinary team work. *Rehabilitation Nursing, 13,* 338–339.

O'Toole, M. (1992). The interdisciplinary perspectives on disability. *International Disability Studies, 13,* 109–110.

Roseman, E. (1985). Collaborative problem solving. *Medical Laboratory Observer, 17*(2), 59–62.

Rothberg, J. (1981). The rehabilitation team: Future directions. *Archives of Physical Medicine and Rehabilitation, 62*(8), 407–410.

Senge, P. M. (1990). *The fifth discipline: The art and practice of the learning organization.* New York: Doubleday.

Spross, J. A. (1989). The CNS as collaborator. In A. B. Hamric & J. A. Spross (Eds.), *The clinical nurse specialist in theory and practice* (2nd ed., pp. 205–226). Philadelphia: W. B. Saunders.

Weeks, D. (1992). *The eight essential steps to conflict resolution preserving relationships at work, at home, and in the community.* New York: G. P. Putnam & Sons.

CHAPTER 5

Nursing Process and Nurse-Client Relationship
Patricia A. Chin

Key Terms *Change Agent*
Contracting
Counseling
Expected Outcomes
Formative Evaluation
Functional Assessment
Implementation
Long-Term Goals
Movement
Nursing Diagnosis
Nursing Interventions
Nursing Process
Outcome Goals
Outcome-Oriented Rehabilitation
Planning
Prioritization
Refreezing
Short-Term Goals
Summative Evaluation
Unfreezing

Objectives
1. Discuss the five phases of the nursing process and relate their purpose and meaning to the rehabilitation process.

2. Compare the nursing process with the rehabilitation process.

3. Identify the optimum outcomes of the rehabilitation process.

4. Discuss functional assessment and identify selective current functional assessment tools.

5. Discuss outcome-oriented rehabilitation.

6. Identify the criteria for well-written expected outcomes.

7. Identify the benefits of early discharge planning for the rehabilitation client.

8. Compare and contrast formative and summative evaluations.

9. Discuss the nature of the nurse-client relationship in the rehabilitation setting.

10. Describe the role of the nurse as change agent in the rehabilitation setting.

Nursing Process in Rehabilitation Nursing

Goal-directed nursing care requires that the nurse possess and apply critical thinking and problem-solving skills. It requires the nurse to be able to make clinical judgments, and evaluate the effectiveness of interventions and treatment outcomes. The nursing process as currently used in clinical practice is an appropriate tool for developing a comprehensive plan of care for clients in rehabilitative settings. The nursing process provides a dynamic organized method for identifying client problems, while addressing individual client needs, strengths, and limitations. Mutual goal setting assists clients and caregivers to take responsibility for managing physiological and psychological problems and for attaining and maintaining optimal levels of functioning. The purpose of this chapter is not to present an in-depth discussion of the theoretical foundations of the nursing process. Several available texts provide a comprehensive discussion of the nursing process (Berger & Williams, 1992; Ellis & Nowlis, 1994; Potter & Perry, 1993). This chapter addresses specific issues in the application of the nursing process in the rehabilitative setting.

The **nursing process** is a dynamic, ongoing process that is evolving as long as the client and the nurse have interactions directed toward change in the client's physical, psychological, emotional, and behavioral responses to a change in health state. An effective plan of care will reflect the shared belief system of rehabilitation nursing about disability and the rights of individuals with disabling conditions and chronic illness. The plan of care designed for the client by the rehabilitation nurse will also reflect and incorporate the goals of the interdisciplinary team into the plan of care to achieve effectively the outcomes of medical rehabilitation. The plan of care will evolve to accomplish the goals of rehabilitation nursing: assisting the client and family to attain maximum functional ability, maintaining optimal health, adapting to an altered lifestyle, and facilitating independent living.

The rehabilitation process is a planned and orderly sequence of individualized services designed to meet the unique needs of the client. The rehabilitation process and nursing process are similar. The problem-solving approach (American Congress of Rehabilitation Medicine, 1992) used in all rehabilitation settings should include

- A comprehensive interdisciplinary patient functional evaluation
- Identification of all the client's physiological and psychological problems

- The determination of comprehensive treatment goals
- The implementation of the treatment plan
- An evaluation of the outcomes identified in the rehabilitation treatment plan

Assessment in Rehabilitation Nursing

Assessment is the foundation of the nursing process, directly enhancing or limiting the delivery of total care. Comprehensive assessment is the systematic collection of data to determine the client's or family member's current health status, functional abilities and capabilities, and to evaluate the effectiveness of past and present coping strategies. The purpose of assessment is to establish a usable client database. Monitoring and evaluation of the client's progress is contingent on reliable baseline assessment information.

Assessment is a process of continuous information gathering and professional judgment. Client data are gathered in a systematic fashion, classified, and analyzed. Although assessment is the first step in the nursing process, data should be gathered continuously until the client is no longer involved in the rehabilitation process. The function and health state of the client will constantly be evolving over the course of the rehabilitation process.

Functional Assessment

Rehabilitation assessment is performed within the framework of **functional assessment.** The assessment of functional performance is of central importance in providing direction for the planning, performing, and evaluation of restorative nursing care. Functional assessment is an extension of the usual components of nursing assessment. It is more useful for meeting rehabilitation process goals than the traditional systems or disease-oriented approaches to gathering data. The purposes of the functional assessment are to determine physical functional status, to identify and document the need for interventions, and to monitor the client's progress. The purposes of functional evaluation in rehabilitation nursing as identified by Dittmar (1984) are to

- Systematically identify functional limitation
- Recognize a client's learning needs
- Document feedback about progression toward goal accomplishment
- Coordinate care
- Provide a means to gather objective data for the analysis of cost, benefits, use of resources, and quality of care
- Facilitate client discharge planning and placement decisions
- Assist accreditation bodies with program evaluation
- Systematically research and evaluate activities

The concept of functional assessment is grounded in disability theory and a functional limitations framework.

Functional limitation (Nagi, 1965) consists of four categories: (1) pathology, (2) impairment, (3) functional limitation, and (4) disability. Within this framework *pathology* refers to disease. *Impairment* refers to physiological abnormalities. *Functional limitation* is described as sensorimotor inability, and *disability* is defined as an inability or limitation in performance of expected roles and activities associated with family, work, education, community, or society membership. Functional assessment is a multidimensional method for describing abilities and limitations to measure a client's use of a variety of skills. These skills are included in performing tasks necessary to daily living, leisure activities, vocational pursuits, social interaction, and other behaviors necessary to lead a productive and meaningful life.

A variety of functional assessment scales are available for use in the rehabilitation setting (see Table 1). The dimensions of these assessment systems or scales usually include self-care, mobility, cognitive, emotional, perceptual, social, and vocational functioning.

Assessment begins with the initial client contact. This will usually be at the time of admission to the inpatient facility, outpatient setting, or rehabilitation program. The process of assessment usually begins with a screening for impairments and disabilities followed by a detailed formal assessment. The purpose of the screening assessment is to identify how the client would benefit from rehabilitation, and to guide the choice of treatment and of the most appropriate setting for rehabilitation. The formal assessment can be used to validate referrals, formulate treatment goals, confirm the management plan, and provide a baseline for monitoring change. The monitoring and evaluation of client progress is continuous throughout rehabilitation. Monitoring is important to follow the degree of client progress, adjust therapy as needed, and identify developing problems. Reliable, established tools are critical for achieving valid comparisons of client progress. After client discharge from rehabilitation, assessment will involve monitoring of adaptation to the community, maintenance of functional gains, and adjustment to the environment.

Each assessment scale has specific instructions for scoring and for interpreting those scores. Some scales must be administered and evaluated by the member of the interdisciplinary team responsible for each category of the scale (e.g., the Patient Evaluation Conference System).

Diagnosis in Rehabilitation Nursing

In the problem identification phase the nurse uses critical thinking skills to organize data, make inferences regarding the collected data and formulate a **nursing diagnosis.** After the database is established the data are sorted and analyzed, and nursing diagnoses are created (Berger & Williams, 1992; Ellis & Nowlis, 1994; Potter & Perry, 1993). The nursing diagnosis names, or labels, the client's problem. It is important to create nursing diagnoses so that the problem, and the eti-

Table 1
Selected Established Assessment Measures

Measure	Title of Measure	Ref.	Description
Disability measures	Barthel Index	Mahoney & Barthel (1995)	Ordinal scale, weighted items: feeding, bathing, grooming, dressing, bladder bowel control, toileting, chair/bed transfer, mobility, and stair climbing
	Kenny Self-Care Scale	Schoening & Iversen (1968)	Ordinal scale of 17 with 6 activities: bed activities, transfers, locomotion, personal hygiene, dressing, and feeding
	Functional Independency Measure (FIM)	Granger, Hamilton, & Sherwin (1986)	Ordinal scale areas of assessment: feeding, self-care, sphincter control, mobility, locomotion, communication, and social cognition
	Patient Evaluation Conference System (PES™)	Harvey & Jilinek (1981)	Ordinal scale to evaluate total dependence/independence, physical mobility, ADL,* communication, medications, device utilization, finances, social issues, therapeutic recreation, nutrition, pain, pulmonary function
Activities of daily living scales	Functional Health Status	Rosow & Breslau (1966)	Guttman scale determining ascending dependency, global assessment
	Philadelphia Geriatric Center Morals Scale	Lawton (1972)	Guttman scale measuring broad spectrum of independent living skills, shopping, walking, food preparation, laundry, housekeeping, transportation, etc.
	Katz Index of ADL	Katz (1963)	Dichotomous Guttman rating scale of independence and dependence including bathing, dressing, toileting, transferring, continence, feeding
Cognitive scale	Mini-Mental State Examination	Folstein & McHugh (1975)	Measures seven dimensions of cognition including orientation, registration, calculation, recall, language, visual construction
Affective scale	Center for Epidemiologic Studies of Depression	Radloff (1977)	Measures severity of depression
Quality-of-life scale	Medical Outcome Study	Ware & Sherbourne (1992)	Assesses eight domains: physical and social activities, mental health, general health, perceptions, vitality, and discomfort
	Sickness Impact Profile	Carter, Bobbitt, Bergner, Gibson (1976)	Measures ambulating, self-care, emotions, alertness, habits, home and recreation environments, vocation, and social interactions

* ADL, Activities of daily living.

ology (or *causative factors*), are obvious. This core of the nursing diagnosis (problem and etiology) establishes the focus for appropriate nursing interventions. Nursing actions are identified to overcome or mitigate the effects of the causative factors for the identified problems. Sound nursing care in rehabilitative nursing practice is the recognition and identification of patterns of client physical, emotional, psychological, behavioral, and spiritual responses to illness, injury, disease, or disability and existing unmet health needs. It is important that adequate assessment data be available to support any identified nursing diagnosis.

After compiling a comprehensive client problem list the next step is **prioritization:** that is, problems are prioritized, or organized in order of importance. Highest priority is given to problems that are life threatening; next are problems that are likely to cause destructive damage or complications if not addressed and lowest priority is assigned to those problems related to normative or developmental experiences. (Berger & Williams, 1992; Ellis & Nowlis, 1994; Potter & Perry, 1993).

Outcome Identification and Planning in Rehabilitation Nursing

Nursing care is goal directed and outcome oriented. In the **planning** phase interventions are established to eliminate, prevent, reduce, or monitor the client's problems. The purpose of planning is to design the strategy for achieving the established goals of the interdisciplinary rehabilitation team. Nursing goals are established to assist the nurse in providing direct care, identifying the desired outcomes of care, and measuring the effectiveness of team interventions (Berger & Williams, 1992; Ellis & Nowlis, 1994; Potter & Perry, 1993). Goals help team members in promoting the retention and transferral of skills learned in therapy sessions to the nursing unit during inpatient care, and to community settings.

A variety of schemes have been proposed to conceptualize nursing process goals. Theoretically speaking, goals are statements of desired outcomes. Three types of goal seem most logical for the rehabilitation setting:

Long-term goals: Global statements of desired outcome, developed for each aspect of the treatment program
Short-term goals: Specific statements of desired outcomes, which are related to the achievement of long-term goals. Short-term goals will assist the client in progressing toward the accomplishment of the long-term goals and outcome goals
Outcome goals: Statements reflecting the anticipated status of the client at discharge

In the rehabilitation setting goals are set for the client, and the nursing interventions would include strategies or actions taken by the nurse to assist the client in reaching the goals.

Examples of Levels of Client Goals

Short-term goal: The client will call the nurse for assistance before attempting to get out of bed.
Long-term goal: The client will be free from injury related to falls.
Outcome goal: The client will prevent injury to self in the work place.

Criteria do exist to facilitate creating outcomes that are attainable (Redman, 1993). Outcome goals that can be evaluated indicate exactly what to do, how and how often to do it, with what degree of proficiency it is to be done, and when and where it is to be done. To accomplish this, goals should be

- Client oriented: Meaningful to client and family members
- Observable
- Measurable, verifiable, and related to projected outcomes
- Time limited
- Mutual
- Realistic

The optimal outcomes of actions to meet the needs of clients in rehabilitation or with disabilities are (Kemp, Brummel-Smith, & Ramsdell, 1990)

1. Stabilization of the client's primary problems
2. Prevention of secondary complication or increased dysfunction
3. Restoration of lost functional abilities
4. Promotion of the adaptation of the client and family
5. Adaptation of the environment to meet the needs of the client

Each member of the rehabilitation team contributes and is accountable for supporting and enhancing the client's rehabilitation program.

Clinical Outcomes

A rehabilitation program driven by *expected outcomes* has a variety of benefits for both the client and the treatment team. With care designed around outcomes, clients in any phase of rehabilitation from acute injury or illness through complete integration into society can be described and classified. Outcome-driven planning allows for the cost accounting of resources to various areas of care and for the allocation of resources. Outcomes link specific treatment paths to resource utilization (DeJong & Sutton, 1995).

Clinical *outcome-oriented* medical rehabilitation represents basic domains that clients include in their lives. These domains include health, personal maintenance, home management, community activity, and productivity. With catastrophic illness or injury the clients usually become disabled to varying degrees in relation to each of the domains. Rehabilitation clients will fall along a spectrum of outcome levels that will indicate the specific treatments and problems at each level. Outcome level is defined by the nature of the typical clinical issues confronting the client and the treatment team (DeJong & Sutton, 1995).

There are six clinical outcome levels (DeJong & Sutton, 1995):

0 = Physiological instability: Patients as they appear just after onset of illness or injury; acute medical diagnostic and management problems

1 = Physiological stability: First and most basic outcome level; major problems are being appropriately managed
2 = Physiological maintenance: Rehabilitation outcomes necessary to preserve the immediate and long-term physiological health of the client are managed
3 = Primary functional goals: Home and residential integration
4 = Advanced functional goals: Community reintegration
5 = Productive activity: Establishing the client in productive activities within capacity

Discharge Planning

Discharge planning is another mechanism for promoting the continuity of care (Joint Commission on Accreditation of Healthcare Organization [JCAHO], 1993). Discharge planning is part of the treatment plan and is incorporated into the nursing care plan early in the rehabilitation process (Povse & Keenan, 1981). Discharge planning is essential for controlling inpatient length of stay and health care costs as well as for facilitating a successful termination of the rehabilitation process.

The benefits of discharge planning are in achieving optimal level of health for the client and decreasing the incidence of disease and complications related to the disability. Client adjustment, adaptation, and reentry into the community are promoted. The number of acute hospital readmissions and physical visits is reduced and appropriate services are available when they are needed by the client. Early discharge planning also prohibits the duplication of services, and cost containment is increased (Povse & Keenan, 1981).

Implementation

The purpose of **implementation** is to initiate and complete those client and nursing actions identified as appropriate to overcome or mitigate the effects of the client's problems on optimal life functioning and to accomplish the defined client outcomes. Nursing *interventions* for facilitating self-care and self-management involve various methods of assisting: doing for or acting for the client, teaching, supporting, guiding and directing, and providing an environment that facilitates client and family development (Orem, 1985).

Evaluation and Modification in Rehabilitation Nursing

Evaluation and modification are the final aspects of the nursing process. The purpose of evaluation is to determine the extent to which goals of care have been achieved. Evaluation of responses provides direction for measuring the progressive movement of the client toward a higher level of function and for giving directions for future care. Two types of evaluation—formative and summative—should be used for evaluation in rehabilitation settings.

Formative evaluation involves reassessment of all aspects of the nursing process. As implementation of the care plan occurs, formative assessment is used to evaluate client responses to nursing intervention. When performing a formative evaluation the adequacy and accuracy of client assessment and established diagnoses are also reviewed. The expected outcomes and planned interventions are examined or discontinued.

Summative evaluation is an evaluation of the entire nurse-client relationship. The summative evaluation is made at the conclusion of the relationship. The review is most beneficial when preparing the client for discharge and is essential for the continuity of care. Information from the formative evaluation is included in the summative evaluation and recommendations for future care are suggested if appropriate. The summative evaluation should include all nursing diagnoses, the client's functional status, recommended actions, and referrals.

Modification is an essential component of the nursing process. Unfortunately, it is the component most often overlooked in practice. Changes in the client's health state or functional status present the treatment team with the need to modify the plan. It may be necessary to modify any aspect of the care plan to facilitate the achievement of expected outcomes.

Nature of the Rehabilitative Nurse-Client Relationship

The nurse-client relationship in rehabilitation nursing practice is like that in other areas of nursing practice: it is a time-limited therapeutic relationship. It begins with the introduction of the client into the rehabilitation setting and terminates with the client's transfer to another rehabilitation setting or reintegration into the community. Unlike nurse-client relationships in other health care settings, the length of the nurse's relationship with the rehabilitation client and family can be extended over a greater span of time and the relationship can be more intense. The nurse-client relationship in the rehabilitation setting is guided by the ethical and professional standards of all therapeutic alliances. The strength of the nurse-client relationship in the rehabilitation setting is mutuality.

The components of the helping relationship in rehabilitation nursing are the same as in other nurse-client relationships. It is important for the rehabilitation nurse to attend carefully to issues of respect for boundaries, caring, empathy, advocacy, acceptance, empowerment, mutuality, authenticity, and trust (Carson & Arnold, 1996; Peplau, 1952). Mutuality is a key building block for the nurse-client relationship in rehabilitation nursing practice.

Mutuality involves inclusion and connection in an equal partnership formed for the purpose of reaching common goals. Mutuality recognizes the separateness, uniqueness, and need for self-growth in all individuals involved but it also acknowledges independence. People can change and take responsibility for themselves when there exists a common understanding regarding the issues involved. In a therapeutic relationship that is founded on mutuality the client presents a view of the situation and the nurse adds additional understanding from the professional perspective. The result is a broader view of the situation. Strategies to enhance mutuality in a therapeutic nurse-client relationship involve searching for common understanding, acknowledging the client's autonomy, creating a shared experience of reality of the situation, pointing out the client's strengths, and commenting on the changes experienced by the client (Carson & Arnold, 1996).

The nurse-client relationship evolves through three phases. The first phase is the *orientation phase,* in which the nurse and client begin to develop reciprocal trust (Peplau, 1952). The tasks of the orientation phase are to establish the relationship, establish role responsibilities, develop rapport, collect and validate assessment data, formulate diagnoses, and develop a therapeutic contract. The primary task of the orientation phase is to develop client trust.

The second phase of the nurse-client relationship is the *working phase.* This is the most active phase of the relationship (Peplau, 1952). The tasks of the working phase are to mutually identify expected outcomes, plan achievable goals, develop realistic solutions to problems, and implement chosen interventions. This phase will be greatly influenced by the client's physiological and psychological states and the motivation and desire to change and grow in self-care and self-management. Resistance at some time during this phase is inevitable. Two intervention strategies to deal successfully with this resistance are (1) *sensitive confrontation* and (2) *immediacy in communication.*

> *An example of sensitive confrontation:* Mr. Jones has been telling the nurse that he desires to get strong enough to go home and is really working hard in therapy. The nurse talks with the physical therapist, who informs her that Mr. Jones has not been working in therapy and has been leaving his sessions early. That evening the nurse asks Mr. Jones how his therapy is going. He responds with his false declarations. The nurse confronts the client: "I talked with the your therapist today, Mr. Jones. I know you have not been working in therapy and have been leaving early. Would you like to talk about this?"

The tone of voice of the nurse is important when using sensitive confrontation. The goal is not to accuse the client or berate him for his behavior. The objective is to bring the behavior out into the open so that it can be addressed and corrected. Immediacy in communication is the direct reflection of the immediate communication process, that is, identifying for the client the messages being sent, and commenting on them.

> *An example of immediacy in communication:* "Mrs. Goldman, you respond to my requests as though I were a drill sergeant . You are resistant and I feel as though you are very angry. I feel as though you want me to leave you alone."

The third phase of the nurse-client relationship is the *termination phase.* This is the resolution phase (Peplau, 1952), or ending, of the relationship. The tasks of the termination phase are to evaluate patient functional performance, evaluate expected outcomes, evaluate future needs, make appropriate referrals, and cope with the behaviors associated with termination. Although termination is described as the final phase of the relationship it should begin during the orientation phase.

Because the nurse-client relationship is a time-limited therapeutic alliance it will come to an end. The client should be prepared for this from the beginning of the relationship. Rehabilitation clients confront multiple losses, and the termination of the nurse-client relationship will add one more. This eventual loss can be used to help clients work through and come to terms with loss and engage in grief work in a safe, guided environment. During the termination phase it is not unusual for the client to demonstrate regressive behavior, anger, withdrawal, and the minimizing of the relationship. Some clients may complain of new and terrible symptoms, in an attempt to remain in the therapeutic alliance.

Ending a therapeutic alliance can create sadness in both the nurse and the client (Carson & Arnold, 1996). The nurse-client relationship confirms the essential nature of another being.

The focus of the role of the nurse in the nature of the rehabilitation therapeutic alliance is very different from the role traditionally assumed in the acute inpatient "nurse-patient" relationship. The goals of nursing and the rest of the interdisciplinary treatment team are to empower the client and family members and move them toward independence and self-management. The expected outcomes for the client involve self-care abilities, capabilities, and self-management. To accomplish this the nursing skills and strategies focused on doing for, or acting for, the client play a minor role in client care. Skills necessary for effective rehabilitative practice include not only physical skill proficiency but those involved in being a teacher and coach, client advocate, supporter (physical and psychological), motivator, change agent, case manager, and consultant.

Nurse as Change Agent

Change is defined as any planned or unplanned alteration in the status quo. Change is a phenomenon experienced by organisms, situations, and processes (Lippitt, 1973). Change is a central concern for nursing (DeFeo, 1990). This is especially true in rehabilitating nursing practice. Rehabilitative nurses regularly interact with clients experiencing great and often overwhelming change. Change in the rehabilitation setting can involve change in knowledge, attitude, behavior, or group organization or functioning. Understanding and facilitating the change process are integral parts of the role of the rehabilitative nurse.

Forces that facilitate or impede the change process are constantly at work. Two types of force at work in the change field are as follows: (1) *driving forces*—forces that facilitate the change process by moving the participant in the direction of a positive outcome, and (2) *restraining forces*—forces that impede the change process (Lewin, 1947). Change occurs when one type of force outweighs the other. The status quo is maintained when the forces are equal: steady state. To be effective as a change agent the nurse must identify both the driving forces and the restraining forces in order to benefit from the power of the driving forces and avert or modify the restraining forces. Permanent change requires alteration of client attitudes as well as behaviors (New & Couillard, 1981).

Types of Change

Planned change: A systematic process directed toward producing improvement in function, output, or for solving a problem. The outcomes of planned change are predictable and deliberate (Bennis, Benne, Chin, & Corey, 1976). Planned change requires problem-solving and decision-making as well as a certain level of interpersonal skill.

Unplanned change or drift: Unplanned change is random, with no effort made by the participants to prepare for the onset of the change process. The outcomes of unplanned change are unpredictable and nondeliberate, but they are not always negative. The change is imperceptible and may be recognized only after it has occurred. The change often occurs as smaller changes that have cumulative effect that is perceived as a rapid, sudden change.

Knowledge changes appear to be the easiest to effect, followed by changes in attitude. Changing a client's behavioral inventory is more time consuming and more difficult to accomplish than changing knowledge or attitudes. Bringing about change in a group of individuals is the most complex and difficult of the fields of change (Hersey & Blanchard, 1988).

Principles Related to the Change Process

Change is difficult for people. Change is especially difficult if the client is stressed, feels out of control or feels powerless, or has suffered an attack on self-esteem or worth. Clients will take part in change to the degree that they participate in the planning of the change. The more participation, the greater the involvement by the client. Clients respond to a gradual shaping of behavior. The consequences of change are likely to be more effective and long-lasting when the change is gradual, or incremental, as opposed to rapid or sudden. Clients require time to extinguish their old behaviors and behavioral patterns while they explore and acclimate the self to the new behaviors (Bushnell, 1979).

Clients will change to the degree that the reward they receive for the change or the benefit to them for changing is greater than the risks or disruption in the status quo. Clients maintain changed behaviors to the degree that those behaviors are rewarded, supported, and satisfying to them (Bushnell, 1979).

Change will be difficult to promote when the client is anxious or in the process of mourning a loss. A person who is highly anxious about, or mourning, a loss created by the change learns or applies little about the desired changes (Bushnell, 1979). A common reaction to change is passive or active resistance. Clients resistant to efforts to facilitate change will oppose, obstruct, or block movement in the change process (Bailey, 1990). Resistance can occur for several reasons. New and Couillard (1981) identified five reasons: threats to self-interest, inaccurate perceptions about the nature or implications of the change, disagreements in understanding of information related to the change, psychological reactance, and feelings of alienation. If the blocker to change is the desire to maintain the status quo the nurse will either have to weaken the restraint forces or strengthen the driving forces (Lewin, 1947).

Behavior is a function of both personality and the environment and the dynamic interaction between them. In the 1940s, Kurt Lewin (1947) used this proposition to develop classical change theory. Lewin (1947) identified three stages of change:

1. **Unfreezing**—Movement from a steady state to a state that is unsteady and amenable to change. Factors leading to a state of unfreezing include: discomfort with the present situation, questioning of the status quo, or establishment of a change relationship. The client recognizes the need for change. In the unfreezing stage the client and family members are helped to identify problems that can be changed and the forces that prevent or promote the change (Bailey, 1990). This stage may be the most difficult for some clients because change requires planning and movement (Laughlin, 1989).
2. **Movement**—Movement to a higher level of behavior. In the movement stage the problem is assessed and labeled, the options and alternatives are identified, goals are established, action is taken, and evaluation is made. In this stage the nurse provides information, support, and encouragement of movement toward change (Farley, 1992).
3. **Refreezing**—Integration and stabilization of learning. In the refreezing stage new responses are integrated into the lifestyle, relationships are modified, and the change is complete. In the final stage nurses work with the client and family members to review the completed change and plan for anticipated future change (Bailey, 1990).

The Change Agent

The **change agent** is defined as a person who deliberately promotes a change process (Mauksch & Miller, 1981). To be an effective change agent the nurse needs to empower the client and family members. An effective change agent is flexible, innovative, and creative. A successful change agent demonstrates self-motivation, sensitivity toward others, and a genuine desire to help others. Change agents are able to deal successfully with ambiguity and adapt to unfamiliar situations, and can model this for the client. They are perceived by others as possessing integrity, optimism, self-confidence, sincerity, and charisma (Lippitt & Lippitt, 1978).

Rogers (1972) identified the functions of the change agent; the change agent

- Develops a need for change
- Establishes the change relationship
- Labels the problem
- Examines the goals and alternative courses of action
- Translates intent into action
- Stabilizes change and attempts to prevent any discontinuance of the changed behaviors
- Facilitates closure

Planned change takes the entire system into account. It takes time to accomplish, and facilities the building for future problem-solving skills. The lack of adequate resources, multiple competing problems, or the inability to detach from perceptions or environmental influences may interfere with, or limit, the individual's movement and capacity to implement changes. Pain, inconvenience, financial constraints and lack of resources, and the desire to maintain the status quo can impede change for rehabilitation clients (Farley, 1992). Change can also be difficult to implement when the rehabilitation client experiences deterioration of vigor, mobility, comfort, erosion of support systems, or the demoralizing effects of day-to-day management of chronic illness (Bailey, 1990).

Counseling

Counseling is related to teaching but it is in fact different. Teaching is viewed as the set of strategies used when providing specific information. Teaching is more structured and instructor-driven whereas counseling is nonstructured and client-driven. Teaching requires a more structured approach to working with the client. Counseling is more an interpersonal intervention process (Janis, 1983). Counseling is appropriate when clients require less structure, can benefit from minimal direction, and can use support and encouragement to apply their own problem-solving skills. The two strategies can be used simultaneously. In counseling the nurse is a facilitator and resource person, allowing the client and family members to independently make their own decisions, after exploring perceptions, feelings, and attitudes and identifying alternatives for coping and meeting goals.

The core elements of counseling are empathy, acceptance, unconditional positive regard, congruency, and genuineness (Janis, 1983; Rogers, 1972). Counseling is an interpersonal strategy that is free from all judgments and coercive pressure (Janis, 1983). Counseling is an advanced practice skill and requires additional education and experience to use successfully.

Contracting

The underlying philosophy of **contracting** is client involvement and the encouragement of self-care and self-responsibility. The use of contracting makes the client a chief partner of the rehabilitative team. Contracting is a useful way to involve clients and families in a collaborative process. A *contract* is a working agreement between two or more people. Contracts should be continuously renegotiable. Contracts should include specific goals, length of contract, clearly stated client and/or family responsibilities, rehabilitation team member responsibilities, specific actions taken to meet the goal, and rewards for meeting goals.

Conclusion

The nursing process is a systematic, dynamic interpersonal interactive framework for problem-solving appropriate in rehabilitative nursing. The nursing process provides an organized method for identifying client problems, while addressing individual client needs, strengths, and limitations. Mutual goal setting assists clients and caregivers to take responsibility for managing physiological and psychological problems and for attaining and maintaining optimal levels of functioning. The nurse-client relationship in rehabilitation nursing represents a unique human encounter. The keys to the successful nurse-client relationship in rehabilitative nursing practice are mutuality and trust. The nurse-client relationship provides an opportunity for the nurse to establish a therapeutic alliance that will move the client and the family toward optimal functioning and productive, meaningful life. In an era of health care delivery that is increasingly dehumanized by bureaucracy, the rehabilitation nurse can function as an active member of an interdisciplinary team to assist clients through traumatic life events while emphasizing the client's and family's humanity.

References

American Congress of Rehabilitation Medicine. (1992). *Guide to interdisciplinary practice in rehabilitation settings.* Skokie, IL: Author.

Bailey, B. (1990). Change agent. In I. M. Bubkin (Ed.), *Chronic illness: Impact and interventions* (pp. 262–278). Boston: Jones & Bartlett.

Bennis, W., Benne, K., Chin, R., & Corey, K. (1976). *The planning of change.* New York: Holt, Rinehart, & Winston.

Berger, K. J., & Williams, M. B. (1992). *Fundamentals of nursing collaborating for optimal health.* Norwalk, CT: Appleton & Lange.

Bushnell, M. (1979). Institution in transition. *Perspectives of Psychiatric Care, 12*(6), 260–265.

Carson, V. B., & Arnold, E. N. (1996). *Mental health nursing: The nurse-patient journey.* Philadelphia: W.B. Saunders.

Carter, W. B., Bobbitt, R. A., Bergner, M., & Gibson, B. A. (1976). Validation of an interval scaling: The Sickness Impact Profile. *Health Services Research, 11,* 516–528.

DeFeo, D. J. (1990). Change: A central concern of nursing. *Nursing Science Quarterly, 3*(2), 88–94.

DeJong, G., & Sutton, J. P. (1995). Rehab 2000: The evolution of medical rehabilitation in American health care. In P. K. Landrum, N. D. Schmidt, & A. McLean (Eds.), *Outcome-oriented rehabilitation: Principles, strategies, and tools for effective program management.* Rockville, MD: Aspen.

Dittmar, S. (1984). Functional assessment in nursing. In C. Granger & G. Gresham (Eds.)., *Functional assessment in rehabilitation medicine* (pp. 194–209). Baltimore: Williams & Wilkins.

Ellis, J. R., & Nowlis, E. A. (1994). *Nursing: A human needs approach.* Philadelphia: J. B. Lippincott.

Farley, A. M. (1992). *Nursing and the disabled across the life span.* Boston: Jones & Bartlett.

Folstein, M. F., & McHugh, P. (1975). Mini-Mental State: A practical method of grading the cognitive state of patients for the clinician. *Journal of Psychiatric Report, 12,* 189–198.

Granger, C. V., Hamilton, B. B., & Sherwin, F. S. (1986). *Guide for the use of the uniform data set for medical rehabilitation.* Buffalo, NY: Uniform Data System for Medical Rehabilitation Project Office.

Harvey, R. F., & Jilinek, H. M. (1981). Functional performance assessment: A program approach. *Archives of Physical Medicine and Rehabilitation, 62,* 456–460.

Hersey, P., & Blanchard, K. (1988). *Management of organizational behavior.* Englewood Cliffs, NJ: Prentice-Hall.

Janis, I. L. (1983). *Short-term counseling guidelines based on recent research.* New Haven, CT: Yale University Press.

Joint Commission on Accreditation of Healthcare Organizations (JCAHO). (1993). *Rehabilitation services: Accreditation manual for hospitals.* Oakbrook Terrace, IL: Author.

Katz, S. (1963). Studies of illness and the aged. The index of ADL, a standardized measure of biological and psychological function. *Journal of the American Medical Association, 185,* 914–919.

Kemp, B., Brummel-Smith, K., & Ramsdell, J. W. (Eds.). (1990). *Geriatric rehabilitation.* Austin, TX: PRO-ED.

Laughlin, J. A. (1989). Rehabilitation: Unlocking the gates to change. In S. Dittmar (Ed.), *Rehabilitation in nursing: Process and application* (pp. 528–535). St. Louis: Mosby.

Lawton, M. P. (1972). Assessment, integration, and environment for older people. *Gerontologist, 10,* 38–46.

Lewin, K. (1947). Frontiers in groups dynamics: Concepts, methods, and reality in social science. *Human Relations, 5*(1), 5–42.

Lippitt, G. L. (1973). *Visualizing change: Model building and the change process.* La Jolla, CA: University Associates.

Lippitt, G. L., & Lippitt, R. (1978). *The counseling process in action.* San Diego, CA: University Press.

Mahoney, F. I., & Barthel, D. (1965). Functional evaluation: The Barthel Index. *Maryland State Medical Journal, 14,* 56–61.

Mauksch, I. G., & Miller, M. H. (1981). *Implementing change in nursing.* St. Louis: Mosby.

Nagi, S. Z. (1965). Some conceptual issues in disability and rehabilitation. In B. M. Sussman (Ed.). *Sociology & rehabilitation* (pp. 100-113). Washington, DC: American Sociological Association.

New, J. R., & Couillard, N. A. (1981). Guidelines for introducing change. *The Journal of Nursing Administration, March,* (8), 7–21.

Orem, D. E. (1985). *Nursing concepts of practice* (3rd ed.). New York: McGraw-Hill.

Peplau, H. (1952). *Interpersonal relations in nursing.* New York: G. P. Putman & Sons.

Potter, P. A., & Perry, A. G. (1993). Fundamentals of nursing concepts, process & practice. St. Louis: Mosby–Year Book.

Povse, S. M., & Keenan, M. E. (1981). Discharge planning for the transition from a health care facility to the community. In N. Martin, N. B. Holt, & D. Hicks (Eds.), *Comprehensive rehabilitation nursing* (pp. 667–689). New York: McGraw-Hill.

Radloff, S. L. (1977). The CES-D Scale: A self-report depression scale for research in the general population. *Applied Psychological Measurements, 1,* 385–401.

Redman, B. (1993). *The process of patient education* (7th ed.). St. Louis: Mosby.

Rogers, C. R. (1972). *On becoming a person.* Boston: Houghton Mifflin.

Rogers, E. M. (1972). Change agents, clients, and change. In G. Zaltman, P. Kotlteer, & I. Kaufman (Eds.), *Creating social change* (pp. 194–213). New York: Holt, Rinehart, & Winston.

Rosow, L., & Breslau, N. (1966). A Guttman health scale for the aged. *Journal of Gerontology, 21,* 556–559.

Schoening, H. A., & Iversen, I. A. (1968). Numerical scoring of self-care status: A study of the Kenny Self-Care evaluation. *Archives of Physical Medicine and Rehabilitation, 46,* 221–229.

Ware, J. E., & Sherbourne, C. D. (1992). The MOS 36 item short form survey (SF-36). Conceptual framework and item selection. *Medical Care, 30,* 473–483.

Suggested Readings

Arnold, E., & Boggs, K. (1995). *Interpersonal relationships: Professional communication skills for nurses.* Philadelphia: W. B. Saunders.

Cotler, M. (Ed.). (1996). Perspectives on chronic illness: Treating patients and delivering care. *American Behavioral Scientist, 39*(6).

Friedman, S. (Ed.). (1993). *The new language of change: Constructive collaboration in psychotherapy.* New York: Guilford Press.

Landrum, P. K., Schmidt, N. D., & McLean, A. (Eds.). (1995). *Outcome-oriented rehabilitation: Principles, strategies, and tools for effective program management.* Rockville, MD: Aspen.

Rice, L. N., & Greenberg, L. S. (Eds.). (1984). *Patterns of change.* New York: Guilford Press.

Sundeen, S. J., Sturat, G. W., Rankin, E. A., & Cohen, S. A. (1994). Nurse-patient interaction: Implementing the nursing process (5th ed.). St. Louis: Mosby.

CHAPTER 6
Client and Family Education:
Issues and Principles

Patricia A. Chin

Key Terms *Adult Learning Principles*
EDICT Model for Designing Teaching Episodes
Learning
Learning Domains
Learning Needs
Learning Style
Readiness to Learn
Teachable Moments
Teaching
Transfer of Learning

Objectives
1. Distinguish between teaching and learning.

2. Identify the goals of client and family teaching in the rehabilitation setting.

3. Discuss four domains of learning essential to the teaching-learning process in rehabilitation nursing.

4. Discuss adult learning principles essential to the teaching-learning process in rehabilitation nursing.

5. Discuss the importance of learning styles to the teaching-learning process in rehabilitation nursing.

6. Discuss factors that will influence client and family learning in the rehabilitation setting.

7. Discuss ways to increase client motivation.

8. Discuss ways to increase the transfer of learning.

9. Discuss issues of teaching session design relevant to the rehabilitation setting.

10. Discuss the assessment of learning needs and learning readiness.

11. Identify nursing assumptions that can negatively influence the teaching-learning process.

12. Discuss the components of the EDICT teaching session design model.

13. Identify methods and tools for effective teaching.

14. Discuss the role of evaluation and documentation in rehabilitation teaching.

Client Education

Client education is the cornerstone for developing self-care and self-management in rehabilitative nursing. The goals of teaching are to increase knowledge, modify attitudes, develop skills, and enhance perceptual abilities (Kopper, 1987). Successful learning is essential to maximize rehabilitation treatment outcomes. Education is an important nursing intervention directed toward assisting clients and families to attain maximum function and reach optimal levels of independent self-care. The educational process is directed toward fostering self-care through the acquisition of new knowledge and the development of new skills. Through education the client and family gain the ability to apply competently new information and skills to functional living activities; develop adaptive behaviors for the management of illness, injury, disease, or disability, and prevent further disability (Deihl, 1989).

The Goals of Health Teaching in Rehabilitation

Health care professionals engage in a variety of teaching activities in their day-to-day practice. This may not be evident because people usually associate teaching and learning in a narrow form involving only formal educational activities. When they think of teaching they envision a formal setting, with one person designated as the "teacher" and the other persons present as the designated "learners." However, in the health care setting, especially rehabilitation settings, teaching is informal, implicit, brief, and learner-directed (Farquharson, 1995). Adults learn best when they are ready and willing to learn (Knowles, 1975). In some instances specific requests for learning may be made of the nurse by the client or family, health care team, friends, or caregivers (Redman, 1988). There are certain moments when people are more open to change. Havighurst (1970) used the term **teachable moments** to describe these teaching opportunities. Nurses need to be alert for these critical opportunities for teaching.

The general long-range goals of education in rehabilitation nursing are

1. To provide information to clients, family members, or caregivers so that they are able to make informed decisions with regard to health and illness
2. To assist clients, family members, and caregivers to participate effectively in the care and treatment of the client
3. To assist clients, family members, and caregivers to adapt to the realities of an illness, injury, disease, or disability and the realities of rehabilitation and treatment

4. To assist clients, family members, and caregivers to experience the satisfaction of seeing their own efforts contribute toward improvements of health (Steiger & Lipson, 1985).

Principles of Teaching and Learning

Meeting client and family member or caregiver educational needs involves principles of both teaching and learning. **Teaching** is the process that facilitates learning. Teaching can be formal (a class for clients who need to learn insulin self-administration) or informal (a nurse discussing childhood immunizations with the mother of a toddler when they are visiting the child's grandfather during visiting hours). The discussion of teaching principles described in this chapter is directed toward formal teaching encounters.

Learning can be conceived as a process of "meaning-making" and learners may be regarded as "meaning-makers" (Postman & Weingartner, 1969; Cranton, 1994). This conceptualization of learning places the client at the center of the learning process. The goal of teaching in this view is to help learners improve their meaning-making abilities. Teaching strategies are directed toward helping the clients learn to deal with what may seem to be "meaningless," to cope with change, and to generate new meanings (Postman & Weingartner, 1969). Learning then is an activity through which clients, family members, and caregivers can reconstruct past health knowledge, experiences, and skills to support healthy behaviors or to change unhealthy behaviors. Knowledge is not something to be acquired or transmitted but a process, being constantly created and recreated (Kolb, 1984).

Human learning involves increasing knowledge, modifying attitudes, developing skills, and enhancing perceptual abilities. Each of these four areas can be considered a separate field of learning activity. Bloom (1956) identified four **learning domains:**

1. Learning that requires the acquisition of new thoughts and ideas (cognitive learning)
2. Learning that involves changes in attitudes or values (affective learning)
3. Learning that involves behaviors (psychomotor skill acquisition)
4. Learning that involves sensation and perception of meaning and performance (perceptual learning)

These domains of learning should be considered as independent of each other but at the same time interdependent. All four domains of learning must be considered when planning any teaching in order to formulate objectives to cover all aspects of learning—and to facilitate the integration of knowledge.

A client may learn (cognitive learning) the techniques of active range-of-motion exercises. She may learn (psychomotor learning) to perform and demonstrate active range-of-motion exercises. However, if she does not learn (affective learning) to value those exercises or see that they are of benefit to her, adherence to a regimen that includes active range-of-motion exercises may be low.

The *cognitive domain* involves activities of knowledge comprehension, reasoning, and processing and recalling information. Example: The client will state four side effects of heparin. The *affective domain* involves activities that focus on feelings, values, and attitudes. Example: The client will make two positive statements about herself. The *psychomotor domain* involves activities of performance, skilled movements, and motor function. Example: The client's wife will demonstrate changing the colostomy dressing. The *perceptual domain* involves awareness and comprehension of symbols and meanings (Kopper, 1987). Example: The deaf client will use a printed script when viewing an educational film.

Adult Learning Principles

Adult learning principles have been identified by Knowles (1975). These principles stress the self-concept of the learners, the accumulated life experiences of the learner, the level and context of learning, and the purpose or application the learner has in mind for the material being learned.

1. The adult learner is self-directed rather than dependent and passive.
2. The adult learner brings a greater quantity and quality of previous experience to new learning situations. The adult learner uses that life experience as a major resource. The adult learner benefits from a highly individualized teaching-learning process.
3. The adult learner's readiness to learn is highly correlated with the perception that new information or skills are necessary for effective performance in some aspect of life.
4. An adult learner's perception of learning is life-centered, task-oriented, or problem-centered.
5. Adult learners are more strongly motivated by internal factors (self-esteem, recognition, quality of life, self-confidence) than external factors (work satisfaction, salary increase).

Using these principles as a foundation, the teacher (rehabilitation nurse) assumes the role of facilitator of learning, and the role of designer and manager of the learning process. The rehabilitation nurse who is mindful of these principles when preparing to teach or during actual teaching opportunities will help the client understand the "new" in terms of the "old," use past experiences to enrich communication between teacher and learner, and make teaching and learning a shared experience (Farquharson, 1995).

Learning Styles

Individuals differ from one another in their ways of conducting learning. Smith (1984) defined **learning style** as the individual's familiar ways of processing information. A model proposed for understanding the process of experiential learning is Kolb's dimensions of learning model (Kolb, 1984). This model suggests that learning style is shaped by two variables: (1) the movement from concrete to abstract (simple to complex) and (2) a shift from active to reflective. Kolb conceptualized four dimensions of learning:

1. Learning from concrete experience, relying on experience-based input
2. Learning from reflective observation, gathering all available data generated by experience
3. Learning from abstract concepts, attempts to explain the data generated
4. Learning from active experimentation

Learners have experiences, they reflect on the cognitive and affective data generated, they use these data to construct an explanation to account for the experience, and they find ways to test the explanations they have formed (Kolb, 1984). Some clients will be stronger in one of the learning dimensions than in the others. Nurses engaged in client education need to assess learning style to adapt and vary teaching strategies. They need to reflect on their own teaching style, and compare that to clients' learning styles. It would be beneficial for both teacher and learner to group individuals with different learning styles together in education sessions. Learners would enhance the session by contributing learning resources for one another. Learning styles must be determined to identify the most appropriate and effective strategies for learning specific tasks (Farquharson, 1995).

Client Factors Influencing Learning

Learning is influenced by a variety of individual characteristics and factors. The learner's physical, psychological, and intellectual developmental level can significantly influence the ability to learn and the selection of strategies used to facilitate learning. Assessment should include the client's vocabulary and communication ability, level of understanding, attention span, memory, and physical ability to perform required tasks (Schuster & Ashburn, 1986). Learning can be significantly influenced by the learner's readiness to learn; physical, emotional, and language barriers; lack of motivation; and the client's family.

Learning is directly related to cognitive abilities. The effectiveness of teaching and degree of learning are directly related to the ability to communicate, the capacity to understand, and attention span. The client must be able to ask questions, verbalize understanding, and clarify and verify information (Schuster & Ashburn, 1986) The ability to attend is also extremely critical. To increase retention and learning, teaching should be planned in segments that accommodate the client's attention span (Schuster & Ashburn, 1986).

Contributing to cognitive abilities are issues of language. Consideration should be given to the client's primary language, the ability to read, to write, and to speak in the teacher's primary language. Supplementary material given to reinforce a teaching session must be available in the client's primary language. Usually these materials are used when the learner does not have access to the teacher for questions and clarification. The teacher must be aware of the use of nursing or medical terminology, slang, or abbreviations that may be unfamiliar to the clients.

Memory plays a major role in learning because learning cannot occur without the ability to retain and recall past experience (Schuster & Ashburn, 1986). Motor skills, both fine and gross, may be necessary to perform certain tasks. When teaching physical skills motor skills should be assessed so that the client has the tools, equipment, or assistance necessary for mastery. Insufficient motor capabilities can frustrate the client and result in a sense of failure for both the teacher and the learner (Schuster & Ashburn, 1986).

Learning is influenced by changes or alterations in sensory modalities. Visual changes can include decreased acuity, sensitivity to light, increased sensitivity to glare, altered color vision, altered depth perception, and a complete or partial loss of sight. Hearing changes can include partial or total loss of hearing. Hearing changes can result in difficulties with speech intelligibility and decreased comprehension. Changes in physical endurance and strength can influence the outcome of learning activities and exercises. The ability to maintain balance should be considered along with determination of activity tolerance.

Readiness to Learn

Learning is influenced by the learner's **readiness to learn.** The educational readiness of clients and families must be initially assessed to establish a client baseline, and to determine capabilities and abilities for learning and understanding the important, and often complex, concepts contained in self-care teaching. Readiness to learn is emotional, involving the motivation to learn. It is also experiential, involving the adequacy of background knowledge; the mastery of specific skills; and the knowledge, attitudes, and values related to learning. Learning readiness depends on the aroused interest or motive of the learner, relevant preparatory training, and physiological maturation (Kaluger & Kaluger, 1984).

Client teaching will usually be directed toward bringing about a permanent behavioral or lifestyle change in the client. Clients demonstrate various stages of learning readiness when behavioral change is involved. To assess the client's initial readiness to learn, ask simple questions: "What have you been told about your condition?" "Do you know what your rehabilitation is going to be like?" This identifies the appropriate targets for teaching.

If the client does not perceive that a problem exists, or states that there is no need for change, education must be focused on raising the client's awareness of the realities of the situation. This may require a review with the client of the benefits of the new knowledge or required change as well as the consequence of not possessing that information or making the change.

Some clients will indicate, or even state, an understanding of the need for education or behavioral change but take no action in that direction. Initial teaching for this client should be focused on reinforcing the understanding that there is a need for learning or behavior modification and on teaching the skills needed to make the change. Once a patient has begun changing behavior on the basis of the teaching-learning process the teaching can be shifted to reinforcing the practice of modified behaviors with modeling and rewards. This is a critical time in the learning process. The client must continue to be motivated to maintain the modified behavior and use the new knowledge that has been gained. This will continue to be the objective of the teaching until the client demonstrates that the modified behavior change or the use of the new knowledge has become a part of the client's typical way of operating. At that time the skills and knowledge are no longer considered a change and so no additional teaching or reinforcement is required.

In family or group learning situations readiness is quite complex and will vary among members. When assessing learning readiness the rehabilitation nurse should work with the family to discover each family member's perceptions and information and skill needs. Readiness to learn can be influenced by grief, pain, medication, or mental and physical conditions experienced by family members, the same as for the client (Farley, 1992).

Caregiver readiness and willingness to invest time in teaching and learning should also be determined. There are indicators of the degree of caregiver readiness; willing caregivers state belief in the client's ability to learn, verbally express willingness to participate in learning, ask questions, involve themselves in record keeping, share observations about the client, and help to set realistic goals for the client and for themselves.

The teaching-learning environment can be hindered by physical, emotional, and motivational barriers. The nurse should be alert for possible physical barriers to learning, which might include pain or other discomfort, limited energy, decreased mobility, nausea, shortness of breath, or decreased sensorimotor skills. Emotional barriers that can hinder learning include denial, depression, feelings of anger and anxiety, low self-esteem, feelings of inferiority or incompetence, and lack of perceived self-efficacy. It is important for the nurse to intervene to remove or mitigate the deleterious effects of any of these barriers.

The source of a lack of client motivation is often difficult for health care providers to understand. Lack of motivation can develop at any time during the rehabilitation process. Even clients who are generally strongly motivated can experience episodic problems with motivation.

Redman (1988) suggested principles that can be useful when attempting to motivate clients.

1. Learning is motivated by incentives.
2. Internal motivation is longer lasting and more self-directed than external motivation.

3. Learning is more effective when the learner feels the need to know.
4. Motivation is enhanced by the organization of the material.
5. Success is a more predictable motivator than failure.
6. Mild anxiety is useful for motivation of individuals.

Family Influence on Learning

Haggard (1989) identified family and significant others as probably the most significant determinant of the success of client teaching. The family contributes to the health and health behaviors of the client. How a family functions also influences how the client reacts to illness. Teaching the client without including the family may result in less than effective teaching. Family members provide the primary source of support for most clients involved in the rehabilitation process. Their reactions and attitude toward the client, the client's health state and status, and the treatment plan will influence the client's ability and desire to learn self-care and self-management. Nurses involved in client education in the rehabilitation setting need to have insight into the client's relationships with family members. The nurse should assess what family members can do for the client and work with them to encourage the client to attempt things that might be perceived as difficult (Falvo, 1985).

Illness, injury, disease, and disability can be stressful and devastating for family members. Family members may respond by being overprotective of the client. This may impede client learning. The client may not feel the need to learn about self-care or self-management because of the family's stepping in and taking over the responsibility for care and learning. The client may not develop a sense of responsibility for care and treatment outcomes. This can also lead to a maladjustment in dependency. Family members who are overprotective may remove the client from decision-making opportunities (see Chapter 12). Overprotectiveness by family members can reinforce the client's perceptions of loss of control over life and the future. Overprotectiveness can also inhibit the development of perceived self-efficacy, and mastery.

Family members may use denial as a coping strategy. They may need time to adjust to the client's change in health state. Family members may deny the realities of the client's life situation even though the client has accepted the illness, injury, disease, or disability. Family denial can be an obstacle to the learning necessary for the implementation and success of the treatment plan. Family denial can also reinforce client denial (Haggard, 1989). Family denial may result in failure to follow up with lifestyle recommendations, failure to keep follow-up examinations and appointments, and deprivation of support for the client (Haggard, 1989).

The purpose of involving family members in client teaching is to gain their support and provide them with necessary information. It is important to remember that family members are not professionals and they are not being prepared to be technicians in client care (Falvo, 1985).

Transfer of Learning

The **transfer of learning** from the artificial environment of the health care facility learning environment to the home environment is of particular importance in the learning process for rehabilitation clients. People recall and apply knowledge best under conditions similar to those in which it was acquired. This includes the internal state of the client as well as the external environment. State-dependent learning theory implies that altered electrolytes, an elevated blood sugar level, and a reduced oxygen concentration could be factors in retention, recall, or application of newly acquired knowledge and skills. It also implies that clients who acquire and practice new knowledge and skills in the health setting might experience difficulty in attempting to apply that knowledge or skill in the home or work place.

Rehabilitation clients, family members, and caregivers are confronted with sustaining learning gains for a very long period of time. Transfer of learning involves the issues and strategies associated with ensuring that learned abilities can be, and are, applied when the learner leaves the learning environment (Fox, 1984). Transfer of learning strategies cannot be introduced at the conclusion of a learning event. When planning teaching strategies the rehabilitation nurse must consider how to transfer learning during assessment, design, implementation, and evaluation phases of teaching (Farquharson, 1995).

It is important to determine and explore how the new learning will fit with the personality of the learner, or with the norms of the learner's family or social network. New learning at odds or inconsistent with the client's values, attitudes, or lifestyle will rapidly fade. Resistance based on an incompatibility between educator's and learner's values, attitudes, lifestyle, or perceived need for education can have serious negative effects on transfer of learning.

Often, health care providers attempt to bring about client change by escalating pressures that push the client in the direction the health care provider prefers. This can lead to resistance or a struggle to maintain the status quo and result in transfer of learning hurdles. Kurt Lewin (1951) determined that it is easier to bring about change by reducing the forces against the change than by increasing the forces to produce the change. He suggested determining what needs are threatened by the proposed change and finding ways to meet those needs even if a change in status quo is introduced.

There are ways to increase the probability that learning will be transferred (Farquharson, 1995):

1. The learning environment should reproduce the setting in which the new behavior will be needed.
2. Provide the learner with the opportunity to demonstrate and perform the actual behaviors that will be required in the home situation.
3. "Overteaching," the repeated practice of new leaning, will produce fluency in situations in which the new learning is needed.

4. Work with the social systems and environments within which the learners will use their new knowledge, skills, or values.
5. Promote conceptual learning rather than information learning.
6. Develop, with the learner, "aids" to help the learner recall desired behavior once the formal learning is completed (e.g., checklists, slogans, posters)
7. Follow up teaching to finetune the application of prior learning.

The Process of Client Education in Rehabilitation

The long-term nature of rehabilitation requires the development and implementation of effective teaching-learning plans that will assist the client and family members to achieve the highest level of self-care functioning possible. Nurses need to be able to recognize client teaching needs, develop and implement effective teaching plans, and critically evaluate the results of those educational programs. The process of client education is similar to the nursing process. The components include assessment and identification of the client's and family's learning needs, establishment of client's and family's learning goals, design of the teaching plan, implementation of the teaching plan, and evaluation of the learning outcomes.

Teaching and education in rehabilitation are geared toward assisting the client and family to engage in self-care, self-responsibility, and self-management. Topics included in the teaching of self-care will involve issues of independent living and functioning as a member of society. To live independently individuals will need to learn skills for maintaining activities of daily life, and for maintaining physical, structural, and functional integrity. Self-care skill development may include feeding, dressing, bathing and grooming, locomotion, toileting, housekeeping, food purchasing and preparation, sight reading, vocational skills, money management, and the use of public transportation. Client, family members, and caregivers may need to become familiar with the use of catheters, bladder and bowel training, colostomy care, sex and reproductive functioning, alternative feeding and eating techniques, ambulating and positioning, or medication administration and storage.

A primary focus in rehabilitation education will be on the development of effective self-care skills. Farley (1992) offered the following suggestions for designing a plan for teaching self-care skills:

- Identify where in the skill sequence to begin.
- Objectively describe the target skills to be taught.
- Identify the rationale for teaching the skills.
- Identify specific behaviors necessary before the target skills can be acquired.
- Determine environmental supports for the target skills.
- Identify the teaching procedures and instructional materials necessary.
- Identify the components of the target skill that are presently intact.
- Conduct a skill analysis.
- Observe and record events antecedent to the skill.
- Identify effective systems for the reinforcement of desired behaviors.

- Specify contingencies for behavior reinforcement.
- Develop a recording system, including the format and guidelines on what to record.
- Implement the plan and collection data.
- Review the data and evaluate the success or failure of the plan.

Identification of Learning Needs

It is necessary to be clear regarding who the learner will be, what his or her **learning needs** are, and who makes those determinations (Vella, 1994). The identification of the client and family learning needs may occur through direct request or by observation of the individuals. Individuals may identify what they "feel" or "perceive" to be their learning needs. But, felt learning needs are not generally an adequate measure of the real needs of adult learners (Brookfield, 1986; Wlodkowski, 1991). Learning needs can be determined by health care providers or by the treatment team on the basis of what they "professionally perceive" to be the need. However, the most effective process by which to identify learning needs is based on an assessment of the measurable difference between the current functioning of the learner and some normative or prescriptive standard (Monette, 1977; Wlodkowski, 1991).

In many cases learning needs and resources will be readily recognized by both the teacher and the learner. There is a mutual perception of need, with the felt need of the learner being consistent with the needs perceived by the teacher. In other cases the teacher will frequently perceive a learning need and the learner will not feel that need. In those situations the teacher must reach out to the learner regarding the need to learn something that the learner may not feel is needed. In still other situations the learner may have a felt learning need not perceived by the teacher. In those situations the learner must make a request to the teacher for the learning. Occasionally the learning need is perceived neither by the learner nor the teacher. In those situations a thorough exploration of needs through mutual reflection is required (Farquharson, 1995).

Clients with cognitive impairments may demonstrate deficits in their ability to discriminate between multiple stimuli because of difficulty in recognizing relevant cues. They will benefit from a reduction in extraneous stimuli and cues that are presented through demonstration, imitation, modeling, and repetition (Farley, 1992). Audiovisual aids are also useful in facilitating learning. Individuals with impaired short-term memories will require one-step directions (Whaley & Wong, 1991).

Behavior modification techniques, especially *shaping* (i.e., using positive reinforcement for desired actions), and *fading* (i.e., gradually decreasing assistance), have proven to be very successful for teaching new tasks.

Nonproductive Nursing Assumptions

Nothing undermines a good teaching plan more than an inaccurate assessment. The learning needs must be identified by information generated about the client, family members, or caregivers—not determined by what the nurse "thinks" the learning needs are for learners. Assumptions about the learner and learning needs can interfere with learning Never assume that the client already has knowledge about and understands the illness, injury, or disease, or about dealing with a disability. This is true even if the client has been living with the illness, injury, disease, or disability and treatment for a long time. Never assume clients understand why they are taking certain medications, or the reason for treatments, or procedures. Never make assumptions about motivation, ability to learn, or adherence on the basis of differences in social, economic, ethnic, racial, cultural, or educational background. Never assume, on the basis of their past history, that clients will remain adherent or nonadherent (Jackson & Johnson, 1988).

Assessment of Learning Needs and Learner Readiness

The assessment component of the client education process involves the physical status of the learner, the psychological state of the learner, the learner's motivation to learn, the capabilities or abilities that the learner brings to the learning task, and the learner's opportunities to implement what is learned. The context in which the learning occurs is almost as important as what is to be taught. Assessment should include the following factors.

Client Factors

- Demographic data: The learner's age, marital status, occupation(s), education, ethnicity, culture, and so on
- The client's physical functioning related to current or past disabilities or limitation
- The degree of disruption to the client's and family's social reality
- Motivation and readiness of the client and family to learn and implement learning
- Psychological disruption for the learner, anxiety and high-stress episodes (i.e., initial stabilization, diagnosis), or shock and denial response stages, depression
- The learner's perceptions of the problem and need for learning and priorities
- The client's and family's attitudes, reactions, and feelings about the client's health state, and health care
- The client's and family's strengths and limitations brought to the learning task
- The client's and family's current level of knowledge or skill development
- Client's level of cognitive functioning and intellectual disruptions

Communication Factors

- Learner's lack of comprehension of the subject matter
- Cultural and language barriers
- Socioeconomic barriers
- Learner's inability to communicate clearly with teacher and others

Situational Factors

- The nature of the environment in which the teaching-learning takes place
- The family's influence on the client's health state, reaction, and adaptation to the illness, injury, disease, or disability
- Timing of the teaching
- Resources available for teaching and application of the learning
- Teaching methods used

Development of the Teaching Plan

The educational plan should be mutually determined by the client, the family, and the treatment team members. A mutual approach assumes that both the client and the health care teacher are equal partners working together to reach a common teaching goal. The client is an active participant in the process, from assessment to evaluation. The role of the teacher is that of a facilitator helping the client, family, or caregivers to help themselves (Falvo, 1985). The plan should be explicit in terms of learning goals and objectives, the educational content to be taught, learning activities to be included, specific desired learning outcomes, and the methods for evaluation and documentation of the effectiveness of the teaching plan.

Several elements must be considered when designing a learning experience. When designing a teaching session key decisions must be made regarding

- Creating both the appropriate physical and psychological learning climate (i.e., furniture arrangement, mutual respect and trust, openness and authenticity, humanness)
- Identifying strategies that include family members and caregivers in the teaching plan
- Mutually planning for the learning experience
- Identifying learning needs
- Formulating learning objectives
- Sequencing learning activities
- Designing and planning each learning episode
- Selecting and developing learning resources

The EDICT Model for Designing Teaching Episodes

Teaching episodes are single teaching interventions that vary in length. In longer teaching interventions several teaching episodes can be linked together. A model that can be used to guide the process of designing a teaching intervention is known as **EDICT** (Farquharson, 1995). Even though the name implies a teacher-centered, directive-based teaching style, the model is actually used in situations that require varying degrees of teacher and learner involvement.

E = Education: Begin by selecting the main ideas to be presented in an episode. Decide how to sequence the explanation and present the information and ideas.

D = Demonstration: Identify how the learner can be assisted to make connections between ideas and information in the education step and events in the real world. Find ways to demonstrate the ideas of information previously presented. This can be done through story telling, brief video, or computer simulations.

I = Involvement: Select ways for the learner to be involved in applying or using the information or ideas previously presented. This can include asking the learner to reflect on the ideas or actually demonstrate the use of the information, idea, or skill. It might also involve role playing, simulation, or problem-solving activities (Farquharson, 1995). The important aspect is that the learner is actively involved in the construction and application of meaning (Meyers & Jones, 1993).

C = Coaching: Following the involvement step the teacher provides feedback to the learner through coaching or corrective feedback. The following guidelines for coaching are use for constructive feedback: (1) Check the learner's self-appraisal; (2) give feedback as soon as possible; (3) present feedback in manageable quantities, giving more positive than negative feedback; (4) give the learner feedback only about things that the learner can change (Farquharson, 1995).

T = Testing: The testing step is important to identify what has been taught and what has actually been learned. Testing can involve checking to see whether teaching has been transferred into changed behavior in the real world (Farquharson, 1995).

Methods and Tools Used for Effective Client Teaching

Success is enhanced when a variety of teaching strategies and aids is combined with opportunities for practicing learned skills in a variety of situations or contexts. Verbal instruction on a one-to-one basis can be used to facilitate individualization of teaching. Group discussion is useful for affective learning. Group discussions can be used to promote the sharing of information about coping, adaptation, and effective management strategies. The lecture format is useful when presenting a great deal of information in a short time frame. Its usefulness in the rehabilitation setting is limited. Its ineffectiveness for skill development is obvious because there is a lack of active participation on the part of the learner. Demonstration, practice, and return demonstration are useful for skill development or behavioral learning. Games are interesting and exciting for the learner. They are most effective as a means of reviewing material presented to the learner.

Resources that can be used in a teaching session or provided to the client to reinforce learning include charts, posters, diagrams, books, self-instruction manuals, instruction sheets, and pamphlets. Audiovisual aids and material to assist in teaching include films, videos, software, mounted illustrations, and models. In future, computer-assisted instruction will be a powerful tool for rehabilitation education. Written aids should be short, easy to read, and present information in a factual, structured manner. They can be used to provide information, reinforce teaching, or supplement instruction. They can be provided to the client or family before or after the teaching session.

Teaching aids are most effective if the client views them as an extension of the teacher. Teaching aids are used to reinforce and illustrate information. They are not meant to replace the nurse. Any teaching aid should be evaluated before use for content and ease of use. Information in the teaching aid should be consistent with, or be complementary to, the information provided in the interaction with the nurse. Each teaching aid should be tailored for each client or family (Falvo, 1985). Teaching aids should not be given to clients without verbal instruction and an explanation of the purpose of the teaching aid.

Implementation of the Teaching Plan

The nurse should attempt to tailor the teaching session to meet individual client and family needs. Teaching sessions should be planned according to client and family member cognitive developmental stage and the learner's ability to focus and concentrate on the material presented for learning. As a rule, teaching sessions should be kept short and involve all sensory modalities. Children learn best in 15- to 20-minute sessions. Adult sessions can be 45 to 60 minutes in length. Both children and adults benefit from the use of visual aids, demonstration, and return demonstration. Tasks should be broken up into logical steps or subtasks progressing from simple to complex. The target date for achieving each specific objective should be identified in the teaching plan.

Some clients with limited or reduced physical strength may learn better in the morning or after rest periods (White, 1989). Learning is most effective when it occurs over a period of time. Environmental settings should be conducive to learning. This means that they are physically comfortable; they are free of distractions, sights, smells, sounds, and extreme temperatures (Whaley and Wong, 1991); and provide adequate lighting to meet the client or family visual needs.

Katz (1997) suggested keeping to the basics when implementing the teaching plan. Katz's suggestions are particularly useful when teaching in the rehabilitation setting, where client comprehension, attention span, or cognitive abilities may be compromised.

1. Get and keep the client's and family's attention.
   a. Make the point clear right from the start of the session.
   b. Vary tone of voice and rate of speech.
   c. Use an assortment of teaching methods and learning aids.
   d. Make the abstract concrete.
2. Stick to the basics.
   a. Remember that less is more; keep it short, simple, and specific.
   b. Be specific about what you want the client to know.
   c. Use simple, everyday language.
3. Make the most use of time.
   a. Incorporate teaching into patient care activities.
   b. Involve family members and friends in the teaching sessions when possible.
   c. Supplement teaching with written materials for the client.
4. Remember that reinforcement is key to retention of learning.
   a. Be a role model for the client and family members.
   b. Provide rewards for success retention of material and accurate demonstration of learning.
   c. Review material over time.
5. Develop a method for testing the client's and family's understanding.
   a. Have the client or family member restate material or demonstrate skills.
   b. Have the client or family members use diaries or schedules to record behavior.
   c. Review written material with the client and family members.

6. Overcome or mitigate the effects of any identified barriers to learning that may exist.
   a. Physical barriers include pain, altered level of consciousness, effects of medications, and so on.
   b. Emotional barriers include stress anxiety, depression, anger, limited perceived self-efficacy, and so on.
   c. Language and culture barriers.
   d. Low reading comprehension level.
   e. Family influences.

Evaluation and Dcoumentation Evaluation

The final phase of the teaching plan is to evaluate the entire process. Evaluation should be summative in nature, involving the continuous monitoring of both implementation and progress. Information should be gathered from the perspective of the learners, teachers, and others involved. It should focus on the learning process and on the achievement of learning outcomes. A plan should be developed to determine to what extent the client, family members, or caregivers have reached the established goals. If the goals are not being attained, what are the factors hindering goal attainment? Using a variety of sources to provide evaluation data allows for the cross-checking of data and for the identification of patterns or inconsistencies in teaching methods and styles (Farquharson, 1995).

A teaching plan is effective if it achieves the goal for which it was designed. Specific outcomes identified during planning should be clearly demonstrated. The methods used to evaluate educational outcomes will vary depending on the nature of the knowledge or skills being developed. Evaluation methods should be simple and efficient in technique. Informal, short-term evaluation may involve conversations with the client or family member (Flavo, 1985). Clients, family members, or caregivers can be asked to perform return demonstration of skills. Paper-and-pencil tests, as well as pretest and posttest examinations, can be administered. Homework assignments can be required. There can be follow-up phone calls to discharged clients. Follow-up calls can be planned at set time intervals and used to review and reinforce learning and to answer questions. Self-appraisal questionnaires can be developed for clients and family members to answer questions regarding the use of learned knowledge and behaviors. Medical records and clinic records can be monitored for successful adherence to treatment regimens. Physical evidence such as laboratory values, medication levels, vital signs, or changes in abilities can be monitored (Haggard, 1989). Whatever evaluation method is used it is important that it measure outcomes that were established in the teaching plan.

The client's and family's evaluation of the teaching plan and the knowledge acquired should also be determined. Have their learning needs been adequately addressed? Do they perceive a need to modify the teaching plan? Necessary revisions to the teaching plan should be clearly articulated to all members of the treatment team who are responsible for client education.

Documentation   A system for documenting client and family education must be developed at the time the treatment plan is developed. Documentation of client teaching assists other members of the treatment team to reinforce information given. It provides an opportunity to further assess learning needs, and to address any problems with the implementation of the teaching plan. The outcomes of the treatment plan should be reflected in the educational plan. A flowchart format of documentation is useful, and it is easy to use and easy to follow. The documentation system should include the topic to be taught, specific learning outcomes, the learning objective established to reach the outcome, the actual plan of teaching (including time line for teaching), the specific teaching strategies to be used, and the evaluation methods. The system should also provide a method for tracking the date of the teaching session, who did the teaching, who was taught, what they were taught in the session, the teaching strategies used, the outcome of the session, and suggestions for modification of the teaching plan.

Conclusion   Client education is the cornerstone for developing self-care and self-management in rehabilitative nursing. The goals of teaching are to increase knowledge, modify attitudes, develop skills, and enhance perceptual abilities. Successful learning is essential to maximize rehabilitation treatment outcomes. In health care settings, especially rehabilitation settings, teaching is informal, implicit, brief, and learner-directed. Adults learn best when they are ready and willing to learn. There are certain moments, "teachable moments," when people are more open to change; nurses need to be alert for these critical opportunities for teaching. In the rehabilitation setting teaching is a client right and a nursing responsibility. Client education does not involve simply giving verbal instruction and handing out printed materials. The client's learning needs and readiness are essential areas requiring nursing assessment before beginning any teaching activities. The nurse in the rehabilitation setting must assess the various factors that may influence or compromise the client's ability to learn and identify the appropriate strategies to overcome, or mitigate, the effects of those factors.

References   Bloom, B. S. (Ed.). (1956). *Taxonomy of educational objectives: The classification of educational goals. Handbook I: Cognitive domain.* White Plains, NY: David McKay Co.

Brookfield, S. (1986). *Understanding and facilitating adult learning: A comprehensive analysis of principles and effective practices.* San Francisco: Jossey-Bass.

Cranton, P. (1994). *Understanding and promoting transformative learning.* San Francisco: Jossey-Bass.

Deihl, L. N. (1989). Client and family learning in the rehabilitation setting. *Nursing Clinics of North America, 24,* 257–264.

Falvo, D. R. (1985). *Effective patient education: A guide to increased compliance.* Rockville, MD: Aspen.

Farley, A. M. (1992). *Nursing and the disabled across the life span.* Boston: Jones & Bartlett.

Farquharson, A. (1995). *Teaching in practice: How professionals can work effectively with clients, patients, and colleagues.* San Francisco: Jossey-Bass.

Fox, R. (1984). Fostering transfer of learning to work environments. In S. Sork (Ed.), *Designing and implementing effective workshops.* San Francisco: Jossey-Bass.

Haggard, A. (1989). *Handbook of patient education.* Rockville, MD: Aspen.

Havinghurst, R. (1970). *Developmental tasks and education.* New York: McKay.

Jackson, J. E., & Johnson, E. A. (1988). *Patient education in home care: A practical guide to effective teaching and documentation.* Rockville, MD: Aspen.

Kaluger, G., & Kaluger, M. (1984). *Human development: The life span.* St. Louis: Mosby.

Katz, J. A. (1997). Back to basics: Providing effective patient teaching. *American Journal of Nursing, 97*(5), 33–36.

Knowles, M. (1975). *Self-directed learning: A guide for learners and teachers.* Chicago: Follett.

Kolb, D. (1984). *Experiential learning.* Englewood Cliffs, NJ: Prentice-Hall.

Kopper, J. A. (1987). Assessing knowledge deficit and establishing behavioral objectives. In C. S. Smith (Ed.), *Patient education nurses in partnership with other health professionals* (pp. 123–158). Philadelphia: W. B. Saunders.

Lewin, K. (1951). *Field theory in social science.* New York: Harper-Collins.

Meyers, C., & Jones, T. (1993). *Promoting active learning: Strategies for the college classroom.* San Francisco: Jossey-Bass.

Monette, M. (1977). The concepts of educational need: An analysis of selected literature. *Adult Education. 27*(2), 116–127.

Postman, N., & Weingartner, C. (1969). *Teaching as a subversive activity.* New York: Dell.

Redman, B. K. (1988). *Process of patient teaching in nursing* (6th ed.). St. Louis: Mosby.

Schuster, C. S., & Ashburn, S. S. (1986). *The process of human development: A holistic approach* (2nd ed.). Boston: Little, Brown.

Smith, R. (1984). *Learning how to learn.* New York: Cambridge University Press.

Steiger, N. J., & Lipson, J. G. (1985). *Self-care nursing: the theory and practice.* Bowie, MD: Brady Communications Co.

Vella, J. (1994). *Learning to listen: The power of dialogue in educating adults.* San Francisco: Jossey-Bass.

Whaley, L. F., & Wong, D. L. (1991). The child with endocrine dysfunction. In L. F. Wang and D. L. Wong (Eds.), *Nursing care of infants and children* (4th ed., pp. 1779-1832). St. Louis: Mosby.

White, B. G. (1989). Teaching learning process. In S. Dittman (Ed.), *Rehabilitation nursing: Process and application* (pp. 63–72). St. Louis: Mosby.

Wlodkowski, R. (1991). *Enhancing adult motivation to learn: A guide to improving instruction and increasing learner achievement.* San Francisco: Jossey-Bass.

CHAPTER 7

Nursing Strategies for Increasing Adherence
Patricia A. Chin

Key Terms
Adherence
Compliance
Contracting
Efficacy Expectations
Health Beliefs Model
Impaired Role
Nonadherence
Noncompliance
Outcome Expectations
Professional Role
Sick Role
Therapeutic Alliance

Objectives
1. Distinguish between client adherence and compliance.

2. Identify desired adherence behaviors.

3. Identify factors influencing client adherence.

4. Discuss the relationship between the health beliefs model and client adherence.

5. Discuss the therapeutic alliance and how to enhance that alliance.

6. Discuss the assessment of the client's explanatory model for rehabilitation, client's worries and concerns about rehabilitation, and client treatment expectations.

Client Adherence and Compliance

The traditional view held by most health care providers is that clients will accept, adopt, and adhere to their suggestions regarding health care. Health care providers frequently identify client adherence as a priority goal for their client interactions. This is true whether the care provided is preventive, curative, or restorative. It would seem logical that a client's well-being would increase if health practices and behaviors were consistent with health care provider recommendations. However, research and experience reveal that there is often a lack of concurrence between what health care providers recommend and the health practices and behaviors that clients actually choose.

Health care providers are frequently suggesting and recommending major changes in client health behaviors and practices. These changes might involve dietary changes, exercises, restrictions in activity, administrations of medications and treatments, or other lifestyle changes that the individual will have to incorporate into daily life. Client behaviors consistent with carrying out health care recommendations and suggestions are referred to by most health care providers as **compliance.** When the individual does not accept, or chooses to ignore, the recommendations of the health care provider the response is labeled a problem of **noncompliance.** Noncompliance is such a predominant client response identified by nurses that it is included among those nursing diagnoses approved by the North American Nursing Diagnosis Association (NANDA)(Carson & Arnold, 1996).

The term *compliance* is generally used to indicate the extent to which clients obey and follow instructions, proscriptions, and prescriptions of health care providers. A negative connotation is attached to the term *compliance* and may imply a prejudicial attitude toward the client. Characterizing a client's response to the suggested treatment regimen as noncompliant implies that the client is passive and lacks autonomy and that the health care provider is coercive and paternalistic. It also conjures up a picture of a person struggling to follow a set of rules prescribed by a dictating professional. A more positive term with which to characterize client responses to health care education, recommendations, and suggestions would be **adherence** (Blevins & Lubkin, 1995, Meichenbaum & Turk, 1987) (Table 1).

Table 1
Comparison of the Terms *Adherence* and *Compliance*

Adherence	Compliance
• Client assumes an active role	• Client assumes a passive role
• Voluntary, collaborative involvement by the client is implied	• Client faithfully follows health care provider's plan of care
• Mutually acceptable course of action to produce preventive and therapeutic results determined by client and care provider	• Client is obedient to health care provider
• Choice is exercised	• Client's behavior coincides with health care provider's advice
• Mutuality in planning and implementation	• Plan of care is developed by the health care provider

The traditional view of the relationship between the client and health care providers has also been to place the responsibility for increasing adherence on the health care providers. However, if the plan of care is to be effective in bringing about the desired goals of both the client and health care providers then the responsibility for increasing adherence belongs to both the providers of care and the recipient of care. Increasing adherence is a mutual activity. This activity must involve the client, the client's family members, the client's support system, any additional caregiver, as well as the members of the rehabilitation team.

Desired Adherence Behaviors

Meichenbaum and Turk (1987) identified those client responses and behaviors that could be considered consistent with being adherent with a treatment regimen.

- The client enters into a health alliance with the health care provider.
- The client continues with the proposed treatment plan.
- The client keeps referrals and follow-up appointments.
- The client correctly consumes prescribed medications.
- The client adopts and follows recommended lifestyle changes.
- The client correctly performs home-based therapeutic regimens.
- The client avoids involvement in health risk behaviors.

Incidence of Nonadherence

Figures on the exact incidence of **nonadherence** are difficult to obtain. Adherence studies are generally disease-specific and the study populations identified by the presence of a particular disease or injury. A wide variety of psychometric measures has been used to measure adherence and nonadherence responses and behaviors. These instruments include interviewing, self-report, self-monitoring, pill counts, refills on medications, behavioral measures, biochemical indicators, records of broken appointments, and clinical outcome improvement (Meichenbaum & Turk, 1987). Each of these measures presents its own unique problems associated with the measurement of adherence or nonadherence behavior. However, even given the methodological difficulties encountered in measuring adherence and nonadherence the research indicates that the client problem of nonadherence is epidemic.

Estimates of treatment nonadherence in America today are reported to range from as low as 4 percent to as high as 92 percent, with the typical range somewhere between 30 and 60 percent (Marston, 1970). Studies indicate that 25 to 50 percent of clients fail to appear for scheduled appointments. This figure does rise to 75 percent adherence when clients make their own appointments (Sackett & Snow, 1979). Among those who are required to self-administer medications, 20 to 60 percent will discontinue prescribed medications before being instructed to do so by a health professional. Nineteen precent of clients will not correctly follow instructions for the administration of the medication, and 25 to

60 percent of clients will make errors in the self-administration of prescribed medication (Stimson, 1974). Vincint (1971) reported that 58 percent of clients seeking medical assistance for glaucoma did not adhere to the directions for installation of eye drop medications often enough to produce the desired therapeutic effect. Clients do seem to adhere to a greater extent when there is a need for direct medication therapy and when there is a high degree of supervision and monitoring of their health-related behaviors. Of particular significance for the rehabilitation nurse is the evidence that adherence rates are lower for clients who have chronic disorders when there is no immediate discomfort, and when prevention or cure is desired as the outcome rather than symptom palliation (Meichenbaum & Turk, 1987).

Problems with adherence are also reported in a number of heath maintenance and preventive health behaviors. These include wearing seat belts, weight reduction, increasing exercise activity, and continuing in psychotherapy. The incidence of relapse following modification efforts for behaviors of smoking, dieting, and substance abuse continues to be a significant health problem (Brownell, Marlatt, Lichtenstein, & Wilson, 1986).

There is some evidence that treatment adherence is higher among health care professionals who need to follow the advice and recommendations of health care providers. Nonadherence rates among psychologists, physicians, pharmacists, nurses, and dentists ranged from 12 to 100 percent, with a median of 80 percent (Levy, 1986).

Adherence is a complex, dynamic phenomenon. A client's degree of adherence to the treatment plan can change over the course of time. Because the client adheres to one aspect of the treatment regimen does not mean that there will be adherence to other aspects of the treatment regimen. The client may even become nonadherent in some aspect of the treatment plan that had not previously been a problem. Evaluation of client, family member, and caregiver adherence must be an ongoing process. There is a need to assess each incident of failure to perform a recommended behavior.

Health care providers must remember that nonadherence to some prescribed treatment might indicate good judgment on the part of the client (Deaton, 1985). It is important that the goal of adherence be balanced against other important client objectives including quality of life, adjustment, and the client's efforts to cope with the illness or injury.

Factors Influencing Client Adherence

All clients have different reactions, experiences, and motives for their behavior (Falvo, 1985). A number of variables have been identified that correlate with treatment nonadherence. These variables can be categorized as patient variables; disease, illness, or disorder variables; treatment variables; and relationship variables. Table 2, which describes these variables, is based on a review of the work of several researchers.

Table 2
Variables Associated with Client Treatment Nonadherence

Variable	Description
Client	• Presence of sensory disabilities and deficits
	• Forgetfulness
	• Lack of understanding regarding the illness, injury, disease, treatment regimen
	• Inappropriate or conflicting health benefits perceived by the client
	• Apathy and pessimism
	• Health beliefs held by the client and/or family members
	• Lack of social support
	• Family instability or disharmony
	• Lack of resources
	• Existence in an environment that supports nonadherent behavior
	• Family member expectations and attitudes toward treatment
	• Lack of insight into the nature of the illness or need for treatment
	• Desire to maintain some control over some aspect of life
	• Sense of fatalism or a paralysis of will
Treatment	• Lack of continuity in care among care providers
	• Scheduling of appointments; long waiting time (more than 1 h)
	• Timing of referrals (more than 1 wk)
	• Availability of transportation for referrals and follow-up appointments
	• Lack of cohesiveness of treatment team members
	• Unfriendly personnel
	• Multiple health care provider interactions
	• Complexity of treatment regimen
	• Uncertainty about the effectiveness of the treatment
	• Impatience with the rate of progress
	• Long duration of the treatment regimen
	• Degree of change and interference with personal lifestyle
	• Inconvenience to the client or family members
	• Expense of prescribed treatment: equipment, medications, therapy
	• Inadequate labels on medications
	• Medication side effects
Relationship	• Inadequate communication with health care provider
	• Perceptions that health care providers are not approachable
	• Failure of health care providers to consider feedback from client regarding care plan
	• Client dissatisfaction with health care providers or the health care delivery system
	• Lack of trust in health care provider
	• Inadequate supervision of the client or caregiver
Disease or disorder	• Chronic condition without overt symptoms
	• Conditions with stable symptoms

Sources: Blevins & Lubkin (1995); Buckalew & Sallis (1986); Caton (1984); Di Matteo & DiNicola (1982); Shelton & Levy (1981).

Although numerous variables promoting nonadherence have been identified, no set of stable characteristics representing the nonadherent client or chronic defaulter has been identified. Even the most unmotivated and uncooperative client is not always the most nonadherent. Every patient is a potential defaulter. Nonadherence can be the response of any client (Seltzer & Hoffman, 1980).

Health Beliefs and Adherence

Clients who perceive that the illness is not especially serious or that the treatment prescribed is ill-advised will forego the treatment regimen sooner than the client who believes that the condition is serious and that the prescribed regimen will be effective and have a positive effect. Clients with personal beliefs, based on past experience, that health care providers have little to offer in the way of treatment will be more reluctant to invest time, energy, or effort in following the plan of care.

The **health beliefs model** has been used to predict client adherence to a plan of care. The model is derived from value expectancy theory. The basic proposal of this model is that behavior is evaluated on the basis of the value of an outcome to the individual and the individual's expectation that the action will be of benefit for reaching the desired outcome (Becker, 1974; 1976). When individuals perceive themselves as susceptible to a change in health state and they perceive that the illness, injury, disease, or disability has a high degree of severity they enter into a state of readiness for taking action. An internal cue (i.e., perception of bodily state; pain, dizziness) or external cue (public news announcement regarding dangers of smoking) to action must be present to trigger the advocated health care practice or behavior. Individuals must value the benefits and efficacy of following the advocated health behavior or fear the negative feature of not engaging in the advocated health behavior. This model proposes that the client is influenced by certain motivators (Table 3); by the value of the reduction of the threat to the individual by the illness, injury, disease, or complications; and by the subjective estimates that the proposed actions are safe and effective for reducing the threat of the illness.

Strategies for Increasing Client and Caregiver Adherence Advancing the Therapeutic Alliance

The manner in which health care providers relate to clients is an important factor influencing client adherence. An *alliance* is a bond, connection, or association among individuals to further common interests. The most effective **therapeutic alliance** will be one that is founded on an empathetic, concerned, compassionate relationship between those providing care and those in need of care. In a therapeutic alliance the client is seen as being knowledgeable, an active ally who participates in the treatment process (Anderson & Kirk, 1982). Planning must be a mutual activity among the various members of the interdisciplinary treatment team and the client. How the members of the team, including the client, per-

Table 3
Health Beliefs Model: Proposed Predictors of Adherence

Predictors indicating readiness to undertake recommended actions

- High value is placed on health
- Cares about health issues in general
- Possesses a positive, healthy lifestyle
- Willing to seek and accept health directions
- Possesses an intention to adhere to regimen
- Probability that action will reduce threat
- High estimate of proposed regimen safety
- High estimate of proposed regimen efficacy to reduce, prevent, delay, or cure
- High estimate of chance of recovery
- Confidence in health care system and care providers

Predictors indicating willingness to modify behavior; enabling factors

- Extremes in age
- Cost, duration, complexity, side effects, and accessibility of regimen
- Need for new patterns of behavior
- Satisfaction with health team members
- Satisfaction with facilities and its procedures and rules
- Quality and type of relationship with team members
- Degree of satisfaction with client feedback to health care team
- Team agreement with client feedback
- Prior experience with health care action, illness, injury, or regimen
- Source of the advice or recommendation given
- Social pressure
- Belief in personal self-efficacy

Source: Becker (1976).

ceive roles can be a significant factor in the effectiveness of the therapeutic alliance.

In 1951 Talcott Parsons, a sociologist, used role theory to describe the relationship between patients and the health care system. Parsons conceived of the patient as fulfilling a **sick role** and of the health care provider as fulfilling a **professional role.** The role of the health care provider in this model is to use knowledge and skills competently to act for the welfare of the patient. The patient complements the professional role by trusting the health care provider, listening to the advice given and following all recommendations. In this model those in the sick role are not to blame for their unhealthy state, and are exempt from their role responsibilities and social duties. They are expected to seek competent medical assistance, are obligated to want to get well, are motivated to return to the healthy state, and are of assistance to those assisting them (Parsons, 1951). According to Parsons this relationship made sense because of the technical competence of the care provider and the emotional need of the patient for direction and guidance. However, the Parsons model fails to consider client values, beliefs, knowledge, and expectations that may differ from those held by the health care provider.

Parson's (1951) "sick role" model does not seem to enhance the therapeutic alliance necessary for positive client outcomes in rehabilitation. Szasz and Hollender (1956) described an alternative to Parson's model. They described three types of health care provider–client relationships that could be adapted to different relationship situations:

Active physician–passive client mode. Apropos for situations in which the client is totally dependent or unable to act on his or her own behalf
Building health care provider cooperating mode. Apropos during most acute conditions or during acute exacerbation of chronic illness
Mutual participating mode. An active partnership apropos for situations in which the role of the health care provider is to assist others to help themselves. It is the mutual participating mode that is most empowering in the rehabilitation setting and will also be most effective for increasing client adherence

Parson's model is valid when the client has an acute illness, and when the prognosis is grave and uncertain. It focuses on recovery. It does not address responses and expectations of those involved in the rehabilitation process. Gordon (1966) identified an **impaired role.** The impaired role is appropriate when the prognosis is known and not considered grave. The impaired role assumes that the individual has a permanent impairment, that the individual does not give up normal role responsibilities and maintains normal behavior, that the individual does not have to want to get well, and that the individual will make the most of remaining abilities and capabilities. The individual must accept the existence of the impairment and recognize limitations imposed by the disability. Activity that facilitates control of the condition, prevents complication, leads to resumption of role responsibilities, and results in realization of potential is acceptable. The impaired role incorporates rehabilitation and maximization of wellness (Wu, 1973).

Improving the Therapeutic Alliance

To improve the therapeutic alliance and increase client adherence it is essential to develop communication skills that demonstrate a respect for the client's intelligence. Health care providers also need to communicate to clients, and their caregivers, that their needs are acknowledged by the health care provider, that their openness with the health care providers is appreciated, and that their feelings are accepted by the health care provider. Perhaps most important is that health care providers develop communication and interpersonal relationship skills that promote client and caregiver collaboration in decision-making (Barnlund, 1976). The rehabilitation team's attitudes and communication style are critical in preventing and remedying nonadherence.

The effective health care provider will also possess *active listening* skills. Health care providers must listen not only to what is said by the client and caregiver, but also to what is not openly stated. It is important to listen to the emotional overtones of the client's statement. Often these overtones are communicated through the client's nonverbal communication. A sensitivity to nonverbal cues is important for increasing the depth of understanding of client messages.

Each message has three components: the experiential component (what is happening), the affective component (how the individual feels about what is happening), and the cognitive component (what the individual thinks about what is happening). The skilled communicator listens to each component of the message and responds to one or all three components of the message. Being a skilled listener requires (1) taking an interest in the message being sent, (2) understanding the meaning of the language of the message, and (3) developing an understanding of the circumstances of the client's message and being sympathetic toward the client. This will result in greater exploration of the client's concerns, and more in-depth comprehension of the lived experience of the client. A commonsense understanding of the client's lived experience is essential to enhancing client adherence.

Improving the therapeutic alliance and increasing client adherence depends on a collaborative approach between the health care provider and the client. There needs to be an open discussion of adherence issues. The health care provider needs to try to see the client's lived experience from the client's perspective. This can be accomplished by investigating the client's and caregivers' major concerns about the change in health state and the treatment regimen. Areas that should be explored with clients include the meaning ascribed to the illness, injury, disease or disability; their representation or explanatory model for their illness, injury, disease, or disability; worries and concerns about the change in health state and the future; and client expectation of the treatment plan and of the health care provider (Meichenbaum & Turk, 1987).

Assessing Client Explanatory Model for Rehabilitation

How the client and/or caregiver perceives or defines the nature of the change in health state and rehabilitation can have a significant influence on adherence. This is especially true if there is incompatibility between how the client and caregiver perceive the situation and how rehabilitation team members perceive the situation. Clients possess their own meaning and perception of health threats and they plan and act according to the accompanying fears and concerns. The rehabilitation team members must assess the client's views of the change in health state and the rehabilitation process, its cause and course, expectation about treatment and rehabilitation, and fears. The perceptions of friends, family, and significant others must also be assessed because those perceptions often significantly influence those held by the client. Assessment questions might include the following:

> What do you call your condition?
> What causes your need for rehabilitation?
> How does your condition affect you?
> What is the problem you are experiencing that requires rehabilitation?
> How ill (disabled, challenged) are you?
> How long will your condition last?
> How long will the rehabilitation process last?
> What is your chief complaint or problem?
> What do you think the rehabilitation period will be like?
> What are you hoping will be the outcome of your rehabilitation process?

Assessing Client Worries and Concerns about Rehabilitation

Often client concerns about the change in health state and rehabilitation are not readily recognized or expressed. Often the client and/or caregiver does not possess the same treatment concerns as the rehabilitation team (i.e., the rehabilitation team's concern is symptom relief and the client's concern is independent living). If concerns are not addressed, unmet expectations can lead to client nonadherence. Exploring for underlying concerns is essential. Most clients are concerned about whether they will be all right, what caused the change in health state or injury, and whether they are responsible for what is happening to them. Assessment questions to determine client concerns might include the following:

> What worries you most about the rehabilitation process?
> Who is most bothered by your condition?
> How does your condition interfere with your life on a daily basis?
> What are some of the things you think, feel, or do about your condition?
> How would you like to change?
> What are some of the ways you have tried to decrease your discomfort?
> On what would the outcome of rehabilitation depend?
> Have you known anyone else with a condition like yours? How did things turn out for them?
> Does anything else worry you about rehabilitation?
> Can you think of any problems rehabilitation might cause you?

Assessing Client Treatment Expectations

A thorough adherence-oriented history is helpful in assessing the client's current expectations about rehabilitation and a good indicator for predicting treatment adherence. If a client failed to adhere to previous treatment regimens there is a strong likelihood of future nonadherence for the rehabilitation treatment plan. Explicitly assessing client expectation is useful for making the distinction between outcome expectations and efficacy expectations.

Outcome expectations are beliefs about whether a given action will lead to given outcomes or individual judgments of the likely consequences such actions will produce. **Efficacy expectations** are beliefs about how capable an individual is of performing the action that leads to those outcomes or individual judgments of capabilities to execute a given level of performance. The greater the client's belief that personal ability can influence outcome the greater the probability that attempts will be made to engage in behaviors or take action (perceived self-efficacy). If the client perceives that he or she does not possess the necessary capabilities or abilities to bring about the desired outcome no attempt will be made to engage in behaviors or to take action. This is especially true when the necessary behaviors or actions are new and not contained in the client's current behavioral inventory.

Outcome and efficacy expectations can be assessed by asking the client and caregiver whether they believe a particular action could be accomplished, and then asking them to rate the strength of their beliefs for accomplishing each act (Bandura, 1986). Other assessment questions might include the following:

How effective do you think rehabilitation will be for you?
Can you think of any problems you might have in following the treatment plan?
What might happen if the rehabilitation plan is not followed?
How likely is it that you will not follow the treatment plan?
Did you ever not follow a treatment plan because you thought it was too strict, difficult, complex, or expensive?
Do you have any questions about your ability to follow the rehabilitation plan?
Does your spouse or other support person understand the rehabilitation plan?
Have the aspects of the rehabilitation plan been explained, the rationale for the plan of care given, benefits of adherence explained, the hazards of nonadherence identified, and do you understand them?

Implications of Practice

Sometimes rehabilitation clients behave in dangerous or risky ways. The fact that clients would engage in behaviors that would make their conditions worse or cause a complication to occur seems illogical. The illogical behavior may be frustrating or puzzling to the treatment team. The foremost objective for the rehabilitation team must be to assess realistically the client's readiness and ability to carry out the proposed plan of care. The objective is to set attainable, feasible goals and actions with which the client, family, and rehabilitation team are comfortable. In planning, consideration must be given to the client's living situation, daily routine, client's other commitments, sources of stress, and community facilities and resources.

The rehabilitation team needs to determine how serious or disabling the condition is felt to be by the client and the family. The team must also determine how the client views the diagnosis and prognosis. Does the client perceive that the prescription for action will be effective or have similar actions in the past been judged by the client or caregiver as being ineffective? Does the client perceive that adherence is of benefit to her or him? An assessment of the client's degree of perceived self-efficacy will be useful for establishing a successful program of skill development.

To address issues related to client adherence in an open way, the rehabilitation team members need to determine what the client perceives as the barriers to taking the advocated actions. Long-term goals may seem unattainable to the client; break goals down into manageable attainable steps and stages. Success in carrying out one action or behavior leads to feelings of efficacy and willingness to try other actions and behaviors (Bandura, 1977). The rehabilitation team members need to understand what role finances will play in the client's ability to adhere with the plan of care.

Contracting is a positive method that can be employed to increase client adherence with the rehabilitation regimen. Contracting is also effective in helping to achieve mutually established treatment goals. Contracting is an active process used to establish goals. Responsibility for achieving goals is shared and all those involved in the process are aware of and understand what can be expected from each other. The contract clearly establishes what is to be done because it reflects specific behaviors to be performed. Contracting focuses on the client's and family's strengths. If difficulties arise the contract can be modified and additional strategies can be considered. Rather than stressing the client's past failures to adhere with health care provider recommendations, contracting emphasizes what has been established.

If a contract is to be effective it must be based on client needs. This includes factors such as the client's current situation. Background information regarding the client's lifestyle and activities helps the nurse gain knowledge about the client's strengths and can be useful to facilitate adherence. Not all clients will be receptive to the idea of contracting and others will find the process of contracting too restricting for practical use.

Treatment objectives might not be attained because of an incorrect diagnosis, an ineffective or incorrect treatment prescription, unclear or partial education or instructions, or nonadherence to instructions. Adherence can be enhanced by tailoring the treatment regimen to the client's daily behaviors, simplifying the regimen, enhancing coping, and contracting for specific goals and methods and explicitly identified incentives.

When substantial changes in the client's health behaviors and practices are required and a great deal of continued effort is needed to maintain relative health stability and daily functioning the tendency to tell the client what to do must be checked. Ultimately, what the clients do about their health and rehabilitation is their decision.

Conclusion

Client adherence in rehabilitation is an important area of consideration for health care providers. Even though many barriers exist to the study of adherence it has been demonstrated to be a significant problem. Self-care and self-management eventually are the responsibility of the client and family. The rehabilitation treatment team must ensure that the client or family has the needed knowledge, motivation, and skills to attain the optimal level of self-care and independent living.

References

Anderson, R. J., & Kirk, L. M. (1982). Methods of improving patient compliance in chronic disease states. *Archives of Internal Medicine, 142,* 1673–1675.

Bandura, A. (1977). *Social learning theory.* Englewood cliffs, NJ: Prentice-Hall.

Bandura, A. (1986). *Social foundations of thought and action.* Englewood Cliffs, NJ: Prentice-Hall.

Barnlund, D. C. (1976). The mystification of meaning: Doctor-patient encounters. *Journal of Medical Education, 51,* 716–725.

Becker, M. H. (1974). A new approach to explaining sick-role behavior in low-income populations. *American Journal of Public Health, 64,* 205–216.

Becker, M. H. (1976). Socio-behavioral determinants of compliance. In D. L. Sackett & R. Haynes (Eds.), *Compliance with therapeutic regimens.* Baltimore, MD: Johns Hopkins University Press.

Blevins, D., & Lubkin, I. (1995). Compliance. In I. M. Lubkin (Ed.), *Chronic illness impact and interventions* (3rd ed., pp. 213–240). Boston: Jones & Bartlett.

Brownell, K. D., Marlatt, G. A., Lichtenstein, E., & Wilson, G. T. (1986). Understanding and preventing relapse. *American Psychologist, 41,* 765–782.

Buckalew, L. W., & Sallis, R. E. (1986). Patient compliance and medication perceptions. *Journal of Clinical Psychology, 42,* 49–53.

Caton, C. (1984). *Management of chronic schizophrenia.* New York: Oxford University Press.

Carson, V. B., & Arnold, E. N. (1996). *Mental health nursing the nurse–patient journey.* Philadelphia: W. B. Saunders Co.

Deaton, A. V. (1985). Adaptive noncompliance in pediatric asthma: The parent as expert. *Journal of Pediatric Psychology, 10,* 1–14.

Di Matteo, M. R., & DiNicola, D. D. (1982). *Achieving patient compliance: The psychology of the medical practitioner's role.* New York: Pergamon Press.

Falvo, D. R. (1985). *Effective patient education: a guide to increase compliance.* Rockville, MD: Aspen.

Gordon, G. (1966). *Role theory and illness: a sociological perspective.* New Haven: College and University Press.

Levy, R. L. (1986). Social support and compliance: Salient methodological problems in compliance research. *Journal of Compliance in Health Care, 1,* 184–198.

Marston, M. V. (1970). Compliance with medical regimens: A review of the literature. *Nursing Research, 19,* 312–323.

Meichenbaum, D., & Turk, D. C. (1987). *Facilitating treatment adherence: A practitioner's guidebook.* New York: Plenum Press.

Parsons, T. (1951). *The social system.* New York: Free Press.

Sackett, D. L., & Snow, J. C. (1979). The magnitude of compliance and noncompliance. In R. B. Hayes, D. W. Taylor, & D. L. Sackett (Eds.), *Compliance in health care.* Baltimore, MD: Johns Hopkins University Press.

Seltzer, A., & Hoffman, B. F. (1980). Drug compliance of the psychiatric patient. *Canadian Family Physician, 26,* 725–727.

Shelton, J. L., & Levy, R. L. (1981). *Behavioral assignments and treatment compliance: A handbook of clinical strategies.* Champaign, IL: Research Press.

Stimson, G. V. (1974). Obeying doctor's orders: A view from the other side. *Social Science and Medicine, 8,* 97–104.

Szasz, T. A., & Hollender, M. H. (1956). A contribution to the philosophy of medicine: The basic models of the doctor-patient relationship. *Archives of Clinical Psychology, 51,* 952–953.

Vincint, P. (1971). Factors influencing patient noncompliance: A theoretical approach. *Nursing Research, 20,* 509–670.

Wu, R. (1973). *Behavior and illness.* Englewood Cliffs, NJ: Prentice-Hall.

PSYCHOLOGICAL AND PSYCHOSOCIAL CONCEPTS

CHAPTER 8
Family Transformations

Patricia A. Chin

Key Terms   *Double ABCX Model*
Family
Family Adaptation
Family Function
Family Development
Family Structure

Objectives   1. Discuss the significance of the family in medical rehabilitation.

2. Describe family responses, adaptation, and adjustment associated with medical rehabilitation.

3. Discuss caregiver burnout and identify strategies for assisting family members who experience burnout.

4. Discuss the implications of medical rehabilitation for the development of the family unit.

5. Discuss the use of the double ABCX model in the rehabilitation setting.

All families go through some type of family transformation as the result of having a family member go through the process of medical rehabilitation. Some degree of family transformation will occur regardless of the nature or severity of the client's illness, injury, disease, or disability that requires rehabilitation care and services. The nature of the family transformation will depend on several factors: family structure and functioning before the onset of rehabilitation, together with the family's communication patterns, values, behaviors, lifestyle, and strategies for adapting and adjusting to stress and crisis. The family will always strive to re-establish equilibrium when confronted with stress. The medical rehabilitative process can seriously affect the family's homeostasis.

Significance of Family in Rehabilitation Care

The rehabilitation client cannot be treated and managed effectively without taking into account the client's family members and the nature of their interpersonal relationships. The role of the family in rehabilitation is crucial. The family can instill hope, empower the client, encourage independence, and help to improve the client's condition. Rehabilitation clients will not make accommodations or adjust to illness, injury, disease, or disability independent of their families. The client's intrapsychic processes will be influenced by family interactions, attitudes, and values. Family members are as important as health care providers to the rehabilitation client. Health care providers are significant for client survival, for providing useful counsel, and for aid in the management of key problems. But, in reality, health care providers tend to be secondary to the client's day-to-day adaptation and adjustment in the face of major illness, injury, disease, or disability.

The family's response to the rehabilitation client may determine the client's motivation to tolerate painful procedures and long-term treatment, face irrevocable losses, and accept major lifestyle changes (Danielson, Hamel-Bissell, & Winstead-Fry, 1993). How family members perform as agents of the client may make a difference in whether the client grows better or worse, or even whether the client survives for very long.

Most family systems will adjust to a crisis fairly well. Adequately organized families will be better prepared to meet the emotional needs of their members and deal with the stress and uncertainty of life than inadequately organized families. They can resolve stress through interfamily actions. They use organized methods to deal with problems, and the members rely on each other for support as they work together toward a return to normalcy. The members of the organized family can temporarily suspend their own personal ambitions to deal with a family crisis, work out new role patterns to carry out family functions, develop collective goals in times of emergency, and work toward accomplishing them cooperatively. Organized families will have had past experiences with success in mediating stress. They have the ability to adapt to change and a family history of meeting problems through discussion and problem solving (Friedman, 1992).

Disorganized families are more vulnerable when confronted with stress. They generally lack the ability to be flexible in the face of change. Family members are less willing to share role responsibilities in an emergency, and there may be less consistent commitment or support for the client. Their interactions with the client and the staff may even thwart rehabilitation success.

The stress of having a family member in rehabilitation, especially when disability is involved, can place the family at risk for psychological problems and marital discord (Vincint and Brown, 1986). The care required by a person in rehabilitation or with a chronic illness or disability can be a very complex and demanding task for other members of the family. Family members may be required to become the agent of the client. They may be confronted with assuming the responsibilities of assisting the client in care; redesigning lifestyles and further goals; and protecting, rescuing, or even controlling the client's behaviors or lifestyle. Arrangements will need to be negotiated among family members to develop basic strategies necessary to reach the client's maximum level of functioning and independence while letting family members attain their own individual development tasks.

Having a family member who has an illness, injury, disease, or disability can be a significant stressor on family structure and functioning. It does not matter whether the illness, injury, disease, or disability is invisible or highly visible to others outside the family unit. The change in health state of one of the family members may not be the actual stressor, or what changes the dynamics of the family's function and structure, but it may serve to magnify the family's strengths and limitations.

Caregivers will also suffer. Caregivers of clients with dementia described feelings of physical exhaustion, feelings of personal loss and the loss of social roles and relationships; and a sense of powerlessness, hopelessness, and endlessness (Farran, Herth, & Popovich, 1995). An awareness of and concern about the unrelenting burdens assumed by family members has focused attention on the issue of respite care for caregivers, advocacy, and funding for supplemental services to augment the care provided by family members.

The family of the client in rehabilitation will be confronted with numerous challenges. They will need support from professionals, their extended family members and friends, and the support of self-help groups. Family members often use interactions with members of the interdisciplinary treatment team as a vehicle for expressing their feelings of grief and loss. The nurse is often the source of information for the family members regarding an illness, injury, disease, or disability and its consequences. The nurse may need to assist the family with issues of parenting, discipline, activities of daily living, recreation, or sex education. Family members may also turn to the nurse for assistance in planning for the future and dealing with the complex issues of placement, guardianship, or other legal matters. Family members will be required to develop the skills needed for the successful use of community resources for the disabled child or adult and to facilitate independent living. It is important to counsel family members not to infantilize the rehabilitation client, but rather to encourage continuing functioning and striving for a productive life.

Nursing care usually emphasizes the physiological well-being of the client. The role of the client's family members should not be underestimated. Nurses in the rehabilitation need to maintain caring and compassionate relationships with the client's family as well as with the client. Nurses need to intervene when the signs and symptoms of caregiver burnout—depression, withdrawal, guilt, fatigue, irrational thinking, irritability, and anger—are observed in family members.

Caregivers need to maintain a balanced perspective of their role in the client's recovery and rehabilitation. They need to be knowledgeable so that they can develop competence and confidence in themselves. They need to be open and creative to new ideas and respect differences in views, personalities, and cultural expressions. They need to develop an awareness that not everything in life can be explained and that there are limits to what they can be expected to accomplish. It is important that they be able to recognize the moments of joy experienced in the struggles of life. Most crucial is that they care for themselves so that they can care for others. They must take advantage of any opportunity to rest, and then begin anew (Fulgrum, 1988; Parse, 1990; Sherwood, 1992). Nursing must assist family members in developing these skills.

Guidelines for the inclusion of the family into an optimal care plan for the rehabilitation client are as follows:

1. The family's involvement in the client's care must begin when the care begins and be maintained throughout all levels of the rehabilitation process.
2. The dynamics of the family must be evaluated, diagnosed, and treated appropriately along with the rehabilitation client's problems.
3. Continuity of treatment must be maintained in the home environment parallel to the rehabilitation client's care and follow-up.

Family

It is important to understand the purpose, structure, and functions of the family system to predict how the family may influence the rehabilitation process and interpret client and family responses to stress and rehabilitation. The basic function of the family is to meet the needs of individual family members and society (Friedman, 1992). For the purposes of this discussion, **family** refers to "two or more persons who are joined together by bonds of sharing and emotional closeness and who identify themselves as being part of the family" (Friedman, 1992, p. 9). The nurse in the rehabilitation setting needs to have an appreciation for a variety of family forms, both traditional and nontraditional, representing all walks of life and lifestyles (Table 1).

Table 1
Current Family Forms

Traditional Family Forms	**Nontraditional Family Forms**
Nuclear dyad	Unmarried parent and child family
Nuclear family	Unmarried couple and child family
Single-parent family	Cohabiting couple
Three-generation extended family	Commune family
Middle-age or elderly couple	Gay/lesbian family
Extended kin network	

Source: Adapted from Macklin (1988); Friedman (1992).

Structure, Function, and Values

How a family is organized, the manner in which members are arranged, and how members relate to each other is referred to as **family structure** (Friedman, 1992). Family structure is based on family form, type of power structure, role structure, value systems, and communication processes. These elements are all interconnected and interdependent. An understanding of family structure, especially relationship patterns, is useful for assisting families adapting to stress. The family's structure and relationship patterns will be dictated by the family's race and culture. An assessment strategy that is helpful in gaining an understanding of the family is the *genogram* or family tree. The genogram is an informative diagram that delineates the family constellation. (For information on developing a genogram, see Friedman, 1992; Wright & Leahey, 1994.) It is important to determine how the client's rehabilitation will disrupt or shift the family's structure, and to what degree the family's role assignments, power structure, or communication process will need to be modified or reorganized. The family's structure promotes the functions of the family.

Family functions are defined as outcomes or consequences of family structure (Friedman, 1992). Family functions are the purpose of the family, or what the family does. Friedman (1992) identifies five basic family functions:

1. *Affective function*—meeting the psychological needs of family members and personality maintenance of each member
2. *Socialization function*—conferring status on family members and socializing children
3. *Reproduction function*—ensuring family continuity over generations
4. *Economic function*—providing sufficient economic resources and allocations
5. *Health care function*—providing of physical needs

In every family each individual is expected to perform a set of socially prescribed personal behaviors identified as *roles.* Each family member assumes a variety of family roles throughout a lifetime. Those roles and how they are actualized are influenced by the family's race and culture as well as the dominant culture in which the family lives. There are formal roles and informal roles. Each role has its own status, set of rules, and expectations regarding how the role should be accomplished. Some roles are lifelong (mother); others can be temporary (follower). When the family is confronted with illness, injury, disease, or disability the potential for role alteration becomes a significant issue. Those expected role behaviors are based on one's personal values and beliefs, as well as on cultural influences. The evaluation of the family's role and relationship patterns focuses on family life processes, work, school, and social activities. Alterations in role performance or relationships can often result in dysfunctional family processes, disturbances in role structures, social isolation, impaired communication patterns, unresolved conflicts, issues of dependency and independence, and relocation syndrome.

One's position in a family structure is temporary in character. Formal roles assigned to members of a family unit include spouse, partner, parent, child, and sibling. There are many informal family roles that are as significant to family functioning as are the formal roles. They include such roles as encourager, harmonizer, initiator, contributor, compromiser, blocker, dominator, blamer, martyr, scapegoat, family caregiver, pioneer, go-between, and bystander (Carson & Arnolds, 1996; Friedman, 1992). Family roles are influenced by age, culture, physical health, and the cognitive abilities of the individuals that make up the family unit. The tasks of the family for maintaining physical well-being, resource allocation, division of labor, reproduction and the nurturing of children, and socialization of children are accomplished through the structure and roles of the family (Friedman, 1992) (Table 2). Illness, injury, disease, and disability can place great strain on the family's ability to accomplish its essential tasks. This is stressful and threatening to the client and all family members.

Values can be defined as a system of ideas and beliefs that binds family members together (Friedman, 1992). Values serve as the general guides to behavior and are influenced by the family's race and culture. The family unit is the basic transmitter of values. Family norms and rules are specific manifestations of the family's values. The family's value system is influenced by ethnicity, religion, social class (most important), rural versus urban locations, and the degree of acculturation by the family of the dominant cultural values. The central configuration of values in the dominant culture today includes productivity, materialism, individualism, work ethic, progress, and education. Conflicts can arise for the family when the results of illness, injury, or disease and the presence of a disability interfere with maintaining the family's norms and roles, or with meeting the dominant cultural values. Those same conflicts can arise between the client and the family and among family members, resulting in strained familial relationships.

The ability to parent and rear children is another family function that can be seriously affected by illness, injury, disease, or disability. The degree of conse-

Table 2
Meeting the Family's Socialization Tasks

Child Stage	Parental Task
Infant	Learning the meaning of cues
Toddler	Learning to accept child's growth and development
Preschool	Allowing children independence
School age	To accept rejection without deserting the child
Teenager	Learning to build a new life for parent

quence of change to the client's ability to parent will depend on the family's stage of development and the age of the individuals who require the assistance of the family for socialization. Socialization is best defined as the training provided by the family to the child for successful functioning in a social environment (Friedman, 1992). The central tasks involved in the socialization of children revolve around teaching children how to function and assume adult roles in society. The primary socialization tasks of the family include: language development; development of sociocultural norms and expectations (right and wrong), sex roles; encouragement of individual initiative and creativity; and the acquisition of health concepts, attitudes, and behaviors (Friedman, 1992)

The presence of an illness, injury, disease, or disability can have a serious impact on the family system, especially on the family's structure and ability to carry out family functions. Illness, injury, disease, and disability can place great strain on the family's value system. The socialization of family members can be challenged depending on the developmental stage of the famly. The effect on family functioning can negatively affect the outcome of rehabilitation. The degree of family disruption experienced by a family is influenced by the seriousness of the change in health state or disability, the status and roles of the client within the family unit, and the developmental state of the family. The impact on the family is most pronounced when the nature of the client's condition is greatly disabling or progressively deteriorating, or when the client is crucial to the family's function.

Family Adjustment

Family adaptation is the general process of adjustment of the family to change. Even the most stable family can be overwhelmed and may become disrupted by the stress involved in caring for the rehabilitation client, especially if a major disability is involved. Some family members may see the need to provide care to a family member during rehabilitation as a means to make amends or atone for past relationship problems or deficiency in caring. Sex and intimacy can be affected. Everyday mood and interpersonal relations can be affected. Visiting friends and relatives and engaging in other leisure time activities can be affected. Conflicts can arise as the result of increasing family expenses coupled with unemployment and the cost of medical and rehabilitation services.

Generally the initial coping and adaptation to a disability is a period of immediate response. The change in family function and structure may be less apparent during this stage. Following stroke, heart attack, accidents, or serious physical trauma family members feel relief that the client did not die. The primary concern is for the client's recovery. During this period the family is vaguely aware of the implication of the illness, injury, or disability for other family members. Family responses during this early phase of rehabilitation care will depend on the relationships within the family (Christopherson, 1962; Danielson, Hamel-Bissell, & Winstead-Fry, 1993).

With the passage of time, and with stabilization of the client's health state and subsequent movement into the rehabilitation phase, however, the influence of the health status change becomes more noticeable (Christopherson, 1962). During reconstruction the client works to regain physical integrity and function and functional abilities and capabilities through the physical-medical regimen. An awareness of the modification (either temporary or permanent) of social, sexual, and economic roles grows. The family begins to struggle with psychological preparation for the future. The family may cling to an unrealistic view of the client's degree of recovery. When all rehabilitation measures have been utilized the plateau stage begins (Christopherson, 1962). This may be the most difficult time for family relationships. All hope for a complete recovery may be gone, emotional and economic resources have been heavily taxed, and decisions regarding client re-entry into the community and independent living may be difficult to face (Christopherson, 1962).

Each of the family members will respond, cope, and adapt in their own way (Table 3). The ability to adjust will be influenced by each member's developmental stage and perception of the world. The individual developmental needs of each family member must be considered to understand the impact of the disability on the family unit.

Families that are very anxious, overprotective, or encourage dependency in the client or each other can prevent accomplishment of rehabilitation goals. If family ties are very close and there are inflexible role patterns client independence may be discouraged. Certain religious and cultural beliefs and values regarding illness and disability may interfere with the family's adherence to the treatment regimen. If the needs of family members are not addressed an additional strain can be placed on the client. The family members may make demands on the client, disrupting the client's emotional equilibrium; demand time from the staff to deal with a family member's problems or crises; or become ill, increasing the strain on the family.

Family members may turn to other activities to avoid the reality of the client's situation. They may become involved in new activities, make changes in the family composition, move to a new residence, change jobs, or spend money on travel or unnecessary purchases. These behaviors indicate denial on the part of the family member.

Problems can develop within the family that can negatively affect client morale. This can occur if other family members take on the client's role on a permanent basis, if the family gives the client mixed messages regarding the continuation of roles, or if the client returns home and finds that roles have been redistributed among family members and none have been assigned to the client. Family members may have opposing views concerning the long-term goals for the client. This can involve teaching, telling the client all information about diagno-

Table 3
Possible Family Responses to Rehabilitation

Positive Family Responses	Negative Family Responses
Willingness to re-establish and maintain the client's values and roles	Overprotection
	Encouragement of client dependency
Involvement of the client in family decision making	Client neglect or neglect in obtaining care for the client
Family understanding of the kind of support useful to the client	Unwillingness to engage in future planning
	Denial of client's health problem, severity of problem, or needs abuse
Active involvement of the family in the client's care, treatment planning, learning, and decision making	Making excessive or inappropriate demands of the client
	Taking punitive actions toward the client
	Rejection, abandonment, or desertion of the client
	Detrimental or interfering actions or decisions related to client's welfare, social economic welfare
	Negative family coping behaviors: blaming or fault finding, aggression, depression, abuse, hostility, stigmatizing
	Inability to maintain and provide diversions or recreational activities or essential services (child care, cleaning, shopping)

ses or prognoses, handling continued crisis, caring for the client at home, making placement decisions, or even the meaning of and value of treatment.

Family, Coping Strategies

Family coping is vitally important because it is the mechanism by which family functions are made possible. One convincing piece of evidence that shows that many families are experiencing problems with adaptation (family coping) is the pervasiveness of mental disorders in our communities. Effective coping by the family during rehabilitation usually occurs when the family has adequate inner and outside resources to draw on; the crisis-provoking event is interpreted in an objective, realistic manner; family bonds and unity exist; and the family has the capacity to shift course and modify roles within the family (Danielson, Hamel-Bissell, & Winstead-Fry, 1993) (Table 4).

Mastery is the end result of functional coping. Mastery will occur when there is repeated success in problem-solving efforts. *Crisis* occurs in the presence of the

Table 4
Factors Enhancing Family Coping and Adaptation

Factors That Enhance Family Coping and Adaptation to Rehabilitation	Factors That Place the Family at Risk for Maladaptation to Rehabilitation
A key factor is the stability of the family before the crisis	The disability is long term and associated with many crisis episodes
A direct approach is used when talking about the client's health state	The family uses denial as a coping mechanism
The family makes good use of medical, educational, and rehabilitative resources	Family members have negative feelings about each other or dysfunctional relationships
The family has an open, direct approach when dealing with the change in health state	The family possesses ineffective coping skills or problem-solving skills
Family members treat the rehabilitation client in a normal manner	The parents are adolescents
There is effective open communication patterns between family members	The family uses dysfunctional communication patterns
The family possesses a strong internal and external support system	The family roles are fixed and rigidly held
There is a high degree of tolerance for differences among family members	There is a family perception of lack of control, helplessness, and hopelessness
There is a deep sense of commitment to the family	There is a weak parental subsystem
There is a strong parental subsystem or a supportive partner	There are scarce available resources, financial, or support systems
The family possesses a strong spiritual belief system	The family system is closed, not allowing any flow of information, resources, or energy outside of the family circle
The client's residence is convenient to shopping, schools, social services, and churches; and transportation is available	

stress and stressors if the family does not possess or fails to use effective adaptive strategies. A family crisis is the result of an imbalance between demands of the family and the family resources or coping efforts (Friedman, 1992). Two factors that will influence the movement to crisis are the perceptions of the event of change and the psychological and physiological resources available to the client and family. Crisis is characterized by family instability and disorganization (Friedman, 1992). If a crisis occurs the family's functioning continues to decline until either the family seeks or receives assistance and begins to deal effectively with the stressor, or the family reaches a low point in family functioning and then stabilizes at this new lower level of family function.

In the period before to exposure to the stressor anticipatory guidance (stress inoculation) is beneficial. Defensive tactics are often necessary adaptive responses during the actual stress period so that physical and psychological resources can be conserved. The family needs to develop effective coping strategies and stress management techniques to accomplish its various developmental tasks and family functions (Table 5).

Double ABCX Model of Family Coping

Family coping is a positive, problem-focused affective response. It also involves perceptual and behavioral responses that families use to resolve a problem or to reduce stress. When the level of coping shifts from the individual level to the family level it becomes more complex. Family coping signifies a group level of analysis (Friedman, 1992; McCubbin, Cauble, & Patterson, 1982; McCubbin & Patterson, 1983). McCubbin and Patterson (1983) created a model for analyzing family coping that is useful in the rehabilitation setting. This model is used as a

Table 5
Common Coping and Adaptive Strategies Used by Families

Strategy	Internal Coping	External Coping
Dysfunctional	Spouse abuse Child abuse Elder abuse Scapegoating Use of threats Triangling Pseudomutuality (false closeness) Authoritarianism (to deal with sense of powerlessness)	
Functional	Role flexibility Family group reliance Use of humor Greater sharing together Normalizing Controlling the meaning of the problem (interpreting or defining reframing) Joint problem solving	Seeking information Maintaining active links with broader community Seeking social support systems Seeking spiritual support

framework to guide interventions and address client issues of adaptation, adjustment, perception, and change. The **double ABCX model** focuses on family adaptation following a crisis and is applicable in the rehabilitation setting.

> *aA* = *Stress and change:* Families are rarely confronted by only one stressor at any one point in time. Rather, there is a pile-up of stressors, particularly in the aftermath of a major stressor. In rehabilitation settings the major stress would be the change in health state or injury. Five broad categories of stressor identified include the initial stressor, transition stressors, prior stressors, the consequences of ineffective family efforts to cope, and ambiguity (McCubbin & Patterson, 1983).
>
> *bB* = *Family resources:* Family resources are the family's capabilities to meet demands. They consist of each family member's personal resources as well as the family system's internal resources. They include education, health, personality characteristics, flexible roles, shared power, clear communication, and family cohesion (McCubbin & Patterson, 1983).
>
> *cC* = *Family perception:* The family's definition and meaning of the situation; the family's positive appraisal or negative interpretation of the stressor (McCubbin & Patterson, 1983).
>
> *xX* = *Family adaptation:* A continuum of outcomes ranging from effective adaptation to maladaptation (McCubbin & Patterson, 1983). Adaptation is a balancing of demands and capabilities, leading to some level of family adaptation.

Assessing the family's multiple demands and stressor(s), coping resources, and perception of the stressor(s) will help the nurse in the rehabilitation setting to help the client and family respond to stressful life events. Intervention strategies based on the assessment data would be used to aid the family to modify perception as necessary to facilitate effective adaptation and to balance the demands made on it with its coping resources and capabilities.

Implications for Family Development

The diagnosis of a life-threatening illness, chronic disorder, or disability can be a devastating experience for even the most stable family. The client and family members may experience feelings of loss of control over life and lack the skills necessary to cope with and adapt to stressful situations and the impending changes in their lives. Farley (1992) suggested that a framework of human development be used in conjunction with the nursing process to facilitate family coping and adaptation.

Farley (1992) identified concerns of families facing disabilities at various stages for **family development.**

Infants

If a disabled infant is born, the family, especially the parents, must deal with the loss of the expected "normal" child. It can be expected that the family will experience a normal grieving process including feelings of shock, anger, guilt, and depression. The family may feel the need to place blame for the event on someone or something. Family bonding with the new family member may be difficult to accomplish because of frequent hospitalizations and separations.

Children and Adolescents

There may be a need to restructure the future goals of the entire family as a unit as well as the future goals and plans for the individual client and/or other members of the family. There may be disruption in marital relationships and the need for significant adjustments among siblings. The cost of health care and rehabilitation may present a serious drain on the family's financial resources. The family may experience actual or perceived social isolation and decreased involvement in kinship and community activities. There will be a need to integrate rehabilitation or treatment into family life. Other family members may experience major disruption in their lifestyles, resulting from the identified client's need for care. If the client has severe cognitive dysfunction there will be concerns regarding sexuality, independence, and the possibility of relocation to living arrangements outside of the family home.

With older children parents may experience anger, but this anger is rarely directed at the disabled child. Parental fear of the child's death and secret wishes for the death of the child combined with guilt can create an overwhelming sense of sadness and helplessness. Self-pity, uncertainty, ambivalence, and spiritual distress can also be experienced by the parents (Farley, 1992). Visible disabilities may cause parental, child, and sibling distress. Parental conflicts can arise over caregiving responsibilities, attention given to the child, and difference in the intensity and expression of grief.

The parental response to disability in adolescence is fear and remorse. Problems can arise in the family when parents are overindulgent with and/or overprotective of the disabled adolescent. Overprotection or overindulgence can deter the adolescent's normal development and sense of control, and result in anger and rebellion (Patterson, 1988). It can also impede the client's progress in self-care development and self-management. Adolescents with disabilities can be caught in a confusing dependent–independent cycle.

Siblings of Disabled Children

Siblings may experience feelings of anger, jealousy, guilt, and resentment related to the increased parental attention focused on a disabled child. Younger and older siblings may experience isolation from parents, other family members, and/or peers. Older siblings may be expected to assume increased role responsibilities within the family or a caregiver role for the disabled family member. If the child has secret thoughts about the disabled person's death or if they have wished for the disabled person to vanish they may react by acceding to every demand made by the disabled individual.

Factors have been identified that correlate with increased risk for physical, emotional, and behavioral problems among siblings of disabled children (Breslau,

1983; Craft and Craft, 1989; Ferrari, 1984; Simeonsson & Bailey, 1986). Factors that have been identified include

1. A current stressor or crisis in their own life
2. Dysfunctional relationships within the family before the onset of the disability
3. The lack of effective coping strategies
4. A limited support system
5. A close relationship with the disabled family member, especially if the sibling is younger or close in age to the disabled child
6. Limited understanding of the disability
7. A need to change residency during hospitalization or rehabilitation of the disabled sibling
8. A perception of parental anger

Adults   Restructuring of future goals and plans may be required. A disability or development of a chronic illness may result in major alterations in lifestyle and role functioning. There may be major changes in household and living arrangements. Clients may experience loss of career opportunities and job flexibility.

Family units can experience reproductive, affective, and socialization difficulties when an adult develops a disability. Marital strain can occur as the result of the care demands of the disabled partner, changes in role functioning and role reversal, financial strain, sexual functioning, and the increased physical and emotional needs of children in the family. Role transfers and transitions may be required that can place any member of the family in role strain or role conflict.

Elderly   Schienle and Eiler (1984) estimated that 85 percent of people older than 65 years of age have at least one disabling condition. In the majority of cases the primary caregivers for these individuals are daughters and daughters-in-law. The spouses of these individuals experience a loss of companionship. The primary caregivers can give up aspects of their own lives. This can result in feelings of frustration, anger, fatigue, exhaustion, and depression. Spouses, partners, and family members may neglect their own health or physical and emotional needs. The phenomenon of caregiver "burnout" can result. Characteristics of the person suffering from burnout include irritability, depression, exhaustion, headaches and other physical symptoms, changes in eating patterns, substance abuse, and abuse of the dependent family member. This is especially true if the primary caregiver is a member of the "sandwiched generation," caring for the needs of partners, children, job, and a disabled parent. There may be a need to restructure retirement plans. Additional strain may be placed on adult children. The primary health care provider may have physical health problems with a complex regimen of care or treatment.

Nursing Process Characteristics and indicators that a family system might be at risk for an actual or potential inability to meet family member needs, carry out family functions, or maintain communication for mutual growth and maturation have been identified (Gordon, 1993). The nurse must remember to assess and reflect on the family and its dynamics within some framework of developmental tasks or stages (Table 6) and under the umbrella of the family's race and culture. Indications of risk are as follows:

- Disorganized, disintegrated, and dysfunctional family processes and dynamics are present.
- There is disruption of structure, role functions, communication patterns, or interpersonal relationships.
- The family demonstrates inadequate emotional problem-solving and decision-making abilities.
- The family lacks an understanding of or willingness to participate in the client's care.
- The family lacks knowledge about the client's condition or prognosis.
- The family engages in impaired health maintenance behaviors.
- The family is unable or unwilling to meet emotional, social, or physical needs of its members.
- The family members lack shared goals.
- There are changes in the effective family patterns of behavior and coping.
- There are changes in roles and responsibilities within the family.
- The family is unable to cope with changes in family structure or function.
- The family is unable to accept and respect the client as part of the family.

Assessment Areas of concern in assessing an actual or potential alteration in family processes are the following:

- The family's developmental stage
- The family's cultural and racial background
- The family's structure and potential disruption to structure
- The family's functional tasks and possible distraction to their ability to meet family tasks
- The family's experience with past crisis or stress
- The family's past coping strategies and the success of those strategies for adapting to change and managing stress
- Initial family reaction to stress during first few weeks of rehabilitation
- Family structure, with an emphasis on family relationships
- The client's position within the family structure
- Family function, with an emphasis on roles and values.
- Family communication patterns

Interventions
- Assisting the client's and family members' expression of feelings appropriate to age
- Encouraging the venting of hidden feelings

Table 6
Developmental Tasks and Possible Effects of Illness, Injury, Disease, or Disability

Stage	Task	Possible Response to Chronic Illness or Disability
Infancy (1 yr)	Trust: Separates from primary caregiver and explores environment	• Separations from parents may affect bonding and parental attachment • Rate of development, temperament, and sociability may be delayed • Parenting demands may differ • Infants may not provide clear cues and may be unresponsive or inattentive • Decreased stimulation and environmental exploration may result in interference with sensory, cognitive, and motor development • Feeding problems may develop
Toddler (2–4 yr)	Autonomy: Feeds self, is toilet trained, has control of motor functioning, and plans and carries out activities	• Delayed or restricted environmental exploration • There may be excessive dependency, separation anxiety, and poor self-image and impulse control • The toddler may lag in linguistic skills • Pain may be viewed as punishment for "bad behavior" • The toddler may use magical thinking to deal with stress of illness or disability
Preschooler	Initiation: Adjusts to school and social areas outside of home and plays cooperatively with others	• Tasks of self-restraint and interest in the ability to develop relationships may not be accomplished • There may be restricted motor and social competency • The child may be fearful and passive • The child may develop a poor self-image • Sex and gender identification may be delayed • The child may believe that good and bad behaviors have an influence over health and disabilities
School-age child	Industry: Demonstrates age-appropriate school performance, follows directions and instructions, completes tasks, participates in organized peer activities, and is responsible for personal hygiene	• The child may experience feelings of inferiority and a loss of control and privacy • School absences and hospitalizations may have a negative effect on academic success • Isolation and withdrawal behavior may be the result of testing or rejection by peers • Poor adjustment behaviors may include dietary and sleeping problems, enuresis and encorpresis, regression or depression, and hypochrondriacal concerns or phobias
Adolescence (13–20 yr)	Identity: Develops peer relationships with both sexes, defines goals in life, selects and prepares for vacation, and gains independence	• The adolescent may develop a sense of "being different" • Normal bodily changes may disrupt the development of a positive self-image • Anxiety may inhibit the development of relationships with members of the opposite sex

Table 6
Developmental Tasks and Possible Effects of Illness, Injury, Disease, or Disability (*Continued*)

Stage	Task	Possible Response to Chronic Illness or Disability
		• Females may be at greater risk for pregnancy because of the desire to be normal • There may be increased anxiety over possible complications, social relationships, future careers, and lifestyle • Some adolescents may use denial as a coping mechanism, resulting in decreased adherence to the treatment regimen, and others may engage in risk-taking behaviors • Some adolescents may have a greater tolerance for stress and life disruptions
Young adult (20–30 yr)	Intimacy: Completes education, achieves economic independence, selects relationship partner and lifestyle, and is socially responsible	• There may be difficulty in developing an intimate relationship with a member of the opposite sex • Social integration may be inhibited by the public's responses to the disabilities • There may be problems in obtaining and maintaining employment • There may be difficulty in accepting the affection of nondisabled persons • There may be disruptions in marital relationships and intimacy • There may be problems with parenting, role functioning, and power functioning in the family.
Middle age (30–60 yr)	Generativity: Stabilizes career, demonstrates concern for next generation, and participates in community activities	• There may be a disruption in the capacity to develop vocationally • There may be a surrendering of the economic role in the family • Involvement in community activities may be curtailed • There may be disruption in sexual functioning and expression • There may be pseudo-intimacy and self-indulgence
Elderly (60 yr–death)	Integrity: Serves as counselor and advisor to younger generations, develops interests and abilities according to physical functioning, and enjoys accomplishments	• Decreased opportunities for socialization • Depression may be masked by physical symptoms • There is an increased risk of suicide

Sources: Erickson (1950, 1982); Farley (1992); Friedman (1992).

- Counseling the family to keep focused on the real crisis
- Helping with limit setting for the client and in understanding and dealing with disruptive client behaviors
- Providing information concerning procedures, simple facts about the injury, and the purpose of treatment methods for illness or disease
- Discussing realistic aspects regarding the future
- Developing a social play area where interpersonal relationships can be strengthened
- Assisting family members to relate to their family member's change in health state
- Assisting the family members to see that their feelings are normal and acceptable
- Creating bridges between the family and community support systems and resources
- Grouping problem-solving sessions combining one or more families that focus on practical and emotional aspects of rehabilitation
- Grouping family sessions of one or more families to focus on encouragement or expression of family member concerns and feelings
- Establishing task-oriented groups of clients and families focused on identifying and practicing new living skills through task assignment within the hospital, rehabilitation setting, and community
- Providing support to the client and family members regarding altered roles and responsibilities
- Including family members in client care
- Including the client and family members in short- and long-term planning
- Providing the client and family privacy within the rehabilitation setting
- Supporting functional communication between the client and the family

Outcomes   Goals of nursing interventions for families with difficulties in coping and adjusting to rehabilitation are to influence the remedial, supportive, and communication skills within the family unit.

Family Expected Outcomes

- The family members express realistic understanding, expectations, and support for each other.
- The family develops realistic goals and means for achieving them through a problem-solving method.
- The family demonstrates positive family coping and decision-making mechanisms.
- The family incorporates family strengths, needs, cultural and spiritual values, and lifestyles into the plan for the future.
- All members are included in the plan of care.
- The family maintains daily activities, wellness, and work activities.
- The family completes stage-related developmental tasks.
- The family is empowered and capable of getting access to resources, making transitions among services and agencies, and allocating resources.
- The family members are active participants in the treatment plan, are knowledgeable about events or conditions, and encourage client self-care and maximum independence.

- The family members resolve their loss and grieving, enabling members to continue with meaningful roles and potential for growth.
- The family members recognize potential problems or changes early and seek preventive assistance from professionals.
- The family members establish adaptive coping for functions, roles, and responsibilities.
- The client communicates effectively regarding goals and activities of family life.

Conclusion

Even the most organized and stable family can be overwhelmed and alienated from the rehabilitation client by the residue of physical injury and long-term progressive and disabling results of illness and disease. Dealing with individuals as if they function in a social vacuum is like treating the proverbial tip of the iceberg (Danielson, Hamel-Bissell, & Winstead-Fry, 1993). Treatment team identification of functional and dysfunctional family dynamics influencing the process of rehabilitation is significant for the accomplishment of treatment goals. All members of the interdisciplinary treatment team must be aware of the behavioral reactions of the family and the impact of those reactions on the health of the rehabilitation client.

This chapter has focused on the family and its importance to rehabilitation nursing. The family is an extremely complex phenomenon, with intricate processes and relationships. How the family copes and adjusts to illness and injury is extremely difficult to discuss in depth within the context of a single chapter in a book focused on rehabilitation care. This chapter presents a broad spectrum of topics and information at a superficial level. It addresses the issues of family from the dominant culture: middle-class American. Several important references (see References and Suggested Readings) provide the reader with sources to increase knowledge in this important and fascinating area of nursing care.

References

Breslau, N. (1983). Family care: Effects of siblings and mother. In G. H. Thompson, I. L. Rubin, & R. M. Bilenger (Eds.), *Comprehensive management of cerebral palsy* (pp. 299–309). New York: Grune & Stratton.

Carson, V. B., & Arnold, E. N. (1996). *Mental health nursing the nurse–patient journey.* Philadelphia: W. B. Saunders.

Christopherson, V. A. (1962). The patient and family. *Rehabilitation Literature, 23*(2), 34–41.

Craft, M. J., & Craft, J. L. (1989). Perceived changes in siblings of hospitalized children: A comparison of sibling and parent reports. *Children's Health Care, 18*(1), 42–47.

Danielson, C. B., Hamel-Bissell, B., & Winstead-Fry, P. (Eds.). (1993). *Families, health & illness: Perspectives on coping and intervention.* St. Louis: Mosby.

Erikson, E. H. (1950). *Childhood and society.* New York: W. W. Norton & Co.

Erikson, S. H. (1982). *The life cycle completed.* New York: W. W. Norton & Co.

Farley, A. M. (1992). *Nursing and the disabled across the life span.* Boston: Jones & Bartlett.

Farran, C. J., Herth, K. A., & Popovich, J. M. (1995). *Hope and hopelessness critical clinical constructs.* Thousand Oaks: Sage.

Ferrari, M. (1984). Chronic illness: Psychosocial effects of siblings: Chronically ill boys. *Journal of Child Psychology and Psychiatry, 25*(3), 249–476.

Friedman, M. M. (1996). *Family nursing theory and practice* (44th ed.). Norwalk, CT: Appleton & Lange.

Fulgrum, R. (1988). *All I really need to know I learned in kindergarten.* New York: Random House.

Gordon, M. (1993). *Manual of nursing diagnoses: 1993–1994.* St. Louis: Mosby–Year Book.

Macklin, E. D. (1988). Nontraditional family forms. In M. B. Sussman & S. K. Steinmetz (Eds.), *Handbook of marriage and the family* (pp. 317–353). New York: Plenum Press.

McCubbin, H. I., Cauble, A. E., & Patterson, J. M. (1982). *Family stress, coping, and social support.* Springfield, IL: Charles C. Thomas.

McCubbin, H. I., & Patterson, M. (1983). Family transition: Adaptation to stress. In H. I. McCubbin & C. R. Figley (Eds.), *Stress and the family: Coping with normative transitions* (pp. 5–25). New York: Brunner/Mazel.

Parse, R. (1990). Essentials for practicing the art of nursing. *Nursing Science Quarterly, 2*(3), 111.

Patterson, J. (1988). Chronic illness in children and the impact on families. In C. S. Chilman, E. W. Nunnally, & F. M. Cox (Eds.), *Chronic illness and disability* (pp. 69–107). Newbury Park, CA: Sage.

Schienle, D. R., & Eiler, J. M. (1984). Clinical interventions with older adults. In M. G. Eisenberg, L. C. Sutkin, & M. A. Jansen (Eds.), *Chronic illness and disability through the life span: Effects on self and family* (pp. 245–268). New York: Springer.

Sherwood, G. (1992). The responses of caregivers to the experience of suffering. In P. Stark & J. McGovern (Eds.), *The hidden dimension of illness: Human suffering.* (pp. 105–113). New York: National League for Nursing Press.

Simeonsson, R. J., & Bailey, D. B. (1986). Siblings of handicapped children. In J. J. Gallagher & P. M. Vietze (Eds.), *Families of handicapped persons: Research programs and policy issues* (pp. 67–77). Baltimore, MD: Paul H. Brookes Publishing Co.

Vincint, L., & Brown, P. (1986). *Impact of having a child with a disability on the family.* Madison, WI: University of Wisconsin, Department of Rehabilitative Psychology and Special Education.

Wright, L. M., & Leakey, M. (1994). *Nurses and families. A guide to family assessment and intervention* (2nd ed.). Philadelphia: FA Davis.

Suggested Readings

Boss, P. G., Doherty, W. J., LaRossa, R., Schumm, W. R., & Stienmetz, S. K. (Eds.). (1993). *Sourcebook of family theories and methods: A conceptual approach.* New York: Plenum Press.

Duval, E. M., & Miller, B. L. (1985). Marriage and family development (6th ed.). Philadelphia: J.B. Lippincott.

Eisenberg, M. G., Sutkin, L. C., & Jansen, M. A. (Eds.). (1984). *Chronic illness and disability through the life span: Effects on self and family.* New York: Springer.

Forman, S. G. (1993). Coping skills interventions for children and adolescents. San Francisco: Jossey-Bass.

Hirschberg, G. G., Lewis, L., & Vaughan, P. (1976). *Rehabilitation manual for the care of the disabled and elderly* (2nd ed.). Philadelphia: J.B. Lippincott.

Minuchin, S. (1974). *Families and family therapy.* Cambridge, MA: University Press.

Rolland, J. S. (1994). Families, illness, and disability: An integrative treatment model. New York: Harper-Collins.

Satir, V. (1964). *Conjoint family therapy.* Palo Alto, CA: Science & Behavior Books.

Stark, P. L., & McGovern, J. P. (Eds.). (1992). *The hidden dimension of illness: Human suffering.* New York: National League for Nursing Press.

Strass, A. L., & Glasser, B. G. (1975). *Chronic illness and the quality of life.* St. Louis: Mosby.

CHAPTER 9
Self-Concept and Self-Esteem

Patricia A. Chin

Key Terms   *Anxiety*
Approach Behaviors
Avoidance Behaviors
Body Image
Cognitive Image
Emotional (Affective) Image
Fear
Locus of Control (LOC)
Perceptual Images
Physical Self
Power
Powerlessness
Psychological Self
Self-Concept
Self-Efficacy
Self-Esteem
Social Identity
Social Self
Spiritual Self
Stigma

Objectives   1. Identify and discuss the dimensions of the self-concept.

2. Identify the characteristics of clients with high-level self-esteem and those with low levels of self-esteem.

3. Identify sources of anxiety encountered during rehabilitation.

4. Discuss Peplau's levels of anxiety and the client behaviors associated with each level.

5. Discuss the concept of powerlessness.

6. Identify common nursing diagnoses associated with disturbances in self-concept.

7. Identify assessment criteria for determining if a rehabilitation client has an actual or potential problem with anxiety, self-esteem, or powerlessness.

8. Identify interventions for assisting the rehabilitation client to cope with an actual or potential problem with anxiety, self-esteem, or powerlessness.

9. Identify outcomes of the nursing interventions for assisting the rehabilitation client to cope with an actual or potential problem with anxiety, self-esteem, or powerlessness.

The psychology of disability is no different than the psychology of being human (Marinelli & Dell Orto, 1984). The disabled client does have to cope with more unusual stimuli than the nondisabled person. These stimuli can be biological, social, or economic. Clients in rehabilitation, and those with disabilities, tend to experience a disproportionately large number of frustrations and difficulties in problem solving; they encounter more situations of nonacceptance, prejudice, and devaluation than the nondisabled; and they can experience difficulty in developing realistic and healthy self-concepts (Marinelli & Dell Orto, 1984). The potential effect of physical impairment on self-concept can occur whether the disability is totally disabling or if the degree of disability is low or moderate (Hamburg, 1974; Marinelli & Dell Orto, 1984). The impact of physical impairment will be strongly related to the premorbid personality of the client. If the client has feelings of low self-esteem and inferiority before the impairment those feelings can be intensified by the change in health state. Several psychosocial needs have been identified as being especially important when caring for those requiring medical rehabilitation services and those with disabilities. These are the problems of alteration in self-concept, body image, anger, dependency, motivation, and grieving over loss.

The Dimension of Self

To know who we are we must first possess knowledge of the "self" and be aware of the "self." **Self-concept** is the term that is used to identify that part of the self that lies within the person's conscious awareness (Arnold & Boggs, 1995). The term *self-concept* includes all that the person perceives, knows, feels, or holds as truth about his or her identity. Self-concept involves feelings of self-worth, perceptions about the body, and feelings about control over personal destiny. Self-concept can be thought of as several dimensions. These dimensions include the physical self (body image), the psychological self (personal identity), the social self (represented by the roles used in interactions with others), and the spiritual self (that which is connected to God and sources of meaning and purpose) (Carson & Arnold, 1996).

Rieser (1992) defined **body image (physical self)** as the mental picture each person creates regarding the physical self. The image of the physical self establishes the boundaries between the person's inner self and the external environment. As the physical self develops people recognize that there are similarities and differences among human bodies. Several factors influence how a person feels about the physical self. Factors that significantly influence the physical self include cultural values and desired norms about the self, natural patterns of growth and development, distinct patterns of physical and emotional maturation, and changes in normal or usual bodily functioning. What the person perceives and feels about the physical self will greatly influence interpersonal relations and interactions with others.

Changes in the physical self can result in anxiety, insecurity, self-consciousness about the body, and preoccupation with the body. How a person adapts to changes in the body depends on the ascribed meaning of the change for both the person experiencing the change and the person's significant others. The onset of illness, traumatic injury, surgery, or disability can create anxieties concerning body integrity, body function, and body image. Even medication and medication side effects can cause an alteration in a person's perception of the physical self.

The **psychological self** (personal identity) includes a person's perceptual, cognitive, and emotional images of the self. **Perceptual images** are affected by early interactions with others, especially parents. These perceptual images are not fixed and can continue to develop in complexity over time. Individuals with healthy perceptual processes view situations in broad terms and can infer alternative explanations for life events. They can evaluate new information and identify that previously held perceptions are no longer valid. They can evaluate the effects of their behavior and revise inappropriate attitudes and actions. They can extend themselves to others and receive assistance from others. They demonstrate a balance between dependency and independence. The perceptual process can be influenced by normal maturation changes; drugs; and physical, psychological, and spiritual suffering. Alterations in the perceptual processes can result in distortion of factual perceptions. Distorted perceptual processes, although resistant to change, can be corrected over time through validation of perceptions or the challenging and exploration of errors in perceptions.

A stable self-identity, or sense of who we are, is necessary to provide continuity through life. However, the self-concept is a dynamic phenomenon that responds to numerous situations encountered during the life span. A person's self-concept begins development during infancy and continues to develop throughout the course of life. The self-concept is formed through interactions with others. The foundation for self-perception is formed early in life and is created by what we are told about ourselves by significant others in our lives. The ability to evaluate objectively what we are told by others, directly and indirectly, is essential when a person must accurately determine true talents, abilities, and self-worth.

Innate intelligence, past experiences and memories, educational experiences, and thinking styles make up the **cognitive image** of the self. Thinking is a creative and active mental activity that involves creating mental images from perceived data, drawing conclusions about the images and the meanings they hold, and organizing the images into thoughts that are both useable and retrievable (Carson & Arnold, 1996). Psychological and physiological factors influence cognitive processes. Disease, trauma, and drugs can significantly impair cognitive processes, resulting in unclear, illogical, and irrational thinking patterns and behaviors. That aspect of the self that permits a self-evaluation of what we can do is called **self-efficacy.** Self-efficacy as defined by Bandura (1977) is the ability to perform certain tasks on the basis of what we perceive about our abilities. A person will engage in behaviors, or take those actions that are perceived as what they can do or perform. If the individual does not believe that he or she can do something they will not engage in the behavior or perform the task. This evaluation of ability may or may not correspond with actual ability.

The **emotional (affective) image** consists of feelings experienced in response to life. Incorporated into the emotional self are self-esteem, self-confidence (feeling that one is competent), and self-respect (feeling that what one does is consistent with the value system held). **Self-esteem** is the term used to represent a person's personal judgment of worth. Self-esteem is how we feel about what we perceive about ourselves and is an important key to our behavior (Carson & Arnold, 1996). Individuals constantly compare their perceived self to an ideal self or the "me" that ought to be. This personal judgment influences thoughts, emotions, desires, values, and goals (Dugas, 1983). There are two categories of self-esteem. *Global self-esteem,* or how much we like and approve of our self as a whole, and *specific self-esteem,* how much we like and approve of certain parts of ourselves (Sanford & Donovan, 1984). Self-esteem is not dependent on wealth, education, social class, occupation, or availability of material assets. Five traits are necessary for the development of self-esteem (Sanford & Donovan, 1984):

1. A sense of significance
2. A sense of competence
3. A sense of connectedness balanced with separateness
4. A sense of realism about ourselves
5. A set of ethics and values

Self-esteem affects all aspects of life and is the key to behavior, feeling, thinking, values, and goals. A positive sense of self-esteem makes it possible for the individual to face life demands with confidence. Individuals who have a high positive level of self-esteem are active self-agents, possess positive perceptions of their skills, appearance, and behaviors, are nondefensive and assertive, perform realistic self-evaluations, and expect people to value them. A negative sense of self-esteem causes doubt regarding one's ability to meet life demands. Individuals with low levels of self-esteem, or negative self-esteem, expect others to be critical of them, are passive self-agents, are defensive, and possess unrealistic expectations about their performance (Carson & Arnold, 1996).

The roles we assume, socially accepted behavior patterns associated with functions in social groups, define our **social self.** Role can be ascribed (i.e., family position, birth order, and gender), or those that we assume or choose (i.e., student, nurse, or friend). Each role has expectations, prescribed functions, and boundaries. People can experience *role strain* (too many role demands) and *role conflict* (conflicting role demands). Some roles are assumed more willingly than others (i.e., parent, spouse, mentor). Other roles imposed on individuals may not be of their own choosing (i.e., widow, single parent, caregiver). With some roles stereotypical expectations and stigma may be involved (disabled person).

The **spiritual self** provides for a sense of God consciousness. The spiritual self allows the individual to interpret life events from the broader perspective of a "bigger picture." The spiritual self seeks meaning in life's events. The spiritual self includes beliefs about the universe and our relationship to the universe (Carson & Arnold, 1996).

Self-esteem exists on a continuum, ranging from a well-formed identity and sense of self, resulting in high value of self, to a nonexistent sense of self, lack of a formed identity, or low self-esteem. Most individuals fall somewhere between these two extremes and the perceived level of self-esteem is relatively static. Self-esteem does fluctuate according to the factors impinging on it at specific times and in specific situations. In rehabilitation settings the nurse will encounter clients whose level of self-esteem has been altered by the characteristics of the situation. The rehabilitation client frequently experiences a sudden drop, perhaps only temporarily, in self-esteem related to the effects of illness, injury, disease, disability, or treatment on the social, moral, and spiritual self.

Behaviors Indicating High-Level Self-Esteem

The client with a high level of self-esteem, or self-appraisal of worth, has two main convictions: (1) I am lovable; I have merit, and (2) I have worth; I have something to offer others. Some of the behaviors associated with high self-esteem include inner confidence, a sense of purpose and involvement, and the ability to manipulate social situations and interpersonal encounters. Clients with high self-esteem are assertive and find gratification in activities with others and also in being alone. Characterlogical qualities include boldness, courage, freedom, spontaneity, trust, and self-acceptance. Usually these individuals possess a variety of coping mechanisms and strategies. The person with high self-esteem can allow for differences in people and does not require all people to think, behave, or believe alike. Individuals with high-level self-esteem can make their needs known to others whom they believe can, and will, assist them.

Behaviors Indicating Low-Level Self-Esteem

The behaviors and characteristics indicating low self-esteem can affect all areas of the client's life or be present only in specific areas. Clients with low self-esteem usually demonstrate a lack of inner confidence, a sense of meaningless drifting, or rigid adherence to roles and tasks. They often view life as ambiguous, the future unpredictable, and have a sense of limited control over life. They have difficulty trusting others and making their needs known. They are uncomfortable with change and attempt to maintain a sameness and rigidity in life. Individuals with low self-esteem are either compliant, passive, feeling isolated, or too weak to overcome life difficulties and challenges, or they are aggressive, domineering, and have a need for power and control.

These individuals may overestimate self-worth and brag and exaggerate about skills and abilities. They persistently seek and value conventionally defined symbols and status. They sense a need to decrease differences around themselves. New theories, ideas, and beliefs make these individuals uncomfortable and they do not know how to respond to them.

Three major behavior patterns observed in individuals with low self-esteem are

1. The use of defensive, aggressive, hostile behaviors
2. The tendency to submit; accepting life in a self-effacing manner
3. The tendency to withdraw; removing one's self from social interactions or retreating into fantasy.

Alterations in Perceptions of Self during Rehabilitation

The self-concept is a dynamic process influenced by the person's current health status, past experiences, social relationships, and the previous view of the self. An awareness of self-perceptions is important for an understanding of the person as a whole and for determining the impact of illness, injury, or disease on the person and on adaptation to change. As a result of the experience of major illness, injury, or disability the client may experience a threat to any dimension of self-concept. Anxiety, insecurity, and self-consciousness may be experienced in any component of the "self." The client may experience this as an altered self-perception, an alteration in body image, loss of social self, feelings of dependence, helplessness, or powerlessness, and concerns about control over personal destiny. Changes that the client may experience can be obvious or subtle. Regardless of the nature of the change or the degree of visibility of the alteration, the individual's perception of self-concept must be a critical issue for the nurse.

In rehabilitation nursing practice the nurse encounters clients experiencing illness, injury, disease, role change, crisis, and new growth. The client's level of self-esteem affects all areas of psychological functioning. For the client it affects psychological and physiological health. For the family system it affects parenting behavior with the child, sibling relationships, adult relationships, and parental relationships. In the community it affects the interactions among the client, family, and the community. All of these are situations that can influence the self-evaluation of worth and merit. The result can be major changes in the perceived level of self-esteem. One of the tasks of nursing is to maintain effective functioning of the system (client, family, or community). If low self-esteem decreases the effective functioning of the system then the maintenance of an adequate level of self-esteem, or the raising of low self-esteem, becomes an area of nursing intervention.

Successful rehabilitation requires the integration of a new view of the self. This involves acknowledgment of bodily changes, changes in levels of functioning and independence, and resolution of multiple losses. Rehabilitative nursing is influential in creating an environment that facilitates re-integration of the self and successful function within the family and reentry into the community. Education and learning, perceived self-efficacy, and self-care capabilities will be strongly influenced by the client's perceptions of self-concept, anxiety, and feelings of powerlessness.

Self-Concept and the Role of Anxiety

Anxiety is a self-protective feeling state that occurs when the client experiences a threat to self-concept. When a person experiences anxiety the threat is vague and nonspecific. There is a sense of anticipation, the threat is future oriented (has not yet been experienced), and generates from an internal source. The client is anxious about the outcome of a surgical interventions. This is the opposite of **fear,** where the threat is external, specific, and exists in the present. The client who cannot maneuver a wheelchair out of the way of an automobile is fearful. Anxiety is a sense of alertness that prepares the client for some type of action.

The source of client anxiety can be conceptualized in a variety of ways. Anxiety can arise from a sense of frustration occurring when the client is unable to reach a desired goal. The inability to reach one goal might make it impossible to reach other desired goals. The result may be feelings of failure and anxiety. Anxiety may be viewed as a drive that is learned as a self-protective response used as an attempt to avoid pain. This drive becomes attached to a particular situation or stimulus and then becomes generalized to other similar situations or stimuli. Anxiety can also be conceptualized as arising from conflict.

Conflict occurs when two opposing forces clash (Kritek, 1994). The individual is forced into a position where a choice must be made between the opposing forces. Four types of conflict have been identified: *approach-approach* (two equally desirable forces), *approach-avoidance* (the individual wants to both pursue and avoid the forces), *avoidance-avoidance* (equally undesirable goals), and *double approach-avoidance* (both positive and negative aspects are seen in both alternatives).

Effects of Anxiety on Patterns of Behavior

Anxiety is an uncomfortable and painful experience. Many different behaviors are used to express or relieve it. Anxiety is so psychologically and physiologically deteriorating that clients will search for any behavior that will provide relief. Client dependency on the behaviors used to relieve anxiety can be long- or short-term in nature. Any and all anxiety-reducing strategies will actually relieve the pain of anxiety. The type of anxiety-reducing strategy used by the client is significant in determining whether the effect will be long-term and "healthy," aimed at attacking or modifying the basic anxiety-producing situation, or short-term and "unhealthy," aimed at avoiding the basic anxiety-producing situation. Actions aimed at attacking or modifying the situation are classified as **approach behaviors.** Those that are aimed at reducing the situation without confronting the issues or modifying the stimulus are classified as **avoidance behaviors.** (See Table 1.)

Stigmatization

In current use, **stigma** is the term used to indicate a mark of shame or discredit (*Webster's Third New International Dictionary,* 1986). A society teaches its members to identify and define the attributes and characteristics that are considered ordinary (Goffman, 1963). Daily activities in the world are what the society establishes as the usual and the expected. Goffman proposed that what we recognize and anticipate when we meet others is the **social identity.** The social identity includes personal attributes, structural attributes, physical activities, professional

Table 1
Anxiety-Related Behaviors

Approach Behaviors	Avoidance Behaviors
Recognizing the situation as anxiety producing	Denial of the situation or some aspect of the situation
Recognizing the situation as threatening and attempting to gather information about the situation: • Talking to others (authorities, friends) • Reading about the situation • Reviewing past experience • Determining a course of action • Following through with the course of action	Distorting some major aspect of the situation Refusing to think about the situation or physically withdrawing from the situation Using repression, rationalization, projection, displacement, intellectualization, reaction formation, fantasy, ritual and compulsions, dependency, anger, aggression, hostility, depression, guilt, and somatic complaints
Using information-seeking, direct action, problem-solving, and reaching-out behaviors, and love	

roles, and the concept of self. Some attributes are often associated with incompetence or qualifying factors such as being deaf, having a physical handicap, or using a wheelchair. Currently, in Western society, a person with a diagnosis of acquired immunodeficiency syndrome (AIDS) has a definite social identity. Even though these social identities are not based on any legitimate criteria, they can be stigmatizing.

Often an individual is unaware of social identity until a situation arises in which personal attributes, structural attributes, or expectations no longer fulfill the social definition of ordinary (Goffman, 1963). The difference between the expected attributes and the actual attributes is the cause of discrepancy that spoils the social identity. Stigma can be defined as the negative perceptions and behaviors expressed by "normal" people, as defined by society, toward individuals who are different from themselves. Stigmata are considered threatening to other members of the society because they create feelings of anxiety and apprehension. This is especially true when they encounter "sick" people. Sick people remind other members of the society that as humans people are vulnerable and mortal. Consequently, normal people will attempt to avoid contact with individuals who have an obvious injury, chronic disease, or disabilities (Katz, 1981). Normal people also may make negative value judgments about people who are ill or disabled.

Those who experience illness, injury, disease, or disability are aware of those feelings and perceptions held by others. Many of those who now are confronted with alterations in social identify have shared those feelings and perceptions about others in the past. Because of this deviance from the norm some individuals are devalued and discredited by the other members of the society. Self-value and worth may become a major issue for the rehabilitation client. The degree of difference may have no correlation with the degree of stigmatization experienced.

Responses to stigmatization vary. Social stigma has consequences for both the affected client and the normal population. The client may respond to feelings of being stigmatized by using withdrawal and isolation behavior; by seeking secondary gains; by *passing* (pretending to have a less stigmatic identity or even a normal identity) (Dudley, 1983); or through attempts to cover up, minimize, or de-emphasize their differences (Goffman, 1963). The stigmatized client is often uncertain about the attitudes possessed by others and may feel the constant need to make a good impression on others. Normal individuals may not know how to respond in the presence of a stigmatized individual. Normal individuals may respond by labeling others, by using negative categories or stereotyping, or by devaluing the person with the stigma.

Assisting clients to manage the effect of stigma is complex. It may not be possible to deal with the issues of stigmatization in a holistic manner. Intervention might include

- Encouraging the client to become involved with a support group. Interacting with like-afflicted individuals (*the own*) enables the stigmatized client to feel more like a

normal person (Goffman, 1963). *Caution:* Clients may believe that they can interact only with *the own.* They should use self-help groups only as sources of interaction
- Encouraging the client to develop supportive relationships with others who do not carry the stigmatizing attribute or characteristic (*the wise*). The wise interact with the stigmatized as if they were normal, they do not make them feel shame, and treat individuals in a normal fashion (Goffman, 1963)
- Encouraging the client to seek advocates who support the rights of clients and speak on behalf of those in need (Sims, 1993)

Selecting one of these interventions and focusing on a particular aspect of reducing stigmatization can produce the most positive results (Saylor, 1995).

Anxiety Encountered during Rehabilitation

During the period of recovery and rehabilitation from illness, injury, disease, or disability there are many stressors and threats to self-concepts and self-esteem that the client can encounter. General sources of anxiety-producing stimuli include (1) the illness, injury, disease, or disability and all of its aspects; (2) the hospital and other medically oriented facilities and other unfamiliar surroundings; (3) the requirements of the sick role or impaired role; (4) significant others; (5) employment or usual role and task responsibilities, and (6) finances. These anxiety-producing sources can occur separately but generally they occur in a variety of combinations.

The client may experience high levels of anxiety as a result of a decreased ability to meet basic needs, threats to self-efficacy, changes in life roles and relationships, and loss of personal control. The client may experience situational crises, changes in health status, disability, and deteriorating function. Rehabilitation clients with cognitive impairments are at risk for anxiety related to distortions in cognitive processing that alter their perception of situations. Even changes in the rehabilitation environment, such as transfers, additions to, or changes in caregiver staff, can cause heightened anxiety for the client.

Clients with disabilities may have to continually deal with personal devaluation experiences, uncertainty about abilities and functioning, independence, and an uncertain future. They can experience serious disruption to their social functioning and their interpersonal relationships. Social acceptance or rejection and feelings of inferiority can be serious problems for these clients during and following the rehabilitation process (Eisenberg, Sutkin, & Jansen, 1984; Farley, 1992; Marinelli & Dell Orto, 1984).

Peplau (1963) identified four levels of anxiety and client responses to those anxiety states (see Table 2).

Power and Powerlessness

Power is the potential or actual ability to influence the thinking, attitudes, behaviors, and/or emotions of oneself or others (May, 1950; Seeman, 1959). Feelings of power are necessary to create the potential for human beings to experience af-

Table 2
The Four Levels of Anxiety

	Responses to Anxiety	
Level of anxiety	Physiological	Behavioral/Emotional
Mild anxiety (+)	Sympathetic nervous system arousal: increased pulse, blood pressure, and heart rate	Alertness, increased problem-solving ability, increased attentiveness, increased vigilance and alertness, awareness of relationship factors in the situation, positive behaviors and feelings, ideal state for learning
Moderate anxiety (++)	Activation of sympathetic nervous system: muscle tension, diaphoresis, pupil dilation, increase in heart rate, respiration, and blood pressure	Tension, attention focused on issue of concern, selective attention, sense of apprehension, concern, expectation, hypervigilance and irritability, negative effect on learning
Severe anxiety (+++)	Generalized sympathetic response: "fight or flight," sweating, palpitations, flushing, pallor, dry mouth, paresthesias, hot and cold flashes, urinary frequency	Distress, trembling, reduced sensory perception, limited ability to focus on details, attention directed to scattered details, hyperactivity, inability to learn
Panic (++++)	Constant generalized sympathetic arousal	Client responds only to internal arousal and distress; feelings of inadequacy, distress, and helplessness; emotionally overwhelmed; use of primitive coping behaviors; feelings of doom or death

Source: Peplau (1963).

firmation and for the assertion of self. **Powerlessness,** by contrast, is the expectation that one's own behavior cannot determine outcomes or obtain what is desired. The feelings that one's own actions will not significantly affect the outcomes of a situation result in feelings of alienation due to loss of control of events and decision making (Seeman, 1959). Powerlessness can lead to apathy, helplessness, hopelessness, and eventually death (Seligman, 1975 & 1991).

Seeman (1959) originally conceptualized powerlessness as a subconcept of alienation. Clients who require rehabilitation for an illness, disease, injury, or disability can experience extreme feelings of alienation and powerlessness. They may feel alienated from family, community, society, and even the self. They may feel powerless to deal effectively with life, with the treatment team and plan, or with the future.

The extent to which clients with a significant change in health state, especially disability, believe that they can control events by their own actions can affect problem solving, decision making, and willingness or ability to learn health management behaviors. Some people perceive that life events are controlled by external forces such as chance, fate, or other people. These people are conceived of as possessing an external **locus of control (LOC).** Other people perceive life as being controlled by their own actions. These people are conceived of as possessing an internal locus of control (Rotter, 1954). Until the last decade LOC was considered a trait characteristic; that is, a characteristic of the personality. However, more recent studies indicate that LOC is state specific; that is, situationally bound. Individuals may have internal LOC in some situations and external LOC in others (Lazarus & Folkman, 1984; Rotter, 1975).

Nursing Process (Anxiety, Powerlessness, and Disturbance in Self-Esteem) Nursing Diagnosis: Anxiety

Anxiety is a vague, uneasy feeling with a nonspecific or unknown source (Townsend, 1997, p. 207). **Characteristics** and indicators that might indicate that a client is at risk for actual or potential problem with anxiety (indicators will be related to level of anxiety experienced by the client):

- The client demonstrates physical symptoms (sympathetic arousal) of anxiety.
- The client expresses feelings of apprehension or tension.
- The client is restless and experiences difficulty in resting and sleeping.
- The client has difficulty concentrating and attending.
- The client focuses on the issues of concern with little attention to other issues.
- The client expresses feelings of inadequacy, distress, or helplessness.

Assessment

Areas to be included when assessing whether the client has an actual or potential problem with anxiety are as follows:

- The client's feelings of anxiety (overt and covert)
- The effects of illness, injury, disease, or disability on the client's ability to meet personal needs and fulfill role expectations

- Stressful situations experienced since the onset of the illness, injury, disease, or disability
- Past methods for dealing with anxiety
- Presence of signs or physiological (sympathetic) arousal (see Table 2)

Interventions

Nursing interventions will be determined by the nature of the client's anxiety and the degree of anxiety experienced by the client. General interventions could include

- Developing a trusting, consistent relationship between client and nurse/staff
- Approaching the client in a reassuring, calm, and nonjudgmental manner
- Creating a relaxed environment with an appropriate level of sensory stimulation
- Encouraging the expression of thoughts and feelings
- Exploring the experience precipitating feelings of anxiety
- Providing feedback regarding the client's behavior indicating anxiety
- Teaching the client and family members problem-solving techniques
- Helping the client and family members to identify long-term coping strategies
- Providing an appropriate amount of information and stimulation given the client's level of anxiety
- Encouraging the client and family members to be involved in social activities, and personal interests and hobbies
- Providing instruction on stress reduction and relaxation techniques
- Encouraging development of assertive communication skills

Outcomes

The long-term outcome of nursing interventions for the client experiencing actual or potential anxiety is that the client will be able to recognize the sources of anxiety, the onset of anxiety, and strategies to manage high levels of anxiety.

Expected Outcomes

- The client will experience a decrease in feelings of anxiety.
- The client and family will be able to identify the sources of perceived threats and stress-inducing situations.
- The client and family will implement adaptive, approach strategies to deal with stress-inducing situations.
- The client will experience increased physiological and psychological comfort.

Nursing Diagnosis: Powerlessness

Powerlessness is a perceived lack of control over a situation and belief that actions will not significantly affect outcome (Townsend, 1997, p. 35). **Characteristics** and indicators that the client might be at risk for actual or potential problems with powerlessness:

- The client expresses a sense of having no control or influence over life events or the course of illness, recovery, or self-care management.
- The client expresses feelings of despair, hopelessness, and helplessness.
- The client is unwilling or unable to participate in decision-making activities or self-care management.
- The client exhibits acting-out behaviors, aggressiveness toward others, hostility, or anger.
- The client expresses feelings of apathy, resignation, and passivity or depression.
- The client does not seek information about care or treatment options.
- The client demonstrates dependency on others.

Assessment

A diagnosis of powerlessness cannot be made from the nurse's perception of the client and the situation. Powerlessness is a subjective experience and can be determined only by assessing the client's perception of power and control. Assessment areas of concern in assessing powerlessness are as follows:

- The client's feelings and perceptions regarding the illness, injury, disease, or disability
- The perceived effects of the illness, injury, disease, or disability on the client's life and lifestyle
- The client's feelings and perceptions of lack of control over life and life events
- The client's locus of control (internal or external) regarding health and health issues
- Those situations that the client thinks can be controlled
- Those situations that the client thinks cannot be controlled
- The client's past methods of dealing with difficulties
- The client's successful coping strategies
- The client's present method of dealing with difficulties brought on by illness or injury

Interventions

Nursing intervention will be determined by the degree of powerlessness being experienced by the client. General interventions could include

- Creating an environment that promotes independent behavior and responsibility
- Creating a sheltered environment to promote client independence
- Promoting client and family participation in care
- Encouraging the client to create a personalized space
- Helping the client to express feelings about health state, concerns, and involvement in self-care managment
- Promoting healthy risk-taking behavior
- Helping to develop decision-making strategies by providing opportunities to make decisions
- Respecting and supporting decisions made by the client

- Helping the client distinguish between situations that can be controlled and those that cannot be controlled
- Setting short-term and long-term goals that are attainable by the client
- Assisting the client in the identification and development of strengths and coping strategies for health management

Outcomes

The outcome of nursing interventions for the client experiencing powerlessness is that the client increases expectations that personal actions and efforts can bring about desired effects and that life events can be controlled.

Expected Outcomes

- The client will be able to identify those factors and events in life that can be controlled.
- The client demonstrates increased control of situations and outcomes.
- The client demonstrates an increased involvement and understanding of care and the treatment regimen.
- The client actively participates in decision-making about care and treatment.
- The client demonstrates health management behaviors.

Nursing Diagnosis: Self-Esteem

Disturbance in self-esteem is a negative self-evaluation and feelings about self-capabilities (Townsend, 1997, p. 300). **Characteristics** and indicators that the client is at risk for an actual or potential disturbance in self-esteem:

- The client expresses a negative self-assessment: He or she evaluates self as unable to deal with events.
- The client has difficulty accepting positive feedback.
- The client minimizes strengths and abilities.
- The client demonstrates a failure to care for self.
- The client expresses feelings of inadequacy, worthlessness, helplessness.
- The client fails to follow through on assignments or tasks.
- The client sets unreasonable, unrealistic standards for self.
- The client has a preoccupation with failure.
- The client is hypersensitive to slights or criticism.
- The client degrades others in an attempt to increase own feelings of self-worth.
- The client is grandiose.
- The client controls others through manipulation.
- The client is unable to communicate directly to have needs met and has difficulty seeking assistance from others.

Assessment

Areas to be included when assessing whether the client has an actual or potential disturbance in self-esteem are as follows:

- The client's perceptions of self since the onset of illness or injury
- The client's perceptions of the impact of illness and injury on previous roles and lifestyle
- The client's assessment of strengths or capabilities

Interventions

Nursing interventions will be determined by the nature of the client's actual or potential disturbance in self-esteem. General interventions could include

- Assisting the client with self-care as necessary and encouraging independent performance of personal responsibilities and decision-making
- Assisting the client in identifying positive aspects of self
- Promoting the client's involvement in self-care
- Negotiating short-term realistic goals that allow the client to experience success
- Acknowledging the client's feelings and supporting the client in confronting fears and undertaking new tasks
- Not allowing the client to ruminate on past failures
- Minimizing negative feedback
- Providing a consistent, respectful, honest approach to promote trust development
- Inspiring reality-based hope
- Promoting humor
- Accepting the client with unconditional positive regard
- Providing the client with information necessary to engage in self-care and self-management
- Encouraging the client's participation in decision-making

Outcomes

The outcomes of nursing interventions for clients experiencing a disturbance in self-esteem are that the client will experience an increase in feelings of self-worth and a decrease in feelings of failure.

Expected Outcomes

- The client will initiate self-care health management activities.
- The client will communicate feelings and needs in an assertive manner.
- The client sets and achieves realistic goals.
- The client demonstrates self-valuing behaviors.
- The client discusses fears of failure.
- The client verbalizes positive aspects of self.
- The client verbalizes thoughts and feelings spontaneously.
- The client participates in social and therapeutic activities.

Conclusion

The psychology of disability is no different than the psychology of being human. The disabled client does have to cope with more unusual stimuli than the nondisabled person. These stimuli can be biological, social, or economic. Clients in rehabilitation, and those with disabilities, tend to experience a disproportionately large number of frustrations and difficulties in problem solving; they encounter more situations of nonacceptance, prejudice, and devaluation than the nondisabled; and they can experience difficulty in developing realistic and healthy self-concepts. Five traits are necessary for the development of self-esteem: a sense of significance, a sense of competence, a sense of connectedness balanced with separateness, a sense of realism about ourselves, and a set of ethics and values.

Self-esteem affects all aspects of life and is the key to behavior, feeling, thinking, values, and goals. A positive sense of self-esteem makes it possible for the individual to face life demands with confidence. Rehabilitative nursing is influential in creating an environment that facilitates reintegration of the self and successful function within the family and reentry into the community. Clients must learn to distinguish between those things that can or cannot be controlled to lessen feelings of helplessness or powerlessness. They must also be assisted in developing a realistic perception of who can and who cannot control events in their lives. Most important, clients must be empowered to have control over their own lives.

References

Arnold, E. N., & Boggs, V. B. (1995). *Interpersonal relationships: Communication skills for nurses.* Philadelphia: W. B. Saunders.

Bandura, A. (1977). *Social learning theory.* Englewood Cliffs, NJ: Prentice-Hall.

Carson, V. B., & Arnold, E. N. (1996). *Mental health nursing: The nurse-patient journey.* Philadelphia: W. B. Saunders.

Dudley, J. (1983). *Living with stigma: The plight of the people who we label mentally retarded.* Springfield, IL: Charles C Thomas.

Dugas, B. (1983). *Introduction to patient care: A comprehensive approach to nursing* (4th ed.). Philadelphia: W. B. Saunders.

Eisenberg, M. G., Sutkin, L. C., & Jansen, M. A. (Eds.). (1984). *Chronic illness and disability through the life span: Effects on self and family.* New York: Springer.

Farley, A. M. (1992). *Nursing and the disabled across the life span.* Boston: Jones & Bartlett.

Goffman, E. (1963). *Stigma: Notes on management of spoiled identity.* Englewood Cliffs, NJ: Prentice-Hall.

Hamburg, D. A. (1974). Coping behaviors in life-threatening circumstances. *Psychotherapy and Psychosomatics, 23,* 13–25.

Katz, I. (1981). *Stigma: A social psychological analysis.* Hillsdale, NJ: Lawrence Erlbaum and Associates.

Kritek, P. B. (1994). *Negotiating at an uneven table: Developing moral courage in resolving our conflicts.* San Francisco: Jossey-Bass.

Lazarus, R. S., & Folkman, S. (1984). *Stress, appraisal, and coping.* New York: Springer.

Marinelli, R. P., & Dell Orto, A. E. (Eds.). (1984). *The psychological & social impact of physical disability* (2nd ed.). New York: Springer.

May, R. (1950). *The meaning of anxiety.* New York: Ronald Press.

Peplau, H. (1963). A working definition of anxiety. In S. Burd & M. Marchall (Eds.), *Some clinical approaches to psychiatric nursing* (pp. 323–327). New York: Macmillan.

Rieser, P. A. (1992). Educational, psychological, and social aspects of short stature. *Journal of Pediatric Health Care, 6*(5), 325–334.

Rotter, J. B. (1975). Some problems and misconceptions related to the construct of internal versus external control of reinforcement. *Journal of Consulting and Clinical Psychology, 43,* 54–67.

Rotter, J. B. (1954). *Social learning and clinical psychology.* Englewood Cliffs, NJ: Prentice-Hall.

Saylor, C. (1995). Stigma. In I. M. Lubkin (Ed.), *Chronic illness: Impact and interventions* (3rd ed., pp. 99–116). Boston: Jones & Bartlett.

Sandford, L., & Donovan, M. E. (1984). *Women and self-esteem.* New York: Penguin Books.

Seeman, M. (1959). On the meaning of alienation. *American Sociological Review, 24,* 783–791.

Seligman, M. (1975). *Helplessness: On depression, development, and death.* San Francisco: Freeman.

Seligman, M. (1991). *Learned optimism.* New York: Alfred A. Knopf.

Sims, A. (1993). The scar that is more than skin deep: The stigma of depression. *British Journal of General Practice, 43*(366), 30–31.

Townsend, M. C. (1997). *Nursing diagnoses in psychiatric nursing: A pocket guide for care plan construction* (4th ed.). Philadelphia: F. A. Davis.

Webster's Third New International Dictionary (1986). Springfield, MA: G. & C. Merriam.

CHAPTER 10
Stress and Coping

Patricia A. Chin

Key Terms
Acute Stress
Anger
Chronic Stress
Coping
Fight-Flight Response
Ineffective Coping
Relaxation Response
Social Isolation
Stress
Stress Appraisal
Stress Inoculation
Stress Management
Stressors
Stress Response

Objectives

1. Discuss the concepts of stress, stress response, and relaxation response.

2. Discuss the various stressors confronting the client and family in the rehabilitation setting.

3. Discuss the concept of coping, strategies to facilitate coping, and stress inoculation.

4. Discuss the relationship between stress and coping in rehabilitation clients.

5. Identify assessment areas for determining if the rehabilitation client or family is at risk for an actual or potential problem with ineffective coping.

6. Identify nursing interventions for assisting the rehabilitation client or family with an actual or potential problem with ineffective coping.

7. Identify expected outcomes of the nursing interventions used to assist the rehabilitation client or family with an actual or potential problem with ineffective coping.

Stress

Stress and adaptation are necessary for life. Not all stress is bad; some degree of stress is necessary for adaptation to the demands of everyday life (Selye, 1956). Selye identified human responses to stress as fight-or-flight reactions. Selye's theory of stress details a set of universal physiological reactions generated when a person is confronted with stimuli involving fear or anxiety. Stress is defined as a nonspecific response of the body to any demand made on it. It does not matter if the demand on the body is pleasant (preparing for a wedding) or unpleasant (preparing for surgery). Stress is the result of factors that cause worry, anxiety, or strain. Stress is present each time a person must adapt or adjust to personal, social, and environmental influence (Pelletier, 1977).

Two kinds of stress were identified by Pelletier (1977): **acute stress,** which occurs when the threat is immediate and the need to respond instantaneous, and **chronic stress,** which occurs when the threat is prolonged and unabated. In the rehabilitation setting clients are exposed to both kinds of stress. Clients are confronted with many stressful situations, increasing the demands for adaptive behavior above and beyond the level required by people not experiencing rehabilitation. The majority of the stressful events are unpleasant. All stress needs to be counterbalanced through adjustment and adaptation to preserve adaptive energy. Brown (1977) pointed out that stress aggravates all types of illness or injuries and that stress can seriously affect recovery from illness.

All people are exposed to general or social **stressors** to some degree. Common stressors in everyday life include living and working conditions, the constant influx of information, the pace of everyday life, and increased social mobility (Pelletier, 1977). Stress of everyday life is critically compounded when the person experiences a change in health state or injury. Exposure to additional stressors will occur throughout the rehabilitation process. Each demand for adaptation and adjustment is associated with varying degrees of stress (Goodwin, 1984; Holmes & Rahe, 1967).

Stress Response

An innate **stress response** is triggered in humans when they are confronted with acute or chronic stress. The **fight–flight response** results in an increase in blood pressure, heart rate, respiratory rate, blood flow to the muscles, and metabolism. These physical responses are what prepares the person for action. What occurs to the body during chronic stress was described by Selye (1956) in the three stages of the general adaptation syndrome. During the *alarm stage,* the body responds to the stressor in the typical manner. If the resistance of the client is diminished, or if the stressor is strong, death may result. If the exposure to the stressor continues and is compatible with adaptation, resistance occurs. This is the *stage of resistance.* If the body must continue to adapt to the stressor, eventually adaptation energy will become exhausted. This is the *stage of exhaustion.*

The signs of the alarm reaction reappear but now they are irreversible and the individual dies (Potter & Perry, 1993; Selye, 1956). The effects of chronic stress on the client will be influenced by factors of heredity, environment, general health habits, behavioral variables, and past illnesses and experiences with stress (Pelletier, 1977).

There is also a **relaxation response,** which serves as an innate physiological response to counterbalance the stress response. The relaxation response can be consciously triggered and can be used to prevent stress and restore the client's adaptive energy. The relaxation response is a protective mechanism against overstress (Benson & Klipper, 1976). The relaxation response results include a decrease in the rate of breathing, heart rate, and metabolism; a reduction in perceived stress, and the return of the body to a healthier balance. Clients can be taught how to trigger the relaxation response. The response can be triggered by consciously engaging in activities such as meditation, yoga, visualization, biofeedback, progressive relaxation, and hypnosis on a daily basis (Goodwin, 1984).

Stress Response in Rehabilitation of Rehabilitation Clients

From the very beginning of illness, injury, disease, or disability the person is in a state of conflict. Stress is present in the onset, development, recovery, and resulting disability of almost every rehabilitation client. Each time the client is confronted with a new need to adjust or adapt he or she will experience stress. Stress is associated with hospitalization, surgery, and the transitions experienced when entering and leaving rehabilitation centers and other settings. Stress can occur when the rehabilitation client is required to seek assistance from rehabilitation agencies. Meeting the demands of agency procedures can pose numerous stress-provoking situations for the client. Social barriers, prejudiced attitudes, and the restriction of mobility caused by architectural barriers also cause stress for the rehabilitation client.

Too much stress is harmful to health. Helping the rehabilitation client to cope with the stress associated with the many demands of physical, social, family, psychological, sexual, and environmental adjustments is an important task for the rehabilitation nurse. The rehabilitation nurse needs to possess skill to assist the client in coping with life's uncertainties and improve the quality of life.

The stress associated with adjustment during rehabilitation also affects family members. In early studies of the effect on the family of stress associated with disability, Marra and Novis (1959) found that among disabled husbands and fathers the principal changes in family relationship were as follows: (1) wives had to assume greater responsibilities for home management; (2) social and recreational activities were reduced; (3) children assumed more household duties; (4) debt was incurred; (5) plans for a larger family had to be changed; (6) wives had to obtain employment; (7) there was increased marital discord; (8) children's educational plans had to be changed; and (9) a change in living accommodations was required. Not all rehabilitation clients or their family members learn to cope and adapt successfully to the stress associated with illness, injury, disease, or disability. The results can include extreme family disruption or even severing of the family unit.

Individuals involved in the rehabilitation process and their families are usually unprepared for the demands and adjustments required of them. These demands can be physical, psychological, social, and/or spiritual. The adjustments and adaptation can be difficult, seemingly unending, and can cause severe physical and emotional pain and discomfort. All of those involved in the rehabilitation process will probably experience frustration, rejections, socially imposed limitations, threats to self-concept, and insecurity. It is the role of the members of the treatment team to assist individuals and their families to deal effectively with these experiences and progress to productive and fulfilling lives.

Stress Appraisal

Stress appraisal refers to the evaluative cognitive processes that intervene between the encountering of stress and the reactions to stress. It is through the use of cognitive appraisal processes that clients evaluate the significance of life events to their well-being. Appraisal processes shape the reaction of the client to any encounter. Lazarus and Folkman (1984) identified three types of cognitive appraisal to stressful events: primary appraisal, secondary appraisal, and reappraisal.

When the client makes a *primary appraisal* of a stressful event a determination is made concerning whether the event is irrelevant, benign-positive, or stressful (Lazarus & Folkman, 1984). There are three forms of stressful appraisals: harm/loss (damage that has already occurred), threat (anticipated harms and losses), and challenge (possibilities for growth and mastery). A *secondary appraisal* is a judgment of what might and can be done (Lazarus & Folkman, 1984). The client judges whether a particular coping option will be useful and evaluates the consequences of using a particular coping option. *Reappraisal* follows appraisals and refers to a changed appraisal that the client makes on the basis of new information from the environment or from others (Lazarus & Folkman, 1984). Clients will take action on the basis of their appraisal of the event for their life. Cognitive appraisal processes are not always conscious and it is not always easy to access or to shape the appraisal processes.

Stress appraisal is influenced and determined by personal factors and situational factors. Personal factors include commitment and belief. Commitment and belief determine what the client judges as important for well-being, for shaping the person's understanding of the event, and for providing the basis for evaluating outcomes. The situational factors influencing appraisal include the novelty of the event or stressor, predictability, uncertainty, ambiguity, and timing of the event or stressor (Lazarus & Folkman, 1984).

Coping

Coping is a dynamic process initiated in response to internal, external, or system changes that alter or place stress on the individual or the ecological system (Lazarus & Folkman, 1984). Stress can be the result of development or situational events. Acute, traumatic, and chronic stressors can elicit differing coping behaviors. A client can be attempting to cope with life stress with multiple combinations of coping behaviors and strategies at the same time. Client's coping mechanisms are dynamic and ongoing, 24 hours per day throughout the life span. The need to cope changes with the client's status or perceptions of life events.

The manner in which the client handles stress and the outcomes to exposure to stressful events will depend on several variables, including family and social support, and the client's individual strengths and needs. Four primary factors influencing the nature of the client's coping strategies are the client's premorbid personality and adjustment strategies; developmental state; meaning of the illness, injury, disease, or disability to the client and family members; and available social supports.

Coping behaviors serve to relieve stress, protect self-esteem, and assist the client in handling problems connected with the stress of illness, injury, disease, or disability (Lazarus & Folkman, 1984). Coping behaviors are manifested through cognitive function, motor actions, effective responses, and psychological defense mechanisms. Coping constitutes all of the ways in which the client attempts to minimize threats to personal integrity and emotional equilibrium while simultaneously maximizing body function (Kahn, 1995; Lazarus & Folkman, 1984). The manner and degree to which coping behaviors are used vary among clients. Some clients need only a few psychological coping mechanisms to deal with a stressful situation, others require a great many coping mechanisms, and some clients will not be able to cope with stress no matter how many coping strategies they attempt to use.

Coping strategies are behaviors the client uses to reduce stress. These can include walking, running, swimming, reading, gardening, yelling, shouting, crying, slamming doors, throwing things, breaking things, speeding while driving a car, painting, praying, taking a hot bath or shower, abusing substances, and so on. The client's health state and functioning in rehabilitation may prohibit the use of the client's previous effective coping strategies. They may need assistance to identify and develop new, alternative coping strategies. Client coping behaviors commonly used fall into one of four behavioral patterns:

- Adaptive growth-producing behaviors that incorporate problem-solving strategies. *Examples:* Information seeking, asking questions

- Withdrawal and avoidance. *Examples:* Denial, social isolation, regression, loneliness, depression, and rejection
- Acting out. *Examples:* Anger, hostility, suspicion
- Somatization. *Examples:* Gastric ulcers, headaches

The last three patterns are considered maladaptive because they will not result in the client's increased management of stress and stressful situations. Acting out, withdrawal and avoidance, and somatic complaint are actually avoidance tactics. Their use will not facilitate client growth or long-term coping (Carson & Arnold, 1996).

Coping strategies and methods are considered to be effective (successful or adaptive) when the discomfort and disturbance associated with the stressor resolves, if the physical integrity of the client is preserved, if the client can maintain relationships and life role, and if a positive self-concept is maintained. Coping strategies are productive if they can facilitate new behavioral responses for effective future problem solving or ways of adapting to change.

Ineffective coping refers to unsuccessful and/or maladaptive coping strategies and methods, such as when essential treatment is delayed or not sought by the client, when coping attempts cause the client more distress than the initial stressor, or when the coping strategies impede activities of daily living or cause the client to abandon usual sources of gratification (Senescu, 1963). Ineffective coping strategies may temporarily alleviate the response to stress; however, client growth will not occur. The inadequacy of previous coping strategies may become the incentive for readiness to change. When unresolved stress occurs clients may regard any change as preferable to the anxiety, fatigue, and sense of powerlessness created by the crisis (Aguilera, 1994). Evaluation of ineffective coping strategies is very subjective and the nurse should not use personal values to judge what constitutes ineffective coping.

Clients can be inoculated against stress. **Stress inoculation** is a cognitive coping intervention. Stress inoculation techniques prepare clients to cope with upcoming stressful situations. Stress inoculation is incorporated into peri-operative teaching. Discussing the various stages of peri-operative care, pain experience, the surgical environment, and wound care and management before an event assists the client to prepare for the upcoming event. It can alter the client's perceptions of the stress and the event. When promoting coping skills during client interactions it is essential to teach the client that growth and change are processes and that coping skills are needed to make lasting changes (Carson & Arnold, 1996). Effective coping behaviors will be easier to develop in individuals who have hardiness characteristics, who have an internal locus of control, and who are undaunted by change (Wallston & Wallston, 1982).

Nursing Process (Ineffective Coping—Individual; Ineffective Coping—Family; Ineffective Coping—Anger; Social Isolation) Nursing Diagnosis: Ineffective Coping—Individual

Ineffective coping (individual) is the impairment of adaptive behaviors and abilities in meeting life's demands and roles (Townsend, 1997, p. 294). **Characteristics** or indicators that might indicate that a client is at risk for actual or potential problems with ineffective individual coping:

- The client demonstrates an inability to meet role expectation.
- The client demonstrates an alteration in societal participation.
- The client demonstrates an inability to solve problems.
- The client demonstrates increased dependency.
- The client demonstrates a change in communication patterns.
- The client demonstrates an inability to meet basic needs.
- The client demonstrates physiological signs of stress.
- The client has an increased vulnerability to illness.
- The client demonstrates an inability to meet age-related role tasks or societal expectations.
- The client demonstrates destructive behaviors toward self or others.
- The client demonstrates the following behaviors: withdrawal, hyperactivity, denial, acting out behavior, avoidance behaviors.

Interventions

Nursing interventions will be determined by the nature of the client's ineffective coping and the degree of stress experienced by the client. General interventions could include

- Maintaining a safe environment for the client
- Assessing the client's coping skills: identifying ineffective coping and the degree of impairment
- Promoting and reinforcing problem-solving and coping behaviors and techniques
- Educating the client about the crisis or stress and its effect on the client
- Reinforcing important decision-making efforts
- Improving the client's self-esteem level and sense of self-efficacy
- Maintaining hope and empowerment
- Promoting strengthening of family and social support systems
- Teaching the client and family members stress management techniques
- Teaching the client and family members techniques to reduce the stress response and trigger the relaxation response:
  Relaxation techniques
  Reframing perceptions
  Participating in previously gratifying activities
  Meditation, yoga, visualization, biofeedback, progressive relaxation, and hypnosis
- Avoiding the reinforcement of client's dependent behaviors
- "Inoculating" the client and family against upcoming stress

Outcomes

The outcome of nursing interventions for clients experiencing ineffective individual coping is that the client will identify, develop, and use effective, growth-producing long-term coping skills.

Expected Outcomes

- The client gives evidence of improvement in coping skills and tolerance for stress.
- The client expresses increased psychological and physiological comfort.
- The client gives evidence of improvement in problem-solving and decision-making skills.
- The client is able to solve problems and fulfill activities of daily living independently.

Nursing Diagnosis: Ineffective Coping—Family

Ineffective coping (family) is when a significant other's behavior disables the client's capacity to address effectively tasks essential to adaptation (Gordon, 1993). **Characteristics** and indicators that might indicate that the family is at risk for an actual or potential problem with ineffective family coping:

- The family neglects the client's basic needs.
- The family denies or avoids assistance, or neglects obtaining care.
- The family rejects, abandons, or deserts the client.
- The family engages in detrimental or interfering actions or decisions related to client welfare.
- The family process is disorganized, disintegrated, and dysfunctional.
- The family experiences disruption of structure, role functions, communication patterns, interpersonal relationships, and socialization function.
- The family demonstrates maladaptive coping behaviors: blaming or fault finding, aggression, depression, abuse, hostility, stigmatizing.
- The family demonstrates a lack of understanding or interest in the treatment plan.
- The family is overprotective.
- The family has closed boundaries and limited or no social support network.

Assessment

Areas to be included when assessing to determine if the family has an actual or potential problem with ineffective coping are as follows:

- The family's communication pattern
- The family's previous experiences with stress and coping strategies used to combat stress
- The family's perceptions of the current stressful event and environment
- The degree of interest and involvement in the client's care and treatment plan
- The nature of relationships among family members
- The nature of the family's social support network

- The impact of the client's change in health state on the various members of the family and on family functions and structure

Interventions

Nursing interventions will be determined by the nature of the family's ineffective coping and the degree of stress experienced by the family. General interventions could include

- Helping the family verbalize perceptions of and knowledge about the stressor
- Encouraging the family to clarify approaches to coping and adaptation
- Encouraging the family's active involvement in the therapeutic treatment plan and the therapeutic alliance
- Identifying family barriers to developing effective coping strategies
- Educating family members in techniques to reduce the stress response and trigger the relaxation response:
  Relaxation techniques, reframing perceptions
  Participating in previously gratifying activities
  Meditation, yoga, visualization, biofeedback, progressive relaxation, and hypnosis
- "Inoculating" the client and family against upcoming stress

Outcomes

The outcome of nursing interventions for the family experiencing ineffective coping is that the family will identify, develop, and use effective, growth-producing long-term coping skills.

Expected Outcomes

- The family expresses realistic understanding, expectations, and support for individual members.
- The family develops realistic goals and means for achieving them through problem-solving techniques.
- The family demonstrates positive family coping.
- The family maintains its functions and structure, modified to adapt to the current life experience.
- Family members attain stage-related developmental tasks.
- The family is empowered and capable of dealing with rehabilitation-related stressors.
- Family members recognize potential problems or changes and seek preventive assistance.
- The family demonstrates techniques to reduce the stress response and trigger the relaxation response:
  Relaxation techniques, reframing perceptions
  Participating in previously gratifying activities
  Meditation, yoga, visualization, biofeedback, progressive relaxation, and hypnosis

Nursing Diagnosis: Ineffective Coping—Anger

Ineffective coping (anger) is a state in which an individual acts out feelings of rage, aggression, and hostility when dealing with stress. **Characteristics** or indicators that might indicate that a client is at risk for an actual or potential problem with **anger:**

- The client demonstrates behaviors of aggression:
  Increased motor activity, agitation, pacing, fidgeting
  Rigid posture, clenched fists and jaw
  Angry facial expression, staring or lack of eye contact
  Extreme quiet
- The client verbalizes anger and aggression:
  Argumentative, shouts profanities
  Repeats demands, requests, complaints
  Makes false accusations, expresses fear of loss of control
- The client engages in pushing and shoving or hitting
- The client slams door, throws or breaks objects

Assessment

Areas to be included when assessing to determine if the client has an actual or potential problem with ineffective coping (anger) are as follows:

- The client's verbalization of feelings of anger or hostility, disappointment, hurt, irritation, or rage
- The client's physiological responses of anger
- How the client handles objects in the environment
- Type of interactions client has with family, friends, and staff

Intervention

Nursing interventions will be determined by the nature of the client's ineffective coping and the degree of stress experienced by the client. General interventions could include

- Providing constructive outlets for energy of anger
- Setting limits on the expression of anger
- Reducing sources of stress and anger
- Acknowledging the client's feelings of anger
- Helping the client to recognize the feelings of anger
- Encouraging the client to describe feelings of anger
- Teaching the client conflict resolution strategies
- Teaching the client anger management strategies
- Teaching the client assertiveness skills
- "Inoculating" the client against upcoming stress

Outcomes

The outcome of nursing interventions for the client experiencing anger is that the client will identify, develop, and use effective, growth-producing long-term coping skills.

Expected Outcomes
- The client will verbalize the use of new coping behaviors.
- The client will describe behavioral signs of anger.
- The client will demonstrate anger management techniques.
- The client will demonstrate techniques to reduce the stress response and trigger the relaxation response:
  Relaxation techniques, reframing perceptions
  Participating in previously gratifying activities
  Meditation, yoga, visualization, biofeedback, progressive relaxation, and hypnosis
- The client will demonstrate effective coping techniques to deal with anger.

Nursing Diagnosis: Social Isolation

Social isolation is a condition of aloneness experienced by the client (Townsend, 1997, p. 214). **Characteristics** and indicators that might indicate that a client is at risk for an actual or potential problem with **social isolation:**

- The client exhibits a sad, dull affect.
- The client expresses loneliness or feelings of rejection.
- The client is uncommunicative and withdrawn, avoids eye contact, stays alone in his or her room.
- The client demonstrates angry, hostile, irritable behaviors.
- The client appears insecure in public.
- The client maintains a low level of contact with family, peers, and staff.
- The client expresses feelings of being different from others.

Assessment

Areas to be included when assessing to determine if the client has an actual or potential problem with social isolation are as follows:

- Client's ability to cope with and adapt to life changes
- Environmental barriers or socioeconomic factors that might not permit socialization
- Feelings of inferiority and rejection
- Level of hardiness and self-esteem
- Client's past coping strategies
- Number of social interactions and nature of those interactions
- Amount of time spent alone
- Symptoms of depression

Interventions

Nursing interventions will be determined by the nature of the client's social isolation and the degree of stress experienced by the client. General interventions could include

- Involving the client and family in setting goals for making decisions about care
- Encouraging activities and interaction through recreational therapy
- Identifying and involving the client with successful role models
- Involving the client with those who have shared interests
- Providing an environment conducive to interpersonal interaction
- Inviting the client and family to support group activities
- Conveying an accepting attitude
- "Inoculating" the client and family against upcoming stress

Outcomes

The outcome of nursing interventions for the client experiencing social isolation is that the client will demonstrate a willingness and desire to interact with others in a meaningful way.

Expected Outcomes

- The client participates in activities that support vocational, educational, recreational, and social needs.
- The client communicates feelings regarding resocialization.
- The client communicates feelings regarding loneliness.
- The client voluntarily approaches others and attends group activities.

References

Aguilera, D. (1994). *Crisis intervention: Theory and methodology* (7th ed.). St. Louis: Mosby–Year Book.

Benson, H., & Klipper, M. Z. (1976). *The relaxation response.* New York: Avon.

Brown, B. (1977). Biofeedback. *Journal of Holistic Health, 2,* 29–32.

Carson, V. B., & Arnold, E. N. (1996). *Mental health nursing: The nurse-patient journey.* Philadelphia: W. B. Saunders.

Goodwin, L. R. (1984). Stress management for rehabilitation clients. In R. P. Marinelli & A. E. Dell Orto (Eds.), *The psychological & social impact of physical disability.* (2nd ed., pp. 339–347). New York: Springer.

Gordon, M. (1993). *Manual of nursing diagnosis 1993–1994.* St. Louis: Mosby–Year Book.

Holmes, T. H., & Rahe, R. H. (1967). The social readjustment rating scale. *Journal of Psychosomatic Research, 2,* 213–218.

Kahn, A. M. (1995). Coping with fear and grieving. In I. M. Lubkin, *Chronic illness impact and interventions.* (3rd ed., pp. 241–260). Boston: Jones and Bartlett Publishers.

Lazarus, R. S., & Folkman, S. (1984). *Stress, appraisal, and coping.* New York: Springer.

Marra, J., & Novis, F. (1959). Family problems in rehabilitation counseling. *Personnel and Guidance Journal, 38,* 40–42.

Pelletier, K. R. (1977). *Mind as healer, mind as slayer: A holistic approach to preventing stress disorders.* New York: Dell/Delta Books.

Potter, P. A., & Perry, A. G. (1993). *Fundamentals of nursing concepts, process & practice*. St. Louis: Mosby–Year Book.

Selye, H. (1956). *The stress of life*. New York: McGraw-Hill.

Senescu, M. E. (1963). The development of emotional complications in the patient with cancer. *Journal of Chronic Diseases, 16,* 813–832.

Townsend, M. C. (1997). *Nursing diagnoses in psychiatric nursing: A pocket guide for care plan construction* (4th ed.). Philadelphia: F. A. Davis.

Wallston, K. A., & Wallston, B. S. (1982). Who is responsible for your health? The construct of locus of control. In G. S. Sanders & J. Suls (Eds.), *Social psychology of health and illness* (pp. 65–95). Hillsdale, NJ: Lawrence Erlbaum and Associates.

CHAPTER 11

Body Image

Patricia A. Chin

Key Terms   *Affective Body Image*
Body Boundaries
Body Image Disturbance
Body Image Reconstruction
Cognitive Body Image
Physical Body Image

Objectives   1. Discuss the concept of body image.

2. Discuss factors influencing the perception of body image.

3. Discuss normal growth and developmental changes on the evolution of body image.

4. Discuss factors influencing body image alteration and adaptation to alteration.

5. Describe the stages of body image reconstruction following an alteration in body image.

6. Identify characteristics or indicators that are indicative of a disturbance in body image.

7. Identify assessment data associated with disturbance in body image.

8. Identify specific nursing interventions appropriate for clients with disturbances in body image.

9. Identify the expected outcomes of the interventions focused on the client problems of disturbance in body image.

Body Image   *Body image* is defined as the conscious and unconscious mental picture that a person has of the shape, the size, and the mass of the body and its parts. As discussed in Chapter 9, body image is one aspect of the individual's concept of self. Body image can exert a strong influence over the other aspects of the self: self-esteem, self-confidence, and personal identity. Body image serves as a subjective frame of reference when relating to others or when relating to the physical and social environment. Body image can influence emotions, attitudes, and personality. The reactions and attitudes that other people have about us can also be influenced by body image (Bramble, 1995).

Body image is the way clients perceive themselves and the way they think others perceive them. Body image involves the client's view of the physical structure of the body. It is a mental snapshot that individuals carry around with them. Unlike a photograph, however, body image is not one-dimensional. It is a multiple-dimensional construct. Body image involves more than just the body's physical appearance. It also involves bodily functioning, bodily sensations, bodily mobility, and feelings and thoughts. Body image is composed of three specific dimensions. The dimensions of body image are as follows:

physical body image—One's perception of being an object in space
cognitive body image—The way one thinks about and evaluates the body
affective body image—One's emotional experience based on beliefs and feelings about the body

The physical, cognitive, and affective body images are formed from the client's past experiences in the physical and social environments. Each aspect of body image is influenced by the perceptions, actions, and reactions of others toward the client as well as developmental conditions, and changes in the body due to health, injury, and illness. Body image develops as a response to sensory input (visual, tactile, proprioceptive, and kinesthetic) from both the client's internal environment and the external environment. Factors that can influence the client's perceived body image include the client's previous perceptions of bodily appearance and intactness, the client's degree of interest in or preoccupation with the care and development of the body, and society's perceptions of beauty and wholeness (Farley, 1992). When any aspect of a client's physical self is altered the fundamental view of the self can change.

Factors Influencing Perception of Body Image

Body image is influenced by perceived body boundaries, the culture into which the individual is socialized, and internal and external factors. Interpersonal relationships with others are also influential in the development of body image.

Body Boundaries. **Body boundaries** determine how the external body is separated from the external environment. Body boundaries are important for movement through the external environment and determination of spatial and temporal relationships between the body and objects in the external environment. Body boundaries establish our territorial space and make it possible for clients to distinguish the inner self from the outside. These imaginary boundaries establish intimate, personal, social, and public distances that clients maintain in interpersonal relationships. Fisher (1974) noted that the more uncertain a person is about the protection provided by body borders the more that person will seek compensatory ways to reaffirm that border. When a client doubts his or her boundaries, attempts may be made to make the boundaries more visually intense. The client may use other means, such as clothing, decoration, or equipment, to emphasize the body.

It is the mental picture of the body and the perceptions of body boundaries that allow clients to navigate and maneuver successfully through the external environment. By reflecting on the body image, the client can determine whether movement can be performed safely and comfortably through a specific space or if an injury or discomfort may occur.

Culture. Culture influences body image by establishing the values, attitudes, and the desired norms and standards regarding physical appearance and behaviors. American culture values youth and beauty. A great deal of emphasis is placed on good looks, flawless complexions, and perfection. The athletic physique with its strength, suppleness, and grace is idolized. There is little tolerance of difference, imperfection, the need for assistive devices, or lack of muscle strength or motor coordination. Clients who perceive that they reflect the desired norms and standards feel good about the self. Those who perceive themselves to be different from what is desired feel inferior and unattractive.

Internal and External Factors. Internal factors include sensations that signal physiological occurrences within the body. Internal factors are signals from the body about its functioning. Most people can tell when they have an increase in body temperature. The internal signaling of sensations can be affected by disease, such as arthritis or diabetes mellitus. Many clients with diabetes mellitus report that they can perceive fluctuations in blood sugar levels. Women have reported an ability to determine the time of occurrence of ovulation. External factors that can influence the mental picture the client forms of the body can include weather conditions, light, clothing, anatomic structures, and topological experiences (e.g., touch, taste, and pain). A client who is required to wear a leg cast will experience an alteration in the perception of distance and movement through space, and bed-bound clients experience an alteration in time perceptions. A 5-minute time period is overestimated by clients who are immobilized.

Interpersonal Relationships. From infancy the attitudes and reactions of others can impact one's perception of self. Those individuals who can exert the most control over the budding body image include parents, caregivers, siblings, significant friends, and peers. Others who might significantly influence the person's body image include teachers, classmates, neighbors, and society as a whole. Unfortunately, many of the person's experiences with these individuals focus on superficial personal qualities (e.g., bodily appearance, weight, and shape). Orr, Reznikoff, and Smith (1989) observed that the more positive the opinions and attitudes held by others, the more likely the individual will be to develop a positive body image.

During the rehabilitation process clients are confronted with situations that will impact on their perceptions of body image. They may experience loss of an anatomical structure, loss of sensation, disfigurement, invasion of body boundaries, or the application of a cast, brace, or prosthetic device. All of these events may require an adjustment or modification in body image. This adjustment may be temporary or permanent, depending on the disease, illness, injury, or disability.

Developmental Issues and the Evolving Body Image

The mental image that the client has of the body serves several functions. Body image functions to provide the client with a sense of personal identity and can serve as a standard that the client uses to measure the ability to perform actions. Body image also functions as a measure to identify and demonstrate mastery of the world (Norris, 1987). Normal growth and development are factors that influence the formation of body image. Body image evolves through the maturational stages of normal development, infancy, childhood, adolescence, adulthood, and advanced age. The rehabilitation nurse needs to be aware of the normal developmental processes and their relationships to body image evolution to effectively assist clients to integrate their sensations, feelings, and perceptions into a realistic mental representation of their bodies that may be affected by illness, injury, disease, or disability.

Beginning in infancy, body image develops and changes over the life span. In infancy body boundaries are vague. At birth newborns have no concrete concept of body image. The body image forms as the infant begins to recognize itself as a distinct and separate being. That image continues to develop through interactions with caregivers and the external environment. Stimulation, especially tactile and kinesthetic, is critical for the development of body image (Cash & Pruzinsky, 1990) at all ages but particularly during infancy.

Childhood is a dramatic period in body image development, during which multiple rapid changes occur. Body image for the child focuses primarily on performance ability, proprioception, movement, and the positioning of body parts. Toddlers are conscious of body parts and body products. Toddlers and preschoolers are very concerned about the integrity and intactness of their bodies (Arnold & Boggs, 1995). For instance, when procedures violate body boundaries the toddler may fear that he or she might "deflate" (Carson & Arnold, 1996). The shape and size of the body can be a major basis on which children receive recognition from adults, as well as their peers. Along with physical growth and development the child is learning to master and refine physical motor skills, language, and social skills. An awareness of sexual differences also occurs.

Adolescence is another period of rapid bodily change and a period of heightened body consciousness. Adolescents can experience high levels of anxiety, insecurity, and self-consciousness about their bodies as they attempt to develop a self-identity. During adolescence the body image is in a constant state of revision as the final stage of physical growth and maturation occurs. Some bodily changes are normal occurrences of the developmental process, such as height and weight increases, acne, and growing pains. Other are important "rites of passage," such as the beginning of menses and the development of secondary sexual characteristics. During this stage a body image forms that integrates the adolescent's role identity. Normal adolescent behavior is often focused on the self and on characteristics of the body. This is true for both genders. Even more significant than the actual changes in bodily characteristics, shape, and functioning is the meaning the adolescent gives to them. Peer group recognition, acceptance, and comparison are especially important during this stage of development. Body image is also influenced by the adolescent's emotional maturity. Once the identity tasks are mastered body image stabilizes.

During adulthood body image is incorporated into the individual's sense of self. Whether the body image is positive or negative, it is maintained and remains relatively static during this stage of development. Change becomes more difficult to perceive because of the slower rate of change and the more subtle nature of the changes that occur. The adult may ignore changes in the body or others' comments regarding bodily changes in order to avoid creating a sense of anxiety within the self over the bodily changes (e.g., male pattern baldness, weight gain, and wrinkles, etc.).

Confronting the gradual changes that occur during the aging process requires a redefinition of body image. Frequently adults find incorporating these changes into a viable body image difficult. Often the real image of the body is quite different from the one perceived by the individual. The mental image of the self does not seem to age at the same rate as the actual physical body. As sensory acuity decreases the adult interactions with the environment also decrease. Bodily functioning also diminishes with aging. For the elderly, body image concerns involve retreat toward the interior of the body structure and are accompanied by a preoccupation with bodily function. This preoccupation increases as the body begins to function differently. All these changes impact body image.

Adaptation to bodily changes will depend on the meaning of the change for the individual as well as on the meaning that significant others ascribe to the changes (Carson & Arnold, 1996). The changes of normal growth and maturation can have a significant impact on the individual. When these issues are compounded by illness, injury, disease, or disability, as occurs for the rehabilitation client, the stress can be heightened and alterations in body image can occur.

Anxiety develops when the client is concerned about body integrity, function, and body image with the onset of illness, surgery, and sudden traumatic events resulting in injury. Medication administration; casts, braces, and prosthesis; and procedures and treatments can cause alterations in the physical self, disrupting body image (Carson & Arnold, 1996). Fluid retention, alterations in gait and

Table 1
Examples of Changes that Can Result in Body Image Alteration

Type of Change	Examples
External changes	Physical disfigurement, scars
	Skin changes
	Lesions
	Liver spots
	Burns
	Loss of a breast
	Joint swelling
	Malocclusion
Functional limitation	Loss of a body part or change in the function of a body part
	Fractures or joint disturbances
	Immobility
	Inability to perform activities
	Diminished sexual response and functioning

posture, paralysis, perceptual problems, and anatomical or functional disruption can disrupt the mental picture of the body (Table 1).

Alterations in Body Image

Which client might experience an alteration in body image? The client who has an amputation, burn, hysterectomy, mastectomy, vasectomy, or colostomy. Clients with chronic obstructive pulmonary disease, diabetes mellitus, myocardial infarction, or stroke. Clients with altered gastrointestinal functioning, renal failure, spinal cord injury, head trauma, or neuromuscular disease. Clients with alterations in vision, hearing, taste and smell, touch, proprioception, and perceptual deficits. Any client is at risk for a disturbance in body image. The nurse cannot predict the extent to which an injury, illness, disease, or disability may alter a client's body image. Buscaglia (1975) determined that it is not the degree of loss of feelings of intactness that is significant in adjusting to a disability. It is the attitude toward the whole self: the self-concept.

Disruptions in body image can be both actual or perceived. Disruptions in body image can occur as the result of developmental influences, chronic illness, or trauma. Disturbances in body image can reflect a view that is not a realistic representation of reality. This would be the case when a client who has experienced a stroke perceives that some body part is not a part of the whole. For example, she might perceive that her paralyzed leg no longer belongs to her. She perceives the leg as being alien. She may have negative feelings about the leg, feeling that it has failed her in some manner. She then gives the leg a name and begins to refer to it as separated from her. When referring to her paralyzed leg she might say, "Boy, Mr. Leg is really giving me trouble today." It is not uncommon during the early stages of rehabilitation for clients with paralyzed body parts to awake from sleep with a "sense" that there is someone else in bed with them.

Changes in body image must be integrated as events occur across the life span to allow perception of body image to remain consistent with reality. Sudden changes in body image, such as those resulting from trauma, are more difficult to integrate than gradual changes. Covert or internal changes (memory loss) are more difficult to manage than overt or external changes (amputation of an extremity in an accident).

Factors Influencing Adaptation to Changes in Body Image

Body image is threatened when the client attaches great importance to the body part changed or lost. Different body parts will have different meanings to clients (Carson & Arnold, 1996; Norris, 1987). A professional athlete probably would experience a greater degree of **body image disturbance** following the loss of a leg to amputation than would a graphic artist. But this may not be the case. Perhaps the most significant factor that determines the degree of disturbance is the symbolic meaning of the change to the client (Thompson, 1990). Another significant factor is the meaning of the treatment or rehabilitation plan for the client. The perceived change in body image is reduced if the client identifies positive benefits to be gained by actively participating in the treatment plan.

Time is also a variable that can influence the degree of body image disturbance a client might experience. When the change is slow and progressive (rheumatoid arthritis) the client has more time to incorporate the new body image and the resulting changes. When changes develop over time the client can anticipate what might occur and has an opportunity to acknowledge and integrate the change. Sudden, traumatic changes (hemiplegia resulting from a stroke) present no warning of events to come. There is little time or opportunity to cope with the change. Sudden alteration can have more of an impact on the client, resulting in difficulty adapting to the changes in body image.

Clients who considered themselves well, or had experienced few physical symptoms before the event that resulted in a body image change, will have more difficulty adjusting to that change than clients who were ill, or experienced symptoms, for a prolonged period of time beforehand. This is especially true if there is immediate improvement in the quality of life. When quality of life is improved the effect on body image could be positive (Morrall, 1990).

The nature of the client's pre-illness body image can also influence the degree of body image disturbance following change. Beeken (1978) reported that clients who possessed positive images of themselves before illness were more likely to continue to maintain that positive view. Those clients who have a negative body image before the onset of illness, injury, disease, or disability were less likely to have a positive view afterward.

The age of the client can also be a significant factor influencing adaptation to changes in body image. Children may find it less difficult to adapt and adjust to changes in body image. In infancy and childhood body images are malleable and body boundaries are hazy. There may not have been as strong a bonding between physical appearance and identity. Body image changes can be devastating for adolescent clients. The adolescent needs to adjust to normal developmental and maturational changes occurring during this time. Additional changes in appearance or functioning related to illness or injury add additional threats. Adults may not find adapting to bodily change any easier than adolescents. Body image for the adult is stable and provides a basis for identity. Changes occurring in adulthood interfere with the well-established self-image. Elderly clients must adapt and cope with a variety of issues; they must deal with change in conjunction with the anticipated changes of aging, their concerns about decreased productivity and value to society, dependency, and society's value on physical attractiveness and youth.

Clients have difficulty adapting to changes associated with "masculine" or "feminine" characteristics. In western society changes that reduce a woman's ability to conceive or bear children would result in a great degree of alteration in body image for a young woman. A man who experiences diminished sexual performance may experience a disturbance in his view of himself as a "man." Women do seem to be more psychologically comfortable with body change whereas men perceive more threat to the self (Fisher, 1986).

Restructuring Body Image

Kolb and Woldt (1976) suggest two strategies that can be used to assist clients in dealing with body image or physical aspects of rehabilitation and disability. The first is to assist the client to engage in contact with their physique through fantasy, self-exploration, psychodrama, and modified body-movement patterns. Clients should be encouraged to handle and observe the body and its functioning. The client with a paralyzed arm should be encouraged to touch that arm with the unaffected arm and move the affected arm through space. This can be accomplished through bathing, dressing, and other activities of daily living. The client can also observe the functioning of the body in a mirror. By focusing on areas where sensation is blocked and where it is capable of being perceived the client can discuss any preconceptions or misconceptions of personal strength and limitation and discuss how these self-images can restrict or enhance client behavior.

The second intervention is to encourage the client to contact another person through mutual body exploration and nonverbal expressiveness. This helps the client to focus on the experience of giving and receiving sensory communication. This can be accomplished during client interactions with staff and significant others.

Lee (1970) proposed a process for assisting clients to restructure and reintegrate an altered body image. This process can be used for both physical and functional changes. Four stages were proposed: the impact stage, the retreat stage, the acknowledgment stage, and the reconstruction stage. As with all stage theories, clients proceed through stages in different ways and may return to the first stage as they revise their body image. Understanding client behaviors and responses typically observed during periods of **body image reconstruction** can be useful for assisting nurses in evaluating client progress and for determining appropriate nursing interventions.

In the *impact stage* the client will focus on the body part, or disease, that causes the change to occur. Energy is directed toward coping with the illness, injury, disease, or disability. Clients may focus on symptom relief rather than on long-term treatment issues. Typical client responses in this stage are shock and disbelief. Both shock and belief serve as coping strategies and are necessary for the client during this stage. Attempts to get the client to "face" reality are inappropriate and should not be considered. Clients will deal with the change when they are psychologically ready. Present reality to the client in short, safe, non-threatening ways in a matter-of-fact manner.

During the *retreat stage* the client's awareness of the body change increases. The client retreats psychologically. This occurs because the client becomes overwhelmed by the reality of the situation, and lacks the emotional energy to deal with the stress of the change. The client may use denial as the major coping strategy during this stage. Feelings expressed by clients may range from indifference to euphoria. This is not necessarily a negative event for the client. During this retreat the client has the opportunity to rest and reorganize forces and strength and prepare for the work of restructuring and incorporating the new body image. The typical client responses in this stage are denial and anger. As in the earlier stage, do not attempt to remove denial as a coping mechanism. Attempts to remove denial as a coping mechanism should be employed only if the denial interferes with the progression of the treatment plan. Allow for the expression of anger in constructive ways, and always limit the amount of energy and period of time that the client can expend on expressing feelings of anger.

When the reality of the body changes and the resulting losses are faced the client enters the *acknowledgment stage.* As the client acknowledges losses, mourning for the idealized body image occurs. The client may need solitude to work through the redefining of the self-image. During this time the client will need to discuss openly the events surrounding the illness, injury, disease, or disability and the resulting physical and functional changes. How others react and respond to the client during this stage is critical for progress toward reconstructing of body image. Client responses during this stage of image reconstruction can vary. The client may experience feelings of fear, guilt, anger, blame, depression, and suicidal thoughts. The nurse must be alert to the client's emotional state and intervene appropriately to the immediate state. When the predominant state of the client is depression the treatment team members must be alert for signs of suicidal ideation. A suicidal assessment is critical. Suicidal thoughts and ideas can turn into concrete action as the client's condition improves and energy levels rise. When the client has greater energy, strength, and physical abilities they are at greater risk for carrying out a suicidal plan.

Reconstruction and acceptance can begin only after the client has successfully acknowledged the body image change and the threats felt by the client. The length of this stage will be largely determined by the amount of energy the client has available for assimilation of the new image and the incorporation into daily activities of living. The client begins the reorganization of life. New goals are developed and new roles explored. The nurse serves as a resource and support agent for the client. The goal of the treatment team is to establish and provide a growth-promoting environment for the client during this stage.

For most clients the reconstruction stage will be a positive experience, resulting in an adjustment to adaptive devices or technical procedures. A reorientation to the social aspect of life will occur. Finally, the client will experience reintegration of the body image and self-concept (Lee, 1970). However, for some, reconstruction many never occur. Adaptation is not always growth-promoting. Some clients will permanently avoid the reality of changes in the body (Murray, 1972).

Clients who experience difficulty in adapting to a change in body image will manifest a variety of physical and psychological symptoms. Physical symptoms may be vague complaints of illness, chronic fatigue, and pain. Psychological symptoms may include anxiety, denial, guilt, anger, and resentment focused on the family or health care providers; depression, and an inability to complete the grieving process. Clients who have difficulty adapting to a body image change may withdraw from previous social, educational, and occupational pursuits. This is especially true for clients with overt physical changes such as major disfigurement (facial scars) or diminished functioning (paralysis).

Adapting to an alteration in body image and incorporating a new self-concept are not static processes. The rehabilitation client will be continually reintegrating a new image of the self. This reintegration may be necessary any time the client is confronted anew with the original change in body image. This can be during periods of exacerbation of an illness or disease, or when the treatment plan produces further alteration of the body or affects functioning. When this occurs clients must rework their body image perceptions.

Nursing Process Nursing Diagnosis—Body Image Disturbance

Body image disturbance is created by negative feelings or perception about the characteristics, functions, or limits of one's body or body parts (Gordon, 1993). **Characteristics** and indicators that might indicate that a client is at risk for experiencing a disturbance in body image:

- The client experiences a loss of body part or body function.
- The client perceives a disfigurement from surgery or trauma.

- The client has a cognitive disturbance that distorts self-perception.
- The client has an uncontrollable debilitating disease.
- The client experiences uncontrollable pain.
- The client is dependent on mechanical devices.
- The client has psychological or drug-induced disturbances.
- The client is unable to integrate disability-related changes into his or her sociocultural environment.
- The client expresses feelings of disgust or negative beliefs about the body or some aspect of the body.
- The client is unable to look at or touch the affected body area.
- The client engages in attempts to hide or overexpose the affected body part.
- The client expresses feelings of helplessness, hopelessness, or powerlessness about the body.
- The client demonstrates a preoccupation with the loss or change of body function.
- The client expresses fear of rejection by others.
- The client refuses to acknowledge the reality of the change.
- The client lacks knowledge about potential abilities or capabilities.

Assessment Areas to be included when assessing to determine if the client has an actual or potential disturbance in body image are as follows:

- The client's and family's feelings about the body following a change in health state or anatomical change
- The client's and family's perception of the current situation
- The significance and meaning that the client and family assign to the altered body part or change in function and the client's attitude toward it
- The client's and family's assessment of strengths and capabilities
- The client's and family's assessment of limitations
- The presence of family or friends to provide the client with support during restructuring and incorporation of body image
- The client's and family's perception of learning needs
- The client's and family's perceptions of how others see the client

Interventions Nursing interventions will be determined by the nature of the client's disturbance in body image and the stage of restructuring of body image. General interventions could include

- Encouraging the expression of feelings about the body and how it has changed
- Supporting the client throughout the grieving process
- Complementing the client on his or her appearance and efforts to attend to personal hygiene and appearance
- Assisting the client with adaptive clothing to enhance appearance
- Encouraging family members to treat the client in a normal manner
- Encouraging the client to manipulate and observe the affected body part

- Encouraging the client to contact another person through mutual body exploration and nonverbal expressiveness
- Educating the client and family members about capabilities for self-care, participation in social activities, and re-owning of health care
- Facilitating goal setting to assume self-care responsibilities
- Providing referrals to self-help groups

Outcomes The long-term outcomes of nursing interventions for clients experiencing an alteration in body image are (1) for the client to adapt successfully to the body image change and (2) for the client to restructure and incorporate a new self-concept.

Expected Outcomes

- The client openly shares feelings about the body and changed body parts.
- The client recognizes negative feelings about himself and identifies affirmations to counteract them.
- The client expresses feelings of sadness, loss, or anger.
- The client performs self-care activities.
- The client uses appropriate adaptive equipment.
- The client dresses and grooms to enhance appearance.
- The client participates in social activities without hiding affected body part(s).

Conclusion

Body image is the conscious and unconscious mental picture that a person has of the shape, the size, and the mass of the body and its parts. Body image is one aspect of the individual's concept of self. Body image serves as a subjective frame of reference when relating to others or relating to the physical and social environment. Factors that can influence the client's perceived body image include the client's previous perceptions of bodily appearance and intactness, the client's degree of interest or preoccupation in the care and development of the body, and society's perceptions of beauty and wholeness. Adaptation to bodily changes will depend on the meaning of the change for the individual as well as the meaning that significant others ascribe to the changes. Any client is at risk for a disturbance in body image. The nurse cannot predict the extent to which an injury, illness, disease, or disability may alter a client's body image. The role of the nurse is to facilitate the successful adaptation to body image change and to assist the client to restructure and incorporate a new self-concept.

References

Arnold, E., & Boggs, K. (1995). *Interpersonal relationships: Professional communication skills for nurses* (2nd ed.). Philadelphia: W. B. Saunders.

Beeken, J. (1978). Body image changes in plegia. *Journal of Neurosurgical Nursing, 10,* 20–23.

Bramble, K. (1995). Body image. In I. M. Lubkin (Ed.), *Chronic illness: Impact and interventions* (3rd ed., pp. 285–298). Boston: Jones & Bartlett.

Buscaglia, L. (1975). *The disabled and their parents: A counseling challenge.* Thorofare, NJ: Charles B. Slack.

Carson, V. B., & Arnold, E. N. (1996). *Mental health nursing: The nurse-patient journey.* Philadelphia: W. B. Saunders.

Cash, T. F., & Pruzinsky T. (Eds.). (1990). *Integrating themes in body image development, deviance and change.* New York: Guilford Press.

Farley, A. M. (1992). *Nursing and the disabled across the life span.* Boston: Jones & Bartlett.

Fisher, S. (1974). *Body consciousness.* New York: Aronson.

Fisher, S. (1986). *Development and structure of the body image.* Hillsdale, NJ: Lawrence Erlbaum and Associates.

Gordon, M. (1993). *Manual of nursing diagnosis 1993–1994.* St. Louis: Mosby–Year Book.

Kolb, C. L., & Woldt, A. L. (1976). The rehabilitation potential of a Gestalt approach to counseling severely impaired clients. In W. A. McDowell, S. A. Meadows, R. Crabtress, & R. Sakata (Eds.), *Rehabilitation counseling with persons who are severely disabled* (pp. 40–56). Huntington, WV: Marshall University Press.

Lee, J. M. (1970). Emotional reactions to trauma. *Nursing Clinics of North America, 4,* 577–587.

Morrall, S. E. (1990). The shock of the new: Altered body image after creation of a stoma. *Professional Nurse, 5,* 529–537.

Murray, R. L. (1972). Body image development in adulthood. *Nursing Clinics of North America, 7,* 617–630.

Norris, C. M. (1987). Body image: Its relevance to professional nursing. In C. Carlson & B. Blackwell (Eds.), *Behavioral concepts and nursing interventions* (pp. 22–33). New York: J. B. Lippincott.

Orr, D. A., Reznikoff, M., & Smith, G. M. (1989). Body image, self-esteem and depression in burn-injured adolescents and young adults. *Journal of Burn Care and Rehabilitation, 10*(5), 454–461.

Thompson, J. K. (1990). *Body image disturbances.* New York: Pergamon Press.

Suggested Readings

Forman, S. G. (1993). *Coping skills: Interventions for children and adolescents.* San Francisco: Jossey-Bass.

Fox, P. D., & Fama, T. (Eds.). (1996). *Managed care and chronic illness: Challenges and opportunities.* Rockville, MD: Aspen.

Hirschberg, G. G., Lewis, L., & Vaughan, P. (1976). *Rehabilitation manual for the disabled and elderly* (2nd ed.). New York: J. B. Lippincott.

Landrum, P. K., Schmidt, N. D., & McLean, A. (Eds.). (1995). *Outcome-oriented rehabilitation: Principles, strategies, and tools for effective program management.* Rockville, MD: Aspen.

Rolland, J. S. (1994). *Families, illness, and disability: An integrative treatment model.* New York: Harper-Collins.

CHAPTER 12
Independence and Dependency

Patricia A. Chin

Key Terms   *Dependency*
Independence
Interdependency
Maladaptive Dependency
Maladaptive Independence
Malingerer
Secondary Gains

Objectives   1. Identify sources leading to conflicts between independence and dependency needs and desires for rehabilitation clients.

2. Discuss the problems that can arise with maladaptive independence or dependency conflicts.

3. Identify characteristics or indicators that are indicative of unresolved conflicts between independence and dependency needs and desires.

4. Identify assessment data associated with actual or potential unresolved conflicts between independence and dependency needs and desires.

5. Identify specific nursing interventions appropriate for clients with actual or potential unresolved conflicts between independence and dependency needs and desires.

6. Identify the expected outcomes of the interventions focused on assisting clients to resolve conflicts between independence and dependency needs and desires.

Nature of Independence and Dependency Conflicts   **Independence** and **dependency** conflicts represent the lack of resolution between the client's need and the desire to be dependent, or independent, with the expectations (therapeutic, maturational, or social) of being dependent or independent (Gordon, 1993). To be independent is to be free of the control of others or not to require or rely on others. To be dependent is to be influenced by or subject to another, or to rely on others for support (Gove, 1973). Clients in rehabilitation can experience severe independence-dependency conflicts. Those conflicts can result in significant difficulties in adjusting to changes in health state and can have a negative influence on self-esteem. They can also become obstacles to effective client teaching and to self-care mastery. The sources of conflict may vary but they generally arise because the client becomes dependent on external mechanisms for meeting needs. Clients can become dependent on medications, machines, equipment, or other people. The need to be dependent can be in direct conflict with the client's previous lifestyle preference or with the personality of the client. This is especially true in Western culture, with its value and emphasis on autonomy, self-sufficiency, and independence.

Being forced into dependent roles may cause feelings of guilt, anger, depression, or frustration, for clients. Clients may respond to this frustration with anger toward the system and those on whom they are dependent. They may also rebel. It is not uncommon for clients frustrated over dependency to refuse treatment, break rules, miss scheduled appointments, or undertake activities or actions that they have been advised against. Forced dependency is especially difficult for adolescents and young adults, who are still struggling with normal developmental issues of independence and personality identity formation.

The elderly are also at risk for independence-dependency conflicts because during rehabilitation they often sense themselves to be in unmanageable situations with little opportunity for control. Clark and Anderson (1967) found that low morale among the elderly was highly correlated with client physical and financial dependency. With elderly clients the approach should be to provide the necessary amount of support and no more. The focus should be on striving to maintain independence to the greatest extent possible. Providing minimal support to the elderly during rehabilitation would involve relying on existing informal support systems, providing in-home service when needed, and helping the elderly client to realistically evaluate and determine the need for institutional care (Schienle & Eiler, 1984).

Healthy psychological functioning requires the client to balance independence from, dependency on, and **interdependency** with others. The sense of balance experienced leads to increased self-esteem, which in turn leads to increased independence, confidence, and mastery of self-care management. Increased self-esteem is a personal characteristic necessary to reach fullest adult maturity (Orem, 1985). Balancing independence and dependency is greatly influenced by the interactions and reactions of family members, friends, employers, educators, and others with whom the client has relationships and interacts.

During rehabilitation change can occur constantly or intermittently over the course of the process. Balancing independence and dependency needs and desires can be difficult to achieve particularly for individuals with disabilities. The client who attempts to be independent without the appropriate level of physical or cognitive skill may experience additional injury and difficulties. Dependency, when expressed as a lack of motivation or involvement, is frequently a problem in the rehabilitation setting. Wright (1960) indicated that motivating children and preventing dependency are major concerns for the rehabilitation team. Lack of client motivation and dependency have sometimes been attributed to the health care system. This is true when the system creates an environment in which the client assumes a passive role rather than an active, involved role (Morgan, Hohmann, & Davis, 1974; Schlesinger, 1963; Vash, 1975). Overprotected clients exhibit a degree of fixation at primitive levels of coping. Denial, regression, and projection are responses often used by overprotected clients in the rehabilitation setting.

Dependency is an inherent characteristic of the sick role (Parson, 1951). Members of Western society hold the expectation that those who are ill want to get well, and are intolerant of those they perceive as malingerers or clients who want to remain ill in order to receive secondary gains. A **malingerer** knowingly wishes to enter or remain in an inappropriate role (i.e., sick role). **Secondary gains** are rewards the client receives for being dependent. Secondary gains are unconscious needs to retain inappropriate role behaviors for other advantages or benefits. Those rewards may take a variety of forms such as attention from loved ones who are normally inattentive, being released from undesirable or unwanted responsibilities, or even to attain solitude. The economic realities of the current health care delivery systems create pressure to move clients toward independent living.

Dependency has been correlated with a sense of powerlessness (Miller, 1992). Rehabilitation is a stressful experience full of uncertainty and unpredictable dilemmas. Even in the postcrisis stage the client may lack both the physical and psychological energy for recovery. Uncertainty about future progress and the course of treatment, the effectiveness of the treatment regimens, and the disruption of previous patterns of living can deplete the client's and family's psychological and spiritual resources. Being aware of the signs and responses of the client facing independence can alert the nurse to maintain dependency until the client is able to return to normal roles and responsibilities, including the responsibilities for self-care.

As the client progresses and improves in physical status, emphasis on the desire to return to normal roles motivates the client to learn about the condition and necessary procedures for maximizing health and self-care ability and capabilities. Maladjustment in independence or dependency can have negative consequences for both the client and the family.

Maladjustment in Independence or Dependency

Clients can present with maladjustment problems with either independence or dependence.

Maladaptive Independence

Maladaptive independence involves the client who overestimates cognitive or physical capabilities and energy level. Safety can become a major concern when working with these clients, because they tend to overestimate their abilities and capabilities. Some clients may be denying the reality of their limitation whereas others may not have the cognitive function, insight, or judgment to determine accurately the degree of independence possible. Overconfidence regarding abilities can lead to impulsiveness. The client experiencing maladaptive independence may avoid sharing decisions with other family members or significant caregivers. The client may refuse to allow family members to participate in decision-making and reject suggestions that they turn role responsibilities over to others.

It becomes difficult for these clients to determine and maintain their optimal level of self-care. They may act in a rejecting manner toward those who offer them assistance. They have difficulty seeking assistance even when they appropriately assess the need for help.

Maladaptive Dependency

Maladaptive dependency can also have serious negative consequences for both the client and family members. The dependent client actually surrenders control to others. Those others can be family members, caregivers, or the treatment team members. This can result in the creation of feelings of resentment by the dependent person because of the loss of self-control. The dependent client may come to rely heavily on other family members or caregivers, burdening them with undesirable responsibilities and roles or forcing them into decision-making roles they do not want or feel capable of assuming. This can create feelings of resentment in the dependent client as well as in those who are forced to accept increased responsibilities and demands.

Maladjustment in dependency reduces the individual's peace and contentment. These clients may experience difficulty achieving success with work, school, or recreation endeavors. Difficulties with dependence will perpetuate a negative cycle of interpersonal dependency and control. The negative cycle sets the client up for failure. This cycle can manifest itself as a "self-fulfilling prophesy." Those clients who state that they cannot accomplish something, or that something will have a negative consequence, often find that the outcome is as predicted. They come to believe in the negative cycle unconsciously, or consciously, and act in ways to make the prophesy come to fruition.

Nursing Process
Nursing Diagnosis

Unresolved independence–dependency conflict is a lack of resolution of the need and the desire to be dependent or independent with expectations (therapeutic, maturational, or social) of being dependent or independent (Gordon, 1993). **Characteristics** and indicators that might indicate that client is at risk for experiencing an unresolved independence-dependency conflict:

Maladaptive Independence
- The client demonstrates an overconfidence or lack of confidence in abilities and capabilities.
- The client uses denial, regression, or projection as a major coping strategy.
- The client demonstrates impulsiveness.

- The client avoids sharing decision-making with other members of the family or with caregivers.

Maladaptive Dependency

- The client shows little interest in activities of daily living that promote independence.
- The client demonstrates difficulty in making independent decisions.
- The client needs or requests frequent and excessive reassurance from family members and the treatment team.
- The client demonstrates passivity and submissiveness.
- The client is hesitant about trying new situations or skills.
- The client gives the perception that he or she is unable to cope with the situation.
- The client demonstrates indicators of powerlessness.

Assessment Areas to be included when assessing to determine if the client is experiencing an actual or potential unresolved maladjustment in independence or dependence are as follows:

- The client's and family's realistic perceptions of client's physical disabilities and limitations
- The realistic perceptions of client with cognitive disabilities and limitations
- The client's age and client's and family's developmental stage
- The client's interest in being involved in care and treatment planning, degree of passivity or submissiveness
- The client's approach to decision-making and problem-solving
- The client's need for reassurance
- The client's expressions of control or lack of control of life events and treatment
- The client's willingness to attempt new procedures or approaches
- The client's and family's work and educational status
- The client's and family's financial status
- The support systems available to the client and the family

Interventions Nursing intervention for conflicts or maladjustment in independence or dependency will depend on the nature of the client's specific problem. General interventions could include

Dependency

- Supporting the client in a realistic examination of assets, capabilities, and abilities
- Supporting the client in a realistic evaluation of the impact of the illness or injury on work, education, family, and social life
- Encouraging resumption of activities associated with daily living
- Supporting the client's ability to make decisions and assume responsibility for making decisions

- Providing the client and family with information regarding resources available that promote independence
- Encouraging communication within the family unit regarding independent, interdependent, and dependent roles
- Encouraging the client's verbalization of concerns regarding being independent
- Encouraging the client to engage in new situations and to use new skills

Independence

- Being alert for situations that could result in client injury
- Providing an environmentally safe environment
- Increasing the client's and family's safety awareness
- Monitoring the client's ability and interest in involvement in self-care
- Monitoring the client's physical, cognitive, and sensory deficits
- Providing the client and family with the appropriate level of supervision
- Modifying the environment to provide the client with opportunities to exercise control
- Assisting the client to formulate realistic expectations and goals based on health state, energy level, and capabilities
- Increasing the client's and family's knowledge about the client's health status and management
- Encouraging the client's verbalization of feelings of concern regarding being dependent
- Encouraging the client to seek assistance as appropriate

Outcomes The long-term outcome for the client experiencing a conflict or maladjustment in independence or dependency is for the client to reach a healthy balance between independence and dependency.

Expected Outcomes

- The client accurately assesses limitation, capabilities, and abilities.
- The client assumes adaptive dependent, interdependent, and independent roles as appropriate to the situation.
- The client performs optimal self-care activities consistent with abilities and capabilities.
- The client performs roles at an optimal level consistent with abilities and capabilities.
- The client is an active participant in the creation and implementation of the treatment plan.
- The client engages in mutual decision-making with appropriate parties.
- The client seeks assistance as necessary.

Conclusion Independence and dependency conflicts represent the lack of resolution between the client's need and the desire to be dependent, or independent, with the expectations (therapeutic, maturational, or social) of being independent or dependent. The sources of conflict may vary but they generally arise because the client becomes dependent on external mechanisms for meeting needs. Balancing independence and dependency needs and desires can be difficult to achieve, particularly for individuals with disabilities. The long-term outcome for the client experiencing a conflict or maladjustment in independence or dependency is for the client to reach a healthy balance between independence and dependency.

References

Clark, M., & Anderson, C. (1967). *Culture & aging.* Springfield, IL: Charles C Thomas.

Gordon, M. (1993). *Manual of nursing diagnosis 1993–1994.* St. Louis: Mosby–Year Book.

Gove, P. B. (Ed.). (1973). *Webster's New Collegiate Dictionary* (8th ed.). Springfield, MA: G. & C. Merriam.

Miller, J. F. (1992). *Coping with chronic illness: Overcoming powerlessness* (2nd ed.). Philadelphia: F. A. Davis.

Morgan, E. D., Hohmann, G. W., & Davis, J. E. (1974). Psychological rehabilitation in VA spinal cord injury center. *Rehabilitation Psychology, 21,* 3–33.

Orem, D. E. (1985). *Nursing concepts of practice.* New York: McGraw-Hill.

Parson, T. (1951). *The social system.* New York: The Free Press.

Schienle, D. R., & Eiler, J. M. (1984). Clinical intervention with older adults. In M. G. Eisenberg, Schienle, L. E. (1963). Patient motivation for rehabilitation: Integrating staff forces. *American Journal of Occupational Therapy, 17,* 5–8.

Sutkin, L. C., and Jansen, M. A. (eds.). *Chronic illness and disability through the life span: Effect on self and family.* (pp. 245–268). New York: Springer.

Vash, C. L. (1975). The psychology of disability. *Rehabilitation Psychology, 22,* 145–163.

Wright, B. A. (1960). *Physical disability—A psychological approach.* New York: Harper & Row.

Suggested Readings

Eisenberg, M. G., Sutkin, L. C., & Jansen, M. A. (Eds.). (1984). *Chronic illness and disability through the life span: Effects on self and family.* New York: Springer.

Lubkin, I. M. (1995). *Chronic illness: Impact and interventions* (3rd ed.). Boston: Jones & Bartlett.

Marinelli, R. P., & Dell Orto, A. E. (Eds.). (1984). *The psychological & social impact of physical disability* (2nd ed.). New York: Springer.

CHAPTER 13

Loss and Grieving
Patricia A. Chin

Key Terms	*Anger*
	Anticipatory Grief
	Bereavement
	Chronic Grief
	Denial
	Grief
	Loss
	Mourning
	Trigger Experiences

Objective

1. Discuss the concept of loss in the rehabilitation setting.

2. Discuss the concept of grieving in the rehabilitation setting.

3. Discuss the necessity of grieving for the rehabilitation client.

4. Discuss the models created to reflect the human process of loss and mourning.

5. Discuss interventions focused on assisting the rehabilitation client through loss, anger, and grieving.

Loss

Loss is a fundamental human experience. Nurses face loss daily and must continually deal with the diverse reactions of clients and their families to loss. People generally think of the loss of a significant other when they think about death. Although death is the ultimate loss for most people, loss comes in all shapes and forms. A client may experience a hearing loss, divorce, loss of memory, loss of personal sense of meaning, or the loss of the ability to have children. Whatever form loss takes it is the experience of deprivation of, or complete lack of, something that was previously present.

The phenomenon of loss embodies both (1) the deprivation of what was previously present and (2) surviving that deprivation. Loss may come gradually or suddenly, it may be unpredictable or predictable, temperate or traumatic. Loss can also be actual or symbolic (Schmale, 1958). An actual loss is concrete, as would be the loss of a body part, separation, or job loss. Symbolic losses are difficult to define but important to recognize (Saunders, 1989). Symbolic losses are imbedded in actual losses, for example, the feelings of loss associated with a loss of role experienced following the loss of a job. How the client perceives the loss will be determined by past experiences with loss; the value and attachment to the lost object felt by the client; the timing of the loss; the situation surrounding the loss; and the cultural, psychological, and family supports available for handling the loss. For the rehabilitation client it will be greatly influenced by the presence of concurrent losses and other stressors.

Clients involved in the rehabilitative process experience varying degrees or levels of loss. These losses often result in alterations of basic needs, cognitive ability, or functional independence. Clients who require assisted care or adaptive devices and equipment to maintain optimal functioning, independence, quality of life, or even survival all will experience loss. The nurse in the rehabilitative setting should never underestimate the significance and intensity of loss for the client. Clients must develop the skills necessary to cope with irreversible, chronic, progressive, or recurrent losses.

Pereira (1984) described the grieving process experienced by disabled adults as a cycle of helplessness, hopelessness, and dependency in which the individual mourns resulting limitations repeatedly. Kowalsky (1987) identified **trigger experiences** causing the re-experience of the grief process in the physically disabled adult. Trigger experiences can be the admission to an acute rehabilitation center, anniversary dates, going home for weekend visits, contemplation of marriage or independent living, hospitalization, job selections, and vocational rehabilitation. The degree of grieving stimulated by trigger experiences will depend on the success of grieving in the earlier episode, residual grief not dealt with by the client, and the client's physical and psychological state at the time of exposure to the trigger experience.

The loss of a significant other, the loss of some aspect of physiopsychosocial well-being, and the loss of personal possessions are the three major categories of loss that clients experience. Rehabilitation clients may have to face continuous loss in all three categories. This chapter focuses on physiopsychosocial losses experienced by adult rehabilitation patients, and strategies for assisting with the work of grief. Several references are provided for the reader (see References and Suggested Readings) to further develop understanding and strategies for assisting the client and family to deal with the complex phenomenon of loss.

Loss of Physiological and Psychosocial Well-Being

Physiological and psychosocial losses for adults include three components: the state of physiological functioning, the client's ideas and feelings about the self, and the client's social roles. Alterations in any one of these components will invariably affect the other components. Loss, like anxiety and stress, is cumulative. Each new loss adds an additional physical and psychological burden to the client's adaptive resources. All three components will need to be assessed for the rehabilitation nurse to determine the magnitude of a loss for the client.

Loss of physiological functions may occur during partial (changes in hearing) or complete failure (liver failure) of the body and may be either temporary or permanent. The removal of a body part (limb) by surgical amputation or the presence of a chronic illness (arthritis) demonstrates a permanent loss. Each client's experience with a form of loss will be different from every other client's response. No matter what form loss assumes, or the degree of lost functioning, all loss is real to the client. Difficulties in accepting the changes that occur in physiological function or appearance connected to a loss may result in the client feeling inadequate and undesirable. Once an individual with a minor disability begins rehabilitation, these feelings of worthlessness and undesirability can dissipate. The feelings of worth and desirability for the client with a major change in health state will fluctuate depending on life situations and events.

The rehabilitation client may experience the loss of love and approval (Miller, 1992). The rehabilitation client may fear that incapacity or increased physical dependence will cause resentment among family members and friends. The client may also fear that they will be rejected or abandoned, and lose the support of others, especially if a debilitating condition is involved. Clients may feel that they no longer possess the personal quality or characteristic that once made them attractive to others. That quality or characteristic may be the ability to earn money for the family, or the loss of a talent that attracted others to them, as in the case of deficits in sensorimotor ability.

Loss of occupation or profession, status in the family unit, position in the community, and one's sexuality are included among physiopsychosocial losses. Depending on the nature of the change or the degree of change resulting from the illness, injury, disease, or disability the client may need to relinquish some involvement in work, family, and community. If total inability to carry out responsibilities occurs as the result of change in health state the client may be totally removed from professional/work, family, or community roles and interactions.

The effects of illness, disease, injury, or disability can affect the client's sexuality. Clients with sexual dysfunction are concerned about loss of their sense of maleness or femaleness, their existing feelings concerning sexual well-being, the effects that gender has on their everyday living, and the presence of reproductivity or fertility. The ability to procreate is a very important issue for most adolescents and young adults.

Many clients with chronic illness fear the ultimate loss of self: death. Families of clients with significant traumatic injuries and chronic illnesses fear the possible death of the clients. The fear of death can lead to a modification of relationships resulting in mutual withdrawal, decreased quality of interactions between the client and family members, and a lessening of support for the client.

Studies provide support for the idea that grieving and crisis resolution are not time limited. Clients can at any point be working though the grief of a loss, only to experience a new stress or be reminded of their loss and have to begin the process all over again. Ongoing studies demonstrate that coping may reflect recurrent or unresolved grieving or chronic sorrow for a perceived loss, or an actual prior loss (Olshansky, 1962; Parad, 1965). Some clients may actually discover that they are dealing with losses experienced years earlier—losses that had not been resolved but have returned to conscious awareness as a result of the current state of stress. The response to loss is grief.

Grief   **Bereavement** is the experiential state endured after realizing a loss (Kastenbaum, 1977). Bereavement is an objective state (Kastenbaum, 1977). It is the term used to describe various emotions, experiences, changes, and conditions taking place as the result of a loss. **Mourning** represents the culturally defined acts performed after a death (Rosenblatt, Walsh, & Jackson, 1976). **Grief** represents the reactions one experiences while in the state of bereavement. Grief is multilayered and can be felt on many levels at once (Saunders, 1989, p. 9). These reactions or symptoms might include anger, guilt, physical complaints, despair, sadness, depression, and others (Saunders, 1989). For the most part grief is a private experience. The intensity of both states, bereavement and grief, will depend on the type of loss, situation surrounding the loss, and the degree of value and attachment to the lost object.

Lindemann (1944) coined the term **anticipatory grief** to explain the absence of a grief response by survivors of loss. Individuals may experience anticipatory grief when faced with the possibility of a life-threatening condition, an early death, or a diagnosis of a chronic disease or disability. Responses to anticipatory grief may include anxiety, depression, and increased concern about the effects of the condition. Recognizing and adapting to the reality of a loss can be instrumental in gaining control of the situation through the identification of strength and responses. Anticipatory grieving can cause conflict in the nurse-client relationship if the client's grief response following the event of loss is diminished. The nurse may feel that the client is not facing the loss or that the intensity of the loss is being denied. What actually has occurred is that the client or family has been able to deal with the impending loss and does not experience the intensity of a new loss at the time the loss actually occurs.

The symptoms of grief can be experienced when a person suffers a major, or even a minor, loss. The intensity of the grief will depend on the client's perception of the value of the lost object. There are differences in responses and the ability to adapt to loss during different developmental stages.

Anger   After the client has relinquished denial, **anger** is a common response. As the client's awareness of the loss, and the consequence of the loss, increases the client begins to realize that certain needs, plans, and goals cannot be fulfilled. Clients may express their anger through sarcastic, abusive, argumentative, or demanding verbal responses. They may also physically act out, using destructive behaviors to express their inner frustration and distress.

Anger is a normal response to loss, and health care providers should not label angry clients as problem clients. Some staff may find caring for the angry client stressful. They will respond to the client with anger, defensiveness, or avoidance. None of these approaches will help the client learn to deal constructively with their anger and may actually serve to increase the client's anger. The client perceives the staff's anger, defensiveness, or avoidance as additional loss and rejection and a refusal to recognize and deal with their feelings. Staff members must be aware of their own feelings and responses toward clients and seek assistance when those feelings or responses interfere with their ability to care therapeutically for the client.

The angry client is trying to be heard (Kahn, 1995). A nondefensive, nonjudgmental, and empathetic response to the client's verbal expression of anger will convey to the client that the feelings are validated and accepted for what they are: expressions of internal anguish. If the angry client has withdrawn from the external environment, it is the role of the nurse to initiate interaction with the client. An appropriate intervention for the client in this situation is to make a simple, nonjudgmental observation of the client's behavior and express a willingness to help (Kahn, 1995). Limits should be set on the client's ability to express openly or act out feelings of anger. These limits should be clearly identified with the client so that no misunderstandings will occur regarding what is appropriate expressive behavior, or when that behavior is considered acceptable. Reducing hostility-provoking stimuli in the environment is also beneficial for both the client and the staff (Kahn, 1995).

Grieving: A Necessity

Rehabilitation clients, both children and adults, must be given the opportunity to experience the healing nature of grief. They will need the support of others to do this. In the face of loss humans must grieve. Grief may be viewed as both a reaction to loss and as a process of recovery (Hughes, 1984). It is loss in the sense that it represents an attempt to return to a previous state of wholeness. If the client is to accept a loss then the stages of coping or grief must be experienced (Table 1). The client needs to recover from the initial shock associated with loss and endure the sadness and sorrow before full acceptance of the reality of loss can be achieved and the process of reconstructing life without the lost object begun.

It has been suggested that grieving for the loss of physical functioning may be more difficult to cope with than loss through death (Hughes, 1984). The client experiencing physical loss may have more difficulty working through the loss because the grief of physical loss may be difficult to share with others. The client with physical loss may be seen by friends and family only in terms of the loss and therefore in a position of inferiority (Hughes, 1984).

Table 1
Stages of Grieving with Common Biological, Emotional, and Social Levels

Stage	Characteristics of the Phase	Physical Symptoms	Psychological Aspects
Shock	Disbelief Confusion Restlessness Feelings of unreality Regression Helplessness State of alarm	Dry mouth and throat Signing Loss of muscular power Weeping, crying, sobbing Trembling Startle response Sleep disturbance Loss of appetite	Egocentric behaviors Preoccupation with the loss Psychological distancing from others
Awareness	Separation anxiety Conflict Acting out Prolonged stress	Yearning Crying Anger, frustration Guilt, shame Sleep disturbance Fear of death	Oversensitivity Search for lost object Disbelief and denial Dreaming Awareness of the loss
Conservation	Withdrawal Despair Diminished social support Helplessness	Weakness Fatigue Increased sleep Compromise of immune system	Withholding behavior Obsessional review of loss Grief work Turning point
Healing	Turning point Assuming control Identifies restructuring Relinquishes roles	Physical healing Increased energy Return to normal sleep pattern Restoration of immune system	Forgetting Forgiving Searching for meaning Hope
Renewal	New self-awareness Accepting of new responsibilities Learning to live without the lost object	Revitalization Functional stability Caring for physical needs	Living for one's self Anniversary reactions Loneliness Reaching out to others

Sources: Parks (1972); Saunders (1989); Worden (1982).

Denial of a loss should not be encouraged among clients in the rehabilitation settings. To disguise the pain of loss the bereaved need to hide emotions. However, in doing this they deprive themselves of the right to grieve openly (Saunders, 1989). If denial is operating as a coping mechanism the client will not be able to accept their change in health state and the healing process of grief will be delayed. The client's use of denial will vary from day to day. Sedation of clients to diminish the discomfort of pain and sadness in the initial stages of loss should be discouraged.

Some denial will serve as an adaptive mechanism for the rehabilitation client. But it can be overused and interfere with treatment process. Attempts to confront the client's denial can cause alienation or even harm to the client. The client will respond with attempts to restore psychological equilibrium. Trying to get a client to confront the reality of the loss can bring about regressive behavior in the client or even premature discontinuance of rehabilitation (Green, 1985). The best way to decrease client denial is to establish a trusting relationship with the client and determine the underlying threat denial is being used to defend against (Kahn, 1995). Assessing the threat involves exploring the client's values and beliefs and how they are affected by the threat. It is also important to determine how significant others are affected by the loss and how they respond to the threat of the loss. Once the threat is assessed, interventions focus on reducing the threat.

Once denial has ceased to serve a purpose for the client and he or she is able to confront the loss, the client should be able to express sadness and depression openly. This is necessary to move on to the next, inevitable step of pining for the lost object (Parks, 1972). The effective rehabilitation nurse will let the client know that depression is understandable.

Grief can be inhibited by five factors (Stuart & Sundeen, 1991). These factors inhibit the process and put the client at risk for depression and unresolved grief: (1) The practical and necessary tasks associated with rehabilitation subsequent to a loss may prevent the client from an awareness of the emotional significance of loss; (2) lack of support or permission for the person to mourn the loss inhibits the grieving process; (3) early training in the control of feelings can influence the client's expression of feelings. Signs of grieving or sadness may be seen by the client as a form of personal weakness; (4) some clients may believe that their feelings are unusual and unique and will not be understood if they communicate those feelings to others; and (5) the administration of medications to relieve the initial psychological pain of loss actually chemically suppresses normal emotional responses.

Depression among rehabilitation clients is a major concern. Often depression will go untreated because it is not recognized in the chronically ill client (Stuart & Sundeen, 1991). Depression must be treated if the grieving client is to accomplish grief work and restructure life.

Chronic grief may be experienced by those with a chronic illness or disability. There is no perception that there will be an end to physical and psychological suffering. The individual may experience continuous exposure to feelings of helplessness, hopelessness, and dependency. This recurrent grief is often experienced when the client must face new limitations or experiences (Servoss, 1984). An individual who experiences persistent grief may become apathetic and lose interest in normal life and care activities. There may be nutritional and sleep pattern disturbances, feelings of constant sadness, and the client may appear irritable and hostile (Graham, 1989).

For the client in rehabilitation following illness, injury, disease, or disability there must first be the realization that he or she is grieving and that grieving can be as difficult to work through as coping with death. The client needs to face the reality of the loss, avoid prolonged denial, express sadness and anger, and begin to restructure life. This process was first described by Freud (1917) as "the work of mourning" and was later coined "grief work" by Lindemann (1944).

Models of Grief and Loss

Since Lindemann (1944) first described the symptoms observed in adult individuals grieving the loss of loved ones, several models have been developed that attempt to represent the experiences of loss, grieving, death, and dying (see Table 2). Freud (1917) proposed the first intrapsychic theory of grieving. He viewed mourning as a response in the normal course of life. He was primarily interested in the depression that accompanied loss and mourning.

Lindemann (1944) studied the families of people who had been killed in the devastating Coconut Grove fire. He described grief as somatic distress occurring in repeated waves. The individuals experienced feelings of throat tightness, choking with shortness of breath, sighing, an empty feeling in the abdomen, lack of muscular power, and an intense subjective distress described as tension and mental pain. Individuals reported a strong preoccupation with feelings of guilt. Lindemann found that a grieving person may display a loss of warmth in relationships with others, tend to be irritable and angry, and not want to be bothered by others. The person experiencing grief may be extremely self-centered. They may appear to caregivers to be confused, disorganized, apprehensive, and poorly focused. Some individuals may display hyperactivity, restlessness, and searching behavior, and appear to engage in purposeless activity.

Engel (1961) described coping behaviors associated with grieving associated with illness, loss of limb or body part, threats to self-concept, and major alterations in lifestyle. Engel categorized responses to loss and grief into six stages: shock and disbelief, developing awareness, restitution, resolution, idealization, and the outcome. During shock and disbelief the mourner needs time to process the event of the loss. In the second stage the fight–flight pattern is activated and the mourner acts out the emotions being experienced. In restitution the recovery process is initiated as the reality of the death is acknowledged. Finally, the mourner resolves the loss.

Parks (1972), in a study of widows, concluded that grief was similar to a physical injury more than any other type of illness. This study reported feelings of numbness, searching, pining, depression, and recovery. Parks also conceived of loss as being closely aligned with the body's fight–flight response. The symptoms of grieving were the body's attempt to deal with the stress associated with the loss.

Table 2
Theoretical Foundations of Bereavement Theories

Theorist	Theory Classification	Theory Tenets	Bereavement Response
Freud (1917)	Intrapsychic	Normal response to everyday life Primary interest depression Interference with grief potentially harmful Object loss, empty ego	
Fenichel (1945)	Intrapsychic	Ambivalent interjection is an adaptive response Guilt is evident in all grief Interjection acts as a buffer to preserve the relationship while the process of relinquishment takes place	1. Establishing interjection 2. Releasing the interjected object 3. The greater the ambivalence the greater the self-reproach, the greater the grief
Sullivan (1956)	Interpersonal concept of relationships, social interdynamics	Interpersonal situation not the individual Social dimension to grief theory Grief valuable and protective device Relies on early socialization Key: nature of relationship and the depth of the attachment bond threat to security throws person into anxiety	1. Opportunity to extricate from the attachment bond 2. Acknowledging loss obliterates the object of obsession 3. Strengthening hold on reality neutralizes clinging to lost object
Pollock (1961)	Ego-adaptive processes	Mourner struggling to renew an internal balance while adjusting to a threatening external environment	Stability through homeostasis • Shock—ego equilibrium • Grief—inability to discharge energy • Separation—internal object decathexis • Reparation—lasting adaptation
Bowlby (1980)	Attachment and information processing	Separation anxiety and defensive exclusion Need to redefine the self Need to develop new skills and discard old ones	Stages • Numbing • Yearning and searching • Disorganization and despair • Reorganization To reconcile quality of belief and disbelief

Table 2
Theoretical Foundations of Bereavement Theories (*Continued*)

Theorist	Theory Classification	Theory Tenets	Bereavement Response
Engel (1961)	Biological model of response	Grief is an adaptive central nervous system response 1. Fight and flight—anxiety 2. Conservation—withdrawal	Stages • Shock and disbelief • Developing awareness (fight-flight pattern) • Restitution (ritualization) • Resolving loss • Idealization • Outcome (year or more)
Parks (1972)	Physical injury	Changes in body function under control of sympathetic nervous system Energy reserves are mobilized Reluctance to give up possessions, people, status, expectation is basis of grief	Stages • Numbness minutes to days • Searching, restless hyperactivity, inability to concentrate, ruminations, loss of interest, pining • Depression, fruitless efforts, anger • Recovery modes of thinking and assumptions are relinquished
Saunders (1989)	Integrative theory	Inclusion of the idea of motivation Emotional/social/biological levels	Stages • Shock • Awareness of loss biological needs • Conservation-withdrawal • Healing decision to survive • Renewal

Saunder's Levels of Bereavement

Phase	Emotional	Biological	Social
Shock	Impact	Trauma	Egocentric
Awareness	Anxiety	Acute stress	Regression
Conservation	Despair	Chronic stress	Withdrawing
Healing	Gaining control	Healing	Identify
Renewal	New level of functioning	Recovery	Restructuring Renewal

Sources: Bowlby (1980); Engel (1961); Freud (1917); Fenickel (1945); Lindemann (1944); Parks (1972); Pollock (1961); Saunders (1989); Sullivan (1956); Worden (1982).

Kübler-Ross (1969) identified stages of coping with one's own impending death or the death of a loved one. She identified five behavioral themes: denial and isolation, anger, bargaining, depression, and acceptance. This is not a stage theory. The themes identified by Kübler-Ross are based on observable client behavior. Clients rarely progress through a specific pathway of predetermined response behaviors. This is especially true for clients in rehabilitation, who experience multiple concurrent losses and fluctuations in their feelings and perceptions regarding loss.

Worden (1982) discussed similar feelings and behaviors observed by other researchers. The behaviors identified by Worden include shock, numbness, helplessness, guilt, and social withdrawal during the grieving process. He also described the four tasks of mourning. The first task is to accept the reality of the loss. The second task is to experience the pain of grief. The third task is to adjust to the environment in which the valued object is absent. The fourth task is to withdraw emotional energy and reinvest it in another relationship. The skills necessary for the accomplishment of these tasks are the education and foundation of grief counseling.

Saunders (1989) suggested an integrative theory of bereavement. This integrative theory considers both internal and external variables. Saunders proposed that each of the psychological forces operating during the grief process has a biological counterpart that determines the physical well-being of the individual. Saunders viewed the change and awareness of grief as a progression toward resolution and homeostasis. Bereavement is adaptive rather than debilitating, and represents growth rather than regression.

The variability experienced by clients dealing with loss must be considered by the health care providers. Behavioral responses to grief and loss can provide direction for nursing care, and interventions should be designed according to the individual responses as they occur. The rehabilitation client's adjustment to loss is highly individualistic and seldom progresses in a smooth linear fashion from the beginning of the loss to its resolution. Individuals may vacillate between stages of grief before they finally come to acceptance and begin to adapt to the loss.

Hope is a coping strategy that makes life tolerable. Hope can be a positive and a negative factor in the rehabilitative process. When hope is used positively it adds meaning to life. If an individual holds onto unrealistic hope, he or she may experience an inhibition in the resolution of grief and loss. Hope provides a mechanism for denying the existence of a problem. Individuals who are hopeful can maintain a relatively normal life, and gain strength to deal with disabilities and limitations without becoming immobilized. Many individuals with disabilities or chronic illness hope for the magic cure that will take away their suffering and pain.

Interventions for Assisting Adult Clients to Cope with Loss

A plan of nursing interventions for assisting with loss and grieving will need to be individualized for each client. Specific interventions will be dictated by the nature of the client's loss, the client's behaviors and response to the loss, the client's developmental stage, and the stage of grief work that the client is ready to handle. The client should set the tone and the pace of grief work. The following are general intervention strategies based on the four tasks of mourning suggested by Worden (1982) and the integrative theory of bereavement proposed by Saunders (1989).

Worden (1982) suggested ten principles and procedures that make grief work effective:

- Help the client to actualize the loss.
- Help the client to identify and express feelings.
- Assist the client in developing abilities to live without the lost object.
- Facilitate the client's emotional withdrawal from the lost object.
- Provide the client with time to grieve.
- Interpret the client's grief behaviors as normal.
- Allow for individual differences in grief reactions, responses, and behaviors.
- Provide the client with continuing support.
- Help the client examine the coping defenses and styles being used to cope with the loss and reinforce those that are growth effective; explore other coping strategies to increase the client's perceptions of control.
- If complication with grief work arises refer to a professional grief counselor.

Other nursing interventions (Saunders, 1989) include the following:

- Provide the client with nonjudgmental support.
- Be an empathetic listener. The bereaved client needs to be heard repeatedly. This helps to establish the reality of the loss.
- Offer subjective understanding to the client. Focus on modifying maladaptive thinking (Kahn, 1995, p. 254). It is important to intervene in any client perceptions of inadequacy, worthlessness, or pessimism regarding the future.
- Allow the client to use denial as a coping strategy as long as it does not interfere with the therapeutic alliance and place the client at risk.
- Maintain a safe environment for the client in shock and disbelief (stage of grief) and manipulate the environment to maintain the usual activities of daily living.
- Provide the client in shock and disbelief with the basic needs and attend to maintaining physical well-being.
- Encourage the client's developing awareness of the reality of the loss, to take greater responsibility for grief work and self-management.
- During awareness assist the client in the expression of feelings, especially the constructive expression of anger.
- Identify and correct self-defeating behaviors (Kahn, 1995).
- Provide the client with positive social experiences that will reinforce the client's sense of self-esteem and worth (Kahn, 1995).
- Assist the client in finding new meaning in the absence of the lost object.

Goals of Grief Counseling

The overall goal of grief interventions is to help the client complete unfinished business following the loss and to be able to move on with living without the lost object.

Expected Outcomes

1. The client will be able to accept the reality of the loss.
2. The client will cope with expressing feelings about the loss.
3. The client will develop skills for coping with loss.
4. The client will make an emotional withdrawal from the lost object and feel comfortable about reinvesting energy in restructuring life.
5. The client will successfully adapt self-care capabilities and personal abilities following the loss.
6. If the client must relinquish roles, negotiate for shared responsibilities among others who will be assuming the role. Allow the client to be involved in the discussion if possible.

Conclusion

All rehabilitation clients will confront loss. This is true whether the loss is temporary or permanent. Grief is an individual happening. Grief is multilayered and can be felt on many levels at once. Grieving is a process rather than a state. It is not a linear process, because grief has so many ebbs and flows for the client. In many cases the client can become "stuck" in a phase for a long period of time. The rehabilitation nurse should never underestimate the significance of a client's loss, or the depth of the accompanying grief. Grief requires a particular type of growth that demands the formulation of personal identity (Saunders, 1989). Loss and grieving are culturally influenced and client responses will differ according to developmental stages. This chapter has focused on the loss experience common to the process of rehabilitation for the adult client.

References

Bowlby, J. (1980). *Attachment and loss: Loss sadness and depression* (Vol. 3). New York: Basic Books.

Engel, G. L. (1961). Is grief a disease? A challenge for medical research. *Psychosomatic Medicine, 23,* 18–23.

Fenickel, O. (1945). *The psychoanalystic theory of neurosis.* New York: Norton.

Freud, S. (1917). *Mourning and melancholia.* London: Hogarth Press.

Green, S. A. (1985). *Mind and body: The psychology of physical illness.* Washington, DC: American Psychiatric Press.

Hughes, F. (1984). Reactions to loss: Coping with disability and death. In R. Marinelli & A. E. Dell Orto (Eds.), *The psychological & social impact of physical disability* (2nd. ed., pp. 131–136). New York: Springer.

Kahn, A. M. (1995). Coping with fear and grieving. In I. M. Lubkin (Ed.), *Chronic illness: Impact and interventions* (2nd ed., pp. 241–260). Boston: Jones & Bartlett.

Kastenbaum, R. J. (1977). *Death, society and human experience.* St. Louis: Mosby.

Kowalsky, E. L. (1987). Grief: A lost life-style. *American Journal of Nursing, 78*(3), 418–420.

Kübler-Ross, E. (1969). *On death and dying.* New York: Macmillan.

Lindemann, E. (1944). The symptomatology and management of acute grief. *American Journal of Psychiatry, 101,* 131–148.

Miller, J. F. (1992). *Coping with chronic illness: Overcoming powerlessness.* Philadelphia: F. A. Davis.

Olshansky, S. (1962). Chronic sorrow: A response to having a mentally defective child. *Social Casework, 43,* 190–193.

Parad, H. J. (1965). *Crisis intervention: Selected readings.* New York: Family Service Association of America.

Parks, C. M. (1972). *Bereavement: Studies of grief in adult life.* New York: International University Press.

Pereira, B. (1984). Loss and grief in chronic illness. *Rehabilitation Nursing, 9*(2), 20.

Pollock, G. N. (1961). Mourning and adaptation. *International Journal of Psychoanalysis, 43,* 341–361.

Rosenblatt, P. C., Walsh, R. P., & Jackson, P. A. (1976). *Grief and mourning in cross-cultural perspective.* New Haven, CT: Human Relations Area Files Press.

Saunders, C. M. (1989). *Grief: The mourning after: Dealing with adult bereavement.* New York: John Wiley & Sons.

Servoss, A. (1984). Depression and suicide in the disabled. In D. Krueger (Ed.), *Rehabilitation psychology.* Rockville, MD: Aspen.

Schmale, A. H. (1958). Relationship of separation and depression to disease. *Psychosomatic Medicine, 20,* 259–277.

Stuart, G. W., & Sundeen, S. J. (1991). *Principles and practice of psychiatric nursing.* St. Louis: Mosby.

Sullivan, H. L. (1956). The dynamics of emotion. In H. L. Sullivan (Ed.), *Clinical studies in psychiatry* (Chapter 5). New York: W. W. Norton & Co.

Worden, J. W. (1982). *Grief counseling and grief therapy: A handbook for the mental health practitioner.* New York: Springer.

Suggested Readings

Cotler, M. (Ed.). (1996). Perspectives on chronic illness: Treating patients and delivering care. *American Behavioral Scientist, 39*(6).

Dietrich, D. R., & Shabad, P. C. (Eds.). (1989). *The problem of loss and mourning: Psychoanalytic perspectives.* Connecticut: International Universities Press.

Farran, C. J., Herth, K. A., & Popovich, J. M. (1995). *Hope and hopelessness: Critical clinical constructs.* Thousand Oaks, CA: Sage.

Farley, A. M. (1992). *Nursing and the disabled across the life span.* Boston: Jones & Bartlett.

Forman, S. G. (1993). *Coping skills: Interventions for children and adolescents.* San Francisco: Jossey-Bass.

Rolland, J. S. (1994). *Families, illness, and disability: An integrative treatment model.* New York: Harper-Collins.

Shapiro, E. R. (1994). *Grief as a family process: A developmental approach to clinical practice.* New York: Guilford Press.

Stark, P. L., & McGovern, J. P. (Eds.). (1992). *The hidden dimension of illness: Human suffering.* New York: National League for Nursing Press.

Strass, A. L., & Glasser, B. G. (1975). *Chronic illness and the quality of life.* St. Louis: Mosby.

CHAPTER 14
Meeting Clients' Spiritual Needs

Susan McKeever Smith and *Shila Wiebe*

Key Terms

Empathy
Humor
Imagery
Prayer
Religiosity
Sacraments
Scripture
Spiritual Care
Spiritual Distress
Spirituality
Sympathy
Therapeutic Use of Self

Objectives

1. Define spirituality.

2. Assist the client to find meaning in suffering.

3. Identify meaningful beliefs/relationships that maintain and strengthen hope.

4. Develop a format using key questions to assess the client's spiritual needs.

5. Plan potential strategies to meet the spiritual care needs of the client.

6. Discuss with the client examples of spiritual care interventions and implement those preferred by the client.

7. Identify biblical resources that may be shared with the client to enhance the potential for spiritual well-being.

8. Seek opportunities to use spiritual care interventions.

9. Validate the effectiveness of the spiritual care interventions with the client.

Introduction

Historically, nurses have focused on the care of the whole person—mind, body, and spirit. Caring was evident as early as prehistoric times. The earliest descriptions of nursing care took place within a religious community, and many of the religious practices were intertwined with medical and nursing measures. Certainly the influence of Christianity and the values of charity, service, and sacrifice encouraged individuals to care for the ill, destitute, and dying and expanded the role of the nurse. The New Testament describes an organization of deacons who were given the responsibility of providing for the needy. In the early church these leaders were male. Eventually the deacons established the position of *deaconess*. "The deaconesses carried nursing forward as they ministered to the sick and injured in their homes. Phoebe, a friend of Paul's and the very first deaconess in the young Christian church has been called the first visiting nurse" (Zerwekh & Claborn, 1997, p. 33).

> These deaconesses recognized that caring for others included providing for physical needs. . . . They provided intellectual and spiritual nourishment, clothed individuals who had been forgotten or neglected and [were] no longer cared for and loved, and provided hospitality for people who were homeless or who felt lost in a strange environment. In their ministrations, these nurses saw spiritual meaning in the care they provided for the sick. (Carson, 1989, p. 56)

The word *nursing* comes from the Latin word, *nutricius,* meaning nourishment. Through the centuries nursing care continued to be provided by religious communities as well as secular groups.

In the twentieth century, nursing theorists address nursing's responsibility for holistic care. Yet, frequently, they do not specifically speak of the importance of providing care that meets spiritual concerns.

> The current times are very much secular, and today's society focuses on things that are oriented on the present, materialistic, and tangible. Concerns of the spirit, things that are sacred and eternal, receive far less attention in our world. (Carson, 1989, p. 152)

Carson continues to explore this issue in more depth, in an effort to explain why society pays less attention to spiritual needs. Reasons given include both the positive and negative aspects of humanist philosophy, that technology has become like a god to society, and that the family, which is the original source of spiritual awareness, has broken down. She states last, "the aura of mystery that surrounds the topic of spirituality is often felt to be too personal to explore . . . private and off limits for discussion" (Carson, 1989, p. 153).

Yet there is a quest for many individuals to find meaning and purpose in life. Viktor Frankl, a well-known Viennese psychiatrist, who was in a concentration camp during World War II, writes that "our search for meaning is a primary source in life" (Frankl, 1971, p. xiii). Travelbee (1971) supports this, stating that

> . . . meaning can be found in the experiences of illness, suffering, and pain. When such meaning is found the individual is able to use the experience of illness as an en-

abling life experience, i.e., enabling in the sense that it is possible for the individual to achieve self-actualization and that which lies beyond self transcendence. (1971, p. 157)

What implications does this then have for the nurse? Is spiritual care the responsibility of the nurse or the responsibility of some other member of the health team? Is it not sufficient to assist the client to maintain the highest level of functioning? If a spiritual need is ignored can it be said that holistic care was provided?

The nurse cares for the individual, not a body part. The existence of suffering, whether physical, mental, spiritual is the proper concern of the nurse. It is her responsibility to see to it that the ill person received the assistance he requires. (Travelbee, 1971, p. 159)

What does this mean for the nurse? The nurse must also share this belief, "that illness and suffering can be [a] profoundly meaningful life experience, provided the ill individual also comprehends, or is assisted by the nurse to find, meaning and purpose in these experiences" (Travelbee, 1971, p. 160).

This, then is the challenge in nursing the spiritually distressed person: to listen, to accept, to explore, and finally, to offer no ready answers. This is clearly a difficult task but a rewarding one. In the end, persons who discover their own meaning and their own reason for believing in what they do will usually be the more satisfied. (Burnard, 1987, p. 381)

What are the barriers that prevent the nurse from providing this holistic care? Most of the nursing literature dealing with spiritual concerns stems from one particular religion or denomination. The nurse then needs to expand his or her awareness of other beliefs and ideologies. The focus of spiritual care is to assist the client with his or her spiritual distress, not to proselytize. The broader meaning of spirituality is to find meaning and purpose in life and not necessarily to tie spirituality to religious or denominational needs. Another barrier may be the nurse who is unsure of his or her own beliefs and values and who feels that discussion of religious or spiritual needs is a private and personal issue. "The U.S. orientation to life contributes to the idea that many individuals believe health and happiness are the meaning and purpose of life and are to be sought at all costs" (Granstrom, 1985, p. 42). It is usually not until individuals are confronted with illness and suffering that they are forced to deal with their own humanity and mortality.

. . . nurses must help their clients clarify their experiences of suffering, doubt and fear within a framework of faith, hope and love that bring meaning and purpose, that is self-actualizing, not in spite of this illness and crisis but because of it. (Granstrom, 1985, p. 45)

To assist clients to derive meaning and purpose from suffering and illness, the nurse must have a clear definition of spirituality that is distinct from religiosity.

Spirituality Defined

Reed (1991) separated the concepts of **spirituality** and **religiosity,** although they are sometimes used interchangeably. Religion is the personal or institutional system of organized beliefs, practices or rituals, and/or forms of worship. Reed (1991) stated that a broad conceptualization of spirituality includes an

> . . . expression of the human propensity to find meaning and purpose in life through self transcendence, that is through expanding the conceptual boundaries of the self beyond limits posed by the immediate situation, physical limitations, or otherwise constructed views of life and human potential. (p. 122)

In general, Highfield and Cason (1983) agreed that the spiritual dimension focuses on answering the questions related to the meaning and purpose of life. Still others equate spiritual well-being with a sense of interconnectedness among self, others, nature/environment, and God or Ultimate Other (Hungelmann, Kenkel-Rossi, Klaasen, & Stollenwerk, 1985; Stoll, 1987). Stoll (1989) personalized spirituality to mean "my being, my inner person . . . as me expressed through my body, my thinking, my feelings, my judgments, and my creativity . . . who is motivated and enabled to value, to worship, and to communicate with the holy, the transcendent" (p. 6).

Spirituality is a part of every person and suggests a relationship to a transcendent higher being or God. Most religions have some concept of God whether it be Jesus Christ, Buddha, Mohammed, or other beings but this supreme being, God, may not be central in the beliefs, rituals, or group experiences of a particular religion. Therefore, spirituality and religion are not synonymous. Religion may provide the expression of spirituality or assist in meeting spiritual needs but a person outside a particular religion or religious denomination may experience a relationship to a higher being whether it be an unconscious God, created beings, or a personal God, through other avenues. We are created with a God consciousness.

For the humanist spirituality may refer to the values chosen by the individual and that order one's life. In this model, the chosen values direct the person's choice of lifestyle and coping mechanisms used to achieve goals, needs, and aspirations. "This self actualization focus encourages a person toward a spiritual quest for being on a human plane only" (Stoll, 1989, p. 7).

On the horizontal plane spirituality reflects the relationship with God that is being lived out in daily life and in the interactions with self, others, and the environment. From this horizontal dimension flows the psychosocial need for relatedness, and the spiritual need for purpose and meaning, love, trust, hope, and forgiveness. In the situation of life, spirituality may be tested. It is not always a steady upward climb. How does suffering work to increase spiritual growth? Can illness be used to find meaning and purpose?

Concepts of Suffering

Travelbee (1971) defined nursing as "an interpersonal process whereby the professional nurse practitioner assists an individual, family, or community to prevent or cope with the experience of illness and suffering and, if necessary, to find meaning in these experiences" (p. 7). Christians believe that God is with them as they suffer (Isaiah 43:1–7) and through the resurrection of Jesus Christ, one day suffering will cease (Revelation 21:1–4). He (God) demonstrates his power and his love in the midst of suffering (2 Corinthians 12:7–10). "Suffering, like illness, is a common life experience encountered by every human being" (Travelbee, 1971, p. 61). Romans 5:1–5 and 2 Corinthians 1:3–11 say that our own suffering equips us to help others who suffer. Nurses who identify with these values are able to assist clients find spiritual meaning in their suffering. In quiet sharing of this experience the nurse "helps the person to sustain the burden of suffering" (Donley, 1991, p. 178). "Clients from differing cultures or religious preferences other than Christian can be expected to choose their own explanations for suffering" (Solimine & Hoeman, 1996, p. 629). Individuals may have many and varied explanations as to their cause of suffering, for example, punishment for sinning, for wrong-doing, for failure to perform some action, or perhaps someone or something caused the suffering; "but a careful and complete assessment may lead a nurse to determine the unique nature underlying a particular client's suffering" (Solimine & Hoeman, 1996, p. 629). "When nurses, acting compassionately to alleviate suffering, also search with their patients for a spiritual meaning for the experience, there will be a rebuilding of trust in professional relationships" (Donley, 1991, p. 182).

Assessment of Client's Spiritual Needs

The nurse is the key person to begin to assess the client's spiritual needs. Ross (1994) suggested that "spiritual needs are perhaps more subtle and more difficult to identify than some other needs and that whether or not they are identified may depend on the sensitivity of the nurse" (p. 443). There are numerous tools that may assist in exploring the client's spiritual concerns and available resources for dealing with the injury or loss (e.g., see Carpenito, 1997; Carson, 1989; Fish & Shelley, 1978).

During assessment, the nurse's goal is to learn about the client's religion, source of spiritual strength, and how the present situation affects spiritual well-being. It is important to remember that the assessment must remain focused on the client and should not drift over to trying to convert the client to another religion/denomination. The nurse is gathering information to support the client's faith, not to change his or her commitment. Whatever the client's developmental level in the spiritual journey, the nurse meets the client at his level and comes alongside to uphold and affirm his or her walk of faith.

The assessment begins by noting religious preference, which is usually recorded on the face sheet of the chart. In the client's room look for the presence of religious articles at the bedside—Bible, prayer book, rosary, medals, devotional literature, cards. The presence of visitors—family, friends, clergy—indicates the interpersonal relationships established by the client. These are obvious clues that give information about the spiritual ties of the client and may be obtained without asking any questions. After having gathered this information, the nurse continues the assessment by eliciting information from the client. There are three major categories of information needed: (1) belief system, (2) religious rituals and practices, and (3) effect of present situation on spiritual well-being. The questions that best elicit information about the personal belief system relate to (1) the client's source of spiritual strength (e.g., God, Buddha, church, family, friends, self), (2) the availability of that resource at the present time, and (3) the best way the nurse can assist in upholding this client's system of beliefs.

To ascertain religious practices, it is best to ask the client which religious rituals and practices are meaningful to him or her and how the nurse can facilitate these practices. Possible activities might be to pray, read scripture, assist with rituals and sacraments, call for visits of the clergy, or sing a hymn. For information concerning religious practices of the various religions, see Carpenito (1997).

Last, the nurse needs to know the effect of the present situation on the client's spiritual well-being. Begin by asking how this injury/rehabilitation experience has had an impact on the client's relationship with God and the practice of his or her religion. Then find out who or what is available to support your client through this situation.

The answers to these questions should be correlated to spiritual needs for meaning and purpose, love, forgiveness, and hope. The client's response to the present situation demonstrates the meaning and purpose attached to this particular life experience. Those with intrinsic religiosity usually attach meaning to every experience, even to suffering. Gaining meaning lends hope to the present experience, and helps the client to trust God with the future. The need for love is fulfilled in the context of significant human relationships. The number of visitors will reveal the people who have a relationship with the client; the client will need to validate whether these are significant and valued relationships. Love must also be viewed from the perspective of God's love for people. Even when the client feels unloved or unlovely, God's love is constant and forgiving. Love and forgiveness are a part of the character of God, and therefore the client's beliefs about God will color how he or she experiences God's love and forgiveness. The sensitivity of the nurse is needed to make a correct assessment, and to correlate the findings with the specific needs of the client.

On the basis of the assessment of the client's spiritual needs, a nursing diagnosis of spiritual distress or potential for enhanced spiritual well-being is made. Carpenito (1997) defined the major characteristic for **spiritual distress** as a disturbance in belief system, whereas the potential for enhanced spiritual well-being describes a person who is secure in having the needs for meaning and purpose, love, forgiveness, and hope met.

After making a nursing diagnosis, and validating it with the client, the nurse begins planning **spiritual care** interventions. It is important to know the client's wishes and expectations for spiritual care.

What Is Spiritual Care?

Sodestrom and Martinson (1987) studied the spiritual coping strategies of twenty-five oncology patients from the perspective of both the patient and the nurse. In assisting with their spiritual care, the majority of the patients expected the nurse to recognize that patients "fall back on their religion in times of crisis, and to support the patient's belief as a strength and resource for him, but make it specific to the patient's religious background" (p. 45). In addition, approximately 50 percent of patients reported that nurses served as resources for meeting spiritual needs and assisted with spiritual activities, such as referral to clergy for prayer, communion, or sacraments. In a table, Sodestrom and Martinson (1987) summarized data related to patient expectations of the nurse in terms of spiritual care:

> . . . let the patients talk about their feelings about God and being willing to listen, provide privacy for prayer and assist the patient with praying as requested, respect and acknowledge the patient's religious beliefs, assist the patient with Bible reading as requested, and comfort patients by being positive, kind, gentle, and giving good physical care. (p. 45)

Spiritual activities engaged in by patients consisted of "prayer, asks others to pray for him, asks others to pray with him, religious objects or music, religious television or radio, read the Bible, attend church, read other religious books, memorize Bible verses, request Communion" (Sodestrom & Martinson, 1987, p. 44). In the same study, those called on most often as spiritual resource persons were "family (92%), clergy (76%), friends (68%), nurses (48%), and physicians (24%)" (Sodestrom & Martinson, 1987, p. 44). Forbis (1988) found that elderly clients "want nurses to listen, contact religious representatives and pray" (p. 159). In another study by Reed (1991), of three groups of 100 patients each (terminally ill hospitalized, nonterminally ill hospitalized, and well nonhospitalized), "27% of responses wanted the nurse to arrange a visit with the clergy, 17% wanted the nurse to allow time to pray, 15% to provide time for family, and 14% to talk with you about your beliefs" (p. 125). Although the ranking may differ, there emerges a pattern related to client expectations for spiritual care. Listening and supporting the client's religious beliefs, making referrals to clergy, and allowing privacy and time for prayer by the client alone or with the nurse are important approaches in meeting the spiritual needs of clients. These interventions must emanate from a thorough assessment of the spiritual needs of the client, and the client should be a partner in the development of the intervention plan.

Nursing Interventions: Spiritual Care

The nurse has many resources available to assist in providing spiritual care. Therapeutic use of self, hope, prayer, scripture or other religious literature, and religious rituals are tools that may be used to support the client. Music, humor, and imagery have also been found to be effective interventions. Whether in crisis or in the course of daily activities, these tools are available and have the potential to bring power, comfort, and peace to the individual. These practices are most helpful when they are appropriate to the person's belief system and religion.

Use of Self

The nurse is in an enviable position while caring for clients, as he or she provides care 24 hours per day. As such, one of the most significant and effective interventions is the **therapeutic use of self.** "Personal contact has a physical, emotional and spiritual effect" (Warner, 1996, p. 157). The presence of the nurse or use of self to be effective requires many varied behaviors: listening, empathy, humility, vulnerability, commitment, and touch. This occurs through the development of a personal relationship with the client. Travelbee (1971) stated that "the purpose of nursing is achieved through the establishment of a human-to-human relationship" (p. 5). She goes on to say that the purpose of this relationship "is to assist an individual, family or community to prevent or cope with the experiences of illness and suffering and, if necessary, to find meaning in these experiences" (p. 16). It requires an intellectual approach combined with therapeutic use of self.

Communication is the process that establishes a human-to-human relationship. Nonverbal communication is as critical as verbal communication, and nurses need to focus on both the auditory and visual stimuli. This technique is a process that requires the nurse's energy and concentration. Active listening demonstrates interest in the client, and "fosters a trusting relationship that encourages the client to express feelings and share thoughts" (Antai-Otong, 1995, p. 103). "He who answers before listening—that is his folly and his shame" (Proverbs 18:24, New International Version [NIV]). Techniques that facilitate communication are well known to nurses; those frequently used are open-ended comments or questions reflecting content, feelings, and impressions, and the techniques of sharing perceptions to validate meaning. Silence is another significant technique. One of the barriers to therapeutic communication and spiritual interventions may be the nurses themselves. Many individuals feel that discussing religion or spiritual issues is a private matter. Frequently, nurses may experience discomfort or feelings of inadequacy when confronted with issues with which the clients are struggling. A nurse may be confronting spiritual issues within his or her own life (e.g., anger or disappointment with God) and might communicate these feelings to a client in a way that is not supportive of the client's needs and denies the client the opportunity to express his or her needs. Nurses who do not have strong spiritual beliefs may still be capable of providing spiritual care through caring and concern, empathy, listening, and their presence. Open ended questions are questions that begin with what, which, where, when, how, or who, encouraging clients to clarify their thoughts and feelings. Reflecting is used to reduce miscommunication and misunderstanding; it directs questions, feelings, and ideas back to the client. Clarification helps clients clarify their own thoughts and maximizes understanding between the nurse and client. Silence may serve several purposes—a moment of reflection for both participants, organizing thoughts, and encouraging the client to speak. Letting the client break the silence first, frequently when trust is present, allows the client to share thoughts and feelings that might otherwise have been withheld. A thoughtful silence encourages people to talk; it is a time for contemplation and relaxation. If the silence persists, it may be a clue that the topic is exhausted.

Empathy is the ability to experience the feelings of another. Carson (1989) stated that

> . . . empathy is different from sympathy. Sympathy allows the listener to share in the feelings of the other, but in the process of sharing, the listener loses objectivity and is unable to differentiate between his or her feelings and those of the speaker. (p. 166)

Empathy allows the nurse to be supportive and encouraging and communicates a sensitivity to the client's feelings. When unsure of how to be empathetic, reflecting back on crises they have experienced will enable nurses to identify how they felt and the kind of help they wanted, and will increase their sensitivity to their clients' feelings.

"Nurses who are vulnerable are those who are willing to open themselves up to rejection, criticism, and pain, as well to the joy and praise of other people, as they respond to these people in a caring relationship" (Fish & Shelley, 1978, p. 91). Warner (1996) stated that "a nurse's vulnerability prevents him or her from remaining aloof or judgmental" (p. 158). Romans 12:15 tells us, "rejoice with those who rejoice: mourn with those who mourn" (NIV). Sharing in a person's positive and negative experiences demonstrates caring.

"Probably the greatest tool available to nurses for meeting spiritual needs is their own presence and ability to touch another both physically and spiritually"

(Carson, 1989, p. 164). Cassetta (1993) stated, "Touch creates a caring relation-ship . . . and the purpose of touch is to facilitate the healing process"(p. 18). When clients are separated from their support systems and things that are famil-iar, touch and the time spent providing it create a caring environment and may help lessen the feelings of isolation and anxiety. Sharing in these feelings coupled with touch communicates personal spiritual strength and willingness to care, to listen, and to be available (Carson, 1989, p. 165). Having a hand to hold during a stressful or painful time reminds us that we are not alone and touch communi-cates that there is someone there who cares.

"Commitment is a willingness . . . to share in the solitude, anxiety, suffer-ing and grief of patients" (Fish & Shelley, 1979, p. 93). Warner (1996) ex-panded on this, stating that "to be committed to a nurse–client relationship re-quires that the nurse will be present through all stages of emotional and spiritual growth, and not abandon his or her client when the relationship becomes challen-ging or uncomfortable" (p. 159). If this should occur, the client may hesitate to share spiritual needs with the nurse. Commitment to the client is a reflection of God's commitment to humankind. If the nurse withdraws or abandons clients it may reinforce their belief that God has or will abandon them. One of nursing's goals when dealing with a diagnosis of spiritual distress is to assist the client in es-tablishing or maintaining a relationship with God. "When nurses share them-selves in this manner, they can serve as a human bridge between the client and the client's perception of a divine power" (Carson, 1989, p. 168). "To be truly committed indicates a nurse's inner spiritual strength . . ." (Warner, 1996, p. 159).

The nurse at the bedside cannot help but be changed or affected after caring for clients—clients who are experiencing illness, anxiety, suffering, pain, loneli-ness, and dying. A nurse exposed to the sufferings of mankind begins to clarify his or her own feelings on these issues and realizes what it means to be a human being. With this acceptance nurses are able to accept their own humanity. "In fact, it is through one's limitations and weaknesses that God can most effectively work through an individual to assist others" (Warner, 1996, p. 158). Accepting one's own humanity assists the nurse in accepting the humanity of others. "Tran-scendence in nursing means the ability to get beyond and outside of self in order to perceive and respond to human-ness of the ill, suffering, or dying individual" (Travelbee, 1971, p. 42). Warner (1996) added, "the gift of humility increases the level of faith and trust between nurse and client" (p. 158).

The literature abounds with data on identifying spiritual needs and nursing interventions, but little is found on what the client wants from the nurse. Em-blen and Halstead (1993) designed a descriptive study to collect interview data to determine how patients, nurses, and chaplains currently are defining the phrases *spiritual needs* and *spiritual interventions* (p. 175). Patients saw nurses as offering prayer and scripture as religious spiritual interventions, and under the Values category they identified compassion as that value they saw in nurses. The nurse's presence was the sole behavior identified in the Relationships category, which supports the use of self as one of the most significant nursing spiritual interventions. Talk, touch, and smile were those behaviors selected in the Communication area. Under Other, clients expected nurses to refer, provide physical care, accommodate to treatment needs, and assess needs.

> The way nurse and chaplain caregivers define spiritual needs is related to the interventions they identified. Therefore it is important for a nurse to ask patients how they define spiritual needs and what they want the nurse to do to meet the need. (Emblen & Halstead, 1993, p. 182)

Hope

Hope is a critical concept that creates the foundation for spiritual interventions—hope for a peaceful death, a pain-free life, regained mobility or independence, and God's reassurance that he will sustain one through this experience.

Travelbee (1971) stated that "hope enables human beings to cope with difficult and stressful situations, deprivation, tragedy, failure, boredom, loneliness and suffering" (p. 77). " . . . The role of professional nurse practitioner [is] to assist the ill person to experience hope in order to cope with the stress of illness and suffering" (Travelbee, 1971, p. 77). Haase, Britt, Coward, Leidy, and Penn (1992), in a review of literature on hope, identified four critical characteristics: time, action, goals, and feelings. "The first is a focus on time which emphasizes the future" (Haase et al., 1992, p. 143). Hope is the expectation that future prospects will be positive. Romans 8:24–25 states: "Hope that is seen is not hope. For who hopes for what he sees? But if we hope for what we do not see, we wait for it with patience" (NIV). The "second attribute is an energized action orientation" (Haase et al., 1992, p. 143). Individuals who experience hope do it in a constructive way; unlike the hopeless individual, who appears passive and depressed, the hopeful individual uses positive coping mechanisms, such as reaching out for others, exploring alternative treatment modalities, and taking action to plan goals. The "third attribute is the setting of a positive goal or a desired outcome" (Haas et al., 1992, p. 143). Usually these goals focus on coping with illness, relationships with others, and goals for life. These goals are motivating and seen as being attainable and nursing strategies assist in identifying goals. "However, when goals are unrealistic or not embraced by a client, trust and rapport with the nurse will erode" (Solimine & Hoeman, 1996, p. 640). Thompson (1994) said that clients who have hope identify goals dealing with their illnesses, feel these goals will be achieved, and express positive perceptions of the future (p. 12). Last, the fourth characteristic is the feeling of uneasiness or uncertainty. On the basis of these attributes, Haase et al. (1992) defined hope as "an energized mental state involving feelings of uneasiness or uncertainty and characterized by a cognitive, action-oriented expectation that a positive future goal or outcome is positive" (p. 142). Gaskins and Forte (1995) discussed a study of 126 healthy adults, conducted in 1989, which identified the predictors of hope, mental health, religious beliefs, and social supports (p. 18). Gaskins and Forte's own study (1995) identified three sources of hope in older adults: religious symbols, relationships with others, and activities. "Discussing spiritual needs, important relationships and enjoyable activities with other adults (regardless of the setting) would give health care professionals insight into individuals' sources of hope. Only then, can care be planned that fosters, strengthens, or maintains hope" (Gaskin & Forte, 1995, p. 23). Gewe (1994) stated, "from a Christian perspective, it is essential that hope be based upon truth. False hopes which do not materialize can lead to depression, feelings of helplessness, despair and possibly death" (p. 19). "Since God is the same [yesterday, and today and forever] (Hebrews 13:8), contemporary Christians can continue to have hope in God's promises based upon knowledge of God's character and past actions as communicated in scripture" (Gewe, 1994, p. 19).

Scripture references to hope are found in the Old Testament as well as the New Testament. Psalm 119:81: "My soul faints with longing for your salvation, but I have put my hope in your word." We see the words "hope in your word" also in verses 74, 114, and 147 of Psalm 119 (NIV). In Romans 5:2–5, it can be seen how suffering produces hope:

> . . . rejoice in the hope of the glory of God. Not only so, but we also rejoice in our sufferings, because we know that suffering produces perseverance; perseverance, character; and character, hope. And hope does not disappoint us, because God has poured out his love into our hearts by the Holy Spirit, whom he has given us. (NIV)

Raleigh (1992) also found in her study that whether clients had cancer or chronic illnesses, hope was an important strategy in coping and the sources of hope were the same; family, friends, and religious beliefs. Raleigh (1992) also reported that "a smaller proportion reported that a nonreligious philosophy was helpful in maintaining hope" (p. 447).

> The nurse should be aware of these needs and, whenever possible, should encourage visits by family and close friends, allowing them the privacy to communicate at a meaningful level. If such visits are not possible, the nurse's companionship and willingness to listen may help. (Raleigh, 1992, p. 448)

Post-White, Ceronsky, Kreitzer, Nickelson, Drew, Mackey, Koopminers, and Gutknecht (1996) reported in their study reported that "finding meaning and mobilizing resources were elements common to a sense of hope and sense of coherence. Most participants felt that spiritual beliefs and relationships were important to their hope . . . " (p. 1571). Their implications for nursing practice included the following: "Nurses can influence patients' hope by being present, taking time to talk, giving information, being respectful and honest, and acknowledging resources that support hopefulness" (Post-White et al., 1996, p. 1571).

Use of Prayer

Prayer is communication with God. A person converses with God not only to make requests but to find fellowship with God, to offer praise and thanks, and to share life events and the feelings surrounding them. This dialogue with God serves to let God speak concerning his will for each person and for each person to communicate an array of feelings, thoughts, and requests to him.

The power of prayer is emphasized in scripture. The Bible has numerous references that instruct people how to pray. Following are some instructions given related to prayer. 1 Timothy 2:1: "I urge, then, first of all, that requests, prayers, intercession, and thanksgiving be made for everyone." Ephesians 6:18: "Pray in the Spirit on all occasions with all kinds of prayers and requests. With this in mind be alert, and always keep on praying for all the saints." James 5:16: "The prayer of the righteous is powerful and effective." 1 Thessalonians 5:17–18: "Pray continuously. Give thanks in all circumstances for this is God's will for you in Christ Jesus." Matthew 6:8: "Your Father knows what you need before you ask." Matthew 7:7–8: "Ask and it will be given to you; . . . for everyone who asks receives." Matthew 7:11: ". . . how much more will your Father in heaven give good gifts to those who ask him?" Matthew 18:19: ". . . if two of you on earth agree about anything you ask for, it will be done for you by my Father in heaven." These passages show that God is generous, that we are to pray with others, and that the Holy Spirit ministers for us to the Father when we do not know what to pray. God desires fellowship with men and women, and prayer is the link that connects the Christian to a dynamic, powerful, and loving God. The clients who do not embrace Christianity may select and use the texts for a particular religion, a designated prayer, ritual, or book or other meaningful resources.

Guidelines to the use of prayer should answer the questions: when, what, and how.

When to Pray. The question of when to pray may arise. Some people feel it is very private. Others are comfortable praying only when in a church or chapel. Still others love to pray in groups or even in public. The Bible says to pray continuously (1 Thessalonians 5:17–18), under all circumstances, on all occasions (Ephesians 6:18), privately (Matthew 6:6). The nurse can pray any time, whether alone or with the client. Individual prayer is a powerful tool that the nurse can use to intercede for the client even when the client is not present. Many clients are comforted by the fact that someone is praying for them. But before offering to pray with a client it is important that the nurse gain permission from the client and is sensitive to the possible connotation of the act of praying. For example, there was a zealous nurse who felt that she should pray for every one of her clients who were going to surgery. On this particular morning she was running a bit late, so did not get around to praying until the client was being wheeled down the corridor on the operating room gurney. She stopped the gurney, prayed for the client, supposedly just offering a simple prayer that the surgery would go well. However, the client interpreted this quite differently. He became very upset, and asked if the nurse knew something that he did not about the risks of surgery. The nurse was focused on meeting her own objectives and insensitive to the client. Although appropriate to pray anywhere and at all times, the nurse must be sensitive to the client's needs as well as to the meaning of the prayer to the client.

Prayer is best when the nurse prays in response to a need expressed by the client. This means the nurse must take the time to establish a therapeutic relationship with the client so that there is a bond of trust. Once there is trust, the client is free to share real feelings and needs. Before prayer can be offered with understanding and empathy the nurse must have knowledge of the client's real feelings, the client's needs and goals related to this specific situation, and the priority the client places on them. Trust is integral to any nursing intervention and paramount in the area of spiritual care. When the client trusts the nurse, asking for prayer will be simple. When the nurse has gained the trust of the client, offering to pray will be appropriate and acceptable to the client. In response to verbal and nonverbal cues from the client, the nurse can pray specifically for expressions of fear, anxiety, hopelessness, helplessness, grief, stress, and lack of control. However, there may be physical evidence of a strong faith, such as the presence of a Bible, religious literature, devotional book, rosary, medals, and so on, in the room. For these clients prayer may provide fellowship, with God and with the nurse, and comfort through sharing of similar values or beliefs.

The environment should be as private and quiet as possible. Try to avoid prayer in public places, where there are onlookers. Try to provide privacy by closing a door, pulling a curtain, or going to an empty room or chapel. There is a certain reverence required that is best facilitated by privacy. This does not mean that significant others and family should be excluded, but the nurse must be sensitive as to whether these people are a help or hindrance to the spiritual care of the client.

There are some situations in which anxiety is typically high for clients and prayer can be especially helpful. These times include admission to the hospital, especially the emergency room or critical care units, before surgery; while going through major examinations or tests; and during initial placement of equipment to monitor function, sustain life, or assist with activities of daily living. All of these are frightening processes for the client. Through prayer the nurse can assist the client to focus on the resources available to persevere and experience God's love, comfort, peace, and care during a time of crisis. Remind the client that

God cares for him. In 1 Peter 5:7 God tells us to "cast all your anxiety on him because he cares for you."

Prayer is appropriate at any time but is best when offered in the context of a trusting relationship and in response to the specifically stated needs of the client. The environment should be conducive to prayer, and provided in privacy with an attitude of reverence. Whether in the course of daily care, or at times when the client enters a crisis situation and the outcomes are unknown, the nurse can pray for or with the client.

What to Pray. The content of prayer should be directed toward (1) the specific needs identified by the client, (2) a reflective summary of the conversation with the client, and (3) an affirmation of the power of God to act and a reminder of God's love for each person, no matter what.

When the client identifies his specific needs, prayer should focus on those needs and the client can rest assured that the nurse has heard where help is needed. Sometimes a client will identify an unrealistic goal and demand healing. When this happens, the nurse should refocus the need to assist the client to adapt. Consider the client who is grieving the loss of mobility and self-care owing to a spinal cord injury. It is unlikely that the severed spinal cord will regenerate, but the nurse can pray for a spirit of acceptance and perseverance to make the adjustments, and accomplish optimal rehabilitation for this particular injury. In this way prayer focuses on the specific need, but redirects the client to more realistic expectations.

Summation of a conversation in prayer is another part of the "what" of prayer (Stallwood, 1975). The client may have numerous concerns but is unclear concerning priorities or what needs to be done. In this case the nurse can pray for clarity for the client concerning the priorities, and even assist in setting realistic goals. The prayer can recount the problems that have already been solved as evidence of God's work on behalf of the client. In the case of the spinal cord injury, this might include the admission to the rehabilitation hospital, insurance coverage, family support, and availability of psychological counseling. With these areas under control, the nurse prays that the client's anxieties are decreased so his energy can be used for rehabilitative recovery. This type of summary actively includes God as part of the collaborative rehabilitation team.

Affirmation of God's promises and attributes shifts the focus of prayer from the problems to the one who is able to provide solutions. God promises never to leave us or forsake us (Joshua 1:5). His presence is with us continually. Psalm 46:1 states: "God is our refuge and strength, an ever present help in trouble." God never stops loving us. 1 John 4:9 tells us that God has shown us his love by sending his only son into the world so that we could have life through him. Another promise is Psalm 147:5, "Great is our Lord, and mighty in power; His understanding has no limit."

For those times when you do not know what to pray, turn to Romans 8:26–27, which tells us that ". . . the Spirit himself intercedes for us with groans that words cannot express." God hears the prayer that comes out in a painful groan or a convulsive sob.

The Lord's Prayer is a wonderful prayer and guides us to look to the Father for aid. Most people are familiar with the Lord's Prayer and can join in praying it with the nurse. It also serves as a pattern for prayer. In a magnificent way it affirms God's work in the life of his children, petitions God for those things needed for daily sustenance, and concludes with high praise to God. Use of this prayer fulfills the goal of affirming God's attributes and promises in prayer.

How Should We Pray? Prayers should be authentic, simple, and short. God is not impressed with flowery language or lengthy recitation. Remember that ". . . your Father knows what you need before you ask him" (Matthew 6:8). Whether prayer is formal or informal depends on the religious orientation of the patient and the nurse. Some are more comfortable offering spontaneous prayer, whereas others use written prayers from prayer books. Either is acceptable. If the patient has a favorite prayer in a book or liturgy, the nurse should offer to read it. For a Roman Catholic patient, it could be a special blessing to recite the rosary with a nurse who is familiar with it. Referral to clergy may be used to fill this need as well.

Is there a special stance for praying? Not really. Do you need to kneel, close your eyes, or wear a head covering? Whatever is comfortable and appropriate for the people praying should be used. Is there is special attitude for praying? Yes. One comes to God in an attitude of humility, without hypocrisy, asking for his mercy to intervene on the behalf of specific needs. Do not forget to praise God and thank him for the blessings he has already brought, with the expectation of blessings yet to follow.

Last, a word of caution concerning praying for "magic" or "miracles" of healing. Because we do not know the mind of God, it is best to leave those decisions completely in his hands. If you must pray for physical healing, it is imperative that you clearly ascribe the decision to God and pray, "if it be your will, O Lord." Remember that the ultimate healing is a transformed body that will be changed to be like Jesus's glorious body, when we die and go to be with Jesus (Philippians 3:21). When people pray for healing they are usually referring to physical healing that will maintain life. The nurse must be careful to avoid playing God or setting up expectation of physical healing. God may reward faith and send physical healing, but it cannot be guaranteed. We know that God is more interested in a relationship with his children that comes from being committed to Jesus.

What Is the Pattern for Prayer? The pattern for prayer is found in the Lord's Prayer (Matthew 6:9–13). Jesus taught this prayer to his disciples and it serves to guide our prayers. Studying the phrases in the Lord's Prayer will make the pattern for prayer apparent.

Our Father in heaven, hallowed be your name. First is praise. Begin prayer by giving honor to God through praise and acknowledging his nature. God is righteous, holy, forgiving, powerful, present in all places, possessing all knowledge, and abundant in mercy. As a shepherd cares for his sheep, so God cares for his children. As the Great Physician, God is the source of healing and restoration in his prescription for our health.

Your kingdom come, your will be done on earth as it is in heaven. Second, is to declare God's kingdom is established with Jesus as Lord, and God's people are placed in the kingdom to do his will. This puts everything and everyone in the world under the control and protection of Jesus. Therefore control is with God, and the client becomes submissive, although not passive. It is an act of obedience to commit oneself to God's will.

Give us today our daily bread. Third, is to ask God to provide for daily needs. This request is not limited to the client, but extends to the family and the community. Whatever the need, great or small, share it with the Lord. Ask for what you need. It might be food, or clothing, or peace of mind, or strength to do the physical therapy. Whatever! Ask!

Forgive us our debts as we also have forgiven our debtors. Fourth, ask for forgiveness, which God promises to those who confess their sins. In the Bible, we read of King David, who committed adultery and later had the woman's husband murdered. These are high-order sins. Then in Psalm 51 David confesses his sins to God. Later God identifies a forgiven and repentant David as a man of God. Forgiveness requires a humble and broken heart before God; a real grief over the wrongs that have been done and thought. By asking God to forgive him, the client acknowledges that God is able to forgive, and that his guilt is removed. In the same way, the client must forgive others and release them so they are no longer filled with guilt.

And lead us not into temptation but deliver us from the evil one. Claim victory over temptations and the forces of evil. With Jesus there is power and authority to overcome temptation. Temptation will still be present, but there is power not to succumb to the temptation. As the old saying states, "you can't stop the birds from flying over your head, but you can prevent them from making a nest in your hair." Temptation is real. It will come, but you can escape, and not entertain it. The evil powers in this world can be overcome by the Word and the armor of God, which includes truth, righteousness, peace, faith, and salvation.

For thine is the kingdom, and the power, and the glory forever. Amen. This last phrase is not included in the biblical pattern, but is commonly accepted as a part of it. Last, rejoice that God hears prayer, answers prayer, lifts burdens, meets needs, protects from temptation and evil, and is worthy of glory and honor. His power is great. God is bigger than any problem. He can be trusted. He will go on into eternity. Forever. Rejoice! Amen (so let it be)!

Prayer connects people to God, and to the power available to intervene and solve the client's problems. There are no barriers as to time, content, or form. Scripture supports the use of prayer and the Lord's Prayer provides a pattern. Scripture or other religious literature may be used together with prayer.

Scripture, Religious Literature, and Religious Rituals

The use of **scripture** is a valuable means of drawing strength from God. It is best to use those passages that are meaningful to the client, and that will not be misinterpreted. Psalm 23 is a well-known passage that can be suggested. Books of religious liturgy are rich sources of hope and encouragement as well. Contemporary religious books may be pertinent, especially to the client dealing with a chronic or terminal problem. Those that deal with the will of God or the handling of emotions are most helpful. One religious book that could be recommended is *Joni,* by Joni Eareckson (1976). She writes realistically of her struggles and rehabilitation experiences following a spinal cord injury. Now, more than 25 years later, she is an advocate for the disabled, through an organization she established, and as a speaker, artist, and singer to teach and encourage others.

Religious rituals include the celebration of the Mass or Holy Communion; sacrament of the dying; confession of sin; and prayer by the pastor, priest, or rabbi. These may be requested by the client or family, or offered by the nurse. They should never be imposed on the patient, but the nurse should assist in adapting the patient's schedule to allow time to practice the rituals.

The use of prayer, scripture, religious literature, and religious rituals is appropriate in a rehabilitation setting, keeping in mind the religious orientation of the client, using those tools of spiritual care that are meaningful to the patient, and not imposing them on the client who does not want to receive spiritual care.

Music

Much of Christian and classical music is scripture set to music. In that sense it could be used as scripture. However, here we deal with music as therapy for the client with a chronic illness.

Music plays a major role in every culture. It is used in rituals and celebrations, and for personal expression of emotion. In the Old Testament, David was assigned to play the harp to soothe Saul (1 Samuel 16:23). It is noteworthy that Saul requested someone who could play well! (v. 17). The Psalms are filled with references to music, specifically to singing. See Psalms 16:3, 27:6, 30:4, 33:3, 42:8, 45:8, 47:6,7, 57:7, 59:16, 66:2,4, 71:22–23, 81:1-2, 90:14, 92:1, 96:1–2, 126:2, and 145:7. Psalm 150 makes it plain that music is not limited to singing, but includes instruments—trumpet, harp, lyre, tambourine, strings, flute, cymbals—and dancing. In most cases, music is used to express joy or praise, but in 2 Samuel 1:17 we see that David orders that the bow (stringed instruments) be used to express his grief related to the death of Saul and Jonathan. The whole nation joined in the song of lament. In the New Testament parable of the prodigal son we see that the celebration that followed the return of the younger brother included music and dancing (Luke 15:25). What a good time that must have been!

There is a command to Christians to "speak to one another in psalms, hymns, and spiritual songs. Sing and make music in your heart to the Lord, always giving thanks to God the Father for everything, in the name of our Lord Jesus Christ" (Ephesians 5:19–20). Colossians 3:16 gives a similar instruction. It is clear that music must be a part of life, and it is important for occasions of joy and praise, but also for occasions of grief and loss.

The effect of music was noted by Florence Nightingale (1859 [1992], p. 33):

> The effect of music upon the sick has been scarcely at all noticed . . . wind instruments, including the human voice, and stringed instruments capable of continuous sound, have generally a beneficial effect—while the piano-forte . . . has just the reverse.

Current research indicates that music has a measurable effect on humans. When a client listened to music they liked, Bartlett, Kaufman, and Smeltekop (1993) and Lane (1992) found that the subjects had significant positive immune responses. Further, Bartlett, Kaufman, and Smeltekop (1993) found a significant increase in interleukin 1 and a significant decrease in cortisol in healthy adult subjects who listened to 15 minutes of music followed by 15 minutes of describing or drawing how they felt. Schorr (1993) found that during the time spent listening to music, people's pain threshold was significantly increased. These physiological effects draw attention to the efficacy of music to the human spirit.

In health care, music has been found to be beneficial in the treatment of various ailments. In heart ischemia, Guzzetta (1994) reported that soothing music reduced heart rate, blood pressure, mean arterial pressure, cardiac complications, and anxiety. At the same time, peripheral temperature increased.

In the elderly, music has been shown to lift depression. A nursing home client was disoriented but alert and had numerous complaints. Frequently she would cry and later scream, "I just want to die." Add to this the incessant grinding of her teeth. The nursing student assigned to her used all the therapeutic communication techniques she could remember, but there was no change in the woman's behavior. More to calm her own spirit than to intervene with the client, the student began singing to herself. To her surprise, the patient calmed down, and the grinding stopped. Music had reached into the emotions and soul of the client.

Music is effective in clients with Alzheimer's disease, and even with those who are comatose. A nursing student was assigned to care for a young client who was completely comatose. Because the sense of hearing remains intact, the student was instructed to continue to communicate with the client day after day.

This became an extremely difficult task. For her one-sided conversation, the student chose to share her name and what she was doing, report the events of her life and the major news events, as well as the weather and the conditions in the hospital. She continued by affirming to the client how valuable he was and how he was progressing. She read to him—the newspaper, books, poems, the Bible—and even told him some jokes, but after many weeks this became boring, and she ran out of things to say. In desperation she began to hum and to sing—hymns, spiritual songs, pop songs. The young man never emerged from his comatose state while she cared for him. But years later, now a registered nurse, she was walking down the corridor of a rehabilitation hospital and a voice behind her asked, "Aren't you Miss——, the nurse who sang to me?" She recognized him as the comatose young man, and he began to recount all that she had done for him. But obviously it was the music that set her apart.

Now a story about a 73-year-old client with Alzheimer's disease. She had progressed to the point where she recognized none of her five children, but only her husband who was her caregiver. She was a devout Christian, so the family decided to take her to a worship service. They planned together that they would take her out of the service if she became disruptive. To their amazement, when the hymns were sung, the mother joined in, singing all four verses from memory! How blessed! What a ministry of the Holy Spirit to her spirit through music.

Music *is* therapeutic! So let us discuss a few guidelines. First, you may use your own voice to sing whether you think you have a gift of singing or not. If you can sing in the shower, you can sing at the bedside. Think of how many times you have heard clients comment about a housekeeper who hummed as she cleaned the room. Not once have I heard a negative comment from the client about the quality of the music! Second, use of selected tapes and compact discs is as appropriate as singing. Even the radio may be used. Third, try to select the music that is meaningful to the client. If possible, ask the client to name the types of music, the instruments, and even the names of specific songs that are favorites. Usually 90s rock and roll will not be a favorite for a 90-year-old patient. Make selections from soothing popular, light jazz, classical, spiritual (hymns, psalms, spiritual songs), choral, country, and ethnic music. In most cases do not use music with lyrics. The lyrics will tend to distract the client from the flow of the music. Fourth, modulate the volume of the performance so that it is soothing. If the client is hard of hearing, it will need to be a little louder, but remember to protect the eardrums too. Fifth, music can be used for long periods, but 20–30 minutes is the optimal length of time. There should be rest periods of silence, or use of the time for other spiritual care interventions. Sixth, use music at any time of day—to awaken or to go to sleep, or any time in between. While the client is awake music can soothe the soul.

Usually it takes a little planning to use music. Finding the music or the equipment to play the music is well worth the effort. It can calm the client so he or she can relax, celebrate, and enjoy. Just as music can be used to calm the anxious spirit, so can humor and laughter. The nurse can share humorous stories and laughter to assist in client healing.

Use of Humor and Laughter

There is ample evidence in scripture that love, joy, gladness, merriment, rejoicing, and celebration are part of God's plan for his people. Consider Jesus. His first miracle was to turn water into wine at a wedding celebration. Imagine the surprise (and joy) of the guests who thought they were getting the last dregs of the wine, and then ascertained that this wine was better than any they had ever tasted. They must have been delighted, and Jesus must have had a twinkle in his eye as he observed their response. To his disciples Jesus gave the command to rejoice in all things, even in persecution, affliction, or tribulation (see Matthew 5: 11–12). In the Beatitudes, the word "blessed" can be translated as "happy" (Matthew 5:3–12). In the parables Jesus talks about the lost sheep (Luke 15:3–7), the lost coin (Luke 15:8–10), and the prodigal son (Luke 15:11–31). When the lost is found, there is a call for rejoicing and a grand celebration follows. Obviously Jesus had a spirit of joy that spilled over to all around him, and especially to his disciples.

The prescription for joy is not limited to the New Testament. In Proverbs 17:22, we find "a merry heart does good like medicine, but a broken spirit dries up the bones." A good laugh or a joyful spirit is as effective in healing as medication.

Have you ever started laughing just because someone else was? You were not "in" on the joke, but the laugh was contagious. Maybe you laughed until the tears ran down your face! Norman Cousins has demonstrated the value of laughter in healing his painful degenerative spine disease. After checking out of the hospital he went to a hotel. While there he took ascorbic acid by intravenous drip, and watched *Candid Camera* videos, movies of the Marx Brothers, and Laurel and Hardy films. After 10 minutes of belly laughter he could sleep at least 2 hours without pain (Cousins, 1979, p. 39). Sedimentation rates before and after laughter episodes dropped at least five points, maintained the drop, and were cumulative. The first dose of intravenous ascorbic acid dropped the sedimentation rate nine points. Research has demonstrated the changes in body chemistry that occur with laughter—it pumps the heart, the muscles of the abdomen, chest, shoulders, and neck; it stimulates the brain, ventricles, and lungs; it raises heart rate, blood pressure, respiration, and circulation; it improves immunity; it stimulates the secretion of epinephrine, serotonin, and norepinephrine for up to 12 hours. So if you do not feel like laughing—fake it. Your body will not know the difference.

With all these positive physiological results, the benefits of humor are obvious. But good things can be put to a bad use. Words of caution are in order. To create humor the client must not be the brunt of the joke. Laughter at the expense of others is not acceptable. Instead, one must gain the ability to see **humor** in everyday situations and to laugh at oneself and others. Another caution is to ask permission to make the person laugh, just as you would for any other intervention. Be especially considerate of those who will experience pain when they laugh. A new postoperative patient will tolerate a joke that brings a smile or a small laugh, but one that wiggles the whole abdomen may not be in the best interest of comfort.

Maybe you are not a funny person. If you would like to be, you can change. Actively look for humor. See your life as a sitcom. Listen for the funny experience. When you hear it, give it all the mirth you can muster. Make a habit of repeating jokes you have heard, or at least writing them down for future reference. You might consider collecting them in a personal joke book. Add funny cartoons whenever you find them. Buy a cartoon-a-day calendar. Some people spread humor through wearing fake noses, odd eye glasses, funny flashy buttons, ribbons, or clothes. Clown around a little. Share balloons and stickers.

Even if your humor can only be a smile, it will do your face good. It takes more muscles to frown than to smile. By smiling you have energy left over to be healthy. Remember the song in the *Mary Poppins* movie, "I love to laugh"? By the end, the viewer is smiling, if not laughing.

Imagery Another intervention that is seeing increasing use is that of **imagery.** "People who are under stress taking medical tests, undergoing procedures and surgery are more depressed, require more anesthesia, have lower immune functioning, suffer more complications and take longer to heal . . . than patients who know how to draw on inner resources to calm or energize themselves . . ." (Dossey, 1991, p. 31). According to Dossey, what makes the difference is "the use of imagery . . . imagery involves not just visual awareness but all the senses" (Dossey, 1991, p. 31). Negative images are replaced with positive ones to dispel fear, hopelessness, and anxiety. All imagery techniques begin with relaxation, which is the most important part of the process. This process can be very structured, as discussed by Dossey, by identifying the anxiety-provoking image followed by deep breathing (relaxation), developing images of healing resources, and ending with an image of the desired well-being state. This needs to be done for a period of 20 minutes, two or three times daily (Dossey, 1991, p. 32). Although this process sounds simple, it requires the client's focused concentration (Dossey, 1991, p. 32). Dossey identifies different types of imagery (i.e., receptive, active, concrete, symbolic, process, end-state, and what she describes as general healing imagery). "General healing images also may come in experiences of God" (Dossey, 1991, p. 34). Peterson and Nelson (1987) stated that "clients with anxiety may benefit from relaxation activities that use religious imagery" (p. 38). The nurse determines what might be the most meaningful to the client and incorporates that religious image into a relaxation exercise. Religious music can also be part of this exercise to decrease anxiety. Conrad (1985) found that guided meditation or imagery is a technique that has been used successfully in adults to control pain and provide spiritual support and comfort. Carson (1989) supported this by describing the nurse's role as an "imagery guide (that) . . . take(s) clients through a pastoral setting where they are introduced to God, who offers them support, comfort, and encouragement" (p. 242). It is the nurse's presence that facilitates this intervention as well as the others.

Summary

Meeting spiritual needs begins with a philosophy of person. Each person is conceptualized as a biological, psychosocial, and spiritual being with the spirit at the center. This spiritual core is present in every person, both client and nurse. Whether the spiritual component is acknowledged or connected to a specific religion, it still exists as an integral part of the person.

Therefore, the nurse must be aware of personal strengths, biases, and stereotypes that affect his or her spirituality and how this has an impact on the nurse's perception of the client's spirituality. Before embarking on meeting the spiritual needs of others, the nurse must know his or her self. A knowledge base of other religions or ideologies is helpful.

The key person in providing spiritual care is the nurse. There must be a sensitivity to and awareness of the expression of spiritual needs, verbal and nonverbal. After validating the observations with the client the nurse makes a diagnosis and begins to plan spiritual care. The nurse must choose those interventions that are likely to meet the spiritual needs of the client.

Many of the essential tools needed for meeting spiritual needs are integral to the caring skills of the nurse (i.e., touch, presence, commitment, listening). Laughter and music can be used effectively to provide spiritual care in some situations. Use of prayer, reading scripture, and practicing rituals are interventions available to the nurse or may be referred to clergy. When the nurse feels incompetent or incapable of rendering spiritual care, he or she may seek assistance from others (i.e., clergy, other nurses or doctors, family). Even those who feel inadequate should be reassured that they possess the basic caring skills for spiritual care.

The nurse's own spirituality, coupled with a willingness to share his or her journey of faith with others, is the foundation of meeting spiritual needs. Reaching out to others to offer spiritual care involves a small risk. It might be rejected, but the pain of rejection is small compared to the joy of sharing in spiritual comfort or growth.

References

Antai-Otong, D. (1995). Therapeutic communication. In Debora Antai-Otong (Ed.), *Psychiatric nursing: Biological & behavioral concepts* (pp. 95–188). Philadelphia: W. B. Saunders.

Bartlett, D., Kaufman, D., & Smeltekop, R. (1993). The effects of music listening and perceived sensory experiences on the immune system as measured by interleukin-α and cortisol. *Journal of Music Therapy, 30,* 194–209.

Burnard, P. (1987). Spiritual distress and the nursing response: Theoretical considerations and counseling skills. *Journal of Advanced Nursing, 12,* 337–382.

Carpenito, L. (1997). *Nursing diagnosis: Application to clinical practice* (7th ed.). Philadelphia: J. B. Lippincott.

Carson, V. B. (1989). *Spiritual dimensions of nursing care.* Philadelphia: W. B. Saunders.

Cassetta, R. A. (1993). Healing through caring touch. *The American Nurse, 25*(3), 18.

Conrad, N. L. (1985). Spiritual support for the dying. *Nursing Clinics of North America 20*(2), 415–425.

Cousins, N. (1979). *Anatomy of an illness as perceived by the patient.* New York: W. W. Norton.

Donley, R. (1991). Spiritual dimensions of health care: Nursing's mission. *Nursing and Health Care, 12*(4), 178–183.

Dossey, B. A. (1991). Awakening the inner healer. *American Journal of Nursing, 91*(8), 31–34.

Emblen, J., & Halstead, L. (1993). Spiritual needs and interventions: Comparing the view of patients, nurses, and chaplains. *Clinical Nurse Specialist, 7,* 175–182.

Fish, S., & Shelly, J. A. (1978). *Spiritual care: The nurse's role.* Downers Grove, IL: Inter Varsity.

Forbis, P. A. (1988). Meeting patient's spiritual needs. *Geriatric Nursing,* May/June, pp. 158–159.

Frankl, V. E. (1971). *Man's search for meaning.* New York: Washington Square Press.

Gaskins, S., & Forte, L. (1995). The meaning of hope: Implications for nursing practice and research. *Journal of Gerontological Nursing, 21*(3), 17–24.

Gewe, A. (1994). Hope: Moving from theory to practice. *Journal of Christian Nursing, 11*(4), 18–21.

Granstrom, S. L. (1985). Spiritual nursing care for oncology patients. *Topics in Clinical Nursing, 7*(1), 39–45.

Guzzetta, C. (1994). Soothing the ischemic heart. *American Journal of Nursing, 94*(1), 24.

Haase, J. E., Britt, T., Coward, D. D., Leidy, N. K., & Penn, P. E. (1992). Simultaneous concept of spiritual perspective, hope, acceptance and self-transcendence. *Image: Journal of Nursing Scholarship, 24*(2), 141–147.

Highfield, M., & Cason, C. (1983). Spiritual needs of patients: Are they recognized? *Cancer Nursing, 6,* 187–192.

Hungelmann, J., Kenkel-Rossi, E., Klaasen, L., & Stollenwerk, R. (1985). Spiritual well-being in older adults: Harmonious interconnectedness. *Journal of Religion and Health, 24,* 147–153.

Lane, D. (1992). Music therapy: A gift beyond measure. *Oncology Nursing Forum, 19,* 863–867.

Nightingale, F. (1992). *Notes on nursing: What it is and what it is not* (commemorative ed.). Philadelphia: J. B. Lippincott. (Original work published 1859).

Peterson, E. A., & Nelson, K. (1987). How to meet your clients' spiritual needs. *Journal of Psychosocial Nursing, 25,* 34–39.

Post-White, J., Ceronsky, C., Kreitzer, M., Nickelson, K., Drew, D., Mackey, K. W., Koopminers, L., & Gutknecht, S. (1996). Hope, spirituality, sense of coherence, and quality of life in patients with cancer. *Oncology Nursing Forum, 23*(10), 1571–1579.

Raleigh, E. D. H. (1992). Sources of hope in chronic illness. *Oncology Nursing Forum, 19*(3), 443–448.

Reed, P. (1991). Preferences for spiritually related nursing interventions among terminally ill and nonterminally ill hospitalized adults and well adults. *Journal of Applied Nursing Research, 4*(3), 122–128.

Ross, L. A. (1994). Spiritual aspects of nursing. *Journal of Advanced Nursing, 19,* 439–447.

Schorr, J. (1993). Music and pattern change in chronic pain. *Advances in Nursing Science, 15*(4), 27–36.

Sodestrom, K., & Martinson, I. (1987). Patient's spiritual coping strategies: A study of nurse and patient perspectives. *Oncology Nursing Forum, 14*(2), 41–46.

Solimine, M. A., & Hoeman, S. (1996). Spirituality: A rehabilitation perspective. In S. Hoeman & M. A. Shirley (Eds.), *Rehabilitation nursing: Process and application* (pp. 628–643). St. Louis: Mosby.

Stallwood, J. (1975). Spiritual dimensions of nursing practice. *In* I. Beland & J. Passos *Clinical nursing:* pathophysiological and psychosocial approaches (3rd ed.), (pp. 1086–1098). New York: MacMillan Publishing.

Stoll, R. (1989). The essence of spirituality. In V. B. Carson (Ed.), *Spiritual dimensions of nursing practice* (pp. 4–23). Philadelphia: W. B. Saunders.

Thompson, M. (1994). Nuturing hope: A vital ingredient in nursing. *Journal of Christian Nursing, 11*(4), 10–17.

Travelbee, J. (1971). *Interpersonal aspects of nursing* (2nd ed.). Philadelphia: F. A. Davis.

Warner, C. G. (1996). Family spirituality. In P. J. Bomar (Ed.), *Nurses and family health promotion: Concepts, assessment and intervention* (2nd ed., pp. 139–161). Philadelphia: W. B. Saunders.

Zerwekh, J., & Claborn, J, C. (1997). *Nursing today: Transition and trends.* Philadelphia: W. B. Saunders.

Suggested Readings

Barnason, S., Zimmerman, L., & Nieveen, J.(1995). The effects of music interventions on anxiety in the patient after coronary artery bypass grafting. *Heart & Lung, 24*(2), 124–132.

Bauer, T., & Barron, C. (1995). Nursing interventions for spiritual care: Preferences of the community-based elderly. *Journal of Holistic Nursing, 13*(3), 268–279.

Berggren-Thomas, P., & Griggs, M. (1995). Spirituality in aging: Spiritual need or spiritual journey? *Journal of Gerontological Nursing, 21*(3), 5–10.

Burkhardt, M. (1989). Spirituality: An analysis of the concept. *Holistic Nursing Practice, 1*(3), 69–77.

Clark, C. C., Cross, J. R., Deane, D. M., & Lowry, L. W. (1991). Spirituality: Integral to quality care. *Holistic Nursing Practice, 5*(3), 67–76.

Conco, D. (1995). Christian patients' views of spiritual care. *Western Journal of Nursing Research, 17*(3), 266–276.

Cousins, N. (1989). *Headfirst: The biology of hope.* New York: E. P. Dutton.

Dolan, M. (1994). Rx: Laughter, 15 minutes/day. *RN, 57*(12), 80–82.

Eareckson, J. (1976). *Joni.* Grand Rapids, MI: Zondervan.

Gorman, L., Sultan, D., & Raines, M. (1996). *Davis's manual of psychosocial nursing in general patient care.* Philadelphia: F. A. Davis.

Hanser, S., & Thompson, L. (1994). Effects of music therapy strategy on depressed older adults. *Journal of Gerontology, 49*(6), 265–269.

Holy Bible (New International Version) (1978). Grand Rapids, MI: Zondervan.

Lescheid, H. (1994). Singing in the face of death: Bedside hymns bring hope. *Journal of Christian Nursing, 11*(1), 18–19.

Meyer, M. (1997). Laughter: It's good medicine. *Better Homes and Gardens, 75*(4), 72–76.

Oldnall, A. (1996). A critical analysis of nursing: Meeting the spiritual needs of patients. *Journal of Advanced Nursing, 23,* 138–144.

Pope, E. (1995). Music, noise, and the human voice in the nurse-patient environment. *Image: Journal of Nursing Scholarship, 27*(4), 291–296.

Reed, P. (1991). Toward a nursing theory of self transcendence: Deductive reformulation using developmental theories. *Advances in Nursing Science, 13*(4), 64–77.

Samra, C. (1985). A time to laugh. *Journal of Christian Nursing, 2*(4), 15–19.

Schroeder-Sheker, T. (1994). Music for the dying. *Journal of Holistic Nursing, 12*(1), 83–99.

Stephenson, L. (1988). Even patients love a clown. *Journal of Christian Nursing, 5*(2), 18–21.

Winter, M., Paskin, S., & Baker, T. (1994). Music reduces stress and anxiety of patients in the surgical holding area. *Journal of Post Anesthesia Nursing, 9*(6), 340–343.

Major Neurological Deficits and Common Rehabilitation Disorders

CHAPTER 15
Acquired Brain Injury: Traumatic Brain Injury

Anita Rosebrough

Key Terms *Aphasia*
Apraxia
Closed Head Injury
Cognition
Concussion
Contusion
Diffuse Brain Damage
Disability Rating Scale
Dysphagia
Epidural Hematoma
Focal Brain Damage
Glasgow Coma Scale
Glasgow Coma Outcome Scale
Initiation
Intracerebral Hematoma
Mild Traumatic Brain Injury
Moderate Traumatic Brain Injury
Open Head Injury
Rancho Los Amigos Levels of Cognitive Functioning Scale
Sequencing
Severe Traumatic Brain Injury
Subdural Hematoma
Traumatic Brain Injury

Objectives 1. Describe the basic pathophysiology of traumatic brain injury.

2. Describe the common neurological deficits associated with traumatic brain injury.

3. Describe the Glasgow Coma Scale and its application to traumatic brain injury.

4. Describe the Glasgow Coma Outcome Scale and its application to traumatic brain injury.

5. Describe the Rancho Los Amigos Levels of Cognitive Functioning Scale and its application to traumatic brain injury.

6. Describe the Disability Rating Scale and its application to traumatic brain injury.

7. Identify and describe the levels of recovery from brain injury.

8. Develop a comprehensive teaching/learning plan for a traumatic brain injury survivor and the family caregiver.

9. Identify and describe: mild, moderate, and severe traumatic brain injury.

10. Identify and describe the etiology of traumatic brain injury.

11. Develop a nursing care plan for a client with increased intracranial pressure.

12. Identify and describe nursing assessment during the rehabilitation phase of recovery from traumatic brain injury.

13. Compare and contrast epidural, subdural, and intracerebral hematomas.

14. Describe the stages of recovery from traumatic brain injury.

15. Develop a nursing care plan for a client with cognitive, perceptual, behavioral, and emotional neurological deficits.

Introduction Trauma to the central nervous system is a major cause of death and disability in this country. Two major types of neurotrauma are spinal cord injury and head injury. This chapter focuses on head injury. Head injury or acquired brain injury refers to an impairment of brain functioning due to cerebral vascular lesions, hypoxia, tumor, neurological disease, or a neurological insult such as an open or closed head injury.

Traumatic brain injury (TBI), which includes open and closed head injuries, accounts for one-third of all injury deaths in this country, and is a major cause of disability for persons under the age of 40 years. Approximately 2 million people per year sustain head injuries: 500,000 are severe enough to require hospitalization and each year 50,000 people die from head injuries. Most deaths occur at the time of injury or within 2 hours of hospitalization. About 70,000–90,000 TBI survivors annually incur lifelong debilitating loss of function following head trauma. Males between the ages of 15 and 24 years have the highest head injury rate, and tend to sustain more severe head injuries than do females. The outcome of minor head injuries is favorable. Severe head injuries have a devastating effect on the victim and the family. A brain injury survivor typically faces 5–10 years of intensive services at an estimated cost of $4 million (Centers for Disease Control [CDC], 1996; National Institute of Neurological Disorders and Stroke, 1990; Sosin, Sniezek, & Waxweiler, 1995).

Etiology

The most frequent cause of TBI is motor vehicle accidents. Approximately one-third to one-half of brain injuries requiring hospitalization involve alcohol and/or other drugs. Other causes include falls, occupational accidents, assaults, sports, and recreational activities. The use of helmets, seat belts, air bags, and car seats can significantly reduce the mortality and morbidity associated with traumatic brain injury.

Pathophysiology

Traumatic brain injury refers to damage to brain tissue caused by an external mechanical force, and ranges from very mild to severe. Severe injuries result in skull fractures, subdural and epidural hematomas, and contusions and tearing of brain tissue. There are two major classifications of traumatic brain injury: closed head injury and open head injury. A **closed head injury,** also known as a blunt injury, is a nonpenetrating injury with no break in the skull or dura. It can occur without any external signs of trauma. The majority of the damage in a closed head injury is due to the movement of the brain against the skull, resulting in contusions and concussions. Closed head injuries are more common and produce more diffuse brain damage than open head injuries. An **open head injury,** or penetrating head injury, results in communication between the intracranial structures and the environment. Open head injuries include gunshot wounds, compound fractures of the skull, and lacerations. TBIs involve either **focal brain damage** or **diffuse brain damage.** Both cause tissue hypoxia and ischemia. Contusions (bruising) and penetrating injuries are examples of focal injuries. Focal injuries produce localized damage with localized neurological deficits such as motor problems or alterations in speech. Diffuse injuries are caused by rapid acceleration, deceleration, and rotational forces. These forces cause tearing, shearing, and stretching of nerve fibers, and axonal and blood vessel damage leading to disruptions in neuronal connections. Diffuse damage is widespread or scattered. Consequently, the neurological deficits vary widely with each injury.

At the time of mechanical injury there are tears and/or bruises of the brain, resulting in concussions, contusions, or lacerations causing localized or diffuse damage. The extent of the injury depends on the direction and nature of the forces applied to the skull and brain on impact. **Concussion** refers to a jostling, jarring, or shaking of the brain without bruising. A concussion is usually manifested by a brief loss of consciousness and loss of memory. A **contusion** refers to bruising of the brain and is considered more serious than a concussion. Brain lacerations refer to tears in the cerebral tissue and can occur with almost no damage to the skull.

The mechanical insult is followed by a second phase of injury occurring minutes to hours after the initial insult. This phase includes hematoma formation, cerebral edema, increased intracranial pressure, brain distortion, brain herniation, pain, elevated temperatures, venous obstruction, hypoxia, and ischemia. Systemic factors contributing to secondary brain injury include respiratory failure, cardiac arrest, hypotension, hemorrhage, and emboli. These factors all cause an increase in intracranial pressure, which leads to further brain damage.

Traumatic brain injuries are classified as mild, moderate, and severe. Approximately 80 percent of all head injuries are mild, 10 percent are moderate, and 10 percent are severe. **Mild traumatic brain injury,** also called concussion, is due to direct contact or acceleration/deceleration. Loss of consciousness is brief, 20 minutes or less, and in some cases there is no loss of consciousness. Hospitalization is for 48 hours or less, with a Glasgow Coma Scale score of 13–15. Neuroimaging diagnostic studies with mild head injury are negative, and on examination no neurological changes are observed. Most clients recover within weeks to months without specific treatment. Postconcussion syndrome is common following a mild head injury. Mild head injury survivors frequently complain of headaches, dizziness, poor memory, poor concentration, fatigue, and irritability. The extent and duration vary. Some individuals experience persistent neurological symptoms 3–5 years postinjury. The most common complaints are headaches, sleep disturbances, dizziness, fatigue, and memory disturbances (Alexander, 1995; Levitt, Sutton, Goldman, Mikhail, & Christopher, 1994).

Moderate traumatic brain injury is manifested by a loss of consciousness lasting more than 20 minutes, and a Glasgow Coma Scale score of 9–12. In moderate brain injuries there are multiple small hemorrhages, and some cerebral edema occurs. The client with a moderate brain injury exhibits neurological deficits such as hemiparesis. These individuals require rehabilitation. Return to a preinjury lifestyle is possible, but many experience long-term neurological deficits. **Severe traumatic brain injury** is manifested by a loss of consciousness lasting 6 hours or more, and a Glasgow Coma Scale score of 8 or less. In severe traumatic brain injuries the client sustains cerebral contusions, shearing, and tearing of brain tissue. These individuals require extensive rehabilitation and experience many long-term neurological deficits.

Symptoms of TBI are manifested by alterations in cognitive, perceptual, physical, and behavioral/emotional functioning. Table 1 provides a list of frequently experienced neurological deficits following traumatic brain injury. Figure 1 summarizes the functions of specific lobes of the brain.

Routine Medical Management

During the acute phase of the injury the focus is on medically stabilizing the individual with a moderate or severe traumatic brain injury, and preventing secondary physiological complications. A complication of traumatic brain injury is the development of epidural, subdural, and intracerebral hematomas. An **epidural hematoma** develops as a result of a rapid arterial or venous bleed between the periosteal dura and the skull. Epidural hematomas are often associated with lacerations of the middle meningeal artery releasing large volumes of blood into the epidural space. Prompt intervention usually produces a good outcome. A **subdural hematoma** develops as a result of a slow, gradual buildup of blood between the dura and the arachnoid space. This is often seen in more acute injuries and the prognosis is relatively poor. An **intracerebral hematoma** develops from an extravasation of blood into the cerebral tissue, and is frequently associated with contusions and lacerations. The hematomas act as space-occupying lesions compressing vital brain tissues and increasing intracranial pressure. Intracranial pressure is measured hourly in the intensive care unit. Some clinicians advocate aggressive treatment of increased intracranial pressure to improve long-term prognosis. A variety of drugs are used to decrease intracranial pressure. These include osmotic diuretics, loop diuretics, corticosteroids, anticonvulsants, barbiturates, and neuromuscular blocking agents. Low intracranial pressure readings are associated with more favorable outcomes.

Nursing care during the acute phase includes (but is not limited to) monitoring intracranial pressure, assessing for alterations in levels of consciousness and orientation, assessing Glasgow Coma Scale scores, monitoring vital signs, maintaining the head and neck in good alignment, monitoring intake and output, monitoring for seizure activity, and assessing sensory and motor responses. Figure 2 summarizes motor responses to stimuli.

During the acute inpatient rehabilitation phase the emphasis is on improving physical, cognitive, psychological, and social deficits. Factors to assess and evaluate continually during the rehabilitation recovery process include: assessing the client's ability to respond to external stimuli, to focus on a task, and to ignore distractions; assessing the client's ability to store, retain, and retrieve information; assessing the client's ability to plan and regulate own activities; assessing the client's ability to solve problems, sense of direction, manual dexterity, and position in space; assessing the client's ability to use language for communication and problem solving; and assessing the client's ability to relate to and work effectively with others (Sachs, 1986).

Prognostic Indicators for Recovery from Head Injury

The ability to recover from a traumatic brain injury varies, depending on the severity of the injury and the extent of brain damage. Approximately 65 percent of individuals sustaining severe traumatic brain injuries survive. Their survival, however, is marked by prolonged physical, cognitive, behavioral, and psychosocial neurological sequelae. Thirty-five percent of survivors are moderately disabled; the remainder are severely disabled or remain in a vegetative state (Spettell, Ellis,

Table 1
Neurological Complications, Deficits, and Limitations following Traumatic Brain Injury

Cognitive Symptoms

Difficulty processing information
Decreased speed of information processing
Decreased accuracy of information processing
Decreased consistency of information processing
Shortened attention span
Decreased ability to concentrate
Impaired learning
Inattention to detail
Impaired tracking of message production
Organizational deficits
Inability to abstract
Reduced capacity to learn new information
Impaired decision-making
Inability to follow multiple-step commands
Impaired short-term and/or long-term memory or memory loss
Language deficits
Inability to comprehend or express language
Deficits in auditory processing of language including rate, quantity, and complexity of
    information interpretation
Aphasia
Poor syntax
Word-finding deficits
Inability to generate an understandable message
Impaired message formulation
Decreased initiation of language
Impaired communication interactions
Impaired communication strategies
Inability to inhibit responses
Perseveration on vocabulary activation
Recall deficits
Impaired concrete thinking/reasoning skills
Limited vocabulary

Perceptual Symptoms

Changes in vision, hearing, or touch
Loss of sense of time and space, and spatial disorientation
Impaired smell and taste
Altered sense of balance
Increased pain sensitivity

Table 1
Neurological Complications, Deficits, and Limitations following Traumatic Brain Injury (*Continued*)

Physical Symptoms

Various physical impairments depending on location and extent of brain damage
Persistent headache
Extreme mental or physical fatigue
Disorders of movement (gait, ataxia, spasticity, and tremors)
Seizure disorders
Impaired small motor control
Photosensitivity
Sleep disorders
Paralysis
Impaired speech (dysarthria)

Behavioral/Emotional Symptoms

Apathy
Difficulty in planning and organizing
Irritability
Impatience
Impulsivity
Reduced stress tolerance
Lack of initiative
Denial of disability
Lack of inhibition
Impaired social functioning
Inappropriate sexual behavior
Inflexibility
Flattened or heightened emotional responses
Difficulty maintaining employment
Difficulty maintaining relationships
Fatigue
Emotional lability
Depression
Lack of motivation
Impaired motor control including apraxia, dysarthria, ataxia, contractures, posturing, and spasticity

BRAIN

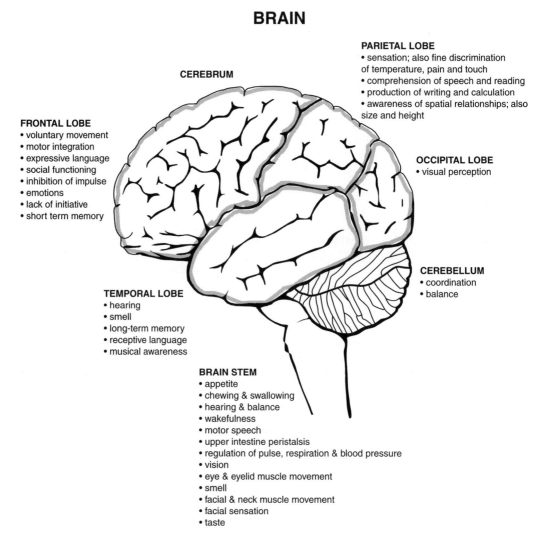

CEREBRUM

PARIETAL LOBE
• sensation; also fine discrimination of temperature, pain and touch
• comprehension of speech and reading
• production of writing and calculation
• awareness of spatial relationships; also size and height

FRONTAL LOBE
• voluntary movement
• motor integration
• expressive language
• social functioning
• inhibition of impulse
• emotions
• lack of initiative
• short term memory

OCCIPITAL LOBE
• visual perception

CEREBELLUM
• coordination
• balance

TEMPORAL LOBE
• hearing
• smell
• long-term memory
• receptive language
• musical awareness

BRAIN STEM
• appetite
• chewing & swallowing
• hearing & balance
• wakefulness
• motor speech
• upper intestine peristalsis
• regulation of pulse, respiration & blood pressure
• vision
• eye & eyelid muscle movement
• smell
• facial & neck muscle movement
• facial sensation
• taste

Fig 1. *Summary of specific brain functions.*

Ross, Sandel, O'Malley, Stein, Spivack, & Hurley, 1991). The most reliable indicator of recovery from traumatic brain injury is the depth and duration of coma. Other factors include age, general health status, support system, type and extent of injury, premorbid personality, motivation, premorbid skills and behavior, history of previous brain injury, and type of hospital and care received. Recovery time will vary. Change and improvement may continue for years. Recovery may

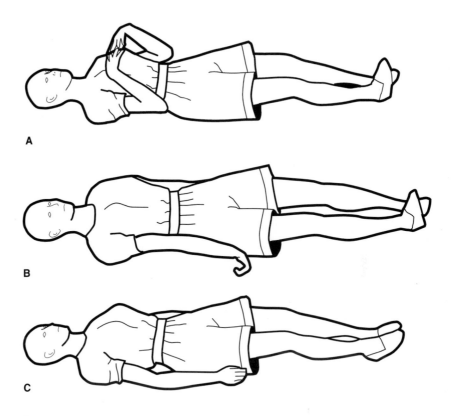

A

B

C

Fig 2.

stop for a time and then resume. No two individuals are alike and each client's recovery will be unique. Many tools have been developed to assist the practitioner in predicting potential recovery. Several of the tools in use today include the Glasgow Coma Scale, the Disability Rating Scale, the Rancho Los Amigos Cognitive Functioning Scale, and the Glasgow Coma Outcome Scale.

The **Glasgow Coma Scale** is a standardized and reliable tool used to assess and describe the level of consciousness and to predict the duration of coma and the outcome of traumatic brain injury (Table 2). It is the international standard for characterizing traumatic brain injury. The scale assesses three areas: eye opening, motor response, and verbal response. Each area is assessed independently and graded numerically by the best response elicited. Scores range from a low of 3 to

Table 2
Glasgow Coma Scale

Parameter	Score
Eye opening	
Spontaneous	4
To speech	3
To pain	2
No response	1
Motor response	
Obeys	6
Localizes	5
Withdraws	4
Abnormal flexion	3
Extensor response	2
No response	1
Verbal response	
Oriented	5
Confused	4
Inappropriate words	3
Incomprehensible sounds	2
No response	1
Total score:	____

Score Interpretation

Severe brain injury score:	3–8
Moderate brain injury score:	9–12
Mild brain injury score:	13–15

a maximum of 15. The results are plotted on a graph to provide a visual representation of changes in the client's condition. The worst score within the first 24 hours of injury is frequently used to predict the severity of the injury. A score of 13–15 indicates a mild head injury. A score of 9–12 indicates a moderate head injury, and a score of 3–8 indicates a severe head injury (Hall & Johnston, 1994).

The **Glasgow Coma Outcome Scale** was developed to assess outcome following traumatic brain injury and scores correlate well with the Glasgow Coma

Scale. It consists of five categories: good recovery, moderate disability, severe disability, persistent vegetative state, and death. Clients in a persistent vegetative state are totally dependent on others for care, are incontinent of bowel and bladder, and are incapable of interpersonal interactions with another person. Severely disabled individuals are capable of some communication, ambulation, and self-care, and frequently require institutionalization. The moderately disabled individual is able to use public transportation and work in a sheltered environment. They experience a variety of residual neurological deficits. Indicators of a good recovery include an average intelligence quotient, nonimpaired communication, and no more than mild behavioral disturbances. A rating of the depth of coma on admission, as determined by Glasgow Coma Scale score, is frequently used to predict outcome. Duration of coma is also used to determine the extent or severity of the brain injury and to predict the outcome. Clients in coma for less than 20 days frequently regain independence in functional activities. Clients in coma for more than 20 days are often profoundly disabled (Spettell, Ellis, Ross, Sandel, O'Malley, Stein, Spivack, & Hurley, 1991).

The **Disability Rating Scale** was developed for use with individuals who had sustained moderate and severe traumatic brain injuries. The tool is used to measure functional status and changes in functional status over time. It can be used throughout the continuum of health care. It can track the TBI survivor from onset of injury to discharge to the community. The Disability Rating Scale consists of eight items. The first three items reflect impairment, items 4–6 reflect level of disability, and items 7 and 8 reflect level of disability. The scale is easy to use and can be completed in approximately 5 minutes (Hall & Johnston, 1994).

The **Rancho Los Amigos Levels of Cognitive Functioning Scale** provides a useful framework for understanding the cognitive recovery process from head injury (Table 3). This scale is used in rehabilitation to assess changes in behavior as the client recovers from brain injury. In this scale clients are categorized into eight stages of recovery ranging from Level I, a comatose individual, to Level VIII, describing an individual capable of independent functioning and living. These levels are the most frequently used descriptors of the cognitive recovery process experienced by persons with traumatic brain injury. Not everyone goes through each level of recovery. Not everyone remains in each level for a specific length of time. Recovery can begin or end at any level, and a person can be in two or more stages at the same time. The levels also describe how the management of the client with a traumatic brain injury differs depending on the client's cognitive level (DiLima & Eutsey, 1996).

Rehabilitation of TBI survivors can be divided into three phases: the stimulation phase, the structured phase, and the reintegration phase. The stimulation phase correlates to Levels I, II, and III of the Rancho Los Amigos Levels of Cognitive Functioning Scale. At these levels the client needs to be stimulated several times daily for periods of 15–30 minutes. As the client starts to respond, the fre-

Table 3
Rancho Los Amigos Head Injury Levels

I. No response
Does not respond to touch, sight, movement, or sound.
The client appears to be in a deep sleep. There is no change in the client's behavior when s/he hears, sees, smells or feels something new

II. Generalized response
There is a physical change observed when the client hears, sees, smells, or feels something new. The earliest response is to pain. The response is inconsistent, nonspecific, nonpurposeful, and may be delayed. Responses may be physiological changes, gross body movements, and/or vocalizations. Common responses include chewing, sweating, increased respiratory rate, moaning, or moving

III. Localized response
The client reacts more specifically but inconsistently to stimuli. The responses are directly related to the type of stimulus presented. The client may blink in response to strong light, or respond to pain by moving away. The client begins to respond to simple commands but the response is inconsistent and may be delayed. Begins to show a vague awareness of self by pulling at nasogastric tube or catheter. Begins to recognize family and friends. Clients may be admitted for rehabilitation at this level

Nursing interventions for cognitive levels II, III, and I are designed to stimulate the client:

1. Introduce smells (food, flowers), touch (warm, cold), auditory (simple commands), and/or visual (light, familiar objects) stimulation. Have family members bring in favorite music, pictures, blankets, and so on
2. Talk in a normal tone of voice
3. Use short, simple phrases
4. Orient frequently to person, place, and time
5. Guide the client to follow simple commands (wink, wiggle fingers or toes). Ask the client to wink, wave, and open mouth
6. Begin to talk to the client about family members and friends. At level III, begin to show pictures of family members and friends
7. Provide rest periods: The client tires easily
8. Allow extra time for response. Response may be incorrect
9. Engage in familiar activities such as listening to favorite music, watching television, reading out loud, putting on lotion, and so on
10. Be careful what you say in front of the client

IV. Confused-agitated
At this level clients may be confused and frightened. Clients do not understand their feelings or what is happening around them. They overreact to what is seen, heard, or felt by screaming, hitting, using abusive language, or thrashing about. The

Table 3
Rancho Los Amigos Head Injury Levels (*Continued*)

client is in a heightened state of activity with a severely decreased ability to process information. The client is alert, very active, aggressive, or bizarre. Behavior is nonpurposeful. Activities are stimulated by internal (self) agitation rather than by commands or comments from others in the environment. The client may cry out or scream out of proportion to stimuli. The client may not understand that people are trying to help and may need to be restrained to prevent injury to him/herself. The client is unable to cooperate with treatment. The client is able to pay attention or concentrate for a few seconds. The client has difficulty following instructions. The client is able to perform simple, routine self-care activities such as feeding with assistance

Nursing interventions at this cognitive level are designed to provide structure:
1. Limit the number of visitors
2. Provide a calm, quiet environment
3. Reorient frequently
4. Reassure the client that s/he is safe
5. Provide physical reassurance (slow rocking, gentle touch)
6. Provide family pictures and familiar objects from home
7. Allow as much freedom of movement as is safe
8. Do not force the client to do things
9. Attempt to point out people, noises, and objects in the room
10. Give breaks and change activities frequently

V. Confused-inappropriate
Client appears alert and is able to respond to simple commands with some consistency. The client is able to pay attention for a few minutes. The client is confused and has difficulty making sense of things outside him/herself. Does not know the date, time, or place. Lacks ability to focus on a specific task. Unable to start or complete activities of daily living without step-by-step directions. Becomes overloaded and restless when tired or overstimulated. Has a poor memory. Long-term memory is better than short-term memory. Attempts to fill in memory gaps by making things up. May perseverate on an idea or activity. Lacks initiation. Client may wander off

Nursing interventions at this cognitive level are designed to provide structure:

1. Use repetition
2. Reorient frequently to person, place, and time
3. Explain why the client is in the hospital
4. Use short and simple comments and questions
5. Assist with activity initiation
6. Show the client pictures and objects that were of interest
7. Talk to the client about who s/he is, where s/he is, and what is happening

Table 3
Rancho Los Amigos Head Injury Levels (*Continued*)

8. Limit the number of visitors
9. Provide frequent rest periods

VI. Confused-appropriate

The client is inconsistent in orientation to time and place. The client occasionally knows where s/he is, the correct date, and is oriented to person. The client can remember what s/he has done that day. The client is able to remember the main points of a conversation, but forgets and confuses the details. The client can pay attention for approximately 30 minutes in a calm, nonstressful environment. Has difficulty concentrating when it is noisy or when an activity involves many steps. The client can perform activities of daily living, such as brushing teeth, getting dressed, feeding, and so on, with assistance. The client knows when s/he needs to use the toilet. The client may do or say things too fast and without thinking first. The client is consistently able to follow simple commands and directions. Still has difficulty with new tasks and skills being taught. Needs cueing for direction. Responses may be incorrect owing to memory problems but are appropriate to the situation. May show beginning awareness of his/her situation. No longer wanders

Nursing interventions at this cognitive level are designed to provide structure:

1. Continue with nursing interventions from level V
2. Use repetition
3. Assist in starting and continuing activities
4. Encourage participation in all therapies
5. Discuss events of the day to help improve memory
6. Work on improving the client's ability to carry on a conversation with one person

VII. Automatic-appropriate

Client is able to perform activities of daily living in a structured and familiar environment without help. Tasks are performed in an automatic, robot-like manner and at a slower than normal rate. Can perform 75 percent of tasks but needs supervision for safety and judgment. Has difficulty in new situations. Gets frustrated and may act without thinking. Has difficulty planning, starting, and completing an activity. The client has difficulty paying attention in distracting or stressful situations. Lacks insight into his/her condition. Does not realize that his/her memory and thinking problems may affect future plans and goals. Does not fully understand the impact of his/her physical and cognitive problems. The client may seem inflexible, rigid, or stubborn; however, these behaviors are related to the brain injury. The client may be able to talk about something, but have difficulty doing it

VIII. Purposeful-appropriate

The client is alert and oriented. S/he is able to recall and integrate the past and recent events. Is aware of and responsive to his/her culture. The client can apply

Table 3
Rancho Los Amigos Head Injury Levels (*Continued*)

new skills taught in therapy into activities of daily living. Client is independent in home and community skills. Realizes that there is a problem with his/her thinking and memory skills and begins to compensate for these problems. Is more flexible and less rigid in thinking. Is able to learn new things but at a slower rate. May continue to show a decrease in premorbid abilities in terms of quality and rate of processing, and abstract reasoning. May still become overloaded in difficult and emergency situations

Nursing interventions at cognitive levels VII and VIII are designed to facilitate reintegration into the community:

1. Ask the client to remember more difficult things from day to day
2. Ask the client to solve problems s/he might encounter at home. For example, "What would you do if you lost the keys to the house?"
3. Treat the individual as an adult
4. Talk with the individual as an adult
5. Provide guidance and assistance in decision making
6. Encourage and allow the client to use his/her judgment, reasoning, and problem-solving skills within the home and safe community settings
7. Help the client to set reasonable goals for the future regarding education and employment
8. Encourage participation in all therapies
9. Discourage the use of alcohol and drugs
10. Encourage the use of memory aids such as note taking
11. Identify situations that make the individual angry and discuss strategies for handling these situations
12. Encourage independent functioning

Source: Reprinted with permission from Rancho Los Amigos Medical Center (Downey, CA), Adult Brain Injury Service.

quency, variety, and length of time of stimuli should be increased. Stimulation should be provided in a variety of ways and should include visual, auditory, olfactory, gustatory, cutaneous, and kinesthetic stimuli.

The structured phase of recovery includes Rancho Los Amigos Levels IV, V, and VI. During this phase clients are confused and agitated, confused and inappropriate, and confused and appropriate. The reintegration phase includes Rancho Los Amigos Levels VII and VIII. Client behavior at this level is automatic/appropriate with minimal confusion, or purposeful and appropriate.

Poor outcomes from TBI are associated with increasing age. TBI outcomes are better for survivors between the ages of 5 and 35 years. In general, children recover faster than the elderly. The presence of multiple injuries also has a negative impact on mortality and morbidity.

Nursing Management of Neurological Complications Cognitive Deficits

A comprehensive multidisciplinary rehabilitation process can improve the TBI survivor's cognitive skills sufficiently to allow some level of independent functioning at home and/or at work. The recovery process differs for each individual, and it is difficult to predict the course of recovery for anyone. For individuals with relatively minor head injuries the recovery process may be quick and complete. In many cases, recovery is rapid in the beginning, and then slows and levels off. Only rarely does the TBI survivor recover to a premorbid level of cognition.

Owing to the diffuse nature of traumatic brain injury there is great variability in the cognitive deficits experienced by survivors. A thorough multidisciplinary evaluation must be conducted to determine the nature and extent of the client's deficits, and to develop an individualized treatment approach. The client's cognitive deficits affect performance in a wide range of activities. It is important that everyone on the multidisciplinary team recognize the cognitive strengths and weaknesses of the individual. It is through cognitive processes that the client understands and remembers directions, solves problems, and performs tasks. **Cognition** involves knowing, thinking, learning, and judging. Impaired cognition hinders skill acquisition during the rehabilitation process.

Shortened Attention Span and Concentration

Attention and *concentration* refer to the client's ability to focus long enough to facilitate understanding and to respond appropriately. Attention requires alertness, effort, and selection. Alertness refers to the readiness of the central nervous system to receive information. Effort is needed for task completion. Selection is the ability to screen out irrelevant stimuli. TBI survivors frequently are unable to attend to or concentrate long enough to understand a task. They are easily distracted by external environmental factors, and frequently are unable to sustain an effort long enough to complete a task.

Nursing Interventions

- Reduce/minimize distractions and stimulation.
- Simplify tasks and procedures; break them down into small steps.
- Allow ample time for task completion.
- Refocus attention as needed.
- Use frequent repetition of new information.
- Encourage simple leisure activities such as card games and puzzles.
- Avoid fatigue.
- Provide frequent verbal, visual, or tactile cues.

Impaired Judgment

Judgment is the ability to understand and determine the consequences of actions taken, and to take action in a safe and appropriate manner. The ability to make even simple everyday choices can be severely impaired by a traumatic brain injury.

Nursing Interventions
- Allow the client to make simple decisions, such as what clothes to wear or what to eat for dinner.
- Involve the client in the decision-making process.
- Provide choices.
- Provide frequent feedback.
- Reduce/minimize distractions.
- Provide ample time.

Impaired Memory

Memory refers to the ability to retain information for retrieval and use at a later time. Memory consists of both short-term and long-term memory. Short-term memory is the ability to retain information for 1 minute to 1 hour. Long-term memory is the ability to retain information for 1 hour or longer. There are almost no limits on long-term memory. Information can be obtained through verbal and visual mechanisms. TBI survivors can have deficits in either verbal or visual memory or both.

Nursing Interventions
- Encourage the use of memory aids such as cards, journals, books, or audiotapes.
- Provide clocks, calendars, television, and radios.
- Structure daily activities.
- Post schedule or daily routine in a highly visible place.
- Use repetition when providing new information.
- Record or write down new information for later review.

Impaired Communication

If the muscles and nerves involved in speech are damaged the client's speech may be impaired. Involvement or damage to the speech centers in the left hemisphere results in expressive, receptive, or global **aphasia.** Speech therapy by a trained speech pathologist is helpful. Nurses must be aware of the plan of treatment and implement any recommendations made by the speech therapist. Patience and persistence are required to ensure that client needs are expressed.

Nursing Interventions
- Speak slowly in a normal tone of voice.
- Use simple words and phrases.
- Ask yes/no questions.
- Provide ample time to process and answer questions.
- Encourage speech efforts.
- Praise speech efforts.

- Encourage the use of gestures.
- Reduce distractions.
- Do not answer or speak for the client.
- Provide clues when appropriate.

Perceptual Deficits

TBI survivors frequently experience perceptual deficits. These include visual field cuts such as hemianopia, impaired figure-ground perception, unilateral neglect, and inability to judge distances correctly.

Nursing Interventions

- Teach the client to scan the environment.
- Provide a full-length mirror.
- Provide verbal or written cues.
- Use multiple teaching modalities.
- Approach the client from his or her unaffected side.
- Incorporate the client's affected side into activities.
- Use color to highlight neglected objects.
- Teach the client to use the affected extremity.

Initiation

Initiation is the ability to start a task and carry it to completion. Some TBI survivors have difficulty beginning or completing tasks. The individual has the motor ability, and the understanding, to perform the task but cannot start or complete the task without cues or reminders.

Nursing Interventions

- Post a readily visible schedule of daily activities.
- Provide memory aids such as strategically placed signs and audiotapes.
- Break tasks down into small, simple steps.
- Provide supervision and support.

Sequencing

Sequencing is the ability to complete a task from start to finish. Frequently, TBI survivors are unable to figure out the proper sequence of steps to take for task completion. They understand the task, can perform the task, and can even begin the task without cues. However, they cannot determine the correct sequence of steps for task completion.

Nursing Interventions

- Break tasks down into simple steps.
- Provide cues for each step of a task.
- Allow the client to complete each step before providing cues for next step.

Behavioral/ Emotional Deficits

The TBI survivor experiences a wide variety of behavioral and emotional difficulties including personality changes, neurotic reactions, changes in coping, denial, depression, lethargy, decreased spontaneity, decreased libido, decreased overt emotions, inability to plan ahead, impulsivity, sexual disinhibition, increased motor activity, inappropriate social irritability, anger, aggression, and agitation. Behavior modification programs are often used for persistent problems. Consistent limit setting and a structured environment are keys to changing undesirable behaviors.

Nursing Interventions for Agitation and Irritability

- Reduce stimulation.
- Provide a safe, structured environment.
- Avoid the use of restraints if possible.
- Remain calm and consistent.
- Provide positive feedback for appropriate behaviors.
- Provide an outlet for restlessness, such as walking or other physical activities.
- Redirect attention.
- Identify triggers and frequency of agitation.

Nursing Interventions for Impulsivity

- Provide immediate feedback for inappropriate behaviors.
- Redirect/refocus attention.
- Provide a safe, structured environment.
- Teach self-control methods by using simple rewards.

Physical Symptoms Bowel and Bladder

Following a traumatic brain injury with prolonged periods of unconsciousness it is not unusual for the individual to experience incontinence. Adequate fluid and dietary intake are essential to managing bowel and bladder programs. The conscious cognitively impaired individual may have difficulty remembering to eat, drink, and toilet. The individual may be unable to sense that the bladder or rectum is full, or may be unable to empty at will. Often continence can be achieved with bowel and bladder retraining programs, and/or medications.

Altered Nutrition

The long-term nutritional needs of an unconscious individual are met via nasogastric or gastrostomy tube feedings. A variety of commercial preparations are available. Gastrostomy tubes are recommended for individuals requiring nutritional support for extended periods of time. It is important that feedings, and all medications, be followed with water to prevent the tube from clogging and to maintain adequate hydration. Residual must be checked before starting feedings and the feeding should be held if the residual is 100 milliliters or more (institutional guidelines may vary).

Following a brain injury the individual may experience loss of appetite associated with weight loss. Offering small, frequent feedings may be a solution to this problem. After the appetite returns the client may want to eat continually. Owing to short-term memory impairment the client may not remember eating or may not have a sensation of fullness.

If the glossopharyngeal and vagus nerves were injured the client may experience swallowing difficulties. For the client with **dysphagia,** swallowing precautions and interventions should be followed to prevent aspiration, and to ensure adequate nutritional intake. See Chapter 18 on chewing, swallowing, and feeding for specific interventions.

Impaired Mobility

Individuals with traumatic brain injuries suffer a variety of motor problems. These include hemiparesis, hemiplegia, monoparesis, monoplegia, incoordination, spasticity, contractures, balance problems, and abnormal gaits and posturing. Range-of-motion exercises should be performed two or three times daily. Braces, splints, slings, and assistive devices are available to promote normal functioning. Physical therapy and occupational therapy are important components of a comprehensive rehabilitation program for the individual with TBI. The goals of therapy are to improve muscle tone, strength, co-ordination, balance, posture, and range of motion.

The TBI survivor may also experience movement **apraxia.** The client with apraxia is unable to perform a movement on command. The individual may be able to perform the movement automatically. There are several types of movement apraxia. The client with constructional apraxia is unable to put things together. The client with constructional apraxia may benefit from drawing simple patterns, and completing simple puzzles. The person with dressing apraxia may put clothes on upside down or put a leg into the sleeve of a shirt. Following the same routine, and laying clothes out in the order they are put on may be helpful. Limb apraxia refers to the inability to plan and perform movements with the upper and lower extremities. The client with oral apraxia has difficulty planning and making movements with the tongue, jaw, and lips.

Altered Sexual Functioning

Individuals with traumatic brain injury often display a variety of inappropriate sexual behaviors. These include loss of inhibition, swearing, and sexual overtures toward staff. The staff must respond to these behaviors with consistent limit setting.

Owing to the young age of TBI survivors, sexual issues are of major concern to them. Nurses must be comfortable in discussing these concerns and making appropriate referrals for counseling. Refer to Chapter 28 on altered sexual functioning for more detailed information.

Self-Care Deficits The TBI survivor will need assistance and retraining with activities of living such as toileting, hygiene, dressing, grooming, feeding, and mobility. Treatment approaches and interventions for these areas are covered in Chapter 25 on functional living skills for self-care.

Seizure Disorders Approximately 7 to 10 percent of individuals with traumatic brain injury will develop seizure disorders within 6–12 months following the injury (National Head Injury Foundation, 1991). TBI survivors may experience petit mal, grand mal, or psychomotor-type seizures. For this reason, they are maintained on anticonvulsant medications such as phenytoin, carbamazepine, or valproic acid postinjury. If the individual remains seizure free for approximately 1 year he or she may be weaned off anticonvulsants. Client and caregiver teaching should include information about anticonvulsants, their action, side effects, and what to do during a seizure. If a seizure should occur, efforts should be made to protect the client from injury. Standard seizure precautions should be followed.

Discharge Planning Many TBI survivors are able to return to their homes. Discharge planning should be initiated at the time of admission to the rehabilitation unit. The options or alternatives for discharge care need to be identified and discussed with the family caregivers. A vital component of effective discharge planning is comprehensive client and family caregiver teaching.

**Teaching/
Learning Needs**

Brain anatomy
Basic function of major brain structures
Cranial nerves
Common cognitive deficits associated with TBI
Management of traumatic brain injury
Management of medication regimen
Management of seizure disorders
Reactions to TBI
Recovery process from TBI
Use of memory aids

**Common Nursing
Diagnosis**

Activity intolerance
Alteration in comfort
Altered family processes
Altered health maintenance
Altered nutrition less than body requirements
Altered respiratory function
Altered urinary elimination
Altered bowel elimination
Altered family processes
Altered sexual functioning

Altered role performance
Altered thought processes
Confusion
Grieving
Impaired communication
Impaired memory
Impaired physical mobility
Impaired swallowing
Knowledge deficit
Risk for impaired skin integrity
Risk for injury
Risk for social isolation
Self-care deficit
Self-concept disturbance
Sensory-perceptual alteration
Sleep pattern disturbance
Spiritual distress
Unilateral neglect

Summary

Traumatic brain injury is a sudden, life-threatening, devastating, and life-changing event for the TBI survivor and family members. Many of the neurological deficits associated with TBI are irreversible and impact all aspects of an individual's life. The sequelae frequently evolve into chronic, long-term problems that present many demands on the individual and family. Recovery is a complex process that requires management by a multidisciplinary team of health care professionals. Nurses are in contact with the TBI survivor and family members during all phases of recovery in a variety of settings.

References

Alexander, M. P. (1995). Mild traumatic brain injury: Pathophysiology, natural history, and clinical management. *Neurology, 45,* 1253–1260.

Centers for Disease Control (CDC). (1996). Epidemiology of traumatic brain injury in the United States (on-line). Available http://www.cdc.gov/ncipc/darrdp/tbi.html.

DiLima, S. N., & Eutsey, D. E. (1996). *Brain injury: Survivor and caregiver education manual.* Gaithersburg, MD: Aspen.

Hall, K. M., & Johnston, M. V. (1994). Outcomes evaluation in TBI rehabilitation. II. Measurement tools for a nationwide data system. *Archives of Physical Medicine and Rehabilitation, 75,* SC-10–SC-18.

Levitt, M. D., Sutton, M., Goldman, J., Mikhail, M., & Christopher, T. (1994). Cognitive dysfunction in patients suffering minor head trauma (on-line). Available http://solaris.Ckm.ucsf.edu:8081/O...als/LevittSutton.Levitt/Sutton.html.

National Head Injury Foundation. (1991). *Head injury fact sheet.*

National Institute of Neurological Disorders and Stroke. (1990).

Sachs, P. R. (1986). A six-factor model for treatment planning and cognitive retraining of the traumatically head-injured adult. *Journal of Cognitive Rehabilitation, 4*(1), 26–30.

Sosin, D. M., Sniezek, J. E., & Waxweiler, R. J. (1995). Trends in death associated with traumatic brain injury, 1979–1992. *JAMA, 273*(22), 1778–1780.

Spettell, C. M., Ellis, D. W., Ross, S. E., Sandel, E., O'Malley, K., Stein, S. C., Spivack, G., & Hurley, K. E. (1991). Time of rehabilitation admission and severity of trauma: Effect on brain injury outcome. *Archives of Physical Medicine Rehabilitation, 72,* 320–325.

Suggested Readings

Armstrong, C. (1991). Emotional changes following brain injury: Psychological and neurological components of depression, denial and anxiety. *Journal of Rehabilitation,* April/May/June, 15–21.

Banja, J., & Johnston, M. V. (1994). Outcomes evaluation in TBI rehabilitation. III. Ethical perspectives and social policy. *Archives of Physical Medicine Rehabilitation, 75,* SC-19–SC-26.

Bombardier, C. H. (1995). Alcohol use and traumatic brain injury. *Epitomes-Physical Medicine Rehabilitation, 162*(2), 150–151.

Bottcher, S. A. (1989). Cognitive retraining: A nursing process approach to rehabilitation of the brain injured. *Nursing Clinics of North America, 24*(1), 193–207.

Brooke, M. M., Patterson, D. R., Questad, K. A., Cardenas, D., & Farrel-Roberts, L. (1992). The treatment of agitation during initial hospitalization after traumatic brain injury. *Archives of Physical Medicine Rehabilitation, 73,* 917–921.

Brooke, M. M., Questad, K. A., Patterson, D. R., & Bashak, K. J. (1992). Agitation and restlessness after closed head injury: A prospective study of 100 consecutive admissions. *Archives of Physical Medicine Rehabilitation, 73,* 320–323.

Cook, E. A., & Thigpen, R. (1993). identification and management of cognitive and perceptual deficits in the rehabilitation patient. *Rehabilitation Nursing, 18*(5), 310–313.

Corrigan, J. D. (1995). Substance abuse as a mediating factor in outcome from traumatic brain injury. *Archives of Physical Medicine and Rehabilitation, 76,* 302–309.

Cowen, T. D., Meythaler, J. M., DeVivo, M. J., Ivie, C. S., III, Lebow, J., & Novack, T. A. (1995). Influence of early variables in traumatic brain injury on functional independence measure scores and rehabilitation length of stay and charges. *Archives of Physical Medicine and Rehabilitation, 76,* 797–803.

DiDonato, B. A., & Schaffer, V. L. (1994). The importance of outcome data in brain injury rehabilitation. *Rehabilitation Nursing, 19*(4), 219–228.

Frost, D., & Barone, S. H. (1996). Functional outcome in elderly patients with traumatic brain injuries. *Rehabilitation Nursing Research, 5*(1), 9–15.

Globus, M. Y.-T., Alonso, O. W., Dietrich, D., Busto, R., & Ginsberg, M. D. (1995). Glutamate release and free radical production following brain injury: Effects of posttraumatic hypothermia. *Journal of Neurochemistry, 65*(4), 1704–1711.

Gorman, L. K., Shook, B. L., & Becker, D. P. (1993). Traumatic brain injury produces impairments in long-term and recent memory. *Brain Research, 614,* 29–36.

Granger, C. V., Divan, N., & Fiedler, R. C. (1995). Functional assessment scales: A study of persons after traumatic brain injury. *American Journal of Physical Medicine and Rehabilitation, 74*(2), 107–113.

Groah, S. L., & Cifu, D. X. (1995). The rehabilitative management of the traumatic brain injury patient with assicuated femoral neuropathy. *Archive of Physical Medicine and Rehabilitation, 76,* 480–483.

Hall, K. M., Karzmark, P., Stevens, M., Englander, J., O'Hare, P., & Wright, J. (1994). *Archives of Physical Medicine Rehabilitation, 75,* 876–884.

Hallett, J. D., Zasler, N. D., Maurer, P., & Cash, S. (1992). Role change after traumatic brain injury in adults. *American Journal of Occupational Therapy, 48*(3), 241–246.

Harrington, D. E., Malec, J., Cicerone, K., & Katz, H. T. (1993). Current perceptions of rehabilitation professionals towards mild traumatic brain injury. *Archives of Physical Medicine Rehabilitation, 74,* 579–586.

Jackson, J. D. (1993). After rehabilitation: Meeting the long-term needs of persons with traumatic brain injury. *American Journal of Occupational Therapy, 48*(3), 251–255.

Johnston, M. V. & Hall, K. M. (1994). Outcomes evaluation in TBI rehabilitation. I. Overview and system principles. *Archives of Physical Medicine Rehabilitation, 75,* SC-2–SC-9.

Kaplan, C. P., & Corrigan, J. D. (1994). The relationship between cognition and functional independence in adults with traumatic brain injury. *Archives of Physical Medicine Rehabilitation, 75,* 643–647.

Katz, D. I., & Alexander, M. P. (1994). Traumatic brain injury: Predicting course of recovery and outcome for patients admitted to rehabilitation. *Archives of Neurology, 51,* 661–670.

Klonoff, P. S., O'Brien, K. P., Prigatano, G. P., Chiapello, D. A., & Cunninham, M. (1989). Cognitive retraining after traumatic brain injury and its role in facilitating awareness. *Journal of Head Trauma Rehabilitation, 4*(3), 37–45.

Mackay, L. E., Bernstein, B. A., Chapman, P. E., Morgan, A. S., & Milazzo, L. S. (1992). Early intervention in severe head injury: Long-term benefits of a formalized program. *Archives of Physical Medicine Rehabilitation, 73,* 635–641.

Mateer, C. A., Soblberg, M. M., & Crinean, J. (1987). Focus on clinical research: Perceptions of memory function in individuals with closed-head injury. *Journal of Head Trauma Rehabilitation, 2*(3), 74–84.

McDougall, G. J. (1996). Predictors of the use of memory improvement strategies by older adults. *Rehabilitation Nursing, 21*(4), 202–209.

Novack, T. A., Bergquist, T. F., Bennett, G., & Gouvier, W. D. (1991). Primary caregiver distress following severe head injury. *Journal of Head Trauma Rehabilitation, 6*(4), 69–77.

Parenté, R., & Hermann, D. (1996). *Retraining cognition: Techniques and applications.* Gaithersburg, MD: Aspen.

Prigatano, G. P. (1991). Disordered mind, wounded soul: The emerging role of psychotherapy in rehabilitation after brain injury. *Journal of Head Trauma Rehabilitation, 6*(4), 1–10.

Rivara, J. B., Fay, G. C., Jaffe, K. M., Polissar, N. L., Shurtleff, H. A., & Martin, K. M. (1992). Predictors of family functioning one year following traumatic brain injury in children. *Archives of Physical Medicine and Rehabilitation, 73,* 899–921.

Scroggs, D. J. (1995). AAC and TBI: Transitioning systems through the phases of recovery (on-line). Available http://kaddath.mt.cs.cmu.edu/scs/95-djs5.html.

Sorensen, S. B., & Kraus, J. F. (1991). Occurrence, severity, and outcomes of brain injury. *Journal of Head Trauma Rehabilitation, 6*(2), 1–10.

Webb, C. R., Wrigley, M., Yoels, W., & Fine, P. R. (1995). Explaining quality of life for persons with traumatic brain injuries 2 years after injury. *Archives of Physical Medicine and Rehabilitation, 76,* 1113–1119.

Wehman, P., Kregel, J., West, M., & Cifu, D. (1994). Return to work for patients with traumatic brain injury: Analysis of costs. *American Journal of Physical Medicine Rehabilitation, 73*(4), 280–282.

Whitlock, J. A., & Hamilton, B. B. (1995). Functional outcome after rehabilitation for severe traumatic brain injury. *Archives of Physical Medicine and Rehabilitation, 76,* 1103–1112.

Willer, B. S., Allen, K. M., Liss, M., & Zicht, M. S. (1991). Problems and coping strategies of individuals with traumatic brain injury and their spouses. *Archives of Physical Medicine Rehabilitation, 72,* 460–464.

Williams, M. H. (1990). The self-help movement in head injury. *Rehabilitation Nursing, 15*(6), 311–315.

Worthington, J. (1989). The impact of adolescent development on recovery from traumatic brain injury. *Rehabilitation Nursing, 14*(3), 118–121.

CHAPTER 16
Acquired Brain Injury: Cerebrovascular Accident

Anita Rosebrough

Key Terms
Anosognosia
Anticoagulant Therapy
Aphasia
Apraxia
Atherosclerosis
Broca's Aphasia
Carotid Endarterectomy (CE)
Cerebrovascular Accident (CVA)
Dysarthria
Dysphagia
Global Aphasia
Hemianopia
Hemiparesis
Hemiplegia
Hemorrhagic Strokes
Homonymous Hemianopia
Intracerebral Hemorrhages
Ischemic Strokes
Lacunar Strokes
Left Cerebral Dominance
Percutaneous Translumenal Angioplasty (PTA)
Reversible Ischemic Neurological Deficits (RINDs)
Subarachnoid Hemorrhages
Thrombolytic Therapy
Transient Ischemic Attack
Videofluoroscopic Modified Barium Swallowing Examination
Wernicke's Aphasia
Yes-No Reliability

Objectives

1. Demonstrate knowledge of the major functions of each lobe of the brain and cerebral circulation.

2. Identify the major sensory and motor deficits experienced after a stroke.

3. Differentiate between transient ischemic attack and a stroke.

247

4. Identify common nursing diagnoses experienced by individuals after a stroke.

5. Differentiate between right and left cerebral hemisphere injury, and discuss the effects of each.

6. Compare and contrast expressive and receptive aphasia.

7. Identify appropriate nursing interventions for the client with Broca's or expressive aphasia.

8. Identify appropriate nursing interventions for the client with Wernicke's or receptive aphasia.

9. Identify appropriate nursing interventions for the client with dysphagia.

10. Identify risk factors associated with cerebrovascular occlusive disease.

11. Differentiate between plaque, thrombus, and embolism.

Introduction   A **cerebrovascular accident (CVA),** or stroke, is a medical emergency that occurs when the blood supply to the brain is interrupted or blocked. The resulting alteration in cerebral perfusion produces acute neurological dysfunction. Signs and symptoms associated with the stroke correspond to the involvement of focal areas of the brain. Strokes have a rapid onset, and the neurological deficits associated with a completed stroke persist for more than 24 hours (Margolis & Preziosi, 1996; National Institute of Neurological Disorders and Stroke [NINDS], 1995).

According to the Agency for Health Care Policy and Research (AHCPR), stroke mortality has declined steadily since the 1940s. However, stroke remains the third leading cause of death. It is the most common disease affecting the nervous system and is a major cause of long-term disability in the United States. Approximately 550,000 people sustain strokes each year, and 150,000 of these die from stroke-related causes. In the United States, there are approximately 3 million people living with varying degrees of neurological dysfunction due to brain damage from strokes. The estimated annual economic cost of providing medical care and lost income for stroke survivors is $25 billion to $30 billion. Stroke mortality ranges from 17 to 34 percent during the first 30 days and from 25 to 40 percent during the first year after a stroke (AHCPR, 1996). Mortality from strokes is on the decline owing to advances in technology, improved acute care, reduced stroke severity, management of modifiable risk factors, and early diagnosis.

Etiology   Interruptions in cerebral blood flow that produce strokes are either ischemic or hemorrhagic in origin. Approximately 75–80 percent of all strokes are due to ischemia. Ischemia refers to the lack of oxygenated blood perfusing cerebral tissue. Ischemia occurs whenever the blood supply to the brain is interrupted or obstructed. In **ischemic strokes,** neurons are damaged by the lack of oxygen and by the buildup of toxins such as glutamate, glycine, and nitric oxide. Both the degree and the duration of the ischemia determine whether neurological impairment is temporary or permanent. The manifestation of neurological deficits is directly related to the area of the brain perfused by the involved artery. The mildest form of a stroke is almost unnoticeable; the most severe forms can result in coma and even death (AHCPR, 1996; Margolis & Preziosi, 1996; National Stroke Association [NSA], 1992a,b).

Many things can cause cerebral ischemia. However, the two most common causes are cerebral thrombosis and cerebral embolism. Cerebral thrombosis accounts for approximately 53 percent of all strokes. Thrombotic strokes arise from arterial occlusions caused by *thrombi* (blood clots) formed in the arteries supplying the brain. Clots often form in arteries already narrowed by atherosclerotic plaque formation, such as in the carotid or vertebral arteries. The development of cerebral thrombosis is most frequently attributed to atherosclerosis and inflammatory diseases, which damage the arterial walls. Conditions that cause inadequate cerebral perfusion, such as dehydration, hypotension, and prolonged vasoconstriction, increase the risk of thrombus formation. However, the most common cause is **atherosclerosis.** If a complete occlusion occurs, irreversible damage to the brain occurs within 4–6 minutes. Thrombotic strokes have a gradual onset, evolving over several minutes to hours. They are not associated with activity (AHCPR, 1996; Margolis & Preziosi, 1996).

Less common are **lacunar strokes,** which occurs when thrombi occlude small arterioles. Lacunar strokes account for 10–23 percent of cerebral infarctions. They occur in deeper regions of the brain and brainstem and are most common in the internal capsule, pons, putamen, caudate nucleus, and the thalamus (Biller & Love, 1991). These strokes result in degeneration of cerebral tissue, which produces cavities or *lakes* visible on magnetic resonance imaging (MRI). The symptoms associated with lacunar strokes are mild owing to microatheroma of a single small vessel. Lacunar strokes are frequently associated with hypertension or diabetes mellitus (AHCPR, 1996; Margolis & Preziosi, 1996; NSA, 1992a,b).

Cerebral embolism is the second most common cause of stroke and accounts for approximately 20 percent of all strokes. Occlusion of a cerebral vessel can be caused by particles or fragments of substances such as clots, tumors, fat, bacteria, or air. Embolic strokes often occur in the middle cerebral artery and are frequently of cardiac origin. The embolus travels to the brain and becomes lodged in a small artery. Embolic strokes have a sudden onset with immediate and maximum neurological deficits. Prognosis is fair to good (Margolis & Preziosi, 1996).

Hemorrhagic strokes account for 20 percent of all strokes. They are due to the rupture of a cerebral artery. The blood escapes into the brain or into the space between the skull and the brain. Hemorrhagic strokes have a variety of causes, with hypertension being the most common cause of **intracerebral hemorrhages.** The hemorrhages vary in size from petechia to massive bleeds several centimeters in diameter. The blood may diffuse or form into hematomas. The hematomas lead to compression of cerebral tissue, causing further neurological damage. Surgical evacuation of the hematoma may be necessary. The prognosis for hemorrhagic stroke is poor. Massive bleeds are usually fatal. A hemorrhagic stroke occurs suddenly, usually while the person is active (AHCPR, 1996; Margolis & Preziosi, 1996; NSA, 1992a).

Seven to 10 percent of strokes are due to **subarachnoid hemorrhages.** The most common cause of these hemorrhages is intracranial aneurysms. The aneurysms generally tend to occur in the circle of Willis. The highest incidence of rupture is in patients between the ages of 35 and 65 years. Symptoms include a sudden, excruciating headache and altered level of consciousness. Other causes of hemorrhagic strokes include trauma, tumors, vascular malformations, and blood dyscrasias (AHCPR, 1996; Margolis & Preziosi, 1996; NSA, 1992a).

Stroke Risk Factors

The association of specific risk factors with stroke development is well documented. Factors that increase the risk of stroke are separated into two groups: modifiable and nonmodifiable. Nonmodifiable risk factors are those over which an individual has no control. These are age, sex, family history, previous history of stroke or heart attack, and ethnicity. The frequency of stroke increases with age and doubles every 10 years after the age of 55 (Dyken, Barnett, Bergen, Hass, Kannel, Kuller, Kurtzke, & Sundt, 1984). Seventy-two percent of strokes occur in people older than 65 years of age. Strokes tend to run in families and are more frequent in men than in women. The mortality rate from stroke is the same for men and women. African-Americans, Asian-Pacific Islanders, and Hispanics have a higher incidence of strokes. African-Americans have two times the risk of death from stroke relative to Caucasians. Thirteen percent of stroke survivors will have a second stroke within 1 year after having their first stroke (AHCPR, 1996).

The modifiable risk factors are hypertension, smoking, diabetes, alcohol abuse, obesity, sedentary lifestyle, drug abuse, and elevated cholesterol and triglyceride levels. Approximately three-quarters of all stroke clients are hypertensive. Hypertensive individuals have four times the risk of stroke of nonhypertensive people. The risk increases with elevations in either the systolic or diastolic pressures. Hypertension also accelerates the development of atherosclerosis (Bronner, Kanter, & Manson, 1996; Matchar, Douglas, McCrory, Barnett, & Feussner, 1994). Smoking is a major cause of both ischemic and hemorrhagic strokes. The risk is higher for female smokers, and the risk increases with the number of cigarettes smoked per day (Bronner, Kanter, & Manson, 1996). Smoking accounts for one-half of stroke deaths in the 35- to 64-year age range. Cigarette smoking accelerates atherosclerotic plaque formation and leads to severe narrowing of the carotid arteries. The risk of coronary artery disease decreases 14 percent within 2 years of smoking cessation (Nurses' Health Study, 1996). Individuals with diabetes have a two to three times greater incidence of ischemic strokes. Women with diabetes are at even greater risk. Research shows that diabetics are more prone to atherothromboembolic infarctions, are at increased risk for intracranial vascular disease, and are at increased risk for lacunar infarctions. Diabetics have more severe cerebral ischemic events and a higher mortality rate after stroke than nondiabetics (Biller & Love, 1991). Alcohol consumption in moderate doses decreases the risk of heart attack and ischemic stroke. However, even a moderate intake of alcohol increases the risk of hemorrhagic stroke. Obesity increases the risk of stroke 50–100 percent. The latest research studies show that even women of average weight are at increased risk of coronary artery disease (Nurses' Health Study, 1996). Regular exercise lowers the risk of stroke for both men and women. Exercise decreases platelet aggregation, weight, and blood pressure, and increases insulin sensitivity and high-density lipoprotein levels (Bronner, Kanter, & Manson, 1996). Drugs, such as cocaine and amphetamines, can cause strokes even in young individuals. High levels of cholesterol and triglycerides contribute to and accelerate atherosclerotic plaque formation. Approximately two-thirds of all ischemic strokes are due to atherosclerosis (AHCPR, 1996; Margolis & Preziosi, 1996).

The risk of stroke increases as the number and the severity of the risk factors increase. It is recommended that people take action to decrease or eliminate risk factors from their lifestyles. Research shows that risk factor modification dramatically reduces stroke risk (AHCPR, 1996; NINDS, 1995; NSA, 1994).

Transient Ischemic Attacks

Approximately 20–30 percent of strokes are due to carotid artery stenosis. Strokes due to carotid artery stenosis are frequently preceded by **transient ischemic attacks** (TIAs). TIAs refer to transient cerebral ischemia with temporary episodes of neurological dysfunction, and are caused by thrombotic particles producing intermittent blockages in cerebral circulation. These blockages usually occur in the carotid artery or vertebrobasilar systems (see Figure 1). TIAs begin rapidly and resolve completely. Their duration is usually a matter of 2–15 minutes but they can last as long as 24 hours. If the neurological deficits associated with a TIA last more than 24 hours but resolve completely in 48 hours, they are termed **reversible ischemic neurological deficits (RINDs).** Common neurological deficits associated with TIAs and RINDs are weakness or numbness of an extremity; alterations in speech, such as slurred speech; and visual problems. Between episodes, the client experiences normal neurological functioning. TIAs and RINDs

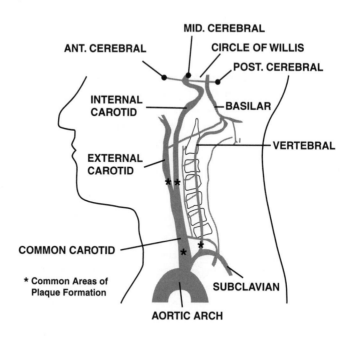

Fig 1. *Cerebral circulation and atherosclerotic plaque formation.*

are warnings of an underlying pathological condition and should not be left untreated. Approximately 35 percent of thrombotic strokes are preceded by TIAs. Most patients experiencing TIAs will have a stroke within 2–5 years (Bronstein, Popovich, & Stewart-Amidei, 1991; Kelly, 1995; Moore & Trifiletti, 1994).

Treatment of TIAs and Stroke Prevention

The treatment of strokes and TIAs is preventive in nature and involves risk factor reduction. Current medical treatments include carotid endarterectomy surgery, percutaneous translumenal angioplasty, anticoagulant therapy, and thrombolysis.

Carotid endarterectomy (CE) surgery is used to remove atherosclerotic plaques from the carotid arteries. Data from four large-scale clinical trials demonstrated that CE reduces the risk of ipsilateral stroke 55 percent in asymptomatic clients with a 60 percent or greater carotid artery stenosis. It is noteworthy that 69 percent of men benefit from the procedure, and only 16 percent of women benefit (Toole, Baker, Castaldo, Chambless, Moore, Robertson, Young, & Howard, 1995).

Percutaneous translumenal angioplasty (PTA) has been approved as treatment for extracranial artery stenosis due to atherosclerosis. Its use for intracranial vessels is still under investigation (Clark & Bamwell, 1995). During PTA, atherosclerotic plaques in the carotid arteries are flattened against the arterial walls by inflating and deflating a balloon-tipped catheter several times. The catheter is then removed. The plaques remain compressed, which improves cerebral circulation and decreases the risk of stroke and TIAs.

Anticoagulant therapy prevents the formation of clots in patients at risk for or with a history of clot formation. Three drugs are currently available to prevent clot formation and strokes: aspirin, ticlopidine hydrochloride, and warfarin. Aspirin blocks prostaglandin synthesis and thrombaxane, thereby decreasing platelet aggregation. No research evidence supports its use for stroke prevention in women. Recommended dosages for men range from 325 to 1300 milligrams per day. Owing to the high incidence of gastric irritation, enteric-coated or buffered tablets are preferred (Bellavance, 1993).

Ticlopidine hydrochloride (Ticlid), a platelet antiaggregant drug, is effective in preventing strokes by reducing/preventing ischemic neurological episodes. It is more effective than aspirin in preventing strokes of noncardioembolic origin. Ticlopidine reduces the incidence of stroke by 48 percent during the first year of therapy. The therapeutic effect of ticlopidine is achieved within 24 to 48 hours. Research shows ticlopidine to be most effective in clients of African-American origin, women, and clients with vertebrobasilar disease. This drug can cause neutropenia and thrombocytopenia, which develop anywhere from 2 days to several weeks after taking the drug. The neutropenia resolves quickly once the drug is discontinued. It is recommended that a complete blood count be done every 2 weeks for the first 3 months of therapy. Ticlid increases the effect of aspirin and should not be taken with heparin or warfarin (AHCPR, 1996; Bellavance, 1993; Bronstein & Chadwick, 1994; Chimowitz, 1995).

Warfarin (Coumadin) anticoagulant therapy reduces the risk of stroke in patients with thrombi of cardiac origin. Clients on anticoagulant therapy should have their coagulation status closely monitored by a physician. For maximum therapeutic effect, it is recommended that the International Normalized Ratio be between 2 and 3 (AHCPR, 1996).

The most common cause of ischemic stroke is a thromboembolic occlusion. In June 1996, the Food and Drug Administration (FDA) approved tissue plasminogen activator (t-PA) for the treatment of acute stroke. t-PA is a thrombolytic agent (clot buster) that acts to break up or dissolve blood clots interrupting blood flow to the brain. Clients treated with t-PA were 30 percent more likely to recover from their strokes (NSA, 1996). The window of opportunity for **thrombolytic therapy** in stroke clients is 3 hours. Time is a critical factor; therefore, for this new treatment to be effective, strokes need to be treated as true medical emergencies (NINDS, 1995).

An emerging field in cerebrovascular therapy is the use of vascular stents. Studies show that stents can be successful in the treatment of carotid artery stenosis and cerebral aneurysms. However, further research is needed to validate their efficacy and also to improve the quality of the stents (American Health Care Consultants, 1996).

The mainstay of stroke prevention is aggressive management of risk factor reduction through client education. Educational programs should place special emphasis on hypertension, smoking, hypercholesterolemia, and recognition of stroke symptoms (AHCPR, 1996; NINDS, 1996; NSA, 1992).

Warning Signs of Stroke

The warning signs of a stroke include the following:

- Weakness, numbness, or paralysis on one side of the body, face, arm, or leg
- Blurred or impaired vision in one or both eyes
- Difficulty speaking or understanding simple statements
- Unexplained dizziness, loss of balance, or coordination (maybe combined with other symptoms)
- Sudden, severe unexplained headache

If any of these symptoms occur, seek help—do not wait!

Stroke Rehabilitation Potential

Stroke rehabilitation should begin when the diagnosis has been made and the client is medically stable. The goals of stroke rehabilitation are to prevent stroke complications, prevent recurrent stroke, mobilize the client, and resume self-care activities. Recovery from stroke is most rapid during the first 3 months and reaches maximum potential within the first 6 months. Some individuals continue to improve up to 1 year after a stroke (AHCPR, 1996; Cifu & Lorish, 1994; Ferrucci, Bandinelli, Guralnik, Lamponi, Bertini, Falchini, & Baroni, 1993). Functional gains made during rehabilitation generally persist after discharge. Clients continue to improve in mobility skills after discharge but tend to lose ground in the areas of dressing and feeding. This may be because families choose to perform these tasks for them (Cifu & Lorish, 1994). Advancing age adversely affects recovery. Bilateral hemisphere involvement has a less favorable outcome than unilateral hemisphere damage. Both advanced age and bilateral hemisphere involvement are associated with lower level functioning on discharge and a lower rate of discharge into the community (Granger, Hamilton, & Fiedler, 1992).

Deficits/Limitations/ Effects of Stroke

The specific neurological deficits experienced by a stroke survivor vary depending on the area of the brain involved and the artery affected (see Figure 2). Variations occur owing to vessel size and flow disruption. The most common and most visible signs of a stroke are paralysis, hemiplegia, or weakness (**hemiparesis**) on one side of the body. The location of the brain injury determines which side of the body is affected. The right hemisphere of the brain controls the left side of the body, and the left hemisphere of the brain controls the right side of the body.

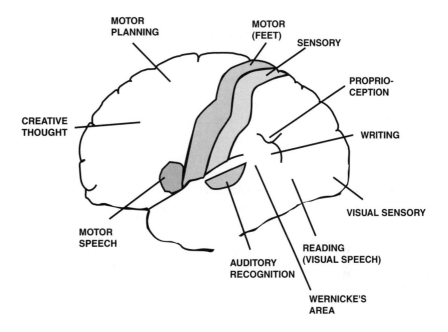

Fig 2. *Brain functions frequently affected by stroke.*

Left CVA/Right Hemiplegia

Hemiplegia is paralysis on one side of the body. When the injury occurs in the left hemisphere of the brain, the right side of the body is affected (see Figure 3). For most people **left cerebral dominance** is the norm—i.e., the left hemisphere of the brain is dominant for speech and language, including left-handed individuals. The client with damage to the left hemisphere often experiences speech and language problems. Although each individual is different, the following characteristics are often observed in individuals with left hemisphere damage:

- Paralysis or weakness on the right side of the body
- Impaired swallowing
- Impaired gag reflex
- Food pocketing
- Aphasia
- Problems with mathematics
- Inappropriate use of yes-no
- Difficulty knowing right from left
- Speech that is jargon, gibberish, or nonsense
- Inability to name objects
- Difficulty recognizing familiar faces
- Inappropriate laughing or crying

- Loss of the right visual fields
- Slow, cautious behavior
- Good judgment
- Good motor planning
- Good problem-solving skills
- Decreased attention span
- Difficulty learning new information
- Becoming easily frustrated

Clients with left cerebrovascular accidents approach tasks with anxiety, fear of failure, and frustration. Their actions are slow, cautious, and disorganized. They require cueing and feedback on each step of a task. Do not rush them. Provide them with time to think things through. All tasks need to be broken down into a simple step-by-step process. Furthermore, it is essential that each step be known and strictly followed by all caregivers. Give immediate feedback so clients know that they are on the right track. Simple gestures, such as a pat on the arm, are very effective for providing praise and feedback. Use a normal tone of voice and keep comments simple. Also, verify comprehension. Individuals may pretend to understand to avoid embarrassment (Martin, Holt, & Hicks, 1981).

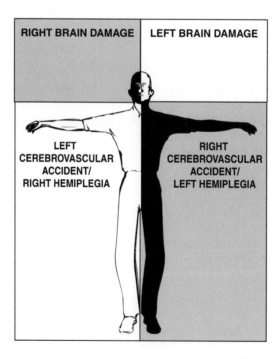

Fig 3. *CVA/Hemiplegia.*

Problems Frequently Associated with a Left Cerebrovascular Accident

Impaired Communication. Understanding and being understood is of primary importance in all human communication. When a stroke damages the left hemisphere of the brain, which is responsible for language and communication, the effect can be devastating to the client and family members. A stroke in the left brain produces several types of communication impairments. Some of the more common impairments are aphasia, expressive aphasia, receptive aphasia, global aphasia, dysarthria, and word apraxia.

APHASIA

Aphasia refers to either the total or partial inability to communicate and commonly occurs after damage to the dominant left cerebral hemisphere. There are two basic types of aphasia: sensory and motor. Deficits manifested include difficulty with speech, speech comprehension, verbal expression, gestures, reading, mathematics, and/or writing. Stroke survivors may suffer an impairment in one or more of these areas of communication. The inability to communicate can be both frightening and frustrating (Cochran, Flynn, Goetz, Potts-Nulty, Rece, & Sensenig, 1994).

Broca's Aphasia (Motor Aphasia/Expressive Aphasia)

Broca's area is located on the inferior frontal gyrus of the brain (see Figure 2). Damage to this area results in **Broca's aphasia,** i.e., expressive or motor speech aphasia. Clients struggle to speak. They know what they want to say but are unable to say it. The ability to understand language usually remains intact. The remaining speech may sound telegraphic. For example, the statement, "The flowers on the table are mine" comes out as "table . . . flowers . . . me." Mild Broca's aphasia is characterized by the loss of only one or two words. In the severe form of expressive aphasia, all words are lost. Nursing interventions for clients with expressive aphasia include establishing yes-no reliability, allowing time for clients to respond, and not speaking for clients (Bronstein, Popovich, & Stewart-Amidei, 1991; Cochran, Flynn, Goetz, Potts-Nulty, Rece, & Sensenig, 1994; Dittmar, 1989; Hickey, 1986).

Wernicke's Aphasia (Sensory/Receptive Aphasia)

Wernicke's area is located in the posterior temporal gyrus and angular gyrus in the dominant hemisphere of the brain. Damage to this area results in **Wernicke's aphasia,** i.e., difficulty interpreting sensory input. Clients can hear sounds and words but are unable to make sense of them. In other words, clients can hear what is said but cannot understand what is being said, much like a foreign language. In its mildest form, only one or two words sound garbled. In the most severe form, clients are unable to understand or interpret all words. The ability to read can also be affected. Clients with receptive aphasia may speak normally and articulate well, or one word may be used for many things. They do not listen to themselves; therefore, jargon or meaningless words are used. Nursing interventions for clients with receptive aphasia include listening carefully and trying to make sense out of what is being said, using demonstration, and gesturing (Bronstein, Popovich, & Stewart-Amidei, 1991; Dittmar, 1989; Hickey, 1986).

Global Aphasia

Global aphasia is a severe communication disorder. Clients with global aphasia experience difficulty with both speech and understanding and exhibit qualities of both expressive and receptive aphasia. They may be unable to make any sounds or use meaningless phrases, such as "I was a was a was" repetitively. Clients do not understand more than one or two words and are unable to put words together. These people have lost all communication skills and present a real challenge for the health care worker. Nursing interventions for clients with global aphasia include establishing yes-no reliability, allowing clients time to respond, using demonstration, and gesturing (Cochran, Flynn, Goetz, Potts-Nulty, Rece, & Sensenig, 1994).

Poststroke survivors may also exhibit speech that is fluent but incoherent. The words and phrases have no meaning. The clients do not realize that the words are meaningless to others. Some experience a loss of written language. They are unable to interpret words, letters, numbers, and even pictures. Some experience word apraxia; that is, they are unable to transform thoughts into meaningful language. Clients know what they want to say and the word to use; however, they are unable to make the muscles of the tongue, lips, and jaw move together to form the word (Bronstein, Popovich, & Stewart-Amidei, 1991; Hickey, 1986).

DYSARTHRIA

Dysarthria is a defect in articulation due to slow or weak muscle coordination. There are several different types of dyarthrias (flaccid, hypokinetic, hyperkinetic, spastic, ataxic, and mixed dysarthria). Clients with dysarthria have difficulty with co-ordination of or an alteration in the muscle tone of the speech musculature. Dysarthria can affect breathing, the voice, the tongue, the lips, the cheeks, the jaw, and the nose (Dittmar, 1989; Hoeman, 1995).

YES-NO RELIABILITY

Whenever working with clients who are experiencing impaired communication, it is important for nurses to determine **yes-no reliability**—i.e., whether the clients' "yes" and "no" responses are appropriate and reliable. This is accomplished by asking questions to which the answers are known: for example, "Is this your husband/wife?" or "Did you eat breakfast?" Allow clients time to respond. The response may be a verbal attempt or a gesture. It usually requires several questions over a week's time to establish yes/no reliability (Martin, Holt, & Hicks, 1981).

ASSESSMENTS FOR IMPAIRED COMMUNICATION

Nursing assessments for impaired communication include the following:

- Ability to name objects
- Fluency patterns
- Speech content
- Prosody of speech
- Grammar
- Ability to repeat words
- Comprehension/understanding
- Yes-no reliability
    Nods "yes" and "no" to same question
- Basic reading skills
    Ability to read single words
    Ability to read sentences
    Ability to read paragraphs
- Basic writing skills
    Ability to write on the right side of the page
    Ability to write own name
    Ability to write single words
    Ability to write sentences
    Ability to write paragraphs
- Ability to make mouth or facial movements on command
- Ability to imitate mouth or facial movements
- Use of nonsense words, jargon, or gibberish
- Stuttering or slurred speech

NURSING INTERVENTIONS FOR IMPAIRED COMMUNICATION

Nursing interventions for impaired communication include the following:

- Consult with a speech therapist or speech pathologist.
- Develop a trusting and therapeutic relationship.
- Face the client and make eye contact.
- Speak in a normal tone of voice—do not raise your voice.
- Allow the client time to respond.
- Acknowledge your lack of understanding.
- Acknowledge the client's frustration.
- Maintain dignity and treat the client at an appropriate developmental level.
- Praise all attempts at communication.
- Use gestures, such as pointing and nodding.

- Use communication aids, such as word boards.
- Speak in clear, short, simple sentences.
- Use common words.
- If the client is able to write or read, use these as alternate forms of communication.
- Point out progress.
- Minimize distractions.
- Explain all procedures.
- Teach the client and family about the communication disorder.
- Assess the client's ability to read, write, and understand English; and access educational level, attention span, and energy level.

Dysphagia

Impaired swallowing or difficulty swallowing (**dysphagia**) is common after a stroke and can lead to aspiration. The incidence of dysphagia following stroke ranges from 50 to 59 percent (Lorish, Sandin, Roth, & Noll, 1994; Lugger, 1994). Dysphagia means that clients have difficulty moving food from the lips to the stomach without getting it into the lungs. Dysphagia occurs because of dysfunction of the mouth, lips, tongue, palate, pharynx, larynx, or upper esophagus. It can occur in any or all stages of swallowing. This is due to muscle weakness, tightness, impaired sensation, or impaired co-ordination. Swallowing difficulties can be complicated by impulsivity and/or poor judgment. These clients are at high risk for aspiration, pneumonia, upper airway obstruction, dehydration, and malnutrition. One-third of dysphagic clients will aspirate, and 40 percent of these will do so silently (Lorish, Sandin, Roth, & Noll, 1994). It is important for the nurse to evaluate clients for potential eating and swallowing difficulties at the time of admission and before starting oral intake. If the nurse determines that a client has swallowing problems, an evaluation by the speech therapist should be ordered. Early assessment and treatment can prevent potential complications (Cole-Arvin, Notich, & Underhill, 1994; Gauwitz, 1995; Holas, DePippo, & Reding, 1994).

In most rehabilitation facilities, nurses monitor clients for swallowing difficulties during meals and with each medication administration. Clients should be assessed for signs of aspiration each time foods or liquids are given. The following is a partial list of potential signs of aspiration and dysphagia:

- Watering eyes
- Reddening face
- Change in respiratory rate
- Difficulty breathing or inability to breathe
- Changes in lung sounds
- Audible breathing
- Wheezing
- Facial grimacing

- Coughing or choking during feedings
- Gagging
- Attempting to clear throat
- Wet, gurgly voice
- Chest pain
- Facial weakness
- Pocketing of food under tongue
- Pocketing of food in cheek
- Excessive tongue movement
- Excessive secretions
- Drooling
- Decreased appetite
- Unexplained weight loss
- High or low back pain
- Inability to talk or talking in a whisper
- Client complains of fullness, tickling, or burning in throat
- Client reports that something is stuck in his or her throat
- Absent or decreased gag reflex

It is the role of the speech-language therapist to diagnose and treat swallowing disorders. A **videofluoroscopic modified barium swallowing examination** is the most accurate method of identifying the specific type and cause of swallowing disorder. A bedside examination including an oral motor assessment and observation of the client during oral intake may also be performed by the therapist. The speech therapist should develop an individualized swallowing program incorporating diet consistency and specific swallowing techniques to prevent aspiration by the client. The following are some general guidelines that nurses can follow until a more specific swallowing program has been developed by the therapist (De-Pippo, Holas, Reding, Mandel, & Lesser, 1994; DiLorio & Price, 1990):

- Check gag reflex.
- Check swallowing reflex.
- Have suction equipment available.
- Have client sit upright during feedings (90° hip angle).
- Progress from thick to thin liquids to client tolerance.
- Use thickening agents.
- Have client flex head slightly forward and tuck chin down.
- Instruct client to think "swallow."
- Place bolus of food on unaffected side of tongue.
- Have client hold breath to swallow.
- Gently stroke side of neck in downward motion.
- Turn head toward the affected side.
- Check for pocketing of food.
- Monitor for coughing or choking.
- Do not use straws

- Give medications in applesauce or puréed foods.
- Limit the size of food bolus.
- Monitor for dehydration.
- Monitor for weight loss.
- Encourage client participation in oral exercises.
- Allow extra time for meals.
- Limit distractions during meals.
- Place food in client's visual field.
- Place food within client's reach.
- Give foods and liquids slowly and in small amounts.
- Keep patient upright 30–45 minutes after meals.
- Use adaptive equipment as needed (special cup, high-rimmed plate, etc.).

In addition to the listed nursing interventions, management of the client with dysphagia frequently includes changes in dietary consistency. Use of dysphagia diet guidelines aids in facilitating swallowing and preventing aspiration. The following diets are commonly recommended by the speech therapist.

DYSPHAGIA DIETS

Texture I: Thick Liquids

- Blended or puréed foods run slowly off the spoon.
- Do not give thin or watery purée.
- No solids or lumps, therefore, no chewing is required.
- Puréed applesauce, cream of wheat, pudding, puréed meat, puréed vegetables.
- Thickened liquids—goal is consistency of honey.

Texture II: Soft Foods with Thick Liquids

- Gelatinous or sticky foods.
- Custards, puddings, yogurt, mashed potatoes, oatmeal.

Texture III: Semisolid with Thick Liquids and Carbonated Beverages

- Semisolid foods stimulate sensation in the mouth and facilitate swallowing.
- Soft fruit, pasta, pancakes, ground meats.

Texture IV: Solids with Thick Liquids

- Firm, chewy, and crispy foods.

Texture V: All Regular Foods

Foods to avoid include very dry, particulate foods, such as toast, crackers, popcorn, and rice, and sticky foods, such as peanut butter (Lugger, 1994; Meehan, 1992).

It is impossible to develop a single management plan for all dysphagic clients. Each client must be evaluated to determine needs. An individualized plan to prevent aspiration and facilitate safe swallowing must be developed and implemented by the interdisciplinary team. It is important for rehabilitation nurses to be aware of their role in treating clients with dysphagia and to understand all phases of the swallowing process. Early assessment is critical to the detection and treatment of dysphagia and the prevention of complications.

APRAXIA

Apraxia is the inability to perform a voluntary learned action on command. Individuals may be able to perform the action spontaneously but cannot do so on command. There are two basic types of apraxia: motor/movement apraxia and word apraxia. Motor apraxia includes dressing apraxia—inability to dress self; limb apraxia—inability to plan and perform movements with arms and legs; and oral apraxia—inability to plan and perform movements with the tongue, jaw, and lips. Word apraxia is the inability to plan and make sounds. Clients know what they want to say but are unable to say it. Apraxia can affect oral movements, speaking, and/or gesturing. Comprehension is intact. Apraxia is often associated with aphasia (Bronstein, Popovich, & Stewart-Amidei, 1991; Dittmar, 1989; Hickey, 1986).

Right CVA/Left Hemiplegia

Clients with damage to the right hemisphere of the brain have difficulty with spatial perceptual tasks, such as the ability to judge distance, size, or position; poor judgment; and impulsive behaviors. Each individual is different but the following characteristics are often observed in individuals with left hemiplegia:

- Paralysis or weakness on the left side of the body
- Shortened attention span
- Loss of the left visual field
- Tendency to eat food only from the right side of the plate or tray
- Poor motor planning
- Poor problem-solving skills
- Poor judgment
- Impulsive behavior and rapid movement
- Inability to cross the midline toward the affected side
- Tendency to overestimate their own abilities
- Lack of awareness of personal limitations
- Difficulty interpreting visual clues
- Impaired ability to retain information
- Tendency to get lost if left alone
- Incessant talking
- Inability to follow more than one instruction at a time
- Altered sensation on the left side
- Difficulty with eye-hand coordination

- Left-sided neglect
- Inappropriate laughing or crying

Clients with a right cerebrovascular accident have a tendency to plunge ahead, totally self-confident and oblivious to safety issues. In general, they are impulsive, unaware of their limitations, inattentive, and exhibit rambling speech. They need constant reminders to slow down and to perform one step at a time. Caregivers should provide immediate feedback in a positive manner regarding inappropriate behaviors, giving only single commands or instructions. Slow down clients if they act too quickly. Use nonverbal cues, such as placing a hand on their arm to stop impulsive behaviors or to silence rambling speech (Martin, Holt, & Hicks, 1981; NSA, 1992a).

Cognition   Cognitive disorders are common after stroke. Cognitive deficits are associated with longer lengths of stay and poorer functional outcomes. Moderate to severe higher level cognitive deficits interfere with clients' abilities to learn new skills during the rehabilitation process. Cognitive deficits are often overlooked or underestimated during routine neurological examinations. It is recommended that simple and well-validated tools be used to assess cognitive functioning in the poststroke client. Frequently used assessment tools include the Barthel Index, the Mini-Mental Status Examination, and the Neurobehavioral Cognition Status Examination (AHCPR, 1996).

Memory deficits affect up to 95 percent of all stroke survivors. Recognition of memory deficits can be complicated by aphasia (Lorish, Sandin, Roth, & Noll, 1994). Some of the more frequently encountered cognitive deficits and their nursing interventions include the following (Hanak, 1992; Hickey, 1986):

1. Memory loss: inability to remember the caregiver's name, day of the week, or the next step in a transfer process
    a. Supply memory aids, such as flash cards or notebooks.
    b. Provide structure, consistency, and repetition.
    c. Emphasize familiar skills.
    d. Pair old information with new information.
2. Shortened attention span
    a. Avoid overstimulation.
    b. Provide short, simple, concrete instructions.
    c. Keep interactions brief.
3. Easily distracted
    a. Simplify environment and minimize distractions.
4. Poor judgment
    a. Teach concept of brain damage and its effects.
    b. Encourage participation in support groups.
    c. Identify problems and work through possible solutions.
    d. Protect from injury.

5. Inability to transfer learning from one situation to another
    a. Provide repetition.
6. Inability to calculate, reason, or abstract
    a. Use multiple teaching modalities.
    b. Teach in a situational environment.
    c. Start with simple tasks and build to more complex ones.

Affective Disorders

Emotional lability, the inability to control one's emotions due to brain damage, and depression are common after an acute stroke. Emotional lability is characterized by inappropriate, uncontrollable bouts of laughing or crying. The bouts occur suddenly, are not related to a particular activity, and resolve suddenly. Most episodes can be easily interrupted by diverting the client's attention.

Depression in the stroke client is due either to brain damage from the stroke or to the client's reaction to the losses associated with the stroke. Signs of depression include lack of interest, decreased energy, decreased appetite, sleep disturbances, agitation, and a feeling of worthlessness. Depression affects the client's participation in rehabilitation and the long-term outcomes of the rehabilitation process. Treatment of depression depends on the cause. Treatment modalities include the use of antidepressant drugs, psychotherapy, and family support (AHCPR, 1996).

Other affective changes experienced by the stroke survivor include loss of self-control and social inhibitions; decreased tolerance of stress; and fear, hostility, frustration, anger, confusion, despair, withdrawal, and isolation (Hickey, 1986).

Visual Deficits

Depending on the location of the brain lesion, strokes can cause a variety of visual deficits, such as double vision, decreased acuity, and hemianopia. **Hemianopia** refers to defective vision or the total loss of one-half of the visual field in each eye. It may be unilateral or bilateral. The most common visual deficit is homonymous hemianopia (see Figure 4). **Homonymous hemianopia** is the loss of vision in the temporal field of one eye and the nasal field of the other eye. The client cannot see out of one-half of each eye. The person sees only one-half of an image or one-half of the environment. It usually occurs on the same side of the body as the paralysis and is caused by damage to the optic tract posterior to the optic chiasm (Dudas, 1986). For example, a client with a right cerebrovascular accident would experience left homonymous hemianopia. The client is often unaware of the visual deficit and ignores what cannot be seen. This places the client at high risk for injury. The problem is of greater significance when it is associated with neglect of the affected side.

Unilateral neglect occurs in strokes affecting the nondominant hemisphere (usually the right hemisphere). Clients with unilateral neglect lack awareness of a specific body part or the affected half of the body. They ignore sensory input from the left half of the environment. Items in the left visual field are ignored,

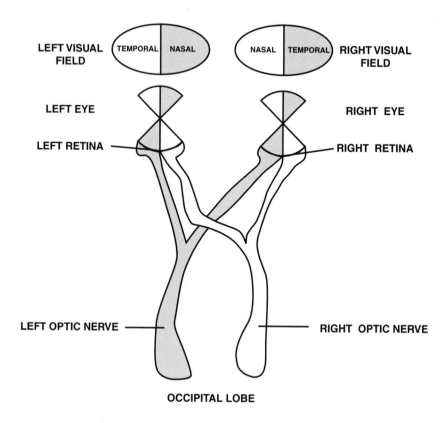

LEFT VISUAL FIELD TEMPORAL NASAL   NASAL TEMPORAL **RIGHT VISUAL FIELD**

LEFT EYE   **RIGHT EYE**

LEFT RETINA   **RIGHT RETINA**

LEFT OPTIC NERVE   **RIGHT OPTIC NERVE**

OCCIPITAL LOBE

Fig 4. *Homonymous hemianopsia.*

such as food. **Anosognosia** occurs when the client denies the affected side of the body and/or refuses to acknowledge that it is paralyzed. The client does not attend to the affected half of the body and may attribute ownership to someone else. These individuals are at high risk for injury. Nursing interventions include teaching the client to scan the environment continuously for potential hazards; and reintegrating the affected side into the body image by teaching the client to look at, touch, and use the affected limb.

Mobility   Immobility is a common problem during the poststroke period. However, the large majority of stroke survivors are able to walk independently 1 year after a stroke. Weakness and paralysis are the most common motor deficits. The client may also experience inco-ordination, clumsiness, involuntary movements, and abnormal postures. Motor deficits influence independent functioning, performance of activities of daily living, physical activity, and endurance. Mobility is a primary focus of rehabilitation nurses and includes assessing and managing abnormal tone and facilitating normal posture, alignment, balance, and movement (AHCPR, 1996; Galarneau, 1993). Clients should be mobilized as soon after admission as possible. Early mobilization helps prevent complications associated with stroke and immobility, such as deep vein thrombosis, contractures, and pneumonia.

Bed mobility refers to the client's ability to move around in bed. It includes rolling and turning from side to side. The client should be positioned on both the affected and the unaffected side. Correct bed positioning and range of motion are important in the prevention of contractures on the affected side. Bed positioning includes placing the client in the supine, side-lying, and prone positions. This minimizes flexion of the hip and knee joints and decreases the risk of developing contractures. It is important to maintain normal anatomic body alignment and support the affected extremities on pillows. Range of motion of the affected extremities should be done one to three times daily. The client should be taught to perform range-of-motion exercises. The exercises can be incorporated into activities of daily living, such as bathing and hygiene. While in bed, the client must be turned every 2 hours. Pressure release techniques are used while the client is in a wheelchair. An order should be obtained for antiembolic stockings and/or a sequential compression device to prevent deep vein thrombosis (Cochran, Flynn, Goetz, Potts-Nulty, Rece, & Sensenig, 1994; Galarneau, 1993).

Clients must be safely transferred from one surface to another, such as when moving from a wheelchair to the bed. Transfer techniques vary according to client ability and the size and expertise of the caregiver. Good body mechanics are essential to avoid back strain and injury. Transfers can be done either standing or sitting. Movement is easier from a higher level to a lower level. Assessment before attempting transfers should include clients' physical abilities, abilities to cooperate, perceptual and sensory deficits, trunk control, height and weight, and equipment needs (Galarneau, 1993; NSA, 1992b). Many devices exist to facilitate safe transfers and include transfer belts, transfer disks, transfer boards, and mechanical slings and chairs.

Many types of adaptive equipment and orthotics are available to assist the client in regaining functional independence, such as by compensating for lack of muscle tone or increased muscle tone. These devices should be used only after a thorough evaluation by the rehabilitation team (NSA, 1992a). Hemislings are used early in the rehabilitation process to protect the flaccid arm. It holds the arm, including the forearm and hand, close to the body to protect it from injury. Shoulder girdle slings hold the shoulder joint in a normal position to prevent subluxation and pain. A resting hand splint is used to place the affected hand into a functional position. It also decreases spasticity and prevents contractures (NSA, 1992a).

Lapboards lie across both arms of the wheelchair. They provide support and proper positioning for the affected arm. They place the affected arm into the client's visual field and help prevent injury. An arm trough attaches to one arm of the wheelchair. It provides support and proper positioning of the affected arm. It is less restrictive than a lapboard (NSA, 1992a).

Orthotics are externally fitted devices that provide support for a specific activity, such as walking. During stroke recovery, the muscles in the lower extremity are usually the last to regain movement and control. An ankle-foot orthosis (AFO) is designed to control the foot and ankle for early ambulation and gait training (AHCPR, 1996; NSA, 1992a). Other adaptive devices to facilitate ambulation include a variety of canes and walkers. A walking aid should allow the client to stand upright with a 15° bend in the elbow (NSA, 1992a).

Wheelchair selection is based on body size, comfort, special needs, and maneuverability. A wheelchair designed for a poststroke client should have a lower base of support and a lowered seat to allow the client to use the unaffected foot to propel the chair (AHCPR, 1996).

Alteration in Urinary Elimination

The AHCPR (1996) defines urinary incontinence as "the involuntary loss of urine sufficient to be a problem, characterized by an inability to restrain or control urinary voiding" (p. 91). The incidence of poststroke urinary incontinence ranges from 38 to 60 percent (Gelber, Good, Laven, & Verhulst, 1993). A poststroke survivor may experience urinary retention, urinary incontinence, or urinary frequency. The three major causes of urinary incontinence in poststroke clients are bladder hyperreflexia with urge incontinence, bladder hyporeflexia with overflow incontinence, or communication and cognitive deficits with normal bladder function (AHCPR, 1996). Clients with impaired communication and cognition frequently are incontinent due to their inability either to recognize the need to void or to communicate that need to caregivers. Impaired cognition has a direct effect on achieving poststroke continence (Owen, Getz, & Bulla, 1995). Clients with poor orientation to time, short-term memory loss, and poor problem-solving skills are less likely to achieve urinary continence by discharge. In many stroke survivors, problems with bladder control and urinary incontinence resolve spontaneously (Brocklehurst, Andrews, Richards, & Laycock, 1985). Approximately 56 to 71 percent of poststroke survivors achieve continence within 3 to 6 months following a completed stroke (Barer, 1989; Borrie, Campbell, Caradoc-Davies, & Spears, 1986).

A poststroke client with normal urinary tract function may also experience functional incontinence. Functional incontinence has a variety of causes. It occurs if the client is unable to get to the toilet independently and in a timely manner, is unable to manage toileting hygiene independently, and is unable to manage lower body clothing independently (Bronstein, Popovich, & Stewart-Amidei,

1991). It is important for nurses to assess both the type and the cause of urinary incontinence before implementing individualized nursing interventions.

During the acute stage and in the acute care setting, urinary problems are frequently managed by insertion of an indwelling Foley catheter. It is recommended that catheters be removed as soon as possible to reduce the incidence of urinary tract infections. Long-term use of indwelling catheters should be limited to clients who do not respond to other treatment modalities. Further, persistent incontinence must be evaluated to determine etiology and appropriate treatment methodology.

Urinary incontinence and frequency are more common than urinary retention in the stroke survivor. Incontinence ranges from occasional to continuous. Frequently, the cause of the incontinence is simply the client's inability to hold the urine long enough to make it to the toilet. The majority of stroke survivors respond to simple nursing interventions to reestablish continence.

In the rehabilitation setting, treatment for poststroke urinary incontinence includes behavioral strategies, such as time voiding, habit training, prompted voiding, and bladder retraining. Before implementing behavioral strategies, the specific technique and its effect should be discussed with the client and the family caregiver.

Nursing interventions for urinary incontinence include the following:

- Provide a means for signaling the need for assistance.
- Establish a timed voiding schedule.
- Note time and volume of each void.
- Monitor fluid intake and patterns of intake.
- Monitor response to specific fluids, such as caffeine.
- Restrict fluid intake after evening meal.
- Maintain adequate hydration.
- Toilet prior to going to bed.
- Assess for effectiveness of bladder stimulation techniques.
- Assess for presence of urological problems, such as urinary tract infection and outlet obstruction.
- Monitor for urinary tract infections.
- Monitor for incontinent episodes and associated activity.
- Assess for impaired mobility and ease of toilet transfer.
- Provide privacy.
- Assess for fecal impaction.
- Monitor skin integrity.

If the stroke damage is extensive or cognition is severely impaired, the client may not respond to bladder retraining programs. Current options available for persistent urinary incontinence include indwelling Foley catheter, external condom catheters, waterproof underpants, pant-liners, and disposable adult diapers.

Client and caregiver education relating to bladder function and management must be included in the discharge planning process.

Alteration in Bowel Elimination

Changes in bowel elimination after stroke are common. Approximately 31 percent of all stroke clients experience alterations in bowel elimination. For the majority, bowel problems resolve spontaneously within 2 weeks (Lorish, Sandin, Roth, & Noll, 1994). Problems most frequently encountered are constipation, fecal impaction, and bowel incontinence. Changes in bowel function may be related to brain damage resulting in loss of cortical inhibition. Clients with an uninhibited bowel experience involuntary stools and are unaware of the need to defecate. Constipation is more common than incontinency (Venn, Taft, Carpentier, & Applebaugh, 1992). If diarrhea occurs, the client should be assessed for fecal impaction.

Before initiating a bowel program, the client's premorbid and current bowel habits should be assessed. A complete physical assessment is conducted to determine the presence of neurological deficits that could contribute to changes in bowel elimination, such as cognitive deficits, memory deficits, decreased attention span, decreased sensation, altered proprioception, and transfer ability. There are several important factors to consider when setting up a bowel care program. Timing is crucial to the success of any bowel program. Establish a regular toileting schedule. If possible, the time should coincide with premorbid habits. Use the gastrocolic reflex by placing the client on the toilet after each meal. Evaluate and maintain adequate hydration. A fluid intake of 2000 to 3000 milliliters per day maintains a soft stool. Encourage good eating habits. Fiber and bulk aid in preventing constipation and hard stools. Exercise promotes a good bowel response. Encourage the client to perform activities of daily living as much as possible. Bowel programs must be individualized and cause-specific. Stool softeners and laxatives may be helpful.

Sexuality

Sexual activity fulfills Maslow's upper level needs of love and belonging. Sexuality can be expressed emotionally and/or physically. Unless the stroke is severe, the client retains the ability to function sexually. However, the vast majority of stroke survivors experience some disruption in their sexual activities. The problems may be directly related to the effects of the stroke or may be side effects of medications used to treat problems associated with the stroke, such as hypertension and spasticity. Both the client and partner need instructions on adapting sexual activity to the stroke survivor's ability (Fraley, 1992; Martin, Holt, & Hicks, 1981; Needham, 1993; Phipps, 1991).

Stroke-related factors affecting sexual performance include the following:

- Inappropriate sexual behaviors or overtures
- Partner "turned off" by client's physical appearance

- Inability to engage in previously meaningful sexual activity
- Fear that sexual activity will cause another stroke
- Decreased ability to sustain an erection
- Decreased or increased libido
- Difficulty with positioning owing to paralysis or spasticity
- Impaired communication due to dysphasia
- Depression
- Loss of self-esteem
- Fatigue and decreased physical endurance
- Immobility and sensory deficits
- Perceptual and visual deficits
- Cognitive and behavioral deficits
- Personality changes
- Emotional lability
- Erection and ejaculation dysfunction
- Decreased vaginal lubrication (Fraley, 1992; Hanak, 1992; Martin, Holt, & Hicks, 1981; Needham, 1993; Phipps, 1991; Rehabilitation Nursing Foundation, 1993).

The AHCPR (1996) recommends that sexual issues be discussed during the rehabilitation process and again after the client has transitioned into the community. It is important for nurses to be comfortable with approaching the issue and granting the client and partner permission to discuss their concerns. Nursing interventions should stress the importance of open communication between partners, instructions for alternate positioning techniques, methods for managing erectile dysfunction, and other adaptive strategies. For more specific nursing interventions, see Chapter 28.

Client and Family Teaching/Learning Needs

Client and family teaching before discharge should focus on those issues most relevant to community reintegration. Teaching must be individualized to the client and family situation. A comprehensive teaching plan may include the following:

- Anatomy and physiology of the brain
- Stroke prevention
- Stroke risk factors
- Signs and symptoms of potential complications
- Medication regimen
- Skin care
- Seizure precautions
- Altered sexual functioning
- Nutrition and hydration
- Bowel and bladder care
- Potential for injury
- Potential for social isolation
- Specific interventions for self-care deficits
- Swallowing techniques for dysphagia

- Gastrostomy feeding tube care
- Home exercises
- Recreational activities
- Vocational activities
- Driving a car
- Safety awareness

Common Nursing Problems include the following:

- Activity intolerance
- Sensory/perceptual alterations
- Altered communication
- Impaired swallowing
- Impaired mobility
- Altered thought processes
- Altered bowel function
- Altered bladder function
- Self-care deficit
- Altered sexual functioning
- Altered self-image
- Altered nutritional status
- Unilateral neglect
- High risk for injury
- High risk for aspiration
- Altered self-concept
- Altered role performance
- Knowledge deficit
- Powerlessness
- Social isolation
- Depression
- Grieving
- Ineffective individual/family coping
- Spiritual distress
- Discharge planning

Pouse and Keenan (1981) define discharge planning as a series of planned events that occur to prepare the client for the orderly transition from one setting to another. The major goal of the discharge planning process is to transition the client back into the community prepared to deal with his or her own health care needs. Discharge planning begins at the time of admission to the rehabilitation facility and continues until the client is discharged. It should be a systematic, co-ordinated, interdisciplinary team process that includes the client and family members as active participants.

A key interdisciplinary team member is responsible for co-ordinating the discharge planning process. In many institutions, nursing is responsible for the discharge planning process. The nurse provides inpatient care and educates the client and the family regarding all aspects of that care. There are many things to consider in the discharge planning process. Some critical factors to consider include the client's functional status, the proposed living arrangements, the need for equipment and supplies, the availability of family support, the availability of financial resources, the need for referral to social and community support systems, the need for homemaking assistance, the need for nursing assistance, the need for vocational rehabilitation, the need for driver's training, and verification of teaching and comprehension of teaching (AHCPR, 1996; Bronstein, Popovich, & Stewart-Amidei, 1991).

There are many benefits achieved through proper discharge planning. Good discharge planning ensures continuity of care, minimizes duplication of services, ensures that client needs are met, and ensures that cost-effective care is provided.

Conclusion

Caring for the stroke survivor is a major challenge for nurses at all levels and in a variety of settings. Each individual has sustained a unique injury with unique neurological deficits. Nursing care must be individualized to meet the special needs of each person. To ensure that the best possible care is provided, nurses must keep abreast with changes in technology and treatment modalities.

References

Agency for Health Care Policy and Research (AHCPR), Public Health Service, U.S. Department of Health and Human Services. (1996). *Clinical practice guideline: Post-stroke rehabilitation.* Gaithersburg, MD: Aspen.

Agency for Health Care Policy and Research (AHCPR), Public Health Service, U.S. Department of Health and Human Services. (1996). *Clinical practice guideline: Urinary incontinence in adults* (on-line). Available http://text.nlm.nih.gov.

American Health Care Consultants. (1996). Angioplasty and stents could revolutionize cerebrovascular therapy (on-line). Available http://www.ticllc.net/~ahcpub/029606.html.

Barer, D. H. (1989). Continence after stroke: Useful predictor or goal of therapy? *Age and Aging, 18*(3), 183–191.

Bellavance, A. (1993). Efficacy of ticlopidine and aspirin for prevention of reversible cerebrovascular ischemic events: The ticlopidine aspirin stroke study. *Stroke, 24*(10), 1452–1457.

Biller, J., & Love, B. B. (1991). Diabetes and stroke. *Clinical Diabetes, 9*(5), 66–79.

Borgman, M. F., & Passarella, P. M. (1991). Nursing care of the stroke patient using Bobath principles. *Nursing Clinics of North America, 26*(4) 1019–1034.

Borrie, M. J., Campbell, A. J., Caradoc-Davies, T. H., & Spears, G. F. S. (1986). Urinary incontinence after stroke: A prospective study. *Age and Aging, 15*(3), 177–181.

Brocklehurst, J. C., Andrews, K., Richards, B., & Laycock, P. J. (1985). The incidence and correlates of incontinence in stroke patients. *Journal of the American Geriatric Society, 33*(8), 540–542.

Bronner, L. L., Kanter, D. S., & Manson, J. E. (1996). Primary prevention of stroke. *The Johns Hopkins White Papers.* Baltimore, MD: The Johns Hopkins Medical Institution.

Bronstein, K. S., & Chadwick, L. R. (1994). Ticlopidine hydrochloride: Its current use in cerebrovascular disease. *Rehabilitation Nursing, 19*(1), 12–24.

Bronstein, K. S., Popovich, J. M., & Stewart-Amidei, C. (1991). *Promoting stroke recovery.* St. Louis: Mosby–Year Book.

Cifu, D. X., & Lorish, T. R. (1994). Stroke rehabilitation 5. Stroke outcome. *Archives of Physical Medicine and Rehabilitation, 75,* S56–S60.

Chimowitz, M. I. (1995a). Atherosclerotic intracranial occlusive disease: Diagnosis, prognosis and treatment: Part I. *Stroke: Clinical Updates, VI*(3), 9–12.

Chimowitz, M. I. (1995b). Atherosclerotic intracranial occlusive disease: Diagnosis, prognosis and treatment: Part II. *Stroke: Clinical Updates, VI*(4), 13–16.

Clark, W. M., & Barnwell, S. T. (1995). Interventional neurovascular therapy in cerebrovascular disease. *Stroke: Clinical Updates, VI*(2), 5–8.

Cochran, I., Flynn, C. A., Goetz, G., Potts-Nulty, S. E., Rece, J., & Sensenig, H. (1994). Stroke care: Piecing together the long-term picture. *Nursing94, 24*(4), 34–41.

Cole-Arvin, C., Notich, L., & Underhill, A. (1994). Identifying & managing dysphagia. *Nursing94,* January, 48–49.

DePippo, K. L., Holas, M. A., & Reding, M. J. (1994). The Burke Dysphagia Screening Test: Validation of its use in patients with stroke. *Archives of Physical Medicine and Rehabilitation, 75,* 1284–1286.

DePippo, K. L., Holas, M. A., Reding, M. J., Mandel, F. S., & Lesser, M. L. (1994). Dysphagia therapy following stroke: A controlled trial. *Neurology, 44,* 1655–1659.

DiLorio, C., & Price, M. E. (1990). Swallowing: An assessment guide. *American Journal of Nursing,* July, 38–41.

Dittmar, S. S. (1989). *Rehabilitative nursing: Process and application.* St. Louis: Mosby.

Dudas, S. (1986). Nursing diagnosis and interventions for the rehabilitation of the stroke patient. *Nursing Clinics of North America, 21*(2), 345–357.

Ferrucci, L., Bandinelli, S., Guralnik, J. M., Lamponi, M., Bertini, C., Falchini, M., & Baroni, A. (1993). Recovery of functional status after stroke. A postrehabilitation follow-up study. *Stroke, 24*(2), 200–205.

Fraley, A. M. (1992). *Nursing and the disabled across the life span.* Boston: Jones & Bartlett.

Galarneau, L. (1993). An interdisciplinary approach to mobility and safety education for caregivers and stroke patients. *Rehabilitation Nursing, 18*(6), 393–398.

Gauwitz, D. F., (1995). How to protect the dysphagic stroke patient. *American Journal of Nursing* (on-line). Available http://www.ajn.org/ajn/5.8/a508034e.1t.

Gelber, D. A., Good, D. C., Laven, L. J., & Verhulst, S. J. (1993). Causes of urinary incontinence after acute hemispheric stroke. *Stroke, 24*(3), 378–382.

Granger, C. V., Hamilton, B. B., & Fiedler, R. C. (1992). Discharge outcome after stroke rehabilitation. *Stroke, 23*(7), 978–982.

Hanak, M. (1992). *Rehabilitation nursing for the neurological patient.* New York: Springer.

Harvard Medical School (1996). Nurses' Health Study Newsletter. Vol. 3, June 1996.

Hickey, J. V. (1986). *The clinical practice of neurological and neurosurgical nursing* (2nd ed.). Philadelphia, PA: J. B. Lippincott.

Hoeman, S. P. (1996). *Rehabilitation nursing: Process and application.* St. Louis: Mosby.

Holas, M. A., DePippo, K. L., & Reding, M. J. (1994). Aspiration and relative risk of medical complications following stroke. *Archives of Neurology, 51,* 1051–1053.

Kelly, M. (1995). Transient ischemic attack: How to identify this precursor to stroke before permanent brain damage occurs. *American Journal of Nursing* (on-line). Available http://ww.ajn.org/ajn/5.9/a509042e.1t.

Lorish, T. R., Sandin, K. J., Roth, E. J., & Noll, S. F. (1994). Stroke rehabilitation. 3. Rehabilitation evaluation and management. *Archives of Physical Medicine and Rehabilitation, 75,* S47–S51.

Lugger, K. E. (1994). Dysphagia in the elderly stroke patient. *Journal of Neuroscience Nursing, 26*(2), 78–84.

Margolis, S., & Preziosi, T. J. (1996). *Stroke: The Johns Hopkins White Papers.* Baltimore, MD: The Johns Hopkins Medical Institution.

Matchar, D. B., & Duncan, P. W. (1995). Cost of stroke. *Stroke: Clinical Updates, V*(3), 9–12.

Matchar, D. B., McCrory, D. C., Barnett, H. J., & Feussner, J. R. (1994). Medical treatment for stroke prevention. *Annals of Internal Medicine, 121*(1), 41–53.

Meehan, M. (1992). Nursing Dx: Potential for aspiration. *RN,* January, 30–34.

Moore, K., & Trifiletti, E. (1994). Stroke: The first critical days. *RN, 57*(2), 22–27.

National Institute of Neurological Disorders and Stroke (NINDS). (1995). NIH announces emergency treatment for stroke. National Institutes of Health (on-line). Available http://www.nih.gov/ninds/whatsnew/presswhn/1995/ntpapr.html.

National Institute of Neurological Disorders and Stroke (NINDS). (1995). *Stroke research highlights 1994.* National Institutes of Health (on-line). Available http://www.nih.gov/ninds/healinfo/disorders/stroke/strokerh.htm#BasicResearch.

National Stroke Association (NSA). (1996). FDA approves first-ever acute stroke treatment. *Be Stroke Smart, 13*(7), 1.

National Stroke Association (NSA). (1992a). *The road ahead: Promoting stroke recovery.* Englewood, CO: Author.

National Stroke Association (NSA). (1992b). *The road ahead: A stroke recovery guide* (2nd ed.). Englewood, CO: Author.

Needham, J. F. (1993). *Gerontological nursing: A restorative approach.* Albany, NY: Delmar.

Phipps, M. A. (1991). Assessment of neurologic deficits in stroke: Acute-care and rehabilitation implications. *Nursing Clinics of North America, 26*(4), 957–969.

Pouse & Keenan. *In* Martin, N., Holt, N., & Hicks, D. (eds.) (1981). *Comprehensive rehabilitation nursing.* New York: McGraw-Hill.

Rehabilitation Nursing Foundation (1993). *The specialty practice of rehabilitation nursing* (3rd ed.). Skokie, IL: The Rehabilitation Nursing Foundation of the Association of Rehabilitation Nurses.

Toole, J. F., Baker, W. H., Castaldo, J. E., Chambless, L. E., Moore, W. S., Robertson, J. T., Young, B., & Howard, V. J. (1995). Endarterectomy for asymptomatic carotid artery stenosis. *JAMA, 273*(16).

Venn, M., Taft, L., Carpentier, B., & Applebaugh, G. (1992). The influence of timing and suppository use on efficiency and effectiveness of bowel training after stroke. *Rehabilitation Nursing, 17*(3), 116–120.

Suggested Readings

Abel, P. M. (1995). Prevention is by far the best treatment of strokes. Cardiovascular Institute of the South (on-line). Available http://www.cardio.com/articles/stroke.html.

American Association of Neurological Surgeons and the Congress of Neurological Surgeons, Joint Section on Cerebrovascular Surgery. (1995). *Carotid endarterectomy update* (on-line). Available http://neurosurgery.mgh.harvard.edu/cea.htm#ACS.

American Heart Association (AHA). (1995). Atherosclerosis. (on-line). Available http://www.amhrt.org/heart/aa24.html.

Axelsson, K., & Asplund, K. (1989). Eating problems and nutritional status during hospital stay of patients with severe stroke. *Research, 89*(8), 1092–1096.

Brandstater, M. E., Roth, E. J., & Siebens, H. C. (1992). Venous thromboembolism in stroke: Literature review and implications for clinical practice. *Archives of Physical Medicine and Rehabilitation, 73,* S379–S389.

Brody, S. J., & Ruff, G. E. (1986). *Aging and rehabilitation: Advances in the state of the art.* New York: Springer.

Carpenito, L. J. (1995). *Nursing diagnosis: Application to clinical practice* (6th ed.). Philadelphia, PA: J. B. Lippincott.

Clagett, C. P., Anderson, F. A., Levine, M. N., Salzman, E. W., & Wheeler, H. B. (1992). Prevention of venous thromboembolism. *Chest, 102*(4), 391S–407S.

DiLima, S. N. (1995). *Stroke rehabilitation: Patient education manual.* Gaithersburg, MD: Aspen.

Dromerick, A., & Reding, M. (1994). Medical and neurological complications during inpatient stroke rehabilitation. *Stroke, 25*(2), 358–361.

Easton, K. L., Zemen, D. M., & Kwiatowski, S. (1994). Developing and implementing a stroke education series for patients and families. *Rehabilitation Nursing, 19*(6), 348–351.

Egelko, S., Simon, D., Riley, E., Gordon, W., Ruckdeschel-Hibbard, & Diller, L. (1989). First year after stroke: Tracking cognitive and affective deficits. *Archives of Physical Medicine and Rehabilitation, 70,* 297–302.

Evans, R. L., Bishop, D. S., & Haselkorn, J. K. (1991). Factors predicting satisfactory home care after stroke. *Archives of Physical Medicine and Rehabilitation, 72,* 144–147.

Evans, R. L., Hendricks, R. D., Haselkorn, J. K., Bishop, D. S., & Baldwin, D. (1992). The family's role in stroke rehabilitation. *American Journal of Physical Medicine and Rehabilitation, 71*(3), 133–139.

Fudge, T. L. (1995). Blocked neck arteries are the major cause of strokes. Cardiovascular Institute of the South (on-line). Available http://www.cardio.com/articles/neck-art.html.

Gent, M., Easton, J. D., Hachinski, V. C., Panak, E., Sicurella, J., Blakely, J. A., Ellis, J. D., Harbison, J. W., Roberts, R. S., Turpie, A. G. G., & the CATS Group. (1989). The Canadian American Ticlopidine Study (CATS) in thromboembolic stroke. *Lancet, 1,* 1215–1220.

Hahn, K. (1987). Left versus right: What a difference the side makes in stroke. *Nursing87, 17*(9), 44–47.

Hajek, V. E., Rutman, D. L., & Scher, H. (1989). Brief assessment of cognitive impairment in patients with stroke. *Archives of Physical Medicine and Rehabilitation, 70,* 114–117.

Hass, W. K., Easton, J. D., Adams, H. P., Pryse-Phillips, W., Molomy, B. A., Anderson, S., & Kamm, B, (1989). A randomized trial comparing ticlopidine hydrochloride with aspirin for the prevention of stroke in high risk patients. *New England Journal of Medicine, 321,* 501–507.

Jorgensen, M. S., Nakayama, H., Raaschou, H. O., Vive-Larsen, J., Stoier, M., & Olsen, T. S. (1995). Outcome and time course of recovery in stroke. Part I. Outcome. The Copenhagen Stroke Study. *Archives of Physical Medicine and Rehabilitation, 76,* 399–405.

Kalra, L. (1994). The influence of stroke unit rehabilitation on functional recovery from stroke. *Stroke, 25*(4), 821–825.

Kalra, L., Yu, G., Wilson, K., & Roots, P. (1995). Medical complications during stroke rehabilitation. *Stroke, 26*(6), 990–994.

Kelly-Hayes, M., & Paige, C. (1995). Assessment and psychologic factors in stroke rehabilitation. *Neurology, 45*(Suppl. 1), S29–S32.

Le, N., Venti, C. R., & Levin, E. R. (1994). Initial assessment of patient cognition in a rehabilitation hospital. *Rehabilitation Nursing, 19*(5), 293–297.

Liebman, M. (1991). *Neuroanatomy made easy and understandable* (4th ed.). Gaithersburg, MD: Aspen.

Lueckenotte, A. G. (1996). *Gerontologic nursing.* St. Louis: Mosby.

Marshall, R. S., & Mohr, J. P. (1993). Current management of ischaemic stroke. *Journal of Neurology and Neurosurgical Psychiatry, 56,* 6–16.

Mitchell, P. H., Hodges, L. C., Muwaswes, M., & Walleck, C. A. (1988). *AANN's neuroscience nursing: Phenomena and practice. Human response to neurological health problems.* Norwalk, CT: Appleton & Lange.

Monga, T. N., Lawson, J. S., & Inglis, J. (1986). Sexual dysfunction in stroke patients. *Archives of Physical Medicine and Rehabilitation, 67,* 19–22.

Morris, P. L. P., Robinson, R. G., Andrezejewski, P., Samuels, J., & Price, T. R. (1993). Association of depression with 10-year poststroke mortality. *American Journal of Psychiatry, 150*(1), 124–129.

Mysiw, W. J., Beegan, J. G., & Gatens, P. F. (1989). Prospective cognitive assessment of stroke patients before inpatient rehabilitation: The relationship of the neurobehavioral cognitive status examination to functional improvement. *American Journal of Physical Medicine and Rehabilitation,* *68*(4), 168–171.

Noll, S. F., & Roth, E. J. (1994). Stroke rehabilitation. 1. Epidemiologic aspects and acute management. *Archives of Physical Medicine and Rehabilitation, 75,* S38–S41.

Oczkowski, W. J., Ginsberg, J. S., Shin, A., & Panju, A. (1992). Venous thromboembolism in patients undergoing rehabilitation for stroke. *Archives of Physical Medicine and Rehabilitation, 73,* 712–716.

Ott, D. J., & Pikna, L. A. (1993). Clinical and videofluoroscopic evaluation of swallowing disorders. *AJR, 161,* 507–513.

Owen, D., Getz, P., & Bulla, S. (1995). A comparison of characteristics of patients with completed strokes: Those who achieve continence and those who do not. *Rehabilitation Nursing, 20*(4), 197–203.

Parikh, R. M., Robinson, R. G., Lipsey, J. R., Starkstein, S. E., Federoff, J. P., & Price, T. R. (1990). The impact of poststroke depression on recovery in activities of daily living over a 2-year follow-up. *Archives of Neurology, 47,* 785–789.

Passarella, P., & Gee, Z. (1987). Starting right after stroke. *American Journal of Nursing,* June, 802–807.

Pierce, L., Rodrigues-Fisher, L., Buettner, M., Bulcroft, J., Camp, Y. G., & Bourguignon, C. (1995). Frequently selected nursing diagnoses for the rehabilitation client with stroke. *Rehabilitation Nursing, 20*(3), 138–143.

Price, M. E., & DiLorio, C. (1990). Swallowing: A practice guide. *American Journal of Nursing,* July 1991, 42–46.

Roth, E. J. (1994). Heart disease in patients with stroke. Part II: Impact and implications for rehabilitation. *Archives of Physical Medicine and Rehabilitation, 75,* 94–101.

Roth, E. J., & Noll, S. F. (1994). Stroke rehabilitation. 2. Comorbidities and complications. *Archives of Physical Medicine and Rehabilitation, 75,* S42–S46.

Salter, J., Camp, Y., Pierce, L. L., & Mion, L. (1991). Rehabilitation nursing approaches to cerebrovascular accident: A comparison of two approaches. *Rehabilitation Nursing, 16*(2), 62.

Sandin, K. J., Cifu, D. X., & Noll, S. F. (1994). Stroke rehabilitation: 4. Psychologic and social implications. *Archives of Physical Medicine and Rehabilitation, 75,* S-52–S-55.

Shah, S., Vanclay, F., & Cooper, B. (1990). Efficiency, effectiveness, and duration of stroke rehabilitation. *Stroke, 21*(2), 241–246.

Solomon, D. H., & Hart, R. G. (1993). Advances in stroke management. *Emergency Medicine,* February 28, 25–37.

Teraoka, J., & Burgard, R. (1992). Family support and stroke rehabilitation. *The Western Journal of Medicine, 157*(6), 665–666.

Vanetzian, E., & Corrigan, B. A. (1995). A comparison of the educational wants of family caregivers of patients with stroke. *Rehabilitation Nursing, 20*(3), 149–154.

Walker, C. M. (1995). The two types of stroke and how they differ. Cardiovascular Institute of the South (on-line). Available http://www.cardio.com/articles/strk-typ.html.

Welte, P. O. (1993). Indices of verbal learning and memory deficits after right hemisphere stroke. *Archives of Physical Medicine and Rehabilitation, 74,* 631–636.

White, M. J., & Holloway, M. (1990). Patient concerns after discharge from rehabilitation. *Rehabilitation Nursing, 15*(6), 318–319.

Whitney, F. (1994). Drug therapy for acute stroke. *Journal of Neuroscience Nursing, 26*(2), 111–117.

Wityk, R. J., Pessin, M. S., Kaplan, R. F., & Caplan, L. R. (1994). Serial assessment of acute stroke using the NIH Stroke Scale. *Stroke, 25*(2), 362–365.

CHAPTER 17

Neurological Deficits Associated with Spinal Cord Injury

Darlene Finocchiaro and *Shari Herzfeld*

Key Terms

Anterior Cord Syndrome
Autonomic Dysreflexia
Brown–Séquard Syndrome
Central Cord Syndrome
Complete Injury
Conus/Cauda Equina Syndrome
Fusion
Heterotopic Ossification (HO)
Incomplete Injury
Laminectomy

Manual Cough
Orthostatic Hypotension (Postural Hypotension)
Paraplegia
Positioning
Posterior Cord Syndrome
Pressure Ulcer
Pulmonary Embolism
Quadriplegia
Spinal Shock

Objectives

1. Describe the physical, social, and economic costs of spinal cord injury.

2. Identify the etiologies and risk factors for spinal cord injury.

3. Describe the pathophysiology of spinal cord injury.

4. Identify the functional abilities at each level of injury.

5. Discuss the effects of spinal cord injury on respiratory function.

6. Discuss the effects of spinal cord injury on skin integrity.

7. Describe autonomic dysreflexia, the causes and necessary intervention.

8. Identify three nursing implications for the SCI client with the unstable spine.

9. Discuss the conservative and nonconservative measures used for the SCI client with an unstable spine.

10. Discuss the etiology, signs and symptoms, and common treatment for the SCI client who suffers from a deep vein thrombosis.

11. Identify at least three methods the nurse can perform in the prevention of a deep vein thrombosis to the SCI client.

12. Discuss the medication management for the client with heterotopic ossification.

13. Discuss the dietary, medication and exercise programs for the SCI client with osteoporosis.

14. Describe correct positioning techniques necessary to prevent contractures.

15. Describe nonsurgical and surgical methods for the control of spasticity.

16. Discuss some of the psychological manifestations experienced by the SCI client.

17. Identify appropriate nursing interventions for the SCI client experiencing denial, anger, depression, hope for a cure, and adaptation to disability.

History

About 5000 years ago, an Egyptian physician said this about a person paralyzed by a spinal cord injury:

> Thou should'st say concerning him. One having a dislocation in the vertebra of his neck while he is unconscious of his 2 legs, and his 2 arms, and he dribbles. An ailment not to be treated. (Gordon & Stevens, 1981)

The situation did not change much until the early 1940s. Before World War II, the life expectancy of a person with a spinal cord injury was less than 2 years. Overwhelming infection or renal failure was generally the cause of early mortality. Medical and surgical advances, most notably the advent of effective antibiotics coupled with the experience gained in caring for a massive number of spinal-injured servicemen, led to advances that today offer the survivor a near normal life expectancy. Progress in specialized, multidisciplinary rehabilitation followed, offering the person with a spinal cord injury the opportunity to resume a meaningful and productive life.

Effects and Etiology of Spinal Cord Injury

Spinal cord injury is one of the most devastating injuries a person can sustain. It affects all aspects of the physical, emotional, and social being. Traumatic spinal cord injuries (SCIs) affect some 177,000 Americans, with approximately 80 percent of these individuals being male and 20 percent being female (Harvey, Rothschild, Asmann, & Stripling, 1990; Stover & Fine, 1987). A traumatic SCI strikes 7000–10,000 people in the United States yearly, with the majority of the victims being 15- to 25-year-old males (Laskowski-Jones, 1993). The most common cause of spinal cord injury is motor vehicle accidents, followed by penetrating wounds (gunshot and stab), falls, and sports accidents.

The aftereffects of a spinal injury include life-long disability, chronic care requirements, and significant loss of earning power. The cost of initial hospitalization, for the average client, is in excess of $50,000.00, and total lifetime cost, including medical care, social services, and lost income, is estimated at $1.5 million (Miller, 1995).

To understand the nature of the injury, it is useful to know how the injury occurred. Regardless of the mechanism of injury, all injuries to the spine should be considered unstable until proven otherwise (Laskowski-Jones, 1993).

The vertebral column is composed of a series of 33 bony rings, the *vertebrae,* which surround the spinal cord. This bony structure provides protection to the spinal cord from direct low-velocity trauma while allowing flexibility. The drawback of this design is the relative weakness of the articulations between the vertebrae, especially when confronted with the types of stress it can be subjected to in vehicles, by high-velocity projectiles, or in sports. If the vertebral column is subjected to severe flexion, extension, or rotation, this can cause contusion, traction, or crushing of the underlying tissue, including the spinal cord and its vascular supply.

Pathophysiology of Spinal Cord Injury

The majority of damage to the spinal cord occurs at the time of injury. The injury can be increased by careless handling of an unstable spine. Thus, any client who sustains any injury to the head, neck, or back should be handled as if the spine were unstable until proven otherwise.

The injury to the spinal cord generally results from disruption of its blood supply. Actual severing of the spinal cord is relatively rare. Loss of blood supply to the spinal cord results in hypoxia and necrosis. Once damaged, the cord is functionally severed. Any healing results in formation of scar tissue, which is nonfunctional neurologically.

Injury to the spinal cord results in loss of all voluntary motor function and sensation below the level of injury, owing to the inability of *afferent* (sensory) and *efferent* (motor) messages to cross the damaged nerve tracts.

Spinal Shock

Immediately after any spinal cord injury, a period of reflex inhibition, or **spinal shock,** occurs. Spinal shock results in areflexia from decreased excitability of neurons below the level of injury. Spinal shock is manifested by loss of bowel and bladder tone, and loss of peripheral vascular tone. Physical findings during spinal shock include bladder distension, paralytic ileus, flaccid paralysis, and hypotension. The return of reflex activity below the level of injury heralds recovery from spinal shock. Flaccid paralysis is replaced by spastic paralysis. It is important not to confuse return of reflexes with voluntary motion.

Complete versus Incomplete Injury

Once spinal shock resolves, an assessment can be made regarding the completeness of the injury. In a **complete injury,** no motor or sensory function is present below the level of injury. Reflexes can occur distal to the injury, as the reflex arc is still intact in the distal stump of the spinal cord.

An **incomplete injury** occurs when some spinal tracts are intact across the injured segment of the spinal cord. Areas innervated by the sacral segments are the most likely to be spared in an incomplete injury; thus, findings of any sensation of voluntary motor function in the perineum are consistent with an incomplete injury. A spinal cord injury is classified as "incomplete" only if one or more of the following three conditions exist:

- Sacral sparing (cervical), in which voluntary contraction of the anal sphincter occurs
- Voluntary toe flexion (motor function is present)
- Intact genital or perianal sensation (sensory)

Although an incomplete injury carries a better prognosis for neurologic recovery, return of function is highly variable. With an incomplete injury, return of function may continue for up to 18 months postinjury. Rapid early neurologic recovery, however, correlates with a greater eventual return of function.

Types of incomplete injury include anterior cord syndrome, central cord syndrome, Brown–Séquard syndrome, posterior cord syndrome (see Figures 1–4) and conus/cauda equina (Figure 5).

With the diagnosis of an **anterior cord syndrome,** the anterior artery is infarcted, stopping blood supply to the anterior two-thirds of the spinal column. Symptoms include loss of voluntary and reflex motor activity and loss of pain and temperature sensations. The ability to sense position, vibration, and light pressure is unimpaired (Laskowski-Jones, 1993) (Figure 1).

The **central cord syndrome** presents damage of the innermost central fibers of the cord, whereas the outermost lateral fibers remain intact. With this syndrome, the upper extremities are affected whereas the lower extremities usually are not (Laskowski-Jones, 1993) (Figure 2).

The client who suffers from **Brown–Séquard syndrome** appears as a stroke client with a hemisection of the cord; one side of the cord is damaged whereas the opposite side of the cord is not (Laskowski-Jones, 1993) (Figure 3).

A **posterior cord syndrome** is rarely seen. This occurs from a severe flexion of the neck. In this situation, the ability to sense position, vibration, and light pressure is affected (Figure 4).

A client with **conus/cauda equina syndrome** has peripheral nerve damage instead of cord damage. There is "root escape" (Figure 5). Symptoms include a loss of motor function in a variety of patterns with asymmetrical involvement. Sensory function is unimpaired. The positive outlook with this diagnosis is that there is root recovery potential, leading to return of function.

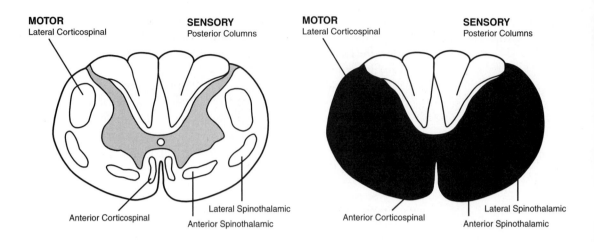

Fig 1. *Anterior cord syndrome (incomplete injury).*

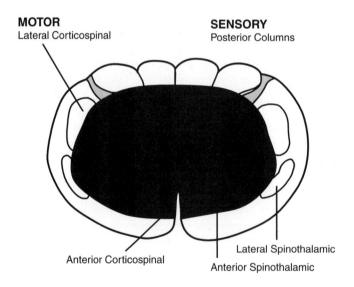

CENTRAL CORD SYNDROME

Fig 2. *Central cord syndrome (incomplete injury).*

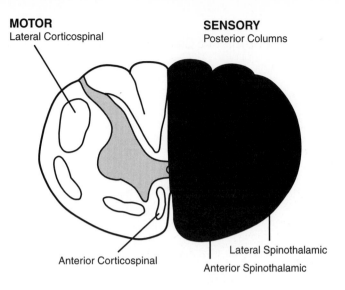

BROWN-SEQUARD SYNDROME (HEMISECTION)

Fig 3. *Brown–Séquard syndrome (incomplete injury).*

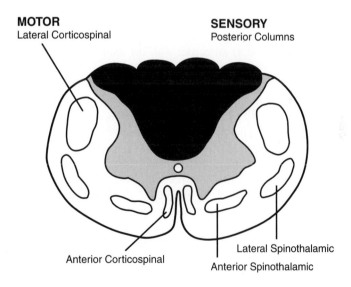

POSTERIOR CORD SYNDROME

Fig 4. *Posterior cord syndrome (incomplete injury).*

Cauda equina injuries:
Peripheral nerve - not cord injuries.
Anatomy of cauda equina area.

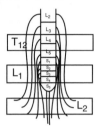

"Root escape"

Fig 5. *Conus/cauda equina (incomplete injury).*

Spinal Anatomy

To understand the effects of a spinal injury, it is necessary to understand the anatomical relationship between the spinal cord and its protective bony support.

The vertebral column consists of 33 bony rings: 7 cervical, 12 thoracic, 5 lumbar, 5 fused as the sacrum, and 4 coccygeal. Each vertebra is named for the spinal region and numbered cephalad to caudal. Superiorly, the first cervical vertebra (C1) articulates with the skull and distally, the sacrum forms the posterior wall of the pelvis. Cartilaginous disks between the vertebral bodies provide cushioning. Ligaments along the length of the vertebral column provide structural support. Foramina, or openings between each bony segment, allow the nerve roots to exit the spinal canal to the periphery (see Figure 6).

The spinal cord extends from the base of the brain, through the spinal canal, the lengthwise "tube" created when the rings of the vertebrae are stacked. Nerves exit between each pair of vertebrae, carrying messages to and from all parts of the body. Early in intrauterine growth, the spinal cord fills the entire length of the spinal canal. By adulthood, the spinal cord ends at the second lumbar vertebra. However, the nerves that exit the spinal cord continue through the spinal canal forming the cauda equina.

The segments of the spinal cord are numbered for the level at which the nerve root exits the bony vertebral column, which is not necessarily the level of that cord segment (see Figure 6). The more caudal, the more significant the discrepancy between the bony and neurological levels. Thus, it becomes critical in describing injuries to the spine to distinguish bony versus neurological levels of injury.

Level of Function

The spine and spinal cord can be injured anywhere along its length, although the areas of intersection between a relatively mobile and relatively rigid section are

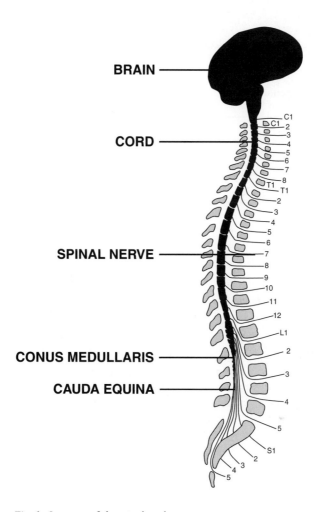

Fig 6. *Segments of the spinal cord.*

most vulnerable. With injury to the spinal cord, functions distal to the area inner-vated by that segment of the spinal cord are affected. When the injury affects the cervical spinal cord, the resulting disability is referred to as **quadriplegia,** in that all four extremities are affected. With injury to the thoracic, lumbar, or sacral spine, the disability is referred to as **paraplegia.** Within these broad categories, there is significant variability in the disability depending on exactly where the le-sion is located. Tables 1 and 2 detail the muscle groups and functional abilities associated with a complete injury at each neurologic level of injury.

Table 1
Spinal Cord Injury Levels of Function: Cervical

Level of Function	Muscle/Action	Functional Goal	Rehabilitation Plan
C1–3	Sternocleidomastoid, upper trapezius/neck stability	Respirator dependent; tongue control electric wheelchair with head support	Positioning, pulmonary toilet, speech therapy, phrenic nerve stimulation. Home adaptations and 24-hour attendant
C4	Trapezius/neck extension Diaphragm/breathing	Chin or tongue control electric wheelchair, direct dependent self-care, desk skills with set-up and assistive devices	Mouthstick for writing, drawing, turning pages, keyboarding, etc.; spasticity management; home adaptations
C5	Deltoid/shoulder flexion, extension, abduction Biceps/elbow flexion Supinators/turn hand palm up	Limited self-care, home skills with set-up and assistive devices; electric wheelchair with hand controls; dependent transfers	Hand control electric wheelchair, limited manual wheelchair mobility with pegs; ratchet or fixed hand splint, adaptive feeding/grooming devices; home adaptations
C6	Extensor carpi radialis/wrist extension, tenodesis	Highest level of injury with potential for functional independence; manual wheelchair; tenodesis (passive) finger pinch; independent sliding board transfer; drive with hand controls	Wrist-driven wrist hand orthosis (WDWHO); tendon transfer surgery to enhance hand function; sliding board transfer; adaptive devices for dressing, light housekeeping, elimination; home adaptations
C7	Triceps/elbow extension Flexor carpi radialis/wrist flexion Finger extensors/finger extension Latissimus dorsi/shoulder internal rotation Pectoralis major/shoulder adduction	Independent bathing, grooming, dressing, elimination program; independent in desk skills, light cooking, shopping, laundry; drive with hand controls and put manual wheelchair into car	Manual wheelchair; WDWHO or built-up handles; adaptive devices for dressing, housekeeping; hand control 2-door car; home adaptations
C8	Flexor digitorum/finger flexion Abductor and adductor pollicis longus/finger abduction and adduction	Independent in self-care, desk skills, home skills, driving	Manual wheelchair, hand control 2-door car; home adaptations

Source: Lewis, Collier, and Heitkemper (1996).

Table 2
Spinal Cord Injury Levels of Function: Thoracic, Lumbar, and Sacral

Level of Function	Muscle/Action	Functional Goal	Rehabilitation Plan
T1–7	Intercostals/chest expansion	Breathe with chest; independent in self-care, desk skills, home skills, driving; wheelchair mobility	Self manual cough; self ROM; manual wheelchair; level transfers; tub/shower seat; hand control 2-door car
T8–12	Abdominals/forceful expiration, trunk control	Functional cough; strenuous wheelchair sports; physiologic walk	Transfer to surfaces of different heights; ambulation trial; "wheelies" to wheel over curbs
L1–2	Siliosoas, sartorius/hip flexion	Functional walk (household); wheelchair community	Long leg braces and crutches; come to stand, swing through gait, fall
L3–4	Quadriceps/extend knee Adductors/adduct thigh	Functional walk (community); hip stability	Short leg braces and crutches
L5–S1	Soleus, gastrocnemius/ankle dorsiflexion Gluteus/hip extension	Ambulate	Push-off gait
S2–4	Bladder detrusor/voiding Anal sphincter/defecation	Bowel, bladder, and sexual function present, but may not be completely normal	Bowel and bladder retraining, sexual counseling

Source: Lewis, Collier, and Heitkemper (1996).

A successful rehabilitation program involves the co-ordinated expertise of the members of a multidisciplinary team, each bringing their respective skills to meet the needs of the spinal cord-injured individual. Making the client and his or her family or significant other a part of goal setting and plan of care is the most important element to a successful rehabilitation process.

Medical Problems/ Complications

Clients with spinal cord injury have the potential for several medical problems. The following problems are discussed, emphasizing the relationship to spinal cord injury, the nursing diagnosis or diagnoses, client goal(s), and appropriate nursing interventions. Medical problems include decreased respiratory function, autonomic dysreflexia, impaired skin integrity, lack of stability, orthostatic hypotension (postural hypotension), deep vein thrombosis, heterotopic ossification, osteoporosis, contractures, spasticity, and psychological manifestations.

Other problems such as bladder, bowel, and sexual dysfunction; self-care deficits; and impaired physical mobility are addressed in other chapters in this book (see Chapter 19 for bladder and bowel functioning; Chapter 28 for sexual functioning; Chapter 25 for self-care deficits; and Chapter 26 for impaired physical mobility).

Respiratory Effects of Spinal Cord Injury

The major innervation for the diaphragm is the phrenic nerve, which originates at C3–C5. Clients with injuries below C5, in which the phrenic nerve is spared, have normal tidal volume (although no intercostal or abdominal muscle innervation) and thus no ability to deep breathe or cough. Injuries involving C5 and above generally require ventilatory support initially, until the diaphragm develops enough strength to maintain oxygenation. Those sustaining injuries to C3 and above may require permanent artificial ventilation (Miller, 1995).

Injuries to the cervical, thoracic, and even lumbar spine cause some degree of accessory muscle paralysis. This interferes with expiratory function, particularly the ability to cough. This can have serious consequences, including the inability to clear the airway of secretions. Also lost is the ability to deep breathe, reducing the individual's reserve capacity.

Nursing Diagnosis
- Ineffective airway clearance related to accessory muscle paralysis

Goals/Outcomes
- The client will maintain clear upper airway breath sounds.

Nursing Interventions
- Assess breath sounds every shift.
- Teach the client and caretaker the **manual cough** technique: Have the client inhale as deeply as possible. Place the flat side of the assistant's closed fist between the client's xiphoid process and umbilicus. Just as the client begins to exhale, the assistant presses sharply inward and upward. Repeat until the airway is clear of all secretions.
- Teach the client to direct another person in this technique.
- Teach the client to self manually cough, using their own hands if possible, or by leaning over the back of a chair.

Paradoxical respirations occur in the client with paralysis of the intercostal muscles. Using only the diaphragm for respirations causes the chest wall to contract with each breath and the abdomen to rise. In the supine position, the weight of the abdominal viscera helps the diaphragm reassume its dome-shaped position on exhalation. When the individual assumes an upright position, the viscera pull down on the diaphragm, thus interfering with passive exhalation.

Nursing Diagnosis
- Ineffective breathing pattern related to dependence on the diaphragm only

Goals/Outcomes

- Client will maintain adequate oxygenation in an upright position as manifested by absence of signs and symptoms of hypoxia (i.e., syncope, cyanosis, lightheadedness).

Nursing Interventions

- Before the client rises, place a corset or scultetus binder around the abdomen, below the rib cage.
- Perform diaphragm-strengthening exercises in collaboration with physical therapy (i.e., place small weights over the abdomen in a supine position for 15 minutes, twice daily; gradually increase the weight to client tolerance). Stay with the client to monitor for signs of respiratory distress.

Autonomic Dysreflexia

Autonomic dysreflexia is a complication unique to spinal cord injuries involving C8 or above. It is also known as *hyperreflexia* (Finocchiaro & Herzfeld, 1990). It results from the loss of communication between the sympathetic and parasympathetic branches of the autonomic nervous system across the damaged section of the spinal cord. Any noxious stimuli below the injury can trigger an episode of autonomic dysreflexia (Finocchiaro & Herzfeld, 1990) (see Figure 7).

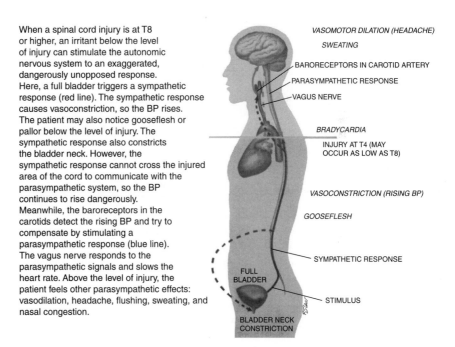

When a spinal cord injury is at T8 or higher, an irritant below the level of injury can stimulate the autonomic nervous system to an exaggerated, dangerously unopposed response. Here, a full bladder triggers a sympathetic response (red line). The sympathetic response causes vasoconstriction, so the BP rises. The patient may also notice gooseflesh or pallor below the level of injury. The sympathetic response also constricts the bladder neck. However, the sympathetic response cannot cross the injured area of the cord to communicate with the parasympathetic system, so the BP continues to rise dangerously. Meanwhile, the baroreceptors in the carotids detect the rising BP and try to compensate by stimulating a parasympathetic response (blue line). The vagus nerve responds to the parasympathetic signals and slows the heart rate. Above the level of injury, the patient feels other parasympathetic effects: vasodilation, headache, flushing, sweating, and nasal congestion.

VASOMOTOR DILATION (HEADACHE)
SWEATING
BARORECEPTORS IN CAROTID ARTERY
PARASYMPATHETIC RESPONSE
VAGUS NERVE
BRADYCARDIA
INJURY AT T4 (MAY OCCUR AS LOW AS T8)
VASOCONSTRICTION (RISING BP)
GOOSEFLESH
SYMPATHETIC RESPONSE
FULL BLADDER
STIMULUS
BLADDER NECK CONSTRICTION

Fig 7. *Autonomic dysreflexia. (Permission granted by AJN.)*

In a neurologically intact individual, the branches of the autonomic nervous system act in a co-ordinated manner to maintain equilibrium. When the feedback between the two branches is absent, sympathetic stimulation below the level of injury leads to an unopposed sympathetic response below the injury. The blood pressure rises, and the urinary sphincter constricts. Above the injury, the baroreceptors in the carotid artery detect the elevated blood pressure and stimulate the parasympathetic response of vasodilation, a message that is received above the level of injury only. This accounts for the typical findings of dysreflexia: pounding headache, profuse sweating and flushing above the level of injury, and nasal congestion. Meanwhile, the parasympathetic system stimulation results in bradycardia. As long as the noxious stimulus that triggered the episode is still present, the blood pressure continues to rise. Removal of the noxious stimulus will result in prompt reversal of the symptoms, with return of the blood pressure to baseline (Finocchiaro & Herzfeld, 1990).

Any person with a spinal cord injury at T8 or above must be taught about the risk of dysreflexia, how to prevent it by avoiding noxious stimuli, and how to respond to an episode. Dysreflexia-prone individuals are encouraged to wear a medical identification bracelet and carry printed material describing dysreflexia and how to manage it.

Nursing Diagnosis

- Autonomic dysreflexia related to a full bladder, full bowel, urinary tract infection, tight clothing, pressure sore

Goals/Outcomes

- The client will be able to describe prevention and management of episodes of dysreflexia.

Nursing Interventions

- Identify clients susceptible to dysreflexia: spinal cord injury at C8 or above.
- Assess for headache, generally described as "pounding."
- Assess for blood pressure elevated 20 mm Hg or more above baseline.
- Assess for the presence of skin flushing or blotching, diaphoresis, bradycardia, goose bumps, nasal congestion, and/or chills without fever.
- Get assistance, as this is a medical emergency and the client should not be left unattended.
- Measure the blood pressure every 2 minutes to monitor the client's response to treatment.
- Elevate the head to lower blood pressure by orthostatic (postural) hypotension.
- Identify noxious stimuli, beginning at the bladder, the most common factor triggering an episode of dysreflexia.

- Verify the free flow of urine:

    Check the drainage system for kinks, an overfilled collection bag, clamps.

    Gently irrigate an indwelling catheter, if present, with no more than 30 cm^3 of normal saline.

    Catheterize the client if not voiding.

- Check for bowel distention if symptoms persist (this is usually the cause, if not the bladder):

    Instill 1 ounce of anesthetic ointment (i.e., dibucaine [Nupercainal]) into the rectum to prevent additional irritation.

    Gently remove, manually, any stool from the rectum.

- Seek any other possible source of irritation that may precipitate dysreflexia (e.g., urinary tract infection, pressure ulcer, instrumentation, sunburn, tight clothing, childbirth labor, any source of pain below the level of injury).
- Call a physician, as antihypertensive medication may be necessary to relieve the episode of dysreflexia when conservative interventions have failed to bring the blood pressure to normal level.
- Have intravenous (IV) insertion equipment and antihypertensive drugs available.
- Once the episode has been resolved, reinforce teaching regarding dysreflexia and the cause of it with the client and caregiver.

Maintaining Skin Integrity

The person with a spinal cord injury is at high risk for impaired skin integrity, particularly **pressure ulcers.** The loss of sensation, immobility, and incontinence that accompany spinal cord injury are the primary factors that increase the risk for developing pressure ulcers (Crenshaw & Vistnes, 1989). Following spinal cord injury, interventions to prevent the development of pressure ulcers should be instituted immediately, and continued throughout the life span of the individual. Only with constant vigilance and attention to prevention can the spinal cord-injured individual maintain the integrity of the skin.

All too frequently, the spinal cord-injured individual develops a pressure ulcer. This is the result of impaired or absent motor and/or sensory ability. In this situation, all preventive interventions must be performed as well as interventions directed at arresting the skin breakdown that has occurred while providing an environment to allow the ulceration to heal. In the case of full-thickness skin loss, healing by primary intention may provide a scar of insufficient strength to provide reliable weight bearing. In this situation, surgical reconstruction is indicated (Pownell, 1995).

Nursing Diagnosis

- High risk for impaired skin integrity (or high risk for skin breakdown) related to sensorimotor deficits secondary to SCI

Goals/Outcomes

- The client will maintain intact skin integrity.

Nursing Interventions

- Inspect the client's skin regularly; inspect all skin surfaces at least once daily. Inspect the skin surface most recently exposed to pressure after each position change, after sitting, and on removal of clothing, shoes, orthoses, or other garments.
- Change the client's position when sitting or lying for any length of time. When lying, turn at least every 2 hours. When sitting, make minor shifts in position every 15 minutes. Clients need to be taught to reposition themselves to alleviate ischial skin embarrassment (RAISE), so as to provide pressure relief. For the client who has strong arm muscles and can perform a depression RAISE from a wheelchair, this should be done frequently, every 15 minutes for 15 seconds. The type of repositioning done (such as a forward RAISE, or side-to-side RAISE) and how frequently it is performed determines the appropriate time to complete. For example, a client who performs a forward RAISE once an hour should stay in this forward position, with assistance from a nurse or other caregiver if necessary, for 60 seconds; if done every 30 minutes, then the RAISE would be done for 30 seconds.
- Use devices to reduce pressure to the skin, such as wheelchair seat cushions, and a pressure-reducing mattress. Be aware of the effectiveness of selected devices as well as possible disadvantages and cost barriers.
- Collaborate with a physical therapist in assuring that a wheelchair is fitted to the spinal cord-injured individual, with attention to weight distribution and pressure relief.
- Use turning, positioning, and transferring techniques and assistive devices that minimize friction and shearing.
- Cleanse the client's skin whenever soiled and at routine intervals, using methods individualized to the needs of the client. Avoid hot water, excess friction, and products that irritate or dry the skin. Avoid "hot tubs" and close contact with fireplaces or hot objects.
- Teach the client to be cautious with pet birds and other animals so as to avoid injury to anesthetic areas of the body.
- Avoid massage over bony prominences.
- Minimize skin exposure to moisture due to incontinence, perspiration, or wound drainage.
- Maintain adequate nutrition. Teach the client to eat a healthy diet with high protein and to drink approximately 2000 cm^3 of fluid daily if the bladder program allows it.
- Teach the client and caregivers about the risk of pressure ulceration, preventive interventions, assessment of skin changes indicative of early breakdown, and how to respond to these skin changes.
- Teach the client how to use, daily, two mirrors in checking skin for irritation or breakdown.

Nursing Diagnosis

- Impaired skin integrity related to sensorimotor deficits, infrequent repositioning, incontinence

Goals/Outcomes

- The client will demonstrate progressive healing of pressure ulcer.

Nursing Interventions

In addition to implementing and/or continuing all interventions listed under high risk for impaired skin integrity,

- Identify the factor causing development of the pressure ulcer and eliminate it.
- Perform an initial assessment of the pressure ulcer, including location, size, stage, necrotic tissue, undermining, drainage, odor, and condition of surrounding skin (Bergstrom, Bennett, Carlson, et al., 1994). Be aware that initial assessment of staging may not be accurate, as necrotic tissue may mask the true depth of the ulceration, dark skin pigmentation makes assessment of color changes difficult, and a red area or small opening may be the superficial manifestation of a large, deep ulceration. Only with complete debridement to healthy tissue can the extent of the ulceration be accurately assessed.
- If the wound contains necrotic tissue, debride to a clean base of granulation tissue. Methods include mechanical, chemical, autolysis, and surgical techniques.
- Once the ulcer has a base of granulation tissue, wound care should be directed at supporting the body's efforts to heal. Use a moist dressing technique.
- For deep full-thickness wounds, surgical repair, including the use of flaps for reconstruction, may be the only way to allow weight bearing over the ulcer site.
- Provide nutritional supplementation to meet the body's baseline needs as well as additional nutritional demands for healing an open wound.
- Reassess the ulcer at least weekly, noting progress, reduction of necrotic tissue, and presence of granulation.

Lack of Stability (Neck or Spine)

Before an SCI client can be moved safely, the status of the spine must be determined. This is generally done by x-ray (Matthews & Carlson, 1987). The stability of the spine must never be assumed. Be sure of the client's condition before raising the head of the bed or turning the client. Usually, the physician will write an order, "Spine is stable," or "Needs cervical collar," or some type of orthosis if the head is to be raised. Check the physician's orders. When in doubt, always log roll, maintaining straight alignment of the spine. If using an orthosis, the nurse must know how to apply it to the client correctly so as to prevent skin breakdown or further instability of the spine.

Regardless of the level of injury, closed or external alignment is generally attempted for cervical injuries. Usually some type of skull tongs and traction is used to align the vertebral column and relieve pressure on neural tissue, such as a halo vest/traction or Gardner–Well cervical tongs (Gordon & Stevens, 1981).

The client with a thoracic injury is placed on bed rest; immobilization with a fiberglass or plastic body cast may be done. For lumbar and sacral injuries, immobilization of the spine is usually accomplished with a brace or corset worn when the client is out of bed (Ignatavicius, Workman, & Mishler, 1995).

If conservative measures are unsuccessful, surgery must be considered, especially if spinal cord compression has occurred. A decompressive **laminectomy** (removal of one or more laminae) allows for cord expansion from edema if other measures such as the use of corticosteroids fail to prevent neurologic deterioration (Ignatavicius, Workman, & Mishler, 1995). An anterior or posterior cervical **fusion** may be done to immobilize the neck if there is hypermobility of the vertebrae that will result in further damage to the spinal column. Additional surgeries to consider include a spinal fusion and the insertion of metal or steel rods, such as Harrington rods, to stabilize thoracic spinal injuries.

Nursing Diagnosis

- Altered (spinal cord) tissue perfusion related to compression, contusion, and/or edema of the spine

Goals/Outcomes

- Client will exhibit no further deterioration in neurologic status (Ignatavicius, Workman, & Mishler, 1995).

Nursing Interventions

- Log roll the client from side to side with the assistance of two or three individuals, as necessary to maintain straight alignment.
- Apply traction or immobilization devices, checking for any skin breakdown.
- Provide postoperative care for clients having surgery:
  Assist client with application of brace, corset, or thoracolumbosacral orthosis (TLSO)
  Assess neurological condition and vital signs every 4 hours
  Monitor for complications such as a hematoma, edema (neurological changes), and cardiovascular instability due to loss of sympathetic innervation.
- Administer corticosteroids for their anti-inflammatory and edema-reducing effects as ordered.

Orthostatic Hypotension

Orthostatic hypotension (postural hypotension) tends to occur with SCI clients with lesions above T6, as a result of interruption of splanchnic control (Matthews & Carlson, 1987). As the client moves from a flat position to a sitting position, the client feels very lightheaded and might pass out. This change of movement is followed by rapid, uninhibited accumulation of blood in the viscera and lower extremities because of disruption in control of splanchnic nerve roots. There is a decrease in blood supply to central veins, decreased return of venous blood, and decreased cardiac output. The blood pressure drops severely and the pulse rises (Guttman, 1976).

Nursing Diagnosis

- Autonomic response: Potential/actual postural hypotension (Matthews & Carlson, 1987)

Goals/Outcomes

- Client will establish and maintain a stable blood pressure after an upright position is assumed.

Nursing Interventions

- Identify clients who are at risk for postural hypotension.
- Apply an abdominal binder and antiembolism stockings. The abdominal binder should extend from the gluteal fold to the waist.
- Assist the client to gradual position level changes, raising the head slowly at intervals, assessing the client's tolerance.
- Monitor for any signs and symptoms of weakness, dizziness, pale color, and blurred vision leading to blackouts or fainting. Also assess for excessive sweating above the level of injury and tachycardia.
- If signs and symptoms of postural hypotension are not present after raising the head of the bed from 30 to 45 degrees to eventually 90 degrees, consider transferring the client to a wheelchair.
- Obtain a recliner wheelchair with elevating foot pedals and have the client begin sitting at an angle that does not cause symptoms of hypotension. Upgrade the wheelchair by 10 degrees as tolerated until 90 degrees is achieved (Matthews & Carlson, 1987).
- Monitor blood pressure before and after transfers. If persistent postural hypotension occurs, the use of ephedrine or sodium chloride might be necessary.

If hypotension occurs (Matthews & Carlson, 1987),

- Take blood pressure and if less than 70/50 or if the client becomes unconscious, stay with the client until the symptoms resolve.
- Safely tip back the wheelchair—if the symptoms do not resolve, place the client in a supine position and notify a physician.
- Continue to monitor vital signs, level of consciousness, and subjective complaints.

Deep Vein Thrombosis

Thrombus (a fibrin network made up of platelets, red blood cells, and granular leukocytes forming in an artery or a vein) formation in a deep vein, with or without inflammation of the vein wall, is known as a *deep vein thrombosis* (DVT) (Fahey, 1989). Most venous thrombi form in the legs, usually in the calves. More than 15 percent of the thrombi that form in the deep veins of the calves migrate upward, above the popliteal vein, increasing the risk of a **pulmonary embolism.** There are three causes of a DVT: stasis of venous blood, intimal damage to the vein wall, and abnormalities of the clotting mechanism (Fahey, 1989). The cause of DVTs for SCI clients is stasis of venous blood return to the heart owing to prolonged immobility or limited mobility. Bed rest can also cause localized trauma of delicate vein structures by the continuous contact or pressure exerted, especially on the lower extremities. Clients with SCI are believed also to be in a state of hypercoagulability, increasing their risk for a DVT (Zejdlik, 1983).

The key sign usually observed first is swelling of the calf, thigh, or entire leg. Other symptoms include redness; warm, hard flesh; low-grade fever; chills; and asymmetrical enlargement of one leg relative to the other. Usually an enlargement in circumference of 2.5 cm or more of one leg is reason for concern. The spinal cord-injured client will not usually experience pain in the leg; however, he or she might complain of increased spasms and cramping in the affected limb and abdominal pain. A positive Homans's sign might occur but this is not advised if a DVT is suspected, as this test can actually cause dislodgment of a clot. Also, an SCI client might not feel any discomfort, and therefore the test response would be unreliable.

Nursing Diagnosis
- Altered peripheral tissue perfusion related to insufficient venous blood flow

Goals/Outcomes
- Client will be able to prevent, recognize the presence of, and obtain medical attention for the occurrence of a DVT.

Nursing Interventions
- Strictly limit the client's activity to prevent clot dislodgment; usually bed rest for approximately 7 days.
- Apply range-of-motion exercises to the *unaffected* leg, not to the affected leg.
- Encourage cough and deep breathing exercises every hour while awake.
- Turn the client without crossing legs.
- Elevate the affected leg, or both legs.
- Apply antiembolism stockings.
- Apply warm moist compresses daily to help reduce swelling.
- Teach the client signs and symptoms of a DVT as previously described.
- Teach the client how to prevent the reccurrence of a DVT:
  Reposition in bed every 2 hours.
  Apply antiembolism stockings.
  Apply range-of-motion exercises to lower extremities (when DVT is no longer present).
  Maintain adequate hydration.
  Avoid smoking (nicotine is believed to cause constriction of the veins, thus slowing venous blood flow).
  Avoid birth control pills.
- Administer heparin, warfarin (Coumadin) (anticoagulants) as prescribed by a physician, monitoring coagulation blood factors (partial thromboplastin time [PTT], prothrombin time [PT]) for effectiveness.
- Monitor the client's vital signs every 4–6 hours.
- In the morning, measure legs for improvement at the knee, 6 inches below the knee, 6 inches above the knee, and 12 inches above the knee and record. Adjust-

ments may be necessary depending on height of client. You are measuring the circumference of the client's calf and thigh, comparing the affected leg with the unaffected leg.
- Assess the client for the complication of a pulmonary embolism (shortness of breath, chest pain, apprehension, cough, hemoptysis, tachypnea, crackles, tachycardia, diaphoresis, and fever).

If there is a massive occlusion that does not respond to medical treatment and the thrombus is of recent onset, surgery will be indicated. Possible surgeries include a thrombectomy or an inferior vena caval interruption.

The occurrence of a DVT is highest for the SCI client within the first 3 months of injury. The nurse can play an important role in its prevention by measuring the legs bilaterally on admission, and twice a week afterward, turning the bedridden client every 2 hours, applying antiembolism stockings, avoiding constrictive clothing, hydrating the client, and monitoring vital signs. Teaching the client signs and symptoms early on can make the difference. The physician will most likely order baseline Doppler studies and either aspirin or heparin subcutaneously as a prophylactic.

Heterotopic Ossification

Heterotopic ossification (HO) is the inflammation of a voluntary muscle around a joint owing to bony deposits, resulting in loss of range of motion and the appearance of localized swelling.

Heterotopic ossification is a pathologic process in which extra-articular bone grows into connective tissue planes (Marinissen, 1993). The onset of HO usually occurs 4 to 12 weeks after injury. HO does not usually appear on x-rays until at least 2 months after injury but laboratory studies will show an elevated serum or alkaline phosphatase (ALP) beginning 2 weeks after injury and lasting about 5 months. ALP is best for an early detection. Treatment may be initiated solely on the basis of an elevated ALP if fracture and deep vein thrombosis are ruled out.

Treatment consists of medication management with etidronate disodium (Didronel) and indomethacin, physical therapy, possible manipulation, and possible surgery. The majority of clients with HO maintain functional joint motion with standard physical therapies, medicines, and (occasionally) forceful manipulations. Only a small percentage require surgery due to frequent recurrences of HO (Garland, 1991).

Didronel is for bone metabolism. It slows the rate of bone turnover, and lowers serum alkaline phosphatase (Wilson & Shannon, 1993). It should be given as a loading dose of 300 milligrams IV over a period of 3 hours daily for 3 days followed by a 5-month course of oral Didronel (Garland, 1991).

Indomethacin (Indocin) is used as a nonsteroid anti-inflammatory drug. Twenty-five milligrams is administered orally three times a week for 6 weeks. It is useful only if administered within 3 months after injury.

Medication may include radiation if it is to prevent or lessen the amount of HO formation after the primary insult or to prevent its recurrence following surgical resection (Garland, 1991).

Physical therapy consists of daily passive range-of-motion (ROM) exercises if related to HO of the hip. If ROM exercise results in discomfort to the client, the use of a continuous passive motion (CPM) machine may be effective. Physical therapy also consists of inhibiting muscle contracture through prolonged stretching. Prolonged stretching is achieved by placing the joint at the end of its ROM for periods to tolerance during the day, followed by positioning (Marinissen, 1993).

Positioning to maintain joint motion is specific to the joint and location of HO and is addressed throughout a 24-hour schedule. Recumbent positions for the hip include the prone position to maintain extension, and the supine position, with hips and knees flexed, to maintain flexion. Seated positioning may include use of custom-made cushions and wedges to maintain whatever ROM is possible (Marinissen, 1993).

Manipulation is considered as a possible treatment but is controversial. Manipulations every 1–2 months might be necessary to achieve the desired results. More than three manipulations is not advised (Garland, 1991).

Surgery excision is indicated when positioning of the limb is inadequate for seating or hygiene activities. Surgery cannot occur until the HO bone is mature, which is at least 1 year after injury in most clients. Indications for HO resection include a decrease in function as a result of decreasing ROM. Surgical intervention should be considered as a last resort for treatment of HO when other measures have been unsuccessful (Marinissen, 1993).

Nursing Diagnosis
- Impaired physical mobility related to limited ROM secondary to heterotopic ossification

Goals/Outcomes
- Client's affected limb or joint will have improved ROM.

Nursing Interventions
- Mobilize joint or limb as soon as possible.
- Perform mild ROM exercises and record limitations of range.
- Teach the client signs and symptoms of HO.
- Encourage sitting with hips and knees bent.
- Administer medications prescribed for HO (as discussed previously).

Osteoporosis

Osteoporosis is a disease in which bone demineralization results in decreased density and subsequent fractures. Usually the wrist, hip, and vertebral column are most affected. Osteoporosis results in irreversible bone mass loss. Owing to the loss of bone substance, the bones become very soft, resulting in fractures. There are several etiologies resulting in osteoporosis: primary causes, which are not associated with an underlying pathologic condition, and secondary causes, which result from an associated medical problem such as prolonged immobilization, excessive inactivity, and paralysis secondary to spinal cord injury.

The SCI client more at risk would include the elderly and especially postmenopausal women. As a rule, a woman's skeleton is smaller than a man's, and so she has less bone to begin with. At menopause, her estrogen level declines, impairing calcium absorption and accelerating the loss of bone mass. The aging process also reduces calcium absorption for both men and women (Beil, 1986).

Diagnostic assessment would include laboratory studies of the client's calcium, vitamin D, phosphorus, and alkaline phosphatase (ALP) levels. Radiographic assessment would include x-rays of the spine and long bones, showing loss of bone density and the presence of fractures. Findings of bone density changes are usually evident only after a 25–40 percent loss of bone has occurred. To detect early bone changes, computed tomography (CT) is a more helpful test, presenting better visualization of changes in cancellous bone (the vertebral column is composed mostly of cancellous bone). Other diagnostic tools include magnetic resonance imaging (MRI), single or dual-photon absorptiometer (densitometer) analysis, and neuron activation analysis (Ignatavicius, Workman, & Mishler, 1995).

Physical assessment would include signs and symptoms of a fracture to an extremity: swelling, change in alignment of an extremity, significant increase in spasticity, hematoma, and crepitation (Matthews & Carlson, 1987).

Nursing Diagnosis
- Impaired physical mobility related to decreased muscle tone and dysfunction secondary to immobility, inactivity of muscles, and paralysis of upper and/or lower extremities

Goals/Outcomes
- Client will recognize the signs and symptoms of fractures.
- Client will have increased muscle tone and physical activity.

Nursing Interventions
- Instruct the client to check all extremities for signs and symptoms of fractures on a routine basis, such as daily or weekly.
- Collaborate with a physical therapist regarding an exercise program to include strengthening exercises and assist the client as necessary.
- Apply assistive and adaptive devices to assist as needed in performance of activities of daily living (ADLs).

- Apply orthotic devises to support the spine, the wrist, or hips as needed, inspecting the skin regularly for any irritation from corset, brace, and so on.
- Teach the client how to keep calcium intake high with dietary supplements.
- Administer medications as ordered by the physician:

Calcium carbonate, 1.0–1.5 grams in divided doses daily with lots of fluids. Give 1 hour before meals. Monitor serum and urinary calcium levels. Observe for signs of hypercalcemia (Ignatavicius, Workman, & Mishler, 1995).

Conjugated estrogen for women, 0.425–1.25 milligrams for 25 days/month. Observe for vaginal bleeding and thrombus formation (Ignatavicius, 1995). Estrogen may not be used owing to the high risk of DVT occurrence to an SCI client.

Vitamin D, 700–800 IU. Observe for signs of hypercalcemia and hyperphosphatemia (Ignatavicius, Workman, & Mishler, 1995).

Other possible drugs include sodium fluoride, androgens, calcitonin, and vitamin D metabolites.

Strengthening exercises for the extremity muscles usually include isometric, resistive, and ROM exercises. The nurse encourages active ROM exercises as the client is able or teaches the family member or significant other to perform ROM exercises to the client, which will improve joint mobility and increase muscle tone.

Dietary management includes keeping calcium intake high through the diet. Milk and other dairy products provide the richest sources of calcium. Three and a half to five cups of milk, three to four cups of low-fat yogurt, or five to seven ounces of hard cheese provide daily recommended amounts. Canned salmon or sardines are also excellent sources to consider. If dietary management is not possible or if the client cannot tolerate milk products, calcium supplements as discussed with medication management will be necessary (Beil, 1986).

Contractures

Contractures occur when there is shortening of muscles due to disuse, making them resistant to stretching and movement; eventually deformity results. Connective tissue changes from disease can produce muscle shortening within 3 days. The development of contractures is not unlikely with the SCI client. Spasticity is a major contributing cause. Other etiologies include immobility, and muscle atrophy.

The muscles a client uses to flex an extremity are stronger than those used to extend the extremity. As a result the paralyzed extremity is more likely to contract in a flexed position (once it is there), than in an extended position (Pires, 1984).

One of the most common contractures in the quadriplegic client is the upper extremity flexion contracture caused by the active elbow flexors, which are innervated at the C6 level. Because innervation to the extensors occurs at T1, contractures tend to develop unless ROM is maintained and good positioning techniques are practiced (Boyink & Straun, 1981).

Contractures can be prevented in an SCI client by keeping the client properly positioned with pillows, performing daily passive ROM exercises, and encouraging self-care activities depending on the client's functional ability.

If contractures are allowed to occur, the client's level of independence to perform ADLs will be affected. For example, hand and arm contractures limit the client's ability to feed, bathe, and dress him- or herself, as well as being able to use hand splints or other adaptive devices. Leg and feet contractures can interfere with the client's comfort while sitting in a wheelchair or even while lying in bed. It can keep the client from wearing shoes or leg braces, complicate dressing and perineal hygiene, and limit positioning options for sexual activity (Pires, 1984).

Nursing Diagnosis
- Disuse syndrome related to limited musculoskeletal inactivity

Goals/Outcomes
- Client will describe how to prevent contractures, performing necessary methods or directing others to implement such methods.

Nursing Interventions
- Provide passive ROM exercises daily to all extremities.
- Implement proper positioning techniques, using pillows or splints as necessary.
- If spasticity is the cause, administer medication as ordered to decrease spasms.

Positioning guidelines for the supine position include the following: Place a small pillow under the client's head for support. Using a bulky pillow or more than one can force the head downward, causing a contracture. Elbows of the paralyzed extremities should be pointed away from the trunk and slightly bent. The lower arms and hands are extended alongside the trunk, about 12 inches away. Change this arm position periodically by extending the elbow. Elevate the lower arms with one pillow and place a small rolled wash cloth or object in the client's paralyzed hands. The object should be removed at intervals, extending the fingers. Align the trunk with the spine, keeping the shoulders aligned at the same level as the hips. Keep the client's legs straight, placing a trochanter roll alongside of the thighs; this is to prevent external rotation of the hip. Avoid placing pillows under the client's knees, which can lead to knee contractures. To prevent footdrop, use a footboard or pillows to support foot alignment at 90 degrees. Other alternatives include the use of Spenco boots or the use of high-top tennis shoes (Redelman, 1984).

The side-laying position is best for preventing contractures. Keep the spine in straight alignment, using a pillow(s) at the back and a pillow at the head for support. Bring the uppermost arm forward in front of the client. Bend the elbow slightly, keeping the wrist extended. Support the arm on a pillow and bring the bottom arm up alongside the face with the palm up. Flex the uppermost leg and bring it forward. Support it on pillows to prevent internal rotation of the hip. Keep the lower leg extended straight and level with the spine. Be sure the client's top leg is not resting on the bottom leg and use pillows against the soles of the feet or shoes as previously discussed to prevent footdrop (Redelman, 1984).

Spasticity

One of the leading causes of contractures is spasticity. Spasticity is abnormally increased muscle tone, causing dysfunctional posture and positioning (Umhauer, 1989). It represents a disturbance in motor function, whose central feature is an increase in tone (Segatore and Miller, 1994). According to Hinderer, Lehmann, Price, White, deLateur, and Deitz (1990), "it is an abnormal, velocity-dependent increase of the resistance to passive movement of peripheral joints" (p. 311). There is an increased stretch reflex at the muscles below the level of injury following some type of stimulus. The occurrence of spasms tends to be present in the SCI client with an upper motor neuron (UMN) lesion, especially those with incomplete UMN lesions.

Having spasms is painful to the client; it is a type of "pain." As such, spasms can interfere with all functional activities, including transfers, toileting, hygiene, dressing, wheelchair mobility, and driving (Segatore and Miller, 1994). However, depending on the degree of spasticity, sometimes they can be an advantage to the client, using them in a positive way to perform transfers and activities. Medication management can aid in decreasing the severity of spasms, therefore making them more manageable and positively useful. Spasms occur usually within 6–10 weeks after injury (Burke & Murray, 1975). They last for about 2 years and gradually decline (Zejdlik, 1983).

Nursing Diagnosis
- Impaired physical mobility related to abnormally increased muscle tone and discomfort of lower extremities.

Goals/Outcomes
- Client will perform mobility activities with greater independence and less discomfort.

Nursing Interventions
- Consider and teach positioning techniques for dressing, toileting, or transferring, so as to "break" the spasm pattern (Zejdlik, 1983).
  Flex the client's hips and knees to avoid extension or place the client in a flexion position in the wheelchair to prevent back extension.
  Curl the client's toes downward to stop the feet from jumping on the foot pedals of the wheelchair.

Teach the client to avoid uneven pressure on limbs, such as pushing the foot hard against the footboard, which will cause jerking movements.

- Teach the client the causes of and differences between spasms and voluntary movement. Spasticity does not mean a return of function.
- Keep the client in a "calm" environment and teach stress management techniques. High stress levels increase spasticity.
- Provide rest periods to decrease episodes of fatigue.
- Teach the client to be aware of contributing factors leading to spasms, such as a bladder infection, pressure ulcer, constrictive clothing, constipation, and ingrown toenails. Teach the client to avoid these causes as much as possible.
- Provide full ROM exercises to joints at least daily. Teach the family member or significant other to give passive ROM exercises at home. Collaborate with the physical therapist regarding appropriate exercises.
- Teach the client and family members to observe for contractures, joint damage, and stiffness; and to maintain correct positioning in wheelchair, bed, and so on.
- Administer antispasmodic drugs as ordered. Most commonly ordered is baclofen (Lioresal). Baclofen is given orally, 5 milligrams three times daily. It may be increased by 5 milligrams per dose every 3 days, with a maximum dose of 80 milligrams daily. Implantable baclofen pumps are also being used with some clients. It is classified as a central acting skeletal muscle relaxant (Wilson & Shannon, 1993). Teach the client to avoid alcohol with this drug, and that withdrawal from it must be done gradually. It is necessary to take baclofen as prescribed. In some clients, baclofen will cause drowsiness.
- Administer Valium if ordered. Valium is sometimes used for control of skeletal spasms. It can be given in conjunction with baclofen.

As an alternative, when medication management and positioning are not effective on their own, several neurological surgical procedures can be done for chronic spasticity. The purpose of the surgeries is to create a lower motor neuron (LMN) lesion. These procedures cut or interrupt reflex arcs, causing flaccid paralysis. Procedures include a *neurectomy* (a peripheral nerve that supplies a localized area is interrupted), *rhizotomy* (nerve roots), or *myelotomy* (spinal cord). These procedures exert negative changes on bowel, bladder, and sexual functioning as well as preserved sensation (Zejdlik, 1983).

A phenol intrathecal nerve block may also be done, which permanently kills the nerve. Before performing this procedure, a xylocaine nerve block can be used as a test.

Psychological Manifestations

The client who suffers from an SCI experiences not only many physical changes but also psychological manifestations. Besides a decreased body image and self-concept, SCI clients most significantly feel a loss of control; powerlessness. To lose control of your bowel and bladder functioning, for example, can result in "accidents" that might make the client feel like a child and be embarrassed. It is important to go beyond the physical needs of the SCI client. Try to imagine what life would be like if you could not feed, dress, or bathe yourself. Imagine if you could not even scratch yourself or shake a fly away that was annoying you. The life of a quadriplegic often is totally dependent on others for the simple activities of everyday life. As the client realizes the changes in his or her life as a result of injury, questions about the future will be a constant inquiry, especially the question about whether he or she will ever walk again.

As the client goes through these changes, he or she typically progresses or goes back and forth through a grief cycle of denial, anger, depression, unrealistic hope for cure, and adaptation to disability. As stated by Christopher Reeve,

> You're sitting here fighting depression, you're in shock, you look out the window and can't believe where you are. The thought that goes through your mind is "This can't be my life, it must be a mistake." (Rosenblatt, 1996, p. 40)

Nursing Diagnosis
- Powerlessness related to lack of independence and loss of body function, secondary to the effects of an SCI.

Goals/Outcomes
See Carpenito (1993):

- The client will identify factors and situations that he or she can control.
- The client will make decisions regarding his or her care, treatment, and future when possible.

Nursing Interventions
- Eliminate or reduce contributing factors if possible, such as lack of knowledge.
- Provide opportunities for the client to make his or her own decisions, such as in choice of clothing, time of bath, and method of bladder management.
- Assess the client's pattern of coping and response to problems. Assist the client with problem-solving skills.
- Encourage the client to participate in therapies and activities, regardless of "state of grief."
- Assist the client in deriving power from other sources such as prayer, clergy, stress reduction techniques, support groups, self-help groups, meditation, and imagery (Carpenito, 1993).
- Initiate health teaching so the client is informed. Remember, knowledge is power.
- Refer to other disciplines as necessary: chaplain, social worker, psychiatric nurse/physician.
- Provide emotional support as able—reassuring the client of his or her importance as a person, emphasizing strengths, instead of weaknesses; praising for positive forward steps; trying to be there for the client when you can or when you said you would be.

- Tell the client what you are doing before beginning. Include the client in the decision-making process.
- During specific stages of grief, consider the following (Pires, 1984):

Denial: Answer all questions truthfully. The client will hear what he or she wants to hear, and when he or she wants to hear it.

Anger: Be understanding and firm, especially when the client is yelling or lashing out. Do not take the client's anger personally. Remember it is the behavior that is unacceptable, not the client. Support the family during this time as well. The client is usually verbally abusive toward them, too. Remind the family that this behavior is temporary.

Depression: Be aware that the client may not want to live as a quadriplegic or paraplegic. He or she might say they want to commit suicide. Encourage the client to express these feelings of despair and grief. Listen actively.

Encourage the client to interact with non-SCI persons in the community and to establish goals for his or her future.

Conclusion

Having an SCI can be an overwelming, devastating condition both physically and psychologically. This chapter has tried to show the many problems SCI clients need to be concerned with and how, with proper care, they can be avoided or at least managed. One of the keys to a successful life postinjury is education. The nurse must spend ample time providing instruction to the client and family on all aspects of care discussed in this chapter. Another necessary ingredient is social support either by supportive friends or family; it has been found to be related to positive desirable outcomes following injury or illness. "For most people, members of their nuclear and extended families are key sources of support" (Rintala, Young, Spencer, & Bates, 1996, p. 67).

Research is another key for the hope of SCI clients. There is much research in progress regarding the management of acute SCI and sequelae. For example, the use of methylprednisolone (MP), which doctors speculate at high doses no longer acts as a steroid but instead inhibits the breakdown of fats into the dangerous free radicals that are like acid to cell tissues, can make a big difference in SCI recovery (Rosenblatt, 1996). A National Institute of Health-supported study showed that if MP was given within 8 hours of an SCI, a client could save about 20 percent more neurons than if the drug were not used (Rosenblatt, 1996). This can have positive effects on respiratory status, the control of bowel and bladder functioning, and movement of extremities. According to Dr. Wise Young of New York University, "It means that you don't have to preserve, restore and regenerate so many axons in order to get functional recovery" (Rosenblatt, 1996, p. 45). What hope for the future! In addition, research is being done worldwide to find a cure for SCI by nerve regeneration. Nurses can and should be involved in this activity.

References   Beil, A. V. (1986). Osteoporosis: How to avoid its crippling effects. *RN, 49*(8), 14–17.

Bergstrom, N., Bennet, M. A., Carlson, C. E., et al. (1994). *Treatment of pressure ulcers. Clinical Practice Guidelines No. 15.* Rockville, MD: U.S. Department of Health and Human Services, AHCPR.

Boyink, M. A., & Strawn, S. M. (1981). Spinal cord injury: Postacute phase. In H. Martin, N. B. Holt, & D. Hicks (Eds.), *Comprehensive rehabilitation nursing.* (pp. 449–491). New York: McGraw-Hill.

Burke, D., & Murray, D. (1975). Introductory presentation of physiology and treatment of spasticity. In D. Burke & D. Murray (Eds.), *Handbook of spinal cord medicine.* (pp. 65–75). London and Basingstoke: Macmillan.

Carpenito, L. J. (1993). *Nursing diagnoses: Application to clinical practice* (5th ed.). Philadelphia: J. B. Lippincott.

Crenshaw, R. P., & Vistnes, L. M. (1989). A decade of pressure sore research: 1977–1987. *Journal of Rehabilitation Research and Development, 26,* 63–74.

Fahey, V. A. (1989). An in-depth look at deep vein thrombosis. *Nursing '89, 19*(1), 86–93.

Finocchiaro, D. N., & Herzfeld, S. (1990). Understanding autonomic dysreflexia. *American Journal of Nursing, 90*(9), 56–59.

Garland, D. E. (1991). A clinical perspective on common forms of acquired heterotopic ossification. *Clinical Orthopaedics and Related Research, 263,* 13–29.

Gordon, D. I., & Stevens, M. M. (1981). Spinal cord injury: Acute phase. In H. Martin, N. B. Holt, & D. Hicks (Eds.), *Comprehensive rehabilitation nursing.* (pp. 418–448). New York: McGraw-Hill.

Guttman, L. (1976). *Spinal cord injuries: Comprehensive management and research* (2nd ed.). Oxford: Blackwell.

Harvey, C., Rothschild, B. B., Asmann, A. J., & Stripling, T. (1990). New estimate of traumatic SCI prevalence: A survey-based approach. *Paraplegia, 28,* 537–544.

Hinderer, S. R., Lehmann, J. F., Price, R., White, O., deLateur, B. J., & Deitz, J. (1990). Spasticity in spinal cord injured persons: Quantitative effects of baclofen and placebo treatments. *American Journal of Physical Medicine and Rehabilitation 69*(6), 311–317.

Ignatavicius, D. D., Workman, M. L., & Mishler, M. A. (1995). *Medical-surgical nursing: A nursing process approach* (2nd ed.). Philadelphia: W. B. Saunders.

Laskowski-Jones, L. (1993). Acute spinal cord injury: How to minimize the damage. *American Journal of Nursing, 93*(12), 23–31.

Marinissen, J. C. (1993). Management of heterotopic ossification following traumatic brain or spinal cord injury. *Orthopaedic Physical Therapy Clinics of North America,* 71–85.

Matthews, P. J., & Carlson, C. E. (1987). *Rehabilitation Institute of Chicago procedure manual: Spinal cord injury—A guide to rehabilitation nursing.* Rockville, MD: Aspen.

Miller, S. M. (1995). Respiratory problems in spinal cord injury. *Resident & Staff Physician, 41*(7), 27–38.

Pires, M. (1984). Spinal cord injuries: Coping with devastating damage. In Urosevich, P. R. (ed.). *Coping with neurologic problems proficiently* (2nd ed.). Nursing '84 Skillbook series. (pp. 99–123). Springhouse, PA: Springhouse.

Pownell, P. H. (1995). Pressure sores. *Selected Readings in Plastic Surgery, 7*(39), 1–27.

Redelman, K. (1984). Dealing with cerebrovascular disease: Providing acute care. In Urosevich, P. R. (ed.). *Coping with neurologic problems proficiently* (2nd ed.). Nursing '84 Skillbook series. (pp. 53–70). Springhouse, PA: Springhouse.

Rintala, D. H., Young, M. E., Spencer, J. C., & Bates, P. S. (1996). Family relationships and adaptation to spinal cord injury: A qualitative study. *Rehabilitation Nursing, 21*(2), 67–74.

Rosenblatt, R. (1996). New hopes, new dreams. *Time, 148*(10), 40–52.

Segatore, M., & Miller, M. (1994). The pharmacotherapy of spinal spasticity: A decade of progress. 1. Theoretical aspects. *SCI Nursing, 11*(3), 66–69.

Stover, S. L., & Fine, P. R. (1987). The epidemiology and economics of spinal cord injury. *Paraplegia, 25,* 225–228.

Umhauer, M. K. (1989). Movement. In Dittmar (Ed.), *Rehabilitation nursing: Process and application.* (pp. 360–406). St. Louis: Mosby.

Wilson, B. A., & Shannon, M. T. (1993). *Govoni & Hayes' Nurses' drug guide 1993.* (pp. 137–139). Norwalk, CT: Appleton & Lange.

Zejdlik, C. (1983). *Management of spinal cord injury.* Belmont, CA: Wadsworth.

CHAPTER 18

Dysphagia: Implication in the Treatment of Clients

Kimberly D. Mory

Key Terms   *Dysphagia*
Esophageal Stage
Pharyngeal Stage
Preparatory Stage
Oral Stage

Objectives   1. The student will be able to define dysphagia.

2. The student will be able to name and define the four stages of swallowing.

3. The student will be able to identify three medical conditions in which dysphagia commonly occurs.

4. The student will be able to name two methods used in the diagnosis of dysphagia.

5. The student will be able to state three techniques for nurses to use while caring for the client with dysphagia.

Introduction   **Dysphagia** is defined as difficulty or inability to swallow. It is not to be confused with *dysphasia,* which is a general term used to describe impairment of language functions. Dysphagia can be present in varying degrees; from difficulty in chewing, to a complete inability to swallow solids and liquids safely. The problem of dysphagia is not to be taken lightly. The effects of dysphagia can be poor nutrition, poor oral hygiene, and aspiration, which can lead to pneumonia and death. It may be difficult to diagnose dysphagia and its cause because the swallowing mechanism is not easily visible without special diagnostic methods. However, once the various stages of swallowing are understood, the cause of the difficulty may be more easily identified and treated.

Stages of Swallowing   The act of swallowing is divided into four stages, with distinct physical actions and anatomy involved at each stage. The four stages are (1) the preparatory stage, (2) the oral stage, (3) the pharyngeal stage, and (4) the esophageal stage. A discussion of each phase follows (Figure 1).

Preparatory Stage   The **preparatory stage** of swallowing is probably the most often overlooked stage, and yet when impaired, can cause significant problems for the client. In

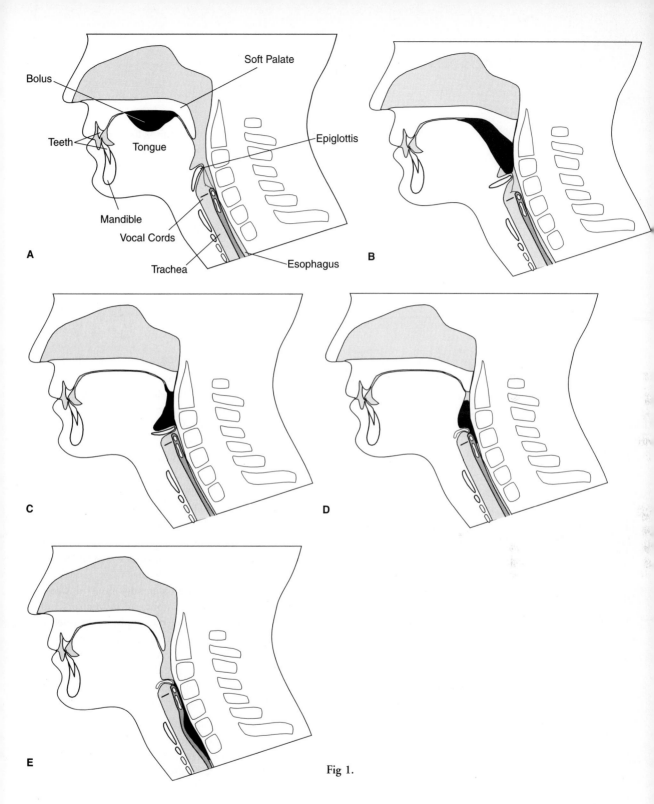

A

Bolus

Soft Palate

Teeth

Tongue

Epiglottis

Mandible

Vocal Cords

Trachea

Esophagus

B

C

D

E

Fig 1.

309

normal swallowing, the individual prepares the mechanism to accept the food or liquid before it even reaches the mouth. The next time you are eating, take notice of what your actions are just before you place a bite of food in your mouth. You will notice that when you begin to eat, your salivary glands produce more saliva in order to break down the food more easily and prepare it for digestion. You'll also notice that as you lift the fork to your mouth, your mouth opens before the food reaches it. The fork does not get all the way to your mouth and then wait for it to open all at once. The same thing happens when you drink liquids. Your lips and mouth begin moving into position to accept the glass and liquid. How fast you drink the liquid depends on the viscosity, temperature, and whether it is carbonated or not.

The preparatory phase is composed of all the actions and movements that occur before the food or liquid enters the mouth.

Oral Stage

The **oral stage** of swallowing (see Figure 1A) begins when the food or liquid enters the mouth. Saliva begins to soften the food, the teeth begin to grind, and the tongue moves the food around to ensure that it is chewed and to form a bolus, in preparation for swallowing. During the consumption of liquids, we rely on sensation to prevent liquid from escaping out of the sides of our lips and mouth.

After the food is ground and formed into a bolus, the front of the tongue must rise up and propel the bolus backward. As the bolus passes the faucial pillars on each side of the oropharyngeal area, the swallowing reflex is triggered, and the bolus enters the third stage of swallowing, the pharyngeal phase.

Pharyngeal Stage

The **pharyngeal stage** (see Figure 1B) consists of moving the food from the oral cavity into the laryngeal area. This is accomplished by peristaltic movement of the lateral and posterior pharyngeal walls. The soft palate rises to prevent the bolus from moving upward into the nasal sinuses. The bolus now moves downward into the laryngeal area (see Figure 1C). A series of complicated movements and split-second timing are required for the bolus to enter the esophagus instead of the trachea. As the bolus moves downward, the vocal folds come together to prevent food and liquid from entering the trachea (see Figure 1D). The epiglottis, a leaf-shaped structure in the larynx, also moves downward to cover the opening into the trachea. This steers the bolus into the esophagus, where it continues to move downward owing to peristaltic movement of the muscles of the esophagus.

Esophageal Stage

The **esophageal stage** is the last phase of swallowing. At the distal end of the esophagus is a sphincter that allows the bolus to pass through, into the stomach. As the bolus moves through the esophagus (see Figure 1E), the individual may be continuing to chew and swallow successive bites of food. This further complicates the delicate timing and sequencing that are required for the swallowing mechanism to perform adequately.

Conditions Impairing Swallowing

We now look at various conditions and how they can impair the ability to swallow. The way in which the swallowing stages are affected will be described in terms of the previous discussion regarding normal swallowing.

Postsurgical Effects

The effects of any type of surgery on a client are often overlooked, as many of the effects are transitory in nature and disappear as the client recovers. However, as a client is coming out of the effects of anesthesia, thin liquids are most often given to the client for hydration without realizing that the client may not be fully conscious and cannot control the swallowing of liquids. Also, the use of endotracheal tubes during surgery can cause severe soreness in the throat and make swallowing very difficult for the client even if the condition is temporary. During the immediate recovery period following surgery, there must be a heightened awareness of the client's control during the intake of food and liquids.

Surgical procedures performed on any of the structures of the mouth, throat, and neck obviously require special precautions when providing hydration and nutrition to the client. Liquids and solids must be carefully and continuously assessed throughout the client's recovery. Typically, a client is started on thin liquids as the first oral intake following surgery. However, thin liquids have been found to be one of the most troublesome substances to swallow owing to the difficulty in forming and controlling the bolus. This increases the risk of aspiration, particularly when respiration may be compromised secondary to anesthesia and surgery. Treatment options are discussed in Diagnosing and Treating Dysphagia (below).

Stroke

One of the most common neurological episodes that can adversely affect a client's swallowing ability is the occurrence of a stroke. Cerebral vascular accidents can impede the integrity of the swallowing mechanism in any number of ways.

Visual deficits, commonly occurring with strokes, may indirectly affect the safe intake of solids and liquids. A client can exhibit signs of visual impairments by closing one eye at a time while trying to focus on an object, squinting, reaching for an object and missing it, or running into walls and objects. Hemianopia is characterized by the client not being able to see half of the visual fields, and visual neglect is displayed by the client not responding to stimuli in the environment, even though the visual fields may be intact. These phenomena can be observed when a client leaves all of the items untouched on one side of the food tray, does not turn his head past midline, or washes or shaves only one side of his face. A client may also have any combination of visual impairments. When visual deficits are present, clients cannot accurately see the texture or the size of bite that they are putting into their mouth. This affects the preparatory stage and does not give accurate information to the client as he anticipates the bite of food, leading to coughing and choking.

It is important to realize that a client exhibiting any type of paresis of the upper and/or lower extremities frequently has unseen weakness in the structures of the face and neck that can significantly affect the stages necessary for safe, oral intake of food and liquids. Weakness of the lips, tongue, or facial muscles make it difficult for the client to chew and move the food or liquid around in the mouth and form it into a bolus. Impairment of the tongue musculature prevents the bolus from being transported backward and triggering the swallowing reflex. Clients with weakness in these structures typically exhibit very slow chewing movements and take an exorbitant amount of time to initiate a swallow. The client may tilt his head backward in an attempt to move the bolus back and make it easier to swallow. Pocketing of food and liquid along the gums on the weakened side is very common and care must be taken that the food is cleaned out of the cheek area immediately after eating to prevent aspiration of material.

A common result of a stroke is a delayed swallowing reflex, secondary to weakness and decreased sensation. The bolus may move backward but not trigger the reflex. If the swallowing reflex does not occur, the epiglottis does not move downward to protect the trachea and the bolus begins to spill over the back of the tongue and trickle down toward the trachea. With decreased sensation, the client may not feel material in the back of the throat and, therefore, not be able to cough the way a person normally would to protect the airway. Weakness of the respiratory muscles may further compromise the client's ability to produce a protective cough.

The client with impaired ability to swallow may complain of not being able to swallow, or describe the feeling of "food being stuck" in his throat. It may take an exorbitant amount of time for the person to eat, or the client may exhibit coughing after each bite of food or drink of liquid. However, very frequently, a client with dysphagia may not complain or show any outward signs or symptoms of any difficulty. This is extremely dangerous because the client may be aspirating without any evidence until he exhibits a fever, one of the first signs of an infection stemming from aspiration.

Impaired cognitive abilities also compromise a client's ability to eat an oral diet safely and successfully. An individual must have sufficient cognitive awareness to be able to have at least a minimal amount of control when eating and drinking. When food or liquid is forced into the mouth of a semiconscious client, there is a high risk of material finding its way into the trachea owing to reasons previously stated. A client exhibiting impulsivity and poor judgment will often put large amounts of food into his mouth successively without chewing, leading to choking and coughing.

Dentures often times do not fit properly after a stroke owing to weakness of the oral–facial structures and atrophy of the gum tissue. This will obviously impede the client's ability to chew foods, and the diet must be altered to accommodate the need for softer foods. During the recovery, the client and family will need to be patient, as it may take several attempts in working with the dentist to get the dentures to fit properly again.

After a stroke, many different factors can negatively impact a client's ability to tolerate an oral diet safely. Most often, it is an astute nursing staff that first recognizes that a client is having difficulty eating or drinking and requests the appropriate referral. This is usually made to a speech pathologist, although a referral may also be made to an otolaryngologist (ENT) to determine the etiology of the difficulty and to develop a treatment plan. There are many other conditions that can cause dysphagia, some of which are discussed in the following sections.

Acquired Brain Injury

Brain injury acquired through trauma or surgical intervention (tumors, aneurysms) can also cause dysphagia secondary to physical, neurological, and cognitive impairments. Many of the deficits may be temporary, but aggressive intervention is often required initially after the injury. If a tracheostomy has been performed, close monitoring and special treatment are necessary to maintain nutrition and facilitate swallowing. Treatment of these clients requires specialized care and is beyond the scope of this chapter. Cognitive deficits are frequently the primary reason to look to alternative methods of administering nutrition in clients who have acquired a brain injury. Clients with cognitive impairments are at just as great a risk for aspiration even though their swallowing mechanism is relatively intact. Brain-injured clients typically have very little control over or recognition of their actions, and are characterized as being very impulsive with little or no awareness of any need for precautions. These clients have been observed to put all sizes and shapes of inedible objects into their mouth and have even been known to swallow different objects. The brain-injured client may cram food into his mouth to such a point that gagging and vomiting ensue, thus further increasing the risk of aspiration. On the other end of the spectrum is the brain-injured client who has no awareness of the feeling of hunger and does not recognize the need or desire for food. Although these clients may not be identified as having any swallowing difficulty, the result of their brain injury and lack of appetite create a very real problem in obtaining adequate nutrition. The resulting weight loss and malnutrition can occur very fast in a client, and require aggressive management to reverse the process.

As in stroke victims, visual perceptual deficits and hemiparesis may also exist in a brain-injured client, impairing the client's ability to eat or drink at any stage of swallowing. Reduced lip, tongue, and jaw movements; delayed swallowing reflex; and reduced peristaltic movement may all be present in varying degrees and each component must be treated to maximize ability.

In a client who has suffered a traumatic brain injury, there may be multiple fractures of the facial bones that require immobilization, and that prevent any movement of the oral structures. As the injuries heal, the treatment will need to be constantly monitored and changed to ensure proper nutrition and to improve the client's ability to eat and drink. Fortunately, a brain-injured client tends to exhibit many of these difficulties temporarily. The client can move through the stages of recovery to a point at which he or she is able to regain the ability to swallow solids and liquids safely, in sufficient amounts for proper nutrition. Compensatory strategies are used to assist the client to regain the ability to swallow. This may occur over a period of a few weeks or a few months.

Other Neurological Conditions

Multiple sclerosis, amyotrophic lateral sclerosis (ALS), and Parkinson's disease are some of the most common neurological conditions that affect the swallowing mechanism. Following is a brief summary of each these disorders.

Multiple sclerosis is considered to be the most common neurologic disease affecting young and middle-aged adults. Demyelination of nerve fibers occurs over a period of time, caused by lesions in the white matter. The neurologic symptoms that are exhibited are due to the interruption of nerve impulses, which can no longer be transmitted owing to the demyelination. There are a wide variety of symptoms that can occur in multiple sclerosis depending on the location of the white matter lesions and resulting demyelination. When the lesions occur in the brainstem, swallowing ability may be affected owing to impairment of the swallowing reflex and reduced peristaltic movement found in the pharyngeal and esophageal stages of swallowing. Multiple sclerosis also affects the motor function of the upper and lower extremities. The most frequent cause of feeding difficulties is severe tremors of the hands, which make it extremely difficult for the client to hold eating utensils and cups. Compensatory strategies such as weighted utensils, scoop bowls, and spoons that can swivel can improve the client's function.

Amyotrophic lateral sclerosis (ALS) is also known in the United States as Lou Gehrig's disease, and is characterized by degeneration of the motor neurons in the central nervous system and the peripheral nervous system. When the degeneration occurs in the cranial nerves, dysphagia is a frequent complaint and is most often accompanied by speech disorders as well. Weakness and muscle fatigue can affect the ability to swallow at any stage. Most often a client will exhibit difficulty in chewing food and getting the tongue to propel the bolus backward to trigger the swallowing reflex. The swallowing of thin liquids may be particularly difficult and clients may avoid drinking liquids, which can lead to dehydration if not carefully monitored. As the disease progresses, diet consistency and positioning strategies can be used to maintain oral feeding for as long as possible.

Parkinson's disease affects the basal ganglia of the central nervous system and is generally a slowly progressive disease. The basal ganglia are involved in carrying out specific motor movements, particularly those involved in automatic motor sequences. It is characterized by resting tremors of the hands and limbs, rigidity of muscle movement, and difficulty with the initiation and execution of motor movement. The disease can cause dysphagia at any stage. Often, it is muscle rigidity of the lips, tongue, and cheeks that creates impairment at the oral stage, exhibited by slowness and ineffectiveness of movement. The tongue frequently moves backward and forward several times in an attempt to form a bolus and propel it backward. Delay in the onset of the swallowing reflex is often exhibited, along with severely reduced peristalsis in the pharyngeal and esophageal stages. The same rigidity can also be apparent in the muscles involved in respiration, making it difficult for the client to coordinate inspiration and exhalation with swallowing. The risk of aspiration increases as the disease progresses, and the client may not be fully aware of the difficulty that is occurring. Oral feeding may need to be discontinued and replaced by tube feeding to provide adequate nutrition.

Diagnosing and Treating Dysphagia

Signs and symptoms of dysphagia may either be easily observed, or be quite difficult to detect. Clients must be observed during meals in order to identify any of the more obvious impairments. A client with visual deficits may eat only items that are on the right or left side of midline. It will appear that the client does not want to eat anymore, but actually the client is not seeing everything on the tray. Depending on where liquids are placed in relation to the visual deficits, the client may not be taking sufficient fluids, leading to dehydration. You cannot depend on the client to be able to tell you that he cannot see well, or that he is still hungry or thirsty. For these clients, ensuring that food and liquid are within their visual field may significantly improve their oral intake.

As mentioned previously, it is frequently the nursing staff that observes a client having difficulty eating and/or drinking and requests an evaluation by the speech pathologist or occupational therapist, depending on which discipline is used in that particular center. The therapist can determine the integrity of the visual fields and whether diplopia (double vision) is also a problem. In stroke and brain-injured clients, different types of apraxia and agnosia can exist in which the client can visually see an object, but has no recognition of what it is or what to do with the item. These clients may require one-on-one feeding until they recover sufficiently to be able to feed themselves.

Clients with hemiparesis of the dominant hand cannot use utensils in the same way they could before the injury. Eating can become a very time-consuming and frustrating event, to such a point that the client avoids eating and drinking. Occupational therapists are known for the many different devices that they use to help the client compensate for reduced strength, poor grip, or impaired motor control. Use of these items and techniques can be important in improving a client's oral intake, as well as in encouraging and increasing the confidence of the client that is so important for overall recovery.

A client exhibiting drooping of the facial muscles, or drooling, suggests decreased sensation and motor control of the oral structures. A bedside swallowing evaluation is usually the first diagnostic method used to determine the actual integrity of the swallowing mechanism, and is primarily completed by the speech pathologist, although it may be a different discipline, again, depending on the center. During a bedside evaluation, the preparatory and oral stages of swallowing are the focus because these stages are most easily observed. Function of the mechanism at the pharyngeal and esophageal stages can only be speculated because it cannot be seen without more intrusive diagnostic methods. The therapist assesses the motor function of the oral structures to include the lips, tongue, and cheeks. Weakness and dysco-ordination of any of these structures will significantly impact the client's ability to eat and drink. If the lips and cheeks (buccal muscles) are weakened, the client will be unable to hold the food or liquid in his or her mouth and it will spill out before he or she can form a bolus and swallow. A tongue affected by weakness is not able to move the food around sufficiently for chewing and forming a bolus, and is unable to propel the food backward to trigger a swallow reflex. This client takes a prolonged period of time to masticate the food, and on having the client open his mouth, the food is spread over all surfaces of the tongue and on all sides of the gums because he cannot form a bolus.

The propulsion ability of the tongue is assessed to determine if it can move the food and liquid backward sufficiently enough to trigger the reflex. It is common for swallowing difficulties to occur at this point in the oral stage. If the tongue cannot propel the bolus to trigger the reflex, the client may give up, complaining of not being able to swallow, and spit the food out. Or, the food and liquid may eventually spill over the back of the tongue and down toward the esophagus and trachea, with a significant risk of aspirating material into the lungs. By placing his or her hand on the client's larynx, the therapist can feel for laryngeal elevation during swallowing to assist in determining when, and if, swallowing is occurring.

The presence of a gag reflex does not ensure that the swallowing mechanism is intake. A client may exhibit a very strong gag reflex and yet aspirate material during the intake of solids and liquids. If the client has a delayed swallowing reflex, the bolus may begin to trickle over the back of the tongue and down toward the larynx. The client generally does not have any sensation of this occurring and does not exhibit any gagging or coughing behavior. The term for this phenomenon is *silent aspiration,* and it can lead to medical complications very quickly.

To assess more completely the function of the swallowing mechanism at the pharyngeal and esophageal stages, various diagnostic tests may be used. Videofluoroscopy is the most common diagnostic method used; it consists of having the client swallow different consistencies of barium as the radiation technician videotapes the x-rays taken successively while the client is moving the material in his mouth and then swallowing. This provides a moving assessment of the dynamics that are occurring, and enables the therapist and the radiologist to determine if aspiration is occurring and if so, at what point in the process. The therapist can also have the client try various positions with his head while swallowing to determine if the swallow can be made easier, or the risk of aspiration decreased. Although the videofluoroscopy study yields a tremendous amount of information, it may not be used if the proper equipment is not available, or if the client is unable to be positioned properly for the study. Also, for the most accurate and helpful results, the client must have sufficient cognitive and language abilities to be able to follow directions.

Other, more complex tests that are not frequently used but may be available combine videofluoroscopy with other procedures such as electromyography and manometry. In these tests, electrodes (electromyography) and sensors (manometry) are used to measure movement of the muscles, and air pressure within the pharynx, to assess further the integrity of the swallowing mechanism. These tests are very time consuming and expensive, as well as being much more intrusive to the client, and are primarily used for very specific disorders.

Treatment   Set-up of the food tray with items placed within the client's visual field, and use of the proper utensils, have been discussed as increasing a client's ability to consume food and liquids. The therapist involved may also recommend that the client, when eating and drinking, use a specific body position to maximize swallowing efficiency. Having the client turn his or her head to the right or left, or to tuck his or her chin down, while swallowing increases protection of the airway and minimizes the risk of aspiration. Once the optimal position is determined, it is imperative that this strategy be followed during the intake of all foods and liquids.

The consistency of food and liquid can also be modified to compensate for poor mastication, or for difficulties in initiating a swallow. Diets can range from a puréed diet and progress to finely chopped foods, mechanical soft foods, a soft diet, and eventually progress to a regular diet. Although thin liquids are the most frequently given form of hydration, thickened liquids are often a better choice for the client. Thick liquids include nectars, or liquids with thickening agents added to them to achieve the desired consistency. A frequent mistake is to give the client water with which to take medication, when the client is restricted to thick liquids. It is important for all members of the treatment team and the client's family to understand the dietary restrictions and adhere to them when giving food or liquids to the client. The client's ability to tolerate foods and liquids can improve with appropriate treatment interventions. The speech pathologist can provide exercises and strategies to increase the strength and range of motion of the oral structures, and can improve the initiation of the swallowing reflex. Treatment addressing cognitive and language deficits can also improve the client's functional abilities by improving attention skills, awareness, and comprehension. Often, non-oral feeding methods are used while treatment continues to focus on improving oral eating skills. Treatment can begin in the inpatient setting and continue through the outpatient or home health setting. An important component of treatment is the followthrough by the caregivers to adhere to the strategies and protocols that have been implemented to improve the swallowing abilities of the client.

Nonoral Feeding

Although it is the desire for all clients to be able to eat orally, it must be recognized that for the client's health there are times when nonoral feeding is the treatment of choice. Owing to cognitive, physical, or physiological impairments, feedings either by nasogastric or gastrostomy tube can sustain nutrition until the client recovers to a more functional level. Gastrostomy tubes, although requiring a minor surgical procedure, are generally considered to be preferential to nasogastric tubes when its use is anticipated to be for more than just a few days. This is because the nasogastric tube can further compromise the structures and function of the oropharyngeal area, and in some cases actually increase the difficulties that the client exhibits. In some of the neurologic disorders, the disease can progress to such a point that oral feeding is no longer appropriate to sustain life and nonoral methods are generally used for the remainder of the client's life. Counseling can be very beneficial for the client and family to understand the need for nonoral feeding and, when appropriate, to comprehend the use of tube feeding as a necessary step in the recovery process.

Goals of Treatment

One need only visit a supermarket or restaurant, or see advertisements on television, to recognize that much of our culture's entertainment and pleasure revolves around food and eating. The most important goal of treatment is to provide the client with the nutrition and hydration necessary for good health. Although the most desirable and functional method is an oral diet, nonoral feedings may actually be more functional and pleasant for the client. If oral feeding is a painstaking and arduous task for the client, with constant admonishments "to eat more," then the goal of treatment may be to initiate tube feedings to maintain nutrition. Frequently, the client can still continue to eat the foods that he or she likes under more pleasant circumstances.

The intake of food and liquids must be functional for the client and the caregiver(s). Fortunately, there are many strategies that can be used to give the client the best opportunity possible to eat and drink orally, and in a safe manner. Recovery from dysphagia can take days, weeks, months, and even years, depending on the severity of the impairment and the overall physical, neurological, and cognitive abilities of the client.

Techniques to Use with Dysphagia Clients

1. Never give liquids or solids to a semiconscious client.
2. Don't give thin liquids to a client restricted to thickened liquids, even if it's just to take medicine.
3. When possible, use a straw to give clients liquids, and control the rate and amount of liquid by pinching the straw. This method is more effective in giving a client liquid in a more controlled manner, and it is easier for the client to drink from the straw than to be given liquid from a cup.
4. During feeding and drinking, have the client in as upright a position as possible, unless contraindicated by other medical issues.
5. Keep the client in an upright position for at least 30 minutes after eating, unless otherwise indicated.
6. Check the client's gum line and cheeks for pocketing of food before the client lays down or goes to sleep.
7. If the client is on a special dysphagia diet (puréed, mechanical soft, chopped), ensure that the client is given the proper diet at each meal and for snacks. Assist with educating and monitoring family members for their compliance with swallowing protocols.
8. Never leave a client alone while he or she is eating and drinking if you are unsure about swallowing competency.
9. If uncertain about a client's swallowing ability, request a dysphagia evaluation.
10. Follow through with strategies and procedures as developed by the therapist(s) for consistency, and to provide as many opportunities as possible to improve swallowing skills.
11. Ask questions if unsure of the procedures to use with a client.

Summary

The problem of dysphagia is not to be taken lightly in the medical management of the client. It must be expected in clients with neurological injuries and specific physical impairments until it is ruled out. It must also be recognized that dysphagia can occur when least expected, such as in the case of postsurgical clients. Because the nursing staff has the most hands-on involvement with the client, nursing is an integral part of treatment, and is vital in the proper diagnosis and successful treatment of the client with dysphagia.

Suggested Readings

Logemann, J. (1983). *Evaluation and treatment of swallowing disorders.* Austin, TX: PRO-ED.

Logemann, J. (1986). *Manual for the videofluorographic study of swallowing* (2nd ed.). Austin, TX: PRO-ED.

Yorkston, K. M., Miller, R. M., and Strand, E. A. (1995). *Management of speech and swallowing in degenerative diseases.* Tucson, AZ: Communication Skill Builders.

CHAPTER 19

Neurogenic Bladder and Bowel Functioning

Darlene N. Finocchiaro and *Michael Finocchiaro*

Key Terms
Areflexic
Automatic
Autonomous
Bulbocavernosus Reflex
Credé's Maneuver
Digital Stimulation
Flaccid
Gastrocolic Reflex
Hypertonic
Hypotonic
Incontinence (Stress, Urge, Functional, Reflex)
Intermittent Catheterization (IC)
Lower Motor Neuron (LMN)
Neurogenic Bowel/Bladder
Reflexic
Saddle Sensation
Strain Voiding
Stress Overflow
Timed Voiding
Triggering Techniques
Uninhibited
Upper Motor Neuron (UMN)
Urinary Diversions

Objectives

1. Discuss the psychosocial impact of incontinence on the client and family.

2. Identify medical diagnoses that can result in a neurogenic bowel and bladder.

3. Discriminate between a normal bladder, an uninhibited neurogenic bladder, a reflex neurogenic bladder, and an autonomous neurogenic bladder.

4. Discriminate between a normal bowel, an uninhibited neurogenic bowel, a reflex neurogenic bowel, and an autonomous neurogenic bowel.

5. Choose the appropriate nursing diagnosis for each type of neurogenic bowel and bladder.

6. Identify nursing interventions for management of the neurogenic bowel and bladder.

7. Describe the effects of medications affecting bladder functioning: cholinergics, anticholinergics, α-adrenergic blockers, adrenergic stimulants, and skeletal muscle relaxants.

8. Describe the effects of medications affecting bowel functioning: suppositories, stool softeners, peristaltic stimulators, and bulk formers.

9. List possible complications resulting from a neurogenic bowel and bladder.

10. Discuss surgical options for a neurogenic bladder: sphincterotomy, transurethral resection of the prostate, suprapubic cystostomy, and urinary diversions.

Introduction   Urinary incontinence is "the involuntary loss of urine sufficient to be a problem" (Urinary Incontinence Guideline Panel, 1992, p. 115). This can be said to be true with bowel incontinence as well. Incontinence, bowel and bladder, is a problem not only for the individual experiencing it, but also for the family, caregivers, and society.

Incontinence is costly in terms of money, time, and personal wellness. Often, the incontinent person will isolate himself or herself socially or give up vocational opportunities because of the fear of "accidents." Incontinence is a problem seen in the rehabilitation setting, often causing delays in the progression of therapy. For this reason, incontinence is a problem that must be dealt with. A team approach to management is necessary, and it is an area where nurses can make a difference.

This chapter discusses bladder and bowel incontinence, focusing on the rehabilitation client with neurogenic dysfunction. Recognizing the different neurogenic bladder and bowel types through a nursing diagnosis and medical classification system is emphasized. Following assessment and diagnosis determination, interventions are described.

Neurogenic Bladder Functioning Process of Micturition

The bladder is a smooth muscular container that is under the control of the autonomic nervous system (Figure 1). Its function is to collect, store, and expel urine. The micturition process begins as the bladder fills and distends or enlarges. It is under reflexic and voluntary control. The reflex voiding center is located at spinal cord sacral segments 2 through 4. As the quantity of urine increases in the bladder, intramuscular sensory fibers are stimulated, causing an urge to void. The fibers send these impulses via the pelvic nerve to the sacral reflex center. The impulses travel up the spinothalamic and posterior columns, transferring the message "urge to void" to the micturition centers in the frontal cortex and brainstem. The impulse message travels down the reticulospinal tract to the pelvic nerves. The wall of the bladder is composed of smooth muscle layers known as the detrusor muscle. The pelvic nerves stimulate detrusor muscle contraction, closure of the urethral orifices, and internal sphincter relaxation (Hanak, 1992). In the bladder neck, muscle fibers converge to form an internal sphincter. The internal sphincter is the first valve in the bladder with an outflow tract at its base. Its function is to keep the bladder neck in the resting (noncontractile) state, maintaining continence (Zejdlik, 1983).

Voluntary control is maintained by the contraction and relaxation phases of the external sphincter and pelvic floor muscles. It is regulated by motor impulses

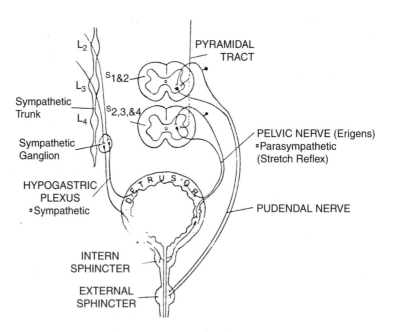

Fig 1. *Autonomic innervation of urinary bladder. (Permission granted by F. A. Davis Co.)*

moving from the frontal cortex down the corticospinal tract to the pudendal nerve. The external sphincter is a striated, skeletal, voluntary muscle surrounding the urethra. It is the second valve in the bladder with an outflow tract. If an individual is near a toileting facility and has the urge to void, the frontal cortex sends a message to the external sphincter to relax and allow emptying. If the time or place is not appropriate for emptying the bladder, the frontal cortex sends a message for the external sphincter to contract instead. For bladder emptying to occur, both urethral sphincters must relax in a synchronous manner.

There is also nervous system stimulation of the bladder. Sympathetic stimulation occurs at spinal cord levels T11 through L2 via the hypogastric nerve. This facilitates a slow filling of the bladder, relaxation of the detrusor muscle (storage of urine), and constriction of the internal sphincter (Pires, 1996). At spinal cord segments S2 through S4, there is parasympathetic stimulation and the final pathway for voluntary motor control. A combination of the nervous systems, along with cerebral control, is necessary for the completion of the micturition process. Cerebral control occurs at the pons and hypothalamus.

A normal bladder has no lesions, uninhibited contractions, or residual urine. The voiding stream is uninterrupted and bladder capacity is approximately 450 cm^3. Intravesical pressure remains fairly constant until bladder volume reaches about 400 cm^3, at which time the urge to void is strong. The first desire to void occurs at about 150 cm^3 (S. Boyarsky, Labay, Hanick, Abramson, & R. Boyarsky, 1979). When there is disruption of the neurological control mechanisms, a normal bladder becomes a **neurogenic bladder** secondary to cortical or subcortical brain lesions, spinal cord lesions, peripheral nerve damage, or abnormalities in the autonomous innervation of the bladder wall (Hanak, 1992).

Urinary Incontinence

Urinary incontinence is the involuntary loss of urine. It may be acute or chronic. Incontinence occurs when there is interference with the following: neural control (cerebrovascular accident [CVA], spinal cord injury), bladder function (inflammatory states, loss of contractility), the urethral sphincter mechanism ("stress" in females, "post-turp" in males), and environmental factors (radiation therapy, medications such as diuretics or anticholingerics). Incontinence is not a disease, but a symptom. It is an abnormal condition that often can be reversed if appropriately assessed and treated. It is a nursing responsibility, but adequate staffing is necessary in hospitals and extended care facilities if interventions other than the use of diapers or changing wet clothes is to occur (McCormick, Scheve, & Leahy, 1988).

The major stressor in caregiving in the home is incontinence (Morishita, 1988), resulting in the second leading cause of institutionalization for the elderly. At least 10 million adult Americans suffer from incontinence (Morishita, 1988). It occurs in 15 to 30 percent of noninstitutionalized people older than 60 and in at least one-half of the 1.5 million nursing home residents. It occurs twice as often in women than in men (Urinary Incontinence Guideline Panel, 1992). If you asked 10 people aged 65 or older if they had a problem with incontinence, five or six of them would state they do (Pires, Lockhart-Pretti, Smith, & Newman, 1991).

The cost for management of urinary incontinence continues to rise yearly. Approximately $7 billion a year is spent on community individuals, and about $3 billion is spent on those living in nursing homes (Pires, Lockhart-Pretti, Smith, & Newman, 1991). According to Hu (1990), direct health care costs were more than $10 billion in 1987, not including the costs for routine care, such as diapers and changing and cleaning of clothes and bedding. These costs are usually not reimbursed by insurance policies or government (Medicaid and Medicare). They are absorbed, instead, by individuals at home or by nursing homes. Direct health care costs can include diagnostic and medical evaluation, treatment for skin irritation, bladder infections, falls, surgical procedures, catheterizations, additional nursing home admissions, and hospital stays.

Beyond financial cost, there is the psychological cost to the individual. Frequently seen behaviors include isolation, loss of dignity, embarrassment, and guilt. Also observed are behaviors of regression, dependence, anger over loss of control, insecurity, and attention seeking (McCormick, Scheve, & Leahy, 1988).

Regardless of what causes incontinence, nurses can respond. Nurses can recommend treatment protocols, such as pelvic floor exercises (Kegel exercises), habit training, and bladder training (Morishita, 1988). The most important intervention that nurses can do is to make a more thorough assessment of a client's bladder functioning status.

Assessment

A thorough assessment should consist of a client interview, tools of measurement, nursing observation, physical examination, and diagnostic laboratory studies.

Start your assessment with open-ended questions. Give your client the opportunity to tell his or her story. Some clients with incontinence do not recognize it as a problem and if asked, "Are you incontinent?" or "Do you have accidents?" the response is "No!" It would be better to ask, "Do you have trouble getting to the bathroom on time?" or "Do you wear pads to catch your urine?" (Wyman, 1988). For someone with neurological problems, you might ask, "Can you tell when you are going to urinate?" or "Can you stop and start your voiding stream?" (Pires, 1996). If the client recognizes that there is a problem, determine what the attitude is about incontinence. Is incontinence perceived as an inconvenience or a disruption of life? Is it seen as "part of aging" and accepted, or a solvable problem?

The following areas must also be included as part of the client interview:

- Usual urinary elimination pattern
- Use of any special assistive devices

- Usual fluid intake
- Recent changes in urinary pattern
- Family and personal medical history
- Use of medications
- Cognition functioning

The usual urinary elimination pattern is determined by asking the client specifics on timing, hesitancy, frequency, nocturia, straining, interruption of stream, amount of urine each voiding, color, odor, and discomfort. Usual voiding patterns range from six to eight times during the day and two or fewer voidings during the night (Abrams, Feneley, & Torrens, 1983). Ask the client what special assistive devices he or she uses to aid with toileting, if any, such as a commode, bedpan, or catheters. Assess what the client's usual fluid intake is and the timing, amount, and types of fluids. Does the client complain of any recent changes in urinary pattern: frequency, urgency, hesitancy, dribbling, retention, or discomfort? Is he or she aware of any known factors for these changes in pattern?

Family and personal history can add further information about the client's condition when it is comprehensive. Ask your client if there is history of renal disease, diabetes, bladder infections, or neurological disorders. Has your client experienced a recent major trauma, sexual problems, infections, or stool impaction? Is she pregnant or experiencing menopause? Perhaps she is incontinent due to lack of postpartum exercise. Does your client have new onset diabetes or a neurological disorder? With women, it is important to determine if voiding after sexual intercourse leads to discomfort, their history of pregnancies, hygiene practices, and method of wiping the perineal area. For men, history of prostate problems needs to be addressed.

Perform a drug history. What medications are being taken by the client (over-the-counter and prescription)? Common causes of transient urinary incontinence include sedative hypnotics, diuretics, calcium channel blockers, anticholinergic agents (antihistamines, antidepressants, antipsychotics, opiates, antispasmodics, antiparkinsonian agents), and α-adrenergic agents (Urinary Incontinence Guideline Panel, 1992).

Interviewing a client can also help determine the cognitive functioning status. The Mini-Mental State Examination measures orientation, registration, attention, and calculation, recall, and language (M. Folstein, S. Folstein, & McHugh, 1975). Clients with cognitive deficits do not always recognize the social significance of remaining dry and, therefore, do not search out toileting assistance on their own.

Tools of measurement include an accurate intake/output record and the client's personal bladder record/voiding diary. These tools can give a better picture of the client's incontinence: the type, frequency, amount, and what leads to the episode each time. Recording of this information should be done for at least 1 week.

Nursing observation is a key to successful assessment. Is your client wearing incontinence pads or were pads brought to the hospital? Is there a foul-smelling odor in the room, suggesting wetness? What position does the client use to facilitate voiding? What environmental factors suggest the potential for incontinence due to limited mobility: high raised toilet seat, grab bars, use of adaptive devices for ambulating? Assess the time required to get to the toilet from a defined starting point, undress, and position on a toilet safely. Assess the client's ability to perform activities of daily living.

Part of nursing observation is a physical examination. This includes assessing abdominal muscle tone, superpubic masses, presence of tenderness, and bladder distention. Examining the genital area includes assessing for any skin breakdown and signs of infection.

Signs of atrophic vaginitis or monilial infection are assessed in women as well. A pelvic examination performed by inserting one or two lubricated, gloved fingers into the vagina can detect the presence of masses, pelvic prolapse, tenderness, or discharge. This would be a good time to ask the woman to squeeze around the examiner's fingers to assess her ability to contract the muscles of the pelvic floor and paravaginal muscle tone (Pires, 1996).

A rectal examination is done to assess for sphincteric tone, stool impaction, masses, contour of the prostate for men, perineal sensation (Figure 2), and the bulbocavernosus reflex. The **bulbocavernosus reflex** (Figure 3) is especially helpful in determining the type of neurogenic bowel and bladder, as it determines reflexic activity of sacral segments 2 through 4. This reflex is stimulated by squeezing the glans penis or glans clitoris while a gloved finger is inserted into the anus. If there is an anal contraction felt by the examiner, a positive bulbocavernosus re-

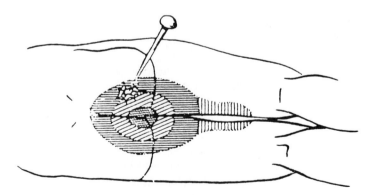

Fig 2. *Pinprick test for perineal sensation. (Permission granted by Rancho Los Amigos Medical Center)*

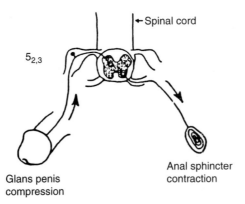

Fig 3. *Bulbocavernosus reflex. (Permission granted by Rancho Los Amigos Medical Center.)*

flex is present. If no anal contraction is felt, there is a negative bulbocavernosus reflex.

On further examination, the presence of edema in the extremities or sacral edema also needs to be assessed. Edema could contribute to the occurrence of nocturia and neurologic conditions that lead to incontinence (Wyman, 1988).

Diagnostic laboratory studies include a urinalysis, urine for culture and sensitivity, and urine for specific gravity and pH balance. Blood tests for blood urea nitrogen (BUN) and creatinine levels might be ordered for clients with possible outlet obstruction, noncompliant bladders, or retention (Pires, 1996). Performing a postvoid residual (PVR) via catheterization is a test frequently given to clients with a neurogenic bladder. It should be done immediately following a voiding episode, determining the amount of urine retained in the bladder. A residual of 50 to 100 cm³ indicates possible disruption in bladder emptying (McCormick, Scheve, & Leahy, 1988). Specialized diagnostic tests include urodynamic testing, endoscopic testing, and imaging.

Urodynamics

Urodynamic testing (UDT) is an important parameter required for complete evaluation of the genitourinary tract. It is a complex of studies that demonstrates mechanical, electrical, and neurological functions of the urinary bladder. Caution must be taken, however, in the interpretation, as it is not equivalent to an EKG in its evaluation.

The following tests are described individually, but a complete set of testing includes

- *Cystometrogram* (*CMG*): Measures the pressure within the bladder and shows with UDT the bladder wall compliance (measurement of compliance change in volume divided by change in pressure when filling study is done). The measurement of intravesical pressure consists of detrusor contractile pressure plus intra-abdominal pressure. As a result, one can measure true voiding pressure if able to distend the bladder adequately and measure it during voiding (Mundy, Stephenson, & Wein, 1984).
- *Intrarectal pressure* (*IRP*): Measures the summation of forces from inherent abdominal wall pressure plus gravitational pressure plus straining pressures within the abdomen (intravesical pressure minus intrarectal pressure equals detrusor pressure).
- *Electromyography* (*EMG*): An EMG of the urethral sphincter shows the electrical activity of the external urethral striated sphincter. (See Figure 4 for a normal versus abnormal urodynamic study tracing.)
- *Urethral pressure profile* (*UPP*): A UPP measures the functional length and pressure of the external urinary sphincter.
- *Fluorourodynamics:* Provides a complete urodynamic study of the bladder performed under fluoroscopic control with use of radiopaque contrast medium as the filling agent. This gives pressure measurements with synchronous micturition cysto-urethrography. With this study, vesicorenal reflux (backflow of urine from the bladder to kidney) can be identified at critical volumes and pressures.
- *Leak point pressure* (*LPP*): The intravesical pressure measured at the moment of fluid leakage during "straining" or Valsalva's maneuver (Urinary Incontinence Practice Guideline Panel, 1992). It can be measured by a simple manometer set up, level to the symphysis pubis.
- *Cystoscopy* is an endoscopic examination of the urethra, bladder, and bladder neck by direct vision through the medium of water. It also gives an examination of the prostatic urethra for the male client. Via instrumentation, biopsies of the bladder or urethral lesions can be obtained.
- *Cystogram:* A radiographic study of the bladder showing its contour, whether reflux is present or absent, and whether bladder stones are present or absent. In the neurogenic client, especially those who have a a spinal cord injury (SCI), it is common to see a classic "Christmas tree"-shaped bladder, which is diagnostic in reflexic disorders.
- *Urethrogram:* Entails the radiographic outlining of the urethra, assessing for strictures, anatomical variation of structure, urethral false passageways, diverticulum, fistulas, abscesses, or extravasation.

Classification System

Assessment can also include the determination of neurogenic bladder type. A classification system groups observed events into categories based on common characteristics. There are several existing classification systems used to name specific types of neurogenic bladders. This book uses the Lapides classification system.

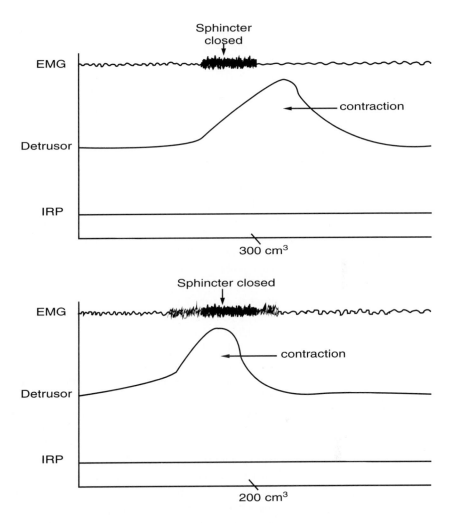

Fig 4. *Normal versus abnormal urodynamic study.* Top: *Normal bladder: Client has urge to void, bladder contracts, and client voluntarily released sphincter to void.* Bottom: *DSD (detrusor–external sphincter dyssynergia): Bladder is contracting but sphincter is closed; urine retained. EMG, electromyogram.*

The Lapides classification system describes the clinical and cystometric (capacity, proprioception, contractility, heat and cold sensation, residual urine) findings associated with many types of neurogenic voiding dysfunction. The Lapides classification system, also known as the classic neuro-urologic classification system, has five categories: the uninhibited neurogenic bladder, reflex neurogenic bladder, areflexic neurogenic bladder, sensory neurogenic bladder, and the motor paralytic bladder (Staskin, 1991).

The *uninhibited neurogenic bladder* results from an injury or disease in the corticoregulatory tract, which has an inhibitory effect on micturition. Damage to this tract results in uninhibited bladder contractions (Staskin, 1991). Clients who are found to have a lesion in the cerebral cortex, spinal motor pathway, or in the cord level before reflex synapse will have an uninhibited neurogenic bladder. A cystometrogram will show that as an uninhibited contraction occurs, the client will have an urge to void; the first urge occurring at approximately 60 cm^3. The perception of fullness occurs at about 160 cm^3. Finally, a strong contraction occurs, pushing urine around the catheter. Bladder capacity is very limited at about 165 cm^3, while frequency and urgency are experienced. The voiding stream is normal, and there is no residual urine (S. Boyarsky, Labay, Hanick, Abramson, & R. Boyarsky, 1979) (Figure 5). Signs and symptoms experienced with an uninhibited bladder include frequency, urgency, urge incontinence, nocturia, and decreased bladder capacity. **Saddle sensation** is present, and the bulbocavernosus reflex is normal (Table 1).

Possible etiology includes head injury or cerebral vascular accident (CVA). If a lesion occurs between the cerebral cortex and the pontine micturition center, an uninhibited bladder will result for the brain injury client. The pontine micturition, which is responsible for the co-ordinated function of the spinal micturition center (S2–4), remains intact. The normal kinesiology of micturition is present but because the client lacks the awareness of "urge to void" and fails to adequately suppress the pontine–spinal loops of micturition, frequent incontinence by reflex occurs (Andrews & Opitz, 1993). The lack of sphincter control following a brain injury is secondary to cognitive and behavioral disturbances in recognition of the basic need to void within acceptable social norms. The client ignores sensory signals or cannot respond appropriately owing to disorientation, agitation, communication, or immobility deficits (Grinspun, 1993).

The CVA client can be seen with three different types of bladder incontinence. One bladder type is hyperreflexia or **uninhibited.** Disruption of the neuromicturition areas and their pathways in the cerebral cortex can lead to loss of inhibitory and modulatory functions, which are necessary for continence. Following a stroke, the detrusor motor area is damaged, resulting in the client not being able to suppress or inhibit the urge to void (Gray, 1993). Hyperreflexia occurs when there is a disruption of the voluntary control by the cerebral cortex of the brainstem and the sacral spine reflex arc (S2–4). A poststroke study (Khan,

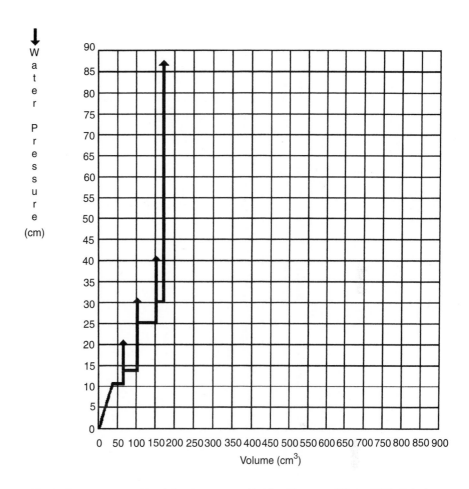

Fig 5. *Cystometrogram: Uninhibited neurogenic bladder. (Courtesy of Nancy Willis-Sukosky, MN, RN, CNA, CRRN.)*

Starer, Yang, & Bhola, 1990) showed that detrusor hyperreflexia was the most common cystometric finding in clients.

Some CVA clients have a normal bladder post-episode, but owing to CVA-related cognitive and language deficits experience incontinence. A small percentage of CVA clients have a hyporeflexic bladder or retention overflow. The cause can be concurrent neuropathy, such as CVA with a history of diabetes or the use of certain medications, such as anticholinergics. A breakdown of bladder function types determined in a study of 51 post-CVA clients (Gelber, Good, Laven, &

Table 1
Neurogenic Bladder Dysfunction and Management

Dysfunction	Level in Neuraxis	Possible Etiology	Voluntary Control	Saddle Sensation	Bulbocavernous Reflex	Signs and Symptoms	Management
Uninhibited neurogenic	Cortical and subcortical	Newborn child, CVA, MS, cerebral arteriosclerosis, brain tumor, pernicious anemia, trauma	Initiation and/or inhibition diminished	Normal	Normal	Frequency Urgency Urge incontinence Nocturia Decreased bladder capacity	Timed voiding Drugs Male: external collection device (condom-type) Female: "Padding"
Reflex neurogenic	Spinal cord above conus medullaris	Trauma, tumor, vascular disease, MS, syringomyelia, pernicious anemia	Absent	Absent or impaired	Hyperactive	Unpredictable voiding Stream starts and stops (may initially appear as areflexic during spinal shock)	Reflex triggering techniques Intermittent catheterization (IC) Drugs Surgery
Autonomous (areflexic) neurogenic, (careflexic)	At conus medullaris or cauda equina	Spina bifida, myelomeningocele, tumor, postoperative radical pelvic surgery, herniated intervertebral disk	Absent	Absent	Absent	Increased bladder capacity High residual Dribbling incontinence No bladder contractions Overflow (stress) Incontinence with straining or compression	Intermittent catheterization (IC) Strain (Valsalva maneuver) Credé's maneuver

| Motor paralytic | Anterior horn cells or S2, S3, S4 ventral roots | Poliomyelitis, herniated intervertebral disk, trauma, tumor | Absent | Normal | Absent | Voiding similar to patients with symptoms of "prostatism" strain to void incontinence rare | Intermittent catheterization Valsalva maneuver (strain) Credé's maneuver |
| Sensory paralytic | S2, S3, S4 dorsal roots or cells of origin or dorsal horns of spinal cord | Diabetes mellitus, tabes dorsalis | Normal initially, becomes impaired with chronic overdistention | Absent | Absent | Voids only 1–3 times daily—overflow incontinence rare | Timed voiding Intermittent catheterization (IC) |

Source: Rancho Los Amigos Medical Center.

Verhulst, 1993) indicated bladder hyperreflexia (37 percent), normal bladder (37 percent), bladder hyporeflexia (21 percent) and detrusor–sphincter dyssynergia (5 percent).

Other medical diagnoses, or causes, resulting in an uninhibited bladder include multiple sclerosis, cerebral arteriosclerosis, brain tumor, senility, infancy, and pernicious anemia.

The *reflex neurogenic bladder* occurs when there is complete interruption of the spinal pathways between the brainstem and sacral micturition center (Staskin, 1991). With a **reflexic** bladder, a neurologic lesion occurs between the pons and the sacrum, which disrupts the relationship between the pontine and sacral micturition centers. As a result, the sacral micturition becomes dyssynergic (Andrews & Opitz, 1993). Dyssynergia refers to various levels or degrees of detrusor and external sphincter contraction. Dyssynergia causes high voiding pressures and incomplete emptying of the bladder, creating a reflexic response (Andrews & Opitz, 1993). A cystometrogram will show many uninhibited contractions leading to a final contraction at about bladder capacity of 250 cm^3. At this strong contraction, urine will be forced around a catheter. The client does not feel any fullness and does not have an urge to void. He or she also has "residual" urine at about 125 cm^3, further decreasing the true capacity. The urinary stream can be weak to strong, but it is involuntary and interrupted. The client has no control over it (S. Boyarsky, Labay, Hanick, Abramson, R. Boyarsky, 1979), (Figure 6). Other signs and symptoms experienced by the client include unpredictable voiding, recurrent bladder infections, and spastic external sphincter; in addition, and the bladder may appear initially areflexic during spinal shock. Saddle sensation is present, and the bulbocavernosus reflex is hyperactive (Table 1).

Possible etiology includes spinal cord injury above the conus medullaris, spinal cord tumor, vascular disease, multiple sclerosis, syringomyelia, and pernicious anemia. With a spinal injury, the damage occurs above the conus medullaris (above the S2–4 segments), keeping the reflex arc intact. Control of the urinary sphincter and the sensation of fullness are absent. The bladder has a high number of detrusor contractions, leading to incontinence (King & Dudas, 1980).

A reflexic neurogenic bladder can also be classified as hypertonic, **automatic,** spastic, or upper motor neuron (above T12 lesion).

The *areflexic neurogenic bladder* occurs when there is complete sensory and motor separation of the bladder from the S2–4 segments of the spinal cord (Staskin, 1991). Damage has occurred to the cauda equina, disrupting pathways that carry sensory impulses from the spinal cord to the detrusor muscle and muscle impulses from the spinal cord to the external sphincter. A neurogenic lesion is present, involving the sacral micturition center or its connections to the bladder and pelvic floor muscle. This results in an underactive bladder and outlet, and an **areflexic** detrusor and external sphincter (Andrews & Opitz, 1993). The characteristics seen on a cystometrogram include absent uninhibited contractions be-

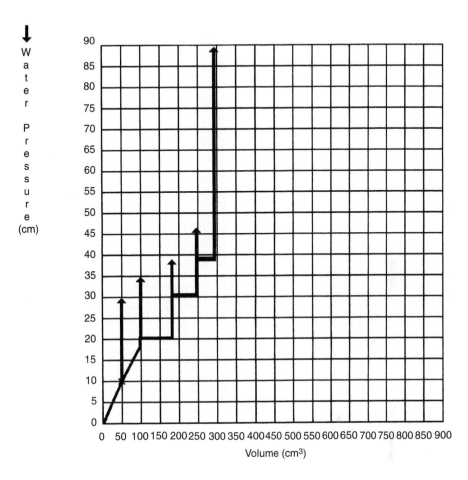

Fig 6. *Cystometrogram: Reflex neurogenic bladder. (Courtesy of Nancy Willis-Sukosky, MN, RN, CNA, CRRN.)*

cause the sacral reflex arc is interrupted, a bladder capacity of about 700 cm³ or greater, a voiding stream that is very weak without some type of suprapubic pressure (Crede's maneuver) applied, and a residual urine of about 150 cm³ following a voiding attempt with applied pressure. The client has no perception of fullness, no uninhibited contractions, and no reflex. Therefore, voiding without suprapubic pressure and possible use of medication management is impossible (Figure 7). Other assessment findings include dribbling incontinence, **stress overflow** incontinence with straining or compression, absent saddle sensation, **flaccid** anal sphincter, and an absent bulbocavernosus reflex (Table 1).

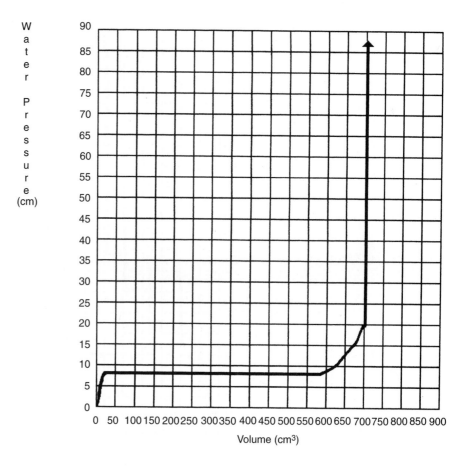

Fig 7. *Cystometrogram: Autonomous (areflexic) neurogenic bladder. (Courtesy of Nancy Willis-Sukosky MN, RN, CNA, CRRN.)*

Etiology resulting in an autonomous neurogenic bladder includes spinal cord injury at the conus medullaris or cauda equina injury, spina bifida, myelomeningocele, spinal cord tumor, status postradical pelvic surgery complication, and herniated intervertebral disk. A spinal cord injury occurring below or at the T12 level results in damage to the conus medullaris (where the S2–4 segments are located) or to the peripheral nerves. The reflex arc is absent. Determining whether the reflex arc is intact is necessary for correct assessment of neurogenic bladder types. Loss of control of the urinary sphincter and the loss of feeling "fullness" lead to retention of urine (King & Dudas, 1980).

The *sensory neurogenic bladder* results from selective interruption of the sensory fibers from the bladder to the spinal cord or from the afferent tracts to the brain (Staskin, 1991). The sensory (afferent) side of the micturition reflex arc is damaged. Characteristics similar to those of the **autonomous** (areflexic) neurogenic bladder are seen. On assessment, the client will show absent saddle sensation and an absent bulbocavernosus reflex. Voluntary control (motor function) is present but, because of chronic overdistention, it becomes impaired. There is a poor or weak **urge** to void, and the client tends to void only two or three times daily—sometimes, or eventually, only once. The most common medical diagnosis for this type of neurogenic bladder is diabetes mellitus (Table 1).

A *motor paralytic neurogenic bladder* is present when there is destruction of the motor innervation to the bladder (Staskin, 1991); the motor (efferent) side of the micturition reflex arc is damaged. Signs and symptoms, which are similar to those of the autonomous (areflexic) neurogenic bladder, include absent voluntary control, absent bulbocavernosus reflex, and a decreased urine stream. The client will experience large residual urine volumes as the detrusor muscle stretches and loses tone. As such, incontinence is rare. Saddle sensation is present, and the client feels "fullness" or "painful retention." Owing to absent motor function, the client will need to "strain" to void and will have difficulty starting the urine stream. Medical diagnoses commonly resulting in a motor paralytic neurogenic bladder include poliomyelitis, herniated intervertebral disk, trauma, tumor, and Guillian-Barré syndrome (Table 1).

The Nursing Process: Nursing Diagnoses, Goals, and Interventions

Once a thorough assessment has been made, a nursing diagnosis, can be formulated. The following nursing diagnoses, which relate to the problem of urinary incontinence, approved by the North American Nursing Diagnosis Association (NANDA), are discussed: stress incontinence, urge incontinence, reflex incontinence, urinary retention, and functional incontinence.

Stress incontinence is defined as "the state in which an individual experiences an immediate involuntary loss of urine upon an increase in intra-abdominal pressure" (Carpenito, 1993, p. 842). There is incompetency of the outlet at the base of the bladder and insufficient resistance of the urethral sphincter to the pressure exerted by the bladder (Palmer, 1990). The client will usually complain of a loss of urine (usually less than 50 cm^3) occurring with increased abdominal pressure from standing, sneezing, coughing, running, laughing, or lifting heavy objects. The urge and voiding frequency will occur more often than every 2 hours (Voith, 1988). Causes include obesity and gravid uterus from high intra-abdominal pressure, multiple pregnancies and bouncing exercises from weak abdominal muscles and structural supports, chronic overdistention (Voith, 1986, 1988), urinary tract anomalies or disorders, estrogen deficiency (Carpenito, 1993), and neurogenic sphincter deficiency (i.e., myelomeningocele) (Urinary Incontinence Guideline Panel, 1992). Diagnostic tests used to confirm the diagnosis include the EMG, stress test for direct visualization, stress cystourethrogram, and dynamic profilometry or leak point pressure (Urinary Incontinence Guideline Panel, 1992).

Nursing Diagnosis
- Stress incontinence related to decreased outlet resistance.

Goals/Outcomes
- Client will have reduced bladder irritability and an increase in tone of supporting structures (Voith, 1986).
- Client will report a reduction or elimination in stress incontinence (Carpenito, 1993).

Nursing Interventions
- Assess cause of incontinence, pattern of voiding, and fluid intake.
- Teach pelvic floor exercises (Kegel exercises).
- Medication management as ordered by physician: the use of α-adrenergics and possible combined treatment with estrogens for women postmenses.

Pelvic floor exercises (Kegel exercises) are performed by instructing the client to voluntarily tighten the pubococcygeus (ring of muscle around the vagina and/or anus) without contracting the legs, buttocks, or abdominal muscles. This should be held for about 10 seconds. This exercise should be repeated 10 times at three intervals daily (McCormick, Scheve, & Leahy, 1998). The pubococcygeus muscle is present in both men and women. "The pelvic floor muscle exercises improve urethral resistance through active exercise of the pubococcygeus muscle. The exercises strengthen the voluntary periurethral and pelvic muscles. The contraction exerts a closing force on the urethra and increases muscle support to the pelvic visceral structures" (Urinary Incontinence Guideline Panel, 1992, p. 31). The exercises should be done before and after situations that lead to leakage. Many clients have reported improved or complete continence (Urinary Incontinence Guideline Panel, 1992).

Biofeedback provides visual feedback about the bladder, abdominal pressures, and external anal sphincter activity so that voluntary sphincter contraction, bladder inhibition, or abdominal relaxation can be taught to the client (McCormick, Scheve, & Leahy, 1988).

Vaginal cone retention may be used in adjunct to pelvic muscle exercise training with women. A series of weighted cones are inserted into the vagina and are kept in place to contract the pubococcygeus muscle. The vaginal cones should be in place for 15 minutes, once or twice daily (Pires, Lockhart-Pretti, Smith, & Newman, 1991).

Electrical stimulation involves stimulating the pelvic viscera, the pelvic muscles, or the nerve supply to these structures (Urinary Incontinence Guideline

Panel, 1992). This can occur internally via a device involving electrical impulses, which is implanted into the pelvic floor musculature, or externally via an external electrical current, which stimulates muscle contraction (McCormick, Scheve, & Leahy, 1988).

Medication management includes the use of α-adrenergics, which promote contraction of the urethral smooth muscle and increase outlet resistance. Drugs, such as pseudoephedrine, imipramine, and phenylpropanolamine, can be used to improve bladder functioning, but can cause delirium or increase the effects of hypertension, cardiovascular disease, and pulmonary disease (Wein, 1990).

Urge incontinence is defined as "the state in which an individual experiences an involuntary loss of urine associated with a strong, sudden desire to void" (Carpenito, 1993, p. 848). Signs and symptoms include uninhibited contractions of the detrusor muscle. There is low bladder volume capacity and frequent voiding urgency leading to incontinence (Palmer, 1990; Carpenito, 1993). The client has the capacity to initiate micturition but cannot inhibit the flow (Dittmar, 1989). Assessment findings and causes are similar to the "uninhibited neurogenic bladder," discussed previously (Figure 8). Other causes include the presence of a bladder infection, holding off "urination," and the use of diuretics (Voith, 1986). Diagnostic testing to confirm this diagnosis includes the use of the "filling" or "simple" CMG (Urinary Incontinence Guideline Panel, 1992).

Nursing Diagnosis
- Urge incontinence related to detrusor instability or irritation.

Goals/Outcomes
- Client will report absence or decreased episodes of incontinence (Carpenito, 1993).

Nursing Interventions
- Assess cause of incontinence, pattern of voiding, and fluid intake.
- Push fluids; limit after dinner.
- Teach client pelvic floor exercises (if cognitive status is not impaired).
- Implement bladder training program or habit training program.
- Supplement habit training program with "prompted voiding."
- Medication management as prescribed by the physician: anticholinergics/spasmodics, musculotropic relaxants, calcium antagonists, tricyclic antidepressants, and β-adrenergic agonists will be considered.

The bladder training, or retraining, program entails taking the client to the bathroom to void at established intervals of time, usually starting at every 1 to 2 hours and then gradually increasing to every 3 to 4 hours. At the intervals, the client is prompted to go to the bathroom. During the interval of time, the client may ask to use the bathroom or may use the bathroom independent of staff. The interval of time may increase or decrease depending on the client's "dryness" status. Relaxation techniques, including deep breathing, can help increase the time

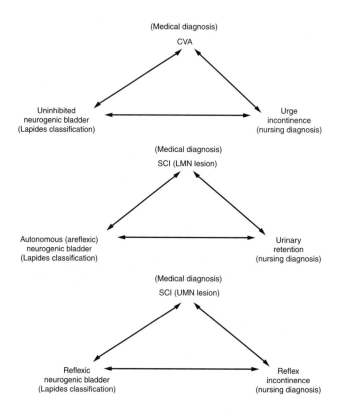

Fig 8. *Comparison of Lapides Classification to nursing diagnoses.*

interval for the client, whenever the urge to void occurs. Client education, scheduled timing, and positive reinforcement are necessary for this intervention to be successful. Praise the client if dry or if he or she urinated in the bathroom on command successfully (Palmer, 1990; Pires, Lockhart-Pretti, Smith, & Newman, 1991). A controlled study by Fantl, Wyman, McClish, Harkins, Elswick, and Taylor (1991) showed that 12 percent of women became continent with the bladder training program and 75 percent improved with a 50 percent decrease in the number of episodes.

The habit training program differs from the bladder training program in that specific times of the day are scheduled for voiding, such as 30 minutes after meals, on awakening, before sleeping, or every 3 hours during the day and perhaps two times during the night. The client is encouraged to use the bathroom or ask for assistance at these specific times. If the client has the urge to void at different times, or intervals, the toileting schedule will need adjustment. Positive reinforcement of desired behavior is necessary with this program as well. The goal is keeping the client dry, asking the client to void at regular intervals, and trying to return to the client's previous regular pattern of voiding (Urinary Incontinence Guideline Panel, 1992; Palmer, 1990; and Pires, Lockhart-Pretti, Smith, & Newman, 1991).

Prompted voiding is a supplement to habit training. It attempts to teach the incontinent client to discriminate his or her incontinence status and to ask for assistance from caregivers. This approach requires monitoring, prompting, and praising (Urinary Incontinence Guideline Panel, 1992).

Medication management usually includes the use of anticholinergics/spasmodics, such as propantheline, imipramine, oxybutynin, flavoxate, and dicyclomine. These drugs decrease bladder contractility. There is also a decreased spasmodic action on smooth muscles, suppressing the parasympathetic responses. Possible side effects include a dry mouth, tachycardia, dizziness, drowsiness, urinary retention, and a changed mental status from an overdose (Wein, 1990; Wyndaele, 1990; Wilson & Shannon, 1993). Oxybutynin chloride (Ditropan) is also classified as a musculotropic relaxant, increasing bladder capacity through its antispasmodic activity. Calcium antagonists decrease bladder contractility, as do tricyclic antidepressants, such as imipramine hydrochloride. Imipramine hydrochloride (Tofranil) also increases outlet resistance. It has a strong systemic anticholinergic effect, but a weak antimuscularimic effect on the bladder smooth muscle. Potential side effects, such as weakness, fatigue, postural hypotension, and hip fractures, are likely to occur in the elderly (Wein, 1990). β-adrenergic agonists, such as terbutaline, increase bladder capacity. Terbutaline increases uterine relaxation, thereby preventing or abolishing high intrauterine pressure (Wilson & Shannon, 1993).

Reflex incontinence is defined as "the state in which the individual experiences an involuntary loss of urine caused by damage to the spinal cord between the cortical and sacral (S1, S2, S3) bladder centers" (Carpenito, 1993, p. 840). Voiding occurs in a potentially predictable pattern because, when the reflex arc controls micturition, voiding will be triggered each time the bladder stretch receptors indicate to the spinal cord that the bladder is distended to a particular degree (i.e., 250 cm^3) (Voith, 1988). Characteristics and causes of reflex incontinence are similar to those described previously for reflexic neurogenic bladder, such as chronic high residuals, lack of feeling "fullness," and no awareness of the bladder filling (Rehabilitation Nursing Foundation, 1995) (Figure 8). Diagnostic tests to determine reflex incontinence include a CMG, EMG, and intrarectal pressure.

Nursing Diagnosis

- Reflex incontinence related to sensory and motor deficits secondary to a spinal cord injury (SCI) above T12.

Goals/Outcomes

- Client will achieve a low-pressure bladder emptying system; client will achieve complete bladder emptying with acceptable postvoid residuals without incontinence (Rehabilitation Nursing Foundation, 1995).
- Client will use triggering methods to initiate reflex voiding (Carpenito, 1993).

Nursing Interventions

- Intermittent catheterization every 4 to 6 hours or external catheterization (bladder emptying methods).
- Teach the client to adhere to a regular schedule for emptying the bladder.
- Instruct the client as to the necessary amount of fluid intake, depending on the bladder emptying method used and postvoid residuals.
- Teach and assist the client with bladder emptying "triggers" to stimulate a reflex response (external catheterization method).
- Indwelling catheter with fluid intake of 2000–2500 cm^3 daily (least desirable method).
- Use a bladder ultrasound or postvoid residuals to determine effectiveness of client's voiding.
- Medication management of α-adrenergic blocking agents and skeletal muscle relaxants. Anticholinergics, such as Ditropan or Banthine may be used if the client is using the intermittent catheterization program for bladder emptying, decreasing bladder spasticity and contractions.
- Prepare the client to handle episodes of incontinence with use of external catheter or absorbent padding.

Intermittent catheterization (IC) on a regular schedule is the preferred method of bladder emptying for the client with reflex incontinence. A regular pattern of catheterization prevents bladder distention and the occurrence of urinary tract infections (Latham, 1994). Intermittent catheterization consists of inserting a clean or sterile tube into the bladder for drainage at scheduled intervals and then removing it (Palmer, 1990). A client receiving intermittent catheterization every 4 hours needs to watch his or her fluid intake carefully. Generally, 100 cm^3 per hour is allowed.

Another option for the client with reflex incontinence is to start bladder training with intermittent catheterization, but gradually to move to an external catheterization program. Initially, every 4 hours the client attempts to void following reflex-stimulating methods, such as suprapubic tapping or tugging on pubic hairs. Measure any amount voided, then catheterize and measure that output. The amount voided (if any) plus the amount obtained by catheterization should not exceed 400 to 500 cm^3 (bladder capacity). When the client begins to void at least 100 cm^3 between periods of catheterization, with a residual urine of 300 cm^3 or less each time, the time interval is changed to every 6 hours with ad libitum intake of fluids allowed. The goal is to obtain a "balanced bladder." When a bladder balance of 50 : 50 is reached (void amount after triggering methods equals the residual urine amount after catheterization), the time interval is changed again to every 8 hours. As bladder balance improves, catheterization is done less frequently (i.e., every 12 hours) and then once daily. Once voiding with triggering methods to stimulate a reflexic response is adequate and postvoid residuals are less than 50 to 75 cm³, the client uses an external catheter for bladder emptying, and urinary output is assessed every shift. Residuals are usually checked weekly and recorded; eventually they are checked only quarterly (Rancho Los Amigos Medical Center, 1987).

Triggering techniques for emptying the reflexic bladder include light tapping, tugging on pubic hair, stroking the inner thighs, running water, drinking warm fluids, and a warm shower (Andrews & Opitz, 1993; Rehabilitation Nursing Foundation, 1995). Suprapubic tapping should be done using a rapid but light approach. Avoid heavy tapping, which can lead to degrees of dyssynergia, increased detrusor contractions, increased residual urine volumes, and increased episodes of bladder infections (Andrews & Opitz, 1993).

Postvoid residuals are done regularly to determine the status of a "balanced bladder." If residuals are too high, more than 100 cm³, the time interval of catheterizations will need to be adjusted "closer" together (i.e., from every 6 hours to every 4 hours). To perform a postvoid residual correctly, have the client void first following triggering methods, record the amount, and then catheterize and record the residual amount.

Clients who choose to use the external catheterization-void by reflex response method for bladder emptying are commonly on α-adrenergic blocking agents (Dibenzyline and Hytrin), which decrease bladder outlet resistance, and skeletal muscle relaxants (Lioresal), which inhibit the reflexes in the skeletal muscles and relax the striated muscle of the external sphincter, allowing urine to flow freely. α-Adrenergic blocking agents lower the blood pressure, which can be helpful for SCI clients who are prone to autonomic dysreflexia. The nurse must watch for postural hypotension, dizziness, headache, faintness, and palpitations. Lioresal can lead to dizziness, drowsiness, and vertigo. It can also increase blood glucose levels. Teach the client not to take these medications with central nervous system (CNS) depressants, such as alcohol (Wilson & Shannon, 1993; Wyndaele, 1990).

The use of an indwelling catheter has its complications, such as chronic bladder infections, bladder stones, and chronic irritation, which can lead to a squamous cell carcinoma of the bladder. "Minimize these complications by ensuring adequate fluid intake, maintaining a catheter changing schedule, and using the smallest lumen or balloon possible" (Rehabilitation Nursing Foundation, 1995, p. 4).

Some clients with a reflexic bladder will need surgical intervention when bladder programs and medication management fail to decrease spasticity of the bladder neck and external sphincter (Menon & Tan, 1992), namely a bladder neck incision and external sphincterotomy.

Urinary retention is defined as "incomplete emptying of the bladder" (Rehabilitation Nursing Foundation, 1995, p. 5). Carpenito (1993) defined it as "the state in which an individual experiences a chronic inability to void followed by involuntary voiding (overflow incontinence)" (p. 851). With overflow incontinence, there is usually obstruction at the outlet of the bladder. This is seen in men who are diagnosed with benign prostate hypertrophy (BPH) or is present when there are disruptions in nerve transmissions leading to insufficient bladder contractions or uncoordinated bladder contraction and urethral sphincter relaxation (Palmer, 1990). The causes and characteristics are similar to those described for the autonomous (areflexic) bladder (Figure 8), including bladder distention, high residual urines, or the absence of urine output. Often, the client will say "I feel like I still need to go more." Possible diagnostic tests to evaluate for overflow incontinence are a postvoid residual, uroflowmetry, voiding CMG (pressure flow), and a cystourethroscopy (Urinary Incontinence Guideline Panel, 1992).

One cause of a nursing diagnosis of urinary retention or overflow incontinence is a spinal cord injury at the conus medullaris where the reflex arc is damaged. However, SCI clients who are in "spinal shock," which occurs immediately following the injury, also encounter urinary retention. During spinal shock, the client has flaccid paralysis, and the bladder is acontractile. The smooth muscle of the detrusor and rectum is affected, resulting in overflow incontinence and constipation. This can last a few days to possibly 2 months (Menon & Tan, 1992). Interventions are as listed below unless or until spinal shock resolves and the client has a reflexic bladder.

Nursing Diagnosis
- Urinary retention related to prostate enlargement.
- Urinary retention related to nonintact sacral reflex arc.

Goals/Outcomes
- Client will have complete emptying with acceptable postvoid residuals (Rehabilitation Nursing Foundation, 1995).
- Client will empty bladder with Crede's and/or Valsalva's maneuvers with residual urines less than 50 cm^3 (Carpenito, 1993).

Nursing Interventions
- Intermittent catheterization every 4 to 6 hours.
- Strain void (Valsalva's maneuver) every 3 to 4 hours.
- Crede's maneuver.

- Fluid intake approximately 2000 cm^3 daily throughout waking hours.
- Instruct client to establish a regular schedule for voiding.
- Instruct client on using bladder emptying triggers previously discussed (tapping over the bladder, tugging on pubic hair, stroking the inner thighs, running water, drinking warm fluids, taking a warm shower or bath).
- Medication management: cholinergic agents and α-adrenergic antagonists.

Triggering mechanisms commonly used for the client with urinary retention include Crede's maneuver and straining (also called Valsalva's maneuver or compression).

The technique of **strain voiding** involves sitting and resting the abdomen forward on the thighs for men and women. To transfer abdominal pressure to the bladder and pelvic floor, hug the knees and legs, which prevents bulging of the abdomen (Andrews & Opitz, 1993). This method would not be advised for someone with a history of cardiac problems.

Crede's maneuver is the exertion of manual pressure over the lower abdomen to express urine from the bladder (Palmer, 1990). The bladder can be compressed using the fist of one hand or using an open-handed approach, which involves placing the thumb of each hand over the area of the left and right anterosuperior iliac spine and fingers over the suprapubic area with slight overlapping of the tips (Andrews & Opitz, 1993). Press downward into the pelvic cavity. Be sure that the client has no history of an abdominal mass or aneurysm which would contraindicate this method. Straining and Crede's maneuver should be done separately, not together.

Cholinergic agents, such as Urecholine (devoid) and bethanechol, are used to increase detrusor contractility. Sometimes α-adrenergic antagonists, such as Hytrin and phenoxybenzamine, are used to decrease bladder outlet resistance as necessary. "Administering bethanechol forty-five minutes before voiding may augment mechanical stimulation of the detrusor" (Andrews & Opitz, 1993, p. 204). Some side effects to watch for include hypotension with dizziness, faintness, flushing, orthostatic hypotension (large doses), mild reflex tachycardia, atrial fibrillation (hyperthyroid clients), and transient complete heart block (Wilson & Shannon, 1993).

Functional incontinence is defined as "the state in which an individual experiences a difficulty or inability to reach the toilet in time due to urgency, environmental barriers, decreased attention to cues and/or physical limitations" (Carpenito, 1993, p. 836). Etiology can be pathophysiologic (brain injury or Alzheimer's disease), treatment related (hypnotics, analgesics), situational (impaired mobility), or maturational (in the elderly, loss of perineal muscle tone). Sensory deficits and limitations in mobility and dexterity tend to result in functional incontinence (Lincoln & Roberts, 1989). These clients have incontinence before or during an attempt to reach the toilet and usually void a large amount at one time.

Nursing Diagnosis
- Functional incontinence related to the inability to reach the toilet quickly.
- Functional incontinence related to disorientation.

Goals/Outcomes
- Client will remove environmental barriers from home (Carpenito, 1993).
- Client will use proper adaptive equipment to assist with voiding transfers (Carpenito, 1993).

Nursing Interventions
- Determine cause of functional incontinence.
- Decrease or eliminate causal factors.
- Promote client motivation to remain "dry" through praise and encouragement to use toilet, commode, or bedpan/urinal.
- Assess for and encourage intact skin integrity and client's personal hygiene habits.
- Orient to unfamiliar settings.
- Limit intake of fluids after dinner and during sleeping hours.
- Keep commode, urinal, or bedpan within close reach.
- Instruct client to wear skid-proof slippers and to use ambulation aides and grab bars as needed.
- Remove environmental barriers to commode or bathroom.

General Nursing Interventions
General nursing interventions for all forms of incontinence include the following instruction to clients:

- Avoid diuretic beverages, such as caffeine and alcohol.
- Maintain a regular pattern of bowel emptying and avoid constipation. Stool in the colon puts back pressure on the bladder, resulting in urgency.

Other Possible Nursing Diagnoses
- High risk for impaired skin integrity related to incontinence.
- Social isolation related to embarrassment from having incontinence episodes.
- High risk for infection related to urinary retention or urinary leakage.

Surgical Interventions The following surgeries are options for clients with a neurogenic bladder to consider: bladder neck incision and external sphincterotomy (BNI&ES) (reflex neurogenic), transurethral resection of the prostate (TURP) for motor paralytic or areflexic-autonomous bladder, suprapubic cystostomy (urinary excretion with appliance), and urinary diversions (externalizing the ureters to bypass the urinary bladder).

BNI&ES is sometimes necessary and the only alternative for the client with cervical traumatic myelopathy with detrusor sphincter dyssynergia (muscular inco-ordination) who is presented with a reflexic neurogenic bladder that is complete. The bladder does not respond well to medication management, has a high pressure (on voiding), or has hydronephrosis. To disrupt the high voiding pressures due to the obstructive dysfunction of the bladder neck and external sphincter dyssynergia, a BNI&ES is performed. This consists of two separate incisions performed with a Kern knife and electrocautery current. It converts the bladder neck and external urinary sphincters from being diaphragmatic ringlike valve muscles into patent arches. In other words, the closing function of the muscles is terminated. The end result should be low voiding pressure and no outlet obstruction.

A TURP is indicated for the client with bladder outlet obstruction due to benign prostatic hypertrophy. This can also be performed for the neurologically compromised client who has a motor paralytic bladder or autonomous areflexic bladder and chooses to "strain void" for bladder elimination. (*Note:* The current method of choice for these clients to empty the bladder is intermittent catheterization.)

This procedure is done with a resectoscope (a large operating scope) and a cutting loop for electrocautery. To illustrate the operation in another perspective, imagine the prostate as a naval orange. Via the naval, the orange meat is removed, leaving orange skin (the surgical capsule) behind. This removes all the obstructive tissue and leaves a wide open space for the urine to bypass. The remaining skin or prostatic gland needs yearly rectal examinations for prostatic cancer. Also seen is a large space as the interior, or the orange skin, leaves some clients with a location for postoperative bleeding. Complications, besides bleeding, can include urethral strictures from trauma of surgery or bladder neck contractures.

Indications for a *suprapubic cystostomy* include urethral strictures or urethral trauma. It is a temporary method for draining urine from the bladder. This can be done either by percutaneous puncture with placement of a Stamey catheter or by surgically opening the bladder and placing a catheter via the abdominal wall into the bladder. If the catheter gets plugged or if the client has bladder spasms, urine will still drain via the urethra.

Urinary diversions use the intestine as a urinary conduit. It is a well known set of procedures indicated in clients, such as some cancer clients, who require removal of the urinary bladder. In neurologically compromised clients, it is often by choice that urinary diversions are performed.

The *ileal cystoplasty* (bladder augmentation) is a procedure in which a segment of the intestine is removed from the intestinal tract, which is then detubularized. The integrity of the intestinal tract becomes re-established. After this occurs, the dome of the bladder is removed in a cup form, the rest of the muscular wall is disrupted, and the detubularized intestine is formed into a patch. Next, it is sutured to the top of the bladder as a replacement noncontractile bladder dome. This converts it into a large, low-pressure, urinary reservoir. An additional procedure that is often done for the ease of performing intermittent catheterization through the abdominal wall is the placement of a Mitrofonoff valve at the umbilicus. "The Mitrofanoff continent catheterizable channel is a surgical option that gives rehabilitation patients who have difficulty gaining access to their urethras for clean intermittent catheterization more independence in self care" (Kurtz, Van Zand, & Sapp, 1996, p. 311).

A *nonrefluxing ileal conduit* replaces the historical ileal conduit, which had the potential complication of renal failure from the occurrence of refluxing urine.

A segment of the small intestine is removed from the intestinal tract and then used to form the conduit. Prior to this occurring, the integrity of the intestinal tract needs to be re-established (rehooked up together). The intestinal segment is then intussuscepted (telescoping one part of the intestine into an adjoining section), forming a valve that allows the urine to drain in only one direction. Ureters are attached to the more proximal end, while the distal end is attached to the skin. The anastomosis is usually stented for a few days to prevent obstruction from edema in the immediate postoperative period (Grossfeld, C. J. Bennett, J. K. Bennett, Martins, Apaydin, & Green 1995).

A *Kock pouch* is a continent bladder replacement to the skin made of small intestine that allows the client to do self-intermittent catheterization to maintain urinary continence. The urinary reservoir maintains large volumes of urine in a low-pressure system without reflux. This is done in cancer clients or those with a severely damaged bladder.

An *Indiana pouch* is a continent bladder replacement to the skin by a low-pressure system made from large and small intestine using the ileocecal valve and the cecum.

Complications that can occur with urinary diversions include wound infection, wound dehiscence, urine leakage from anastamosis sites, urethral obstruction, small bowel obstruction, paralytic ileus, and stomal gangrene. Delayed complications include ureteral obstruction, stomal stenosis, pyelonephritis, and renal calculi.

Neurogenic Bladder Complications

Complications that can result from a neurogenic bladder include frequent bladder infections, pyelonephritis, renal calculi, and autonomic dysreflexia.

Neurogenic Bowel Functioning
Process of Defecation

A combined action of two reflexes is necessary for defecation to occur. The intrinsic reflex is in the colon and is controlled by the myenteric plexus. The pathways of the other reflex are in the sacral segments of the spinal cord (spinal–sacral reflex). The process of defecation usually begins after a meal when a strong peristaltic wave pushes fecal matter into the rectum. The distention in the rectum stimulates a defecation reflex through the myenteric plexus to initiate peristaltic waves in the descending colon and sigmoid, forcing feces through the anus. The peristaltic wave reaches the anus as the internal anal sphincter relaxes. If the external anal sphincter is relaxed, defecation will occur. To have an effective bowel movement, however, rectal distention must also stimulate the "afferent fibers," which transmit impulses to and from the spinal–sacral reflex center (S2–3–4) via the pelvic nerve. These impulses return to the rectum, greatly increasing the strength of the peristaltic waves. Abdominal pressure intensifies, the internal sphincter relaxes, and the defecation reflex is more forceful and effective (Hanak, 1992). Awareness of defecation occurs when there is increased peristalsis and internal sphincter relaxation stimulates the pudendal nerve, which sends impulses up the spinothalamic tract of the spinal cord to the brain. The brain sends the message to "have a bowel movement" down the corticospinal tracts to initiate Valsalva's maneuver. Impulses to and from the sacral reflex center via the pelvic nerve stimulate the parasympathetic nervous system, which promotes defecation by increasing peristalsis. Sympathetic stimulation occurs at T6–L3 of the spinal cord, which inhibits defecation by decreasing peristalsis and contracting the internal anal sphincter. Sympathetic stimulation also inhibits defecation reflexes by inhibiting the external sphincter as well (Hanak, 1992).

Assessment The bowel assessment includes a client interview, tools of measurement, nursing observation, physical examination, and diagnostic laboratory studies.

Using an open-ended approach to questioning the client, the following areas need to be addressed in an interview: diet habits (type of diet, amount eaten, time of meals, appetite, food preferences, and fluid intake/preferences), activity (type of exercise, daily routine, limitations on mobility), bowel habits (color; frequency; consistency; time of day; use of aids such as medications, bran, or prune juice), current problems (constipation, diarrhea, bowel incontinence, and poor awareness of need to defecate), and history of gastrointestinal illnesses (GI) and/or surgeries.

Tools of measurement include evaluating a record of "number of bowel movements (BMs)" per day, per week, and whether written as "small," "moderate," or "large" amount. The record, which could be on a hospital graph form or from a client diary, might also indicate the consistency as "hard," "soft," "formed," and whether and when the client has "accidents."

The nurse should observe for signs of incontinence and other potential problems. Is there skin breakdown at and around the perianal area? Does the client have clothes stained with stool? What is the odor in the room or when in close contact with the client? Is a commode close by, so that immobility is a problem leading to incontinence? Does the client request certain foods or aids, such as prune juice or Metamucil? Does the client have a colostomy? It is also important to observe the client's cognitive status and communication ability. Can the client voice the need to use the bathroom?

Much can be observed from a physical examination. This includes assessing the abdominal contour, listening for bowel sounds, palpating the abdomen, and performing a rectal examination. Is the client's abdominal contour flat or distended? Measure the abdominal girth at the umbilicus. Listen for bowel sounds in all four quadrants. Normally, air and fluid movement through the bowel create irregular bubbling or soft, gurgling noises approximately 5 to 30 times per minute. Assess if the bowel sounds are normal, hypoactive, or hyperactive. Before determining if bowel sounds are absent, listen for 2 to 5 minutes in the right lower quadrant at the ileocecal valve area, because bowel sounds are normally always present there (Jarvis, 1996). Bowel sounds are frequently absent immediately following an injury, such as a brain injury or spinal cord injury. If absent, notify the physician and maintain an NPO (*nil per os,* nothing by mouth) status. A paralytic ileus, obstruction, or peritonitis might be present. Finally, palpate the abdomen for tenderness or tautness. Is the abdomen firm or soft?

During the rectal examination, check for the bulbocavernosus (BC) reflex, voluntary control of the external sphincter, the presence or absence of sensation, presence or absence of stool in the rectal canal, and whether there are any irregularities (such as hemorrhoids) present. When checking for the BC reflex (Figure 3), stimulate the reflex by squeezing the glans penis or glans clitoris while a gloved finger is inserted into the anus. If there is an anal contraction felt by the examiner, a positive BC reflex is present. If no anal contraction is felt, there is a negative BC reflex. The BC reflex helps determine the involuntary response of the external anal sphincter. To determine whether the client has voluntary control of the external anal sphincter, ask the client to clamp down on the gloved finger that has been inserted into the anus, and then have the client release it. This indicates that sacral sparing has occurred. (The connection between the S2–3–4 sacral segments and the brain is intact.)

Perianal sensation is assessed by applying a 25-gauge needle to the perianal area without the client seeing what is being done. If the client can determine the location and the sharpness correctly, perianal sensation is intact.

Diagnostic tests, except possibly a KUB (x-ray of the kidney, ureter, and bladder) or flat plate of the abdomen, are usually not ordered unless there is a history of GI problems or impaction is suspected (Hanak, 1992).

Neurogenic Bowel Dysfunction

The assessment phase helps determine if problems of constipation, diarrhea, or incontinence are present. Looking at the medical history of the client, conditions such as spinal cord injury or a previous CVA might be stated. The problems determined can result from a neurological disorder. A neurogenic bowel results from interruption of neural pathways that supply the rectum, external sphincter, and accessory muscles for defecation (Toth, 1988). Bowel function becomes impaired due to disruption in the neurological control mechanisms secondary to cortical or subcortical brain lesions, spinal cord lesions, or peripheral nerve damage (Hanak, 1992).

Classification of Neurogenic Bowel

Sacral segments 2–3–4, which affect bladder functioning, affect bowel functioning in a similar manner. The approach used to determine the appropriate type of neurogenic bladder, discussed previously, is also used to classify the type of neurogenic bowel (Table 2). Classifications include an uninhibited neurogenic bowel, reflex neurogenic bowel, autonomous (areflexic) neurogenic bowel, sensory paralytic neurogenic bowel, and motor paralytic neurogenic bowel.

An *uninhibited **neurogenic bowel*** occurs when cerebral damage disrupts the inhibitory/facilitory mechanisms in the brain for defecation. Etiology includes CVA, brain injury or tumor, Alzheimer's disease, multiple sclerosis, senility, and infancy. Assessment findings include intact bowel and saddle sensation and intact or increased bulbocavernosus reflex. There is decreased cerebral awareness of the urge to defecate, decreased voluntary control of the anal sphincter, urgency, and incontinence.

A *reflex neurogenic bowel* occurs when there is damage to the **upper motor neuron (UMN)** pathway, which interrupts inhibitory or facilitatory signals from the brain to the external anal sphincter. Because the reflex arc is intact, bowel stimulants or a stimulant response program would be appropriate for bowel management (Carpenito, 1993). Etiology includes spinal cord injury (damage above sacral reflex center), spinal cord tumor, multiple sclerosis, pernicious anemia, vascular diseases, and syringomyelia. Assessment findings include sensory loss of urge to defecate, absent or impaired saddle sensation, inability to control reflex defecation, a positive bulbocavernosus reflex, and automatic bowel emptying.

An *autonomous (areflexic) neurogenic bowel* occurs when there is damage to the **lower motor neuron (LMN)** pathway, which disrupts the defecation reflex and control of the external anal sphincter. Because the reflex is damaged, bowel incontinence can occur without stimulation. Fecal impaction and constipation can also be a problem because the colon contracts, but poorly. Peristalsis is weak, resulting in stool retention. If some stool leaks out, it is soft with much stool still remaining in the rectal vault (Carpenito, 1993). Etiology: Spinal cord injury (damage at the sacral reflex center), spinal cord tumor, cauda equina injury, status postradical pelvic surgery, spinal bifida, herniated intervertebral disk, and myelomeningocele. Assessment findings include absent saddle sensation, absent voluntary control, absent bulbocavernosus reflex, flaccid external sphincter, and fecal incontinence/impacted stool formation.

Table 2
Neurogenic Bowel Dysfunction

Diagnosis	Level of Lesion	Possible Etiology	Pattern of Incontinence	Bowel Program
Uninhibited	Brain	Cerebrovascular accident; multiple sclerosis; brain injury	Urgency: Poor awareness of desire to defecate	Consistent habit and time according to premorbid history; physical exercise; high fluid intake; high-fiber foods; stool softener, suppository as needed
Reflex	Spinal cord above T12 to L1 vertebral level	Trauma; tumor; vascular disease; syringomyelia; multiple sclerosis	Infrequent; sudden; unexpected	Consistent habit and time, physical exercise, high fluid intake, high-fiber foods; suppository program, digital stimulation, stool softener as needed
Autonomous	Spinal cord at or below T12 to L1 vertebral level	Trauma, tumor, spina bifida, intervertebral disk	Frequent; may be continuous or induced by exercise or stress	Consistent habit and time, physical exercise continuous, high fluid intake, high-fiber foods and bulk agents as necessary for firm stool consistency; suppository program, Valsalva's maneuver, manual removal

Source: Mosby–Year Book.

A *sensory paralytic neurogenic bowel* occurs when there is damage to the dorsal roots (sensory afferent side) of the sacral reflex arc. This is commonly seen in the diabetic client. Assessment findings include absent or decreased perianal sensation, impaired awareness or urge, weak bulbocavernosus reflex, and constipation due to decreased awareness of urge. Incontinence rarely occurs unless the diabetic client is in the advanced stages of the disease (Hanak, 1992).

A *motor paralytic neurogenic bowel* occurs when there is damage to the ventral roots (motor efferent side) of the sacral reflex arc. Etiology includes poliomyelitis, herniated intervertebral disk, Guillain-Barré syndrome, trauma, and tumor. Assessment findings include normal perianal sensation, awareness of urge, sphincters intact, absent bulbocavernosus reflex, and constipation due to a decreased bowel tone (Hanak, 1992).

Nursing Diagnoses, Goals, and Interventions

Colonic constipation is defined as "the state in which an individual experiences or is at risk of experiencing a delay in passage of food residue resulting in dry, hard stool" (Carpenito, 1993, p. 158). Characteristics can include decreased frequency of stool, hard dry stool, straining to have a bowel movement, painful defecation, and abdominal distention (Carpenito, 1993). This nursing diagnosis can be seen in clients with neurological disorders, such as spinal cord injury, spinal bifida, head injury, CVA, multiple sclerosis, and Parkinson's disease, when bowel programs established fail to work or are inadequate. Clients with neurological disorders also tend to have impaired mobility and decreased peristalsis secondary to trauma resulting in constipation.

Nursing Diagnosis
- Colonic constipation related to sensorimotor deficits and immobility.

Goals/Outcomes
- The client will achieve regular bowel movements (Rehabilitation Nursing Foundation, 1995).
- The client will demonstrate knowledge of risk factors and methods for preventing constipation (Rehabilitation Nursing Foundation, 1995).

Nursing Interventions
- Instruct and assist the client in establishing a regular bowel program based on client bowel assessment, history of bowel habits, diet, and activity patterns, medical and surgical history, and current medical condition.
- Increase fluid intake.
- Provide for colonic and rectal emptying through use of stimulants or irritant cathartics, bulk-forming agents (to be taken at lease 6 to 8 hours before expected and/or desired emptying); use low-volume enemas or suppositories alone or in conjunction with oral medications for complete emptying (McCourt, 1993).
- Increase bulk and fiber in the diet, depending less and less on laxatives and enemas for bowel regularity.
- Promote use of stool softeners or bulk formers with adequate fluids and food intake to establish a bowel routine until regularity is obtained (McCourt, 1993).
- Use the toilet or commode for emptying bowel, utilizing gravity, unless contraindicated.
- Establish regular times for emptying bowel, such as after breakfast or dinner every day or every other day.
- Instruct the client on risk factors that can lead to constipation and methods to prevent constipation.

- Allow several days between any changes in interventions, changing one intervention at a time.
- Encourage the client to maintain same activity level.

A diet high in fiber with adequate bulk and fluids will stimulate bowel activity as peristaltic action increases. Dietary fiber increases the bulk of the stool, which indirectly stimulates the muscles of the bowel. It works by absorbing water from the intestinal contents. According to Iseminger and Hardy (1982), bran is the most concentrated form of fiber. It is the outer layer of the wheat grain and is not entirely composed of fiber. Bran absorbs fluid, producing softer stools; therefore, increasing fluid intake to 2000 to 3000 cm³/day is necessary. Clients with a limited amount of fiber in their diets tend to "strain" to have a bowel movement and have irregular bowel habits (Burkitt & Meisner, 1979). Bulk-forming foods include bran, whole wheat, cornmeal, breakfast cereals, fruits (cranberries, prunes, figs, dates), graham crackers, and vegetables (leafy lettuce, cabbage, spinach, root-boiled carrots, raw turnips, legumes). Foods that are constipating include white rice, white potatoes, white pasta, cheese, and chocolate. Clients with neurological disorders need to maintain a high-fiber diet and limit their intake of constipating foods.

Establishing a regular schedule (**timed voiding**) of rectal stimulation and toileting increases colon peristalsis and more complete emptying of the lower bowel. The best timing for effective emptying of the bowel is 20 to 40 minutes after a meal, when the gastrocolic reflex is stimulated.

Positioning can also make a difference. Bowel emptying can be more effective if facilitated by gravity. Encourage the client to sit on a toilet or commode with knees higher than the hips. If unable to sit on a toilet or commode, have the client lie on his or her left side (with protection pads on bed). While in a sitting position, support the client in a "leaning over" position. Try abdominal massage or, if the client has strong abdominal muscles, have him or her "bear down" to have a bowel movement. To stimulate peristalsis, abdominal massage should start from the cecal area, following the course of the large intestine in a clockwise fashion (right to left).

Medication management can include the use of suppositories, stool softeners, peristaltic stimulators, bulk formers, stimulant laxatives, and irritant cathartics.

Suppositories are used to set off reflexes that start movement of the lower colon and rectum in the hope of preventing constipation. Glycerin suppositories work by causing dehydration of exposed tissue, which produces an irritant effect, and by absorbing water from tissues, creating more mass, stimulating peristalsis (Wilson & Shannon, 1993). Dulcolax suppositories, when used in conjunction with glycerin suppositories or by themselves, stimulate nerve endings as the suppository comes in contact with the intestinal wall. As the nerve endings are stimulated, peristaltic contractions occur in the colon. Glycerin suppositories have a milder effect than Dulcolax suppositories.

Stool softeners (colace, surfak, dialose) are used to avoid impaction or constipation. They are also useful with clients who must avoid "straining." Detergent action lowers surface tension, permitting water and fats to penetrate and soften stools for easier passage (Wilson & Shannon, 1993). Clients on stool softeners must drink plenty of fluids, 2000 to 3000 cm^3/day to be effective. Two or 3 days of therapy are necessary before results will be noticed. Ideally, the use of stool softeners should be for a limited time, as a high-fiber diet and appropriate fluid intake are established. If stools become too soft, discuss with the physician decreasing or holding the medication.

Bulk laxatives, or formers, such as Metamucil, are often used to prevent constipation. On contact with water, Metamucil produces bland, lubricating, gelatinous bulk, which promotes peristalsis and natural elimination (Wilson & Shannon, 1993). Metamucil not only absorbs water to maintain a soft stool, but also helps control the incidence of loose stools by absorbing excess water. One to 2 teaspoons are administered daily with 8 ounces of fluid. Without abundant water intake, constipation can increase with Metamucil.

Peristaltic stimulators are combination stool softener and laxative, such as Pericolace, Doxidan, and Dialose-Plus. These medications stimulate the normal wave-like movement of the bowel, which propels stool through the bowel. If the client has loose stools or unscheduled bowel movements, stop the medication or decrease the dose following consultation with a physician.

Stimulant laxatives (Senokot, Dulcolax tablets, cascara sagrada) stimulate peristalsis in the colon through direct chemical irritation. The effect usually takes approximately 6 to 12 hours after administration. If a bowel program is scheduled after dinner, a stimulant laxative should be given in the morning or at noon.

Magnesium citrate is an irritant cathartic. It promotes bowel evacuation by causing osmotic retention of fluid, which distends the colon and stimulates peristaltic activity. Magnesium citrate is not recommended for clients with renal disease or those experiencing nausea, vomiting, or diarrhea owing to the side effects of fluid and electrolyte imbalance. It also is not recommended for SCI clients with a T8 or higher level injury, owing to their being prone to autonomic dysreflexia.

Bowel incontinence, as a nursing diagnosis, is defined as "a state in which an individual experiences a change in normal bowel habits characterized by involuntary passage of stool" (Carpenito, 1993, p. 169). Involuntary passage of stool occurs and tends to be present when there is a loss of sphincter control (Carpenito, 1993). Bowel incontinence as a nursing diagnosis can be used for clients who have an uninhibited neurogenic bowel, reflex neurogenic bowel, autonomous (areflexic) neurogenic bowel, motor paralytic neurogenic bowel, or sensory paralytic neurogenic bowel. For the sake of discussing specific goals and interventions for the different types of neurogenic bowel, bowel incontinence as a nursing diagnosis will be stated as three different diagnoses.

Nursing Diagnosis

- Bowel incontinence: uninhibited neurogenic bowel related to diminished sphincter control, damage to UMN, or related to cognitive/perceptual impairment of CNS.

Goals/Outcomes

- Client will achieve a routine of regular, complete bowel elimination with fewer incontinent episodes or without incontinent episodes.

Nursing Interventions

- Push fluids, limit after dinner.
- Encourage high-fiber diet and avoid overly spiced and gas-forming foods.
- Provide privacy.
- Use toilet or commode, utilizing gravity to facilitate bowel emptying.
- Assist to toilet or commode 20 to 40 minutes after a scheduled meal (breakfast or dinner), timing with the gastrocolic reflex.
- Abdominal massage (right to left).
- Medications: cleanse lower bowel on onset. Use stool softeners and bulk formers (gradually eliminating).
- Insert suppositories immediately after a meal, applying directly along the rectal mucosa, and start with a Dulcolax suppository daily, substituting a glycerin suppository daily after bowel has become regulated. *Note:* Following a study of CVA clients, Venn, Taft, Carpentier, and Applebaugh (1992) found that clients receiving suppositories for bowel management in the morning had significantly more efficient results than those receiving suppositories in the evening. Efficiency was also highest when time of program coincided with previous time pattern.
- Encourage the client to use adaptive clothing to ease donning and doffing for toileting (McCourt, 1993).
- Use alternative modalities, such as biofeedback, if indicated, to enhance sphincter tone, thereby increasing continence (McCourt, 1993).
- Maintain a consistent activity/exercise program.

The use of **digital stimulation** daily instead of suppositories for CVA clients is also an approach to bowel care that has been effective. "Digital stimulation is manual stimulation (up to 30 seconds of circular motion against the anal sphincter wall) that increases peristalsis and relaxes the anal sphincter muscle for reflex evacuation" (Munchiando & Kendall, 1993, p. 169). In a study by Munchiando and Kendall (1993), it was found that daily digital stimulation was significantly more effective than every-other-day stimulation for re-establishing continence. For an effective bowel program that works well for CVA clients, see "A Bowel Program that Works" (Figure 9). This bowel program was developed by the nursing and medical staff of the rehabilitation unit, Sacred Heart Hospital (Eau Clair, Wisconsin).

Nursing Diagnosis

- Bowel incontinence: Reflex neurogenic bowel related to lack of voluntary sphincter control secondary to SCI above T11.

Goals/Outcomes

- The client will have regular evacuation of the bowel with no episodes of incontinence.
- The client will evacuate a soft formed stool every day, every other day, or every third day.
- The client will describe and perform (if able) an individual bowel management program.

Nursing Interventions

- Maintain an adequate amount of fluid intake. Increase the amount depending on the bladder program.
- Encourage a consistent amount of a high-fiber diet.
- Medication management of stool softeners and bul formers, peristaltic stimulators, or stimulant laxatives.
- Suppositories: Glycerin and Dulcolax. Depending on each individual client, the combination of both suppositories might be necessary. Some clients have better efficiency with the use of either one glycerin or Dulcolax suppository alone.
- Bowel program consisting of a manual evacuation, followed by the insertion of suppositories (or one suppository). Assess the time required for emptying of stool (usually 20 to 40 minutes). Perform manual evacuation again for any residual, followed by digital stimulation (tolerated well because sensation is impaired or absent). Avoid digital stimulation with clients who have rectal bleeding or hemorrhoids.
- Following insertion of suppositories, while the client is lying on his or her left side, facilitate bowel emptying on a commode or toilet (if possible), utilizing gravity. Encourage the client to lean forward.
- Apply abdominal massage (right to left).
- Provide privacy.
- Schedule the bowel program at the same time every day, every other day, or at least every 3 days, depending on the client's needs for regular complete bowel emptying. Consider the client's independence level and daily schedule (work, school). Initially, clients are put on an every-day program—usually for 5 to 7 days, advancing to every other day and for some clients, every 3 days. This is to ensure that the bowel has been totally emptied before establishing a regular bowel program.
- Maintain a constant activity level.

Following a spinal cord injury, contraction of the internal sphincter is retained, but external sphincter control is absent. This results in unpredictable bowel "accidents," as there is a sudden expulsion of stool (King & Dudas, 1980). The institution of a regulated bowel program, previously described, is what is necessary to prevent the occurrence of "accidents," or at least to limit the

A Bowel Program That Works

Assess the patient's previous time pattern for defecation. If previous bowel habits support an evening regimen, assign a scheduled time for bowel training in the evening within 30 to 40 minutes following the evening meal. If previous bowel habits support a morning regimen or suggest no pattern, assign a scheduled time for bowel training in the morning within 30 to 40 minutes following breakfast.

1. Check the rectum with a gloved, lubricated finger and remove any stool that is present. Insert a bisacodyl (Dulcolax) suppository into the rectum with a gloved, lubricated finger so that it touches the wall of the rectum above the internal sphincter.
2. On the second day and thereafter, give the patient an opportunity to defecate without external stimulation at the scheduled time. If the patient is unable to defecate and if no spontaneous bowel movement has occurred within 4 hours prior to the scheduled time, administer a bisacodyl suppository until a pattern of regular defecation of soft formed stools has occurred for five *consecutive* scheduled times.
3. Once the pattern of regular defecation has been established, a glycerin suppository may be substituted for the bisacodyl suppository. If no bowel movement occurs within 15 to 30 minutes, repeat the procedures using a bisacodyl suppository. Administer a bisacodyl suppository for two consecutive scheduled times. If the bisacodyl suppository has produced results for two consecutive times, the glycerin suppository may be tried again. If no bowel movement occurs within 15 to 30 minutes, repeat the procedures using a bisacodyl suppository. Repeat trials with glycerin suppositories three times. If not effective for these trials, maintain on bisacodyl suppositories.
4. If a strong, consistent pattern of defecation becomes apparent while using glycerin suppositories, attempts should be made to discontinue glycerin to determine if the patient is able to have spontaneous bowel movements without external stimulation.

5. The frequency of the adminsitration of suppositories may be changed to every other day or every third day if a regular pattern of defecation is established and if this timing seems to be a better match for the patient's bowel response.

In cases where a patient is unresponsive to the bisacodyl suppository, the nurse should try the following procedure:

1. If the bisacodyl suppository is ineffective in stimulating defecation after step 1, digital stimulation of the rectum should be performed if this procedure is not painful to the patient or contraindicated by the patient's condition. Insert a gloved, lubricated finger into the rectum and use a gentle circular massage for 1 or 2 minutes. When the internal sphincter relaxes, stop the massage. Wait for 30 minutes for evacuation to occur.
2. If the digital stimulation is not effective, the administration of a bisacodyl suppository and use of digital stimulation may each be repeated once. If these treatments are ineffective, additional assessment is necessary to determine what additional treatment is indicated.

Fig 9. *"A Bowel Program That Works." (Reprinted from* Rehabilitation Nursing, 18*(3), 148–153, with permission of the Association of Rehabilitation Nurses, 4700 W. Lake Avenue, Glenview, IL 60025-1485. Copyright @ 1993. Association of Rehabilitation Nurses.)*

occurrence. In some clients, several weeks are necessary before a regulated, effective bowel program is established, resulting in frustration and embarrassment for the client. Persistence and emotional support are needed while the "right" bowel program is determined. If poor or no results occur after two bowel programs, change only one element of care at a time.

Another approach to the bowel program is to perform digital stimulation 5 minutes after the insertion of a suppository, because the internal sphincter can be relaxed at this time, facilitating bowel emptying (King & Dudas, 1980).

Once regular bowel emptying has been established, digital stimulation alone should be attempted for 15 to 30 seconds every day. If interventions are altered, only one element should be changed at a time, evaluating effectiveness (King & Dudas, 1980).

Which medications are effective for bowel regulation differ with every client. It sometimes becomes "trial and error." Always start with the mildest form of medication. The medication selected depends on action of medication, type of stool (amount and consistency), desired effect on stool, and the actual effect on stool. Even though the use of medications is very helpful and necessary in establishing an effective bowel program, ideally, clients should eliminate medications, one at a time, as results become more satisfactory and predictable. With the proper diet, fluid intake, and activity schedule, clients can decrease the need for medications for bowel management.

Nursing Diagnosis. (appropriate for neurogenic autonomous, sensory paralytic, and motor paralytic bowels)

- Bowel incontinence: Autonomous (areflexic) neurogenic bowel related to lack of voluntary sphincter control secondary to damage of sacral reflex arc.

Goals/Outcomes

- The client will achieve a regular schedule of complete bowel emptying without episodes of incontinence, constipation, or diarrhea.

Nursing Interventions

- Maintain an adequate amount of fluid intake, increasing the amount depending on the individual bladder program.
- Encourage a consistent amount of a high-fiber diet.
- Administer stool softeners daily or twice a day.
- Administer stimulant laxatives or bulk formers every other day or daily.
- Adhere to regular, scheduled time for evacuation, 20 to 30 minutes after a meal daily or every other day. Assess premorbid habits.
- Instruct the client to perform Valsalva's maneuver, "straining" to facilitate bowel emptying while performing abdominal massage and leaning forward. *Do not* teach to clients with a history of cardiac problems. If ineffective, instruct the client to manually remove stool carefully, with a generously lubricated gloved finger.
- After removal of stool from the lower rectum, administer a suppository as high as possible against the rectal wall. This stimulates the colon to empty stool into the rectum for manual removal (Zejdlik, 1992).
- Encourage the client to use a toilet or commode, utilizing gravity to facilitate bowel emptying.
- Maintain privacy.
- Maintain a consistent activity level.
- Assess stool consistency for firmness, but it should not be too hard, which can lead to constipation.

The Use of Enemas. The instillation of enemas is not recommended for clients with a neurogenic bowel. They are not retained well, bowel emptying becomes unpredictable, and high-volume enemas can destroy tone, actually causing incontinence instead of preventing it. According to Hanak (1992), the use of harsh laxatives and enemas should not occur on a regular basis because they can lead to long-term management problems. It can take as long as 3 months to re-establish a regular bowel emptying pattern. The use of high-volume enemas has also been known to cause autonomic dysreflexia in some SCI clients (T8 level or above).

Other possible nursing diagnoses include the following:

- Impaired skin integrity related to bowel incontinence.
- Social isolation related to bowel incontinence.
- Bowel incontinence related to limited mobility in reaching toilet/commode in a timely manner.

Ostomies

Cancer, trauma, or other diseases that will not allow passage of feces through the intestine and anus can necessitate the need for a stoma to be constructed surgically in the abdominal wall (Gender, 1996). Some SCI clients with an autonomous areflexic neurogenic bowel choose an ostomy as an alternative option for bowel management (Saltzstein & Romano, 1996). Bowel diversion ostomies include an ileostomy (opening into the ileum) and colostomy (opening into the ascending, transverse, or descending sigmoid colon).

A regulated bowel program cannot be established with those clients who have an ileostomy or ascending colostomy. Therefore, a bag or pouch will need to be worn at all times. With regular irrigation, a client with a descending and sigmoid colostomy and sometimes a transverse colostomy can regain a regular bowel program. Regulating the diet appropriately for the client can help establish a regular bowel program. Collaborating with an enterostomal therapist to establish regulation of a client's bowel program and obtaining necessary ostomy supplies can also be helpful (Gender, 1996).

The client with an ostomy will need much instruction on how to manage it successfully. Also, the client will need time for psychological adjustment. Assist him or her in enhancing coping skills to deal with this change in body image and hygiene/toileting habits.

Neurogenic Bowel Complications

Possible bowel complications seen in clients with a neurogenic bowel include constipation, impaction, diarrhea, paralytic ileus, and autonomic dysreflexia.

Constipation is probably the most common complication encountered. The client has hard formed stools and irregular bowel movements or has poor or no bowel movements. Other signs and symptoms include decreased bowel sounds, severe flatus, distended abdomen, headache, anorexia, nausea, and/or vomiting (Gender, 1996). Constipation can be caused by decreased mobility, muscle weakness, decreased bowel tone, medications, or a diet limited in fiber. These causes are frequently associated with clients who have neurological disorders (Hanak, 1992). To prevent constipation, a combination of a high-fiber diet, fluid intake, exercise/activity, stool softeners, stimulant laxatives or bulk formers (medications), and prune juice is recommended.

Constipation can lead to *fecal impaction,* which can be relieved by manually removing stool and digital stimulation. Fecal impaction results from one or more bowel programs that have poor or no results.

Diarrhea is the presence of loose, watery stools. It results from rapid movement of fecal matter through the large intestine. Normally, the colon absorbs water from solid wastes received from the small intestine. When something interferes with that absorption or causes the bowel to secrete rather than absorb liquid, or when something speeds the passage of wastes through the bowel so that there is insufficient time to absorb fluid, diarrhea results (Gender, 1996). Treatment consists of determining the cause, decreasing the use of stool softeners, and evaluating diet and fluid intake. It is important to assess electrolyte imbalance.

A *paralytic ileus* is a state of atony of the small bowel with an absence of normal peristaltic movement (Hanak & Scott, 1983). Signs and symptoms include abdominal distention and absent bowel sounds. A paralytic ileus occurs within 24 to 48 hours after SCI and other neurological trauma secondary to sudden cessation of autonomic innervation (Hanak, 1992). It lasts for approximately 1 week. Treatment entails inserting a nasogastric tube, aspirating the contents, and connecting the tube to low suction. Maintain the client on NPO status until bowel sounds return.

Autonomic dysreflexia is a serious, life-threatening complication due to bowel impaction, instrumentation, or disimpaction that SCI clients (T8 level or above) can experience.

Client Education

The time and effort spent developing a bowel program in a hospital will be wasted if the client does not follow through with it after discharge. The client should be acquainted with the use of each bowel medication and how to adjust the dose when necessary. Generic equivalents to brand names and similar medications that can be used as substitutes should be discussed. Client preferences to bowel management need to be considered before discharge. Provide resources for problems and follow-up, such as a nurse consultant, primary care provider, or local pharmacist. It should be explained to the client that bowel accidents are very common during the first few weeks following discharge, owing to activity and diet changes as well as the anxiety that frequently occurs with a new environment. If the bowel program was well established in the hospital, it should stabilize after discharge. A study, however, by Graham and Kunkle (1997) showed that at discharge 66 percent of 114 participants took bowel medications, but 1 month later, only 42 percent did. Half of the clients (50 percent) reduced or discontinued the use of stimulant laxatives.

Conclusion   Neurogenic bladder and bowel functioning requires special attention by the client, the nurse, and the total team. Being aware of the type of neurogenic bladder and bowel and being knowledgeable of the appropriate nursing diagnoses and interventions can make a difference in the quality of life a client has postdischarge. Without being able to manage bowel and bladder functioning successfully, the client will not feel comfortable in a social environment, school or work setting, or in pursuing his or her dreams. Education and support by the nurse is the key!

References   Abrams, P., Feneley, R., & Torrens, M. (1983). *Urodynamics.* New York: Springer-Verlag.

Andrews, K. A., & Opitz, J. L. (1993). Bladder retraining. In M. Sinaki (Ed.), *Basic rehabilitation medicine* (2nd ed.). St. Louis: Mosby–Year Book.

Boyarsky, S., Labay, P., Hanick, P., Abramson, A. S., & Boyarsky, R. (1979). *Care of the patient with neurogenic bladder.* Boston: Little, Brown.

Burkitt, D. P., & Meisner, P. (1979). How to manage constipation with high fiber diet. *Geriatrics, 34* 33–35, 38–40.

Carpenito, L. J. (1993). *Nursing diagnosis: Application to clinical practice* (5th ed.). Philadelphia: J. B. Lippincott.

Dittmar, S. (1989). *Rehabilitation nursing: Process and application.* St. Louis: Mosby.

Fantl, J. A., Wyman, J. F., McClish, D. K., Harkins, S. W., Elswick, R. K., & Taylor, J. R., et al. (1991). Efficiency of bladder training in older women with urinary incontinence. *Journal of the American Medical Association, 265*(5), 609–613.

Folstein, M. F., Folstein, S. E., & McHugh, P. R. (1975). "Mini-Mental State": A practical method of grading the cognitive state of patients for the clinician. *Journal of Psychiatric Research, 12,* 189–198.

Gelber, D., Good, D. C., Laven, L. J., & Verhulst, S. J. (1993). Causes of urinary incontinence after hemispheric stroke. *Stroke, 24*(3), 378–382.

Gender, A. R. (1996). Bowel regulation and elimination. In S. Howman (Ed.), *Rehabilitation nursing: Process and application* (2nd ed.). St. Louis: Mosby–Year Book.

Graham, C., & Kunkle, C. (1996). Do rehabilitation patients continue prescribed bowel medications after discharge? *Rehabilitation Nursing, 21*(6), 298–302.

Gray, M. (1993). *Genitourinary disorders.* St. Louis: Mosby–Year Book.

Grinspun, D. (1993). Bladder management for adults following brain injury. *Rehabilitation Nursing, 18*(5), 300–305.

Grossfeld, G. D., Bennett, C. J., Bennett, J. K., Martins, F., Apaydin, A., & Green, B. G. (1995). The nonreflexing ileal conduit: A new form of urinary diversion. *Journal of Urology, 154* 981–984.

Hanak, M. (1992). *Rehabilitation nursing for the neurological patient.* New York: Springer.

Hanak, M., & Scott, A. (1983). *Spinal cord injury: An illustrated guide for health care professionals.* New York: Springer.

Hu, T. W. (1990). Impact of urinary incontinence on health-care costs. *Journal of the American Geriatrics Society, 38* 292–295.

Iseminger, M., & Hardy, P. (1982). Bran works! *Geriatric Nursing, 3* 402–404.

Jarvis, C. (1996). *Pocket companion for physical examination and health assessment.* Philadelphia: W. B. Saunders.

Khan, Z., Starer, P., Yang, W. C., & Bhola, A. (1990). Analysis of voiding disorders in patients with cerebrovascular accidents. *Urology, 35* 265–270.

King, R. B., & Dudas, S. (1980). Rehabilitation of patients with spinal cord injury. *Nursing Clinics of North America, 15*(2), 226–243.

Kurtz, M. J., Van Zandt, D. K., & Sapp, L. R. (1996). The new technique in independent intermittent catheterization: The Mitrofanoff catheterizable channel. *Rehabilitation Nursing, 21*(6), 311–314.

Latham, L. (1994). When SCI complicates med/surg care. *RN 8*, 26–30.

Lincoln, R., & Roberts, R. (1989). Continence issues in acute care. *Nursing Clinics of North America, 24* 741–754.

McCormick, K., Scheve, A., & Leahy, E. (1988). Nursing management of urinary incontinence in geriatric patients. *Nursing Clinics of North America, 23* 231–264.

Menon, E. B., & Tan, E. S. (1992). Bladder training in patients with SCI. *Urology, 40*(5), 425–428.

Morishita, L. (1988). Nursing evaluation and treatment of geriatric outpatients with urinary incontinence. *Nursing Clinics of North America, 23* 189–204.

Mundy, A. R., Stephenson, T. P., & Wein, A. J. (1984). *Urodynamics: Principles, practice and application.* New York: Churchill Livingstone.

Palmer, M. H. (1990). Urinary incontinence. *Nursing Clinics of North America, 24*(4), 919–934.

Pires, M. (1996). Bladder elimination and continence. In S. P. Howman (Ed.), *Rehabilitation nursing: Process and application* (2nd ed.). St. Louis: Mosby–Year Book.

Pires, M., Lockhart-Pretti, P. A., Smith, D. A., & Newman, D. K. (1991). *Continence: Every nurse's responsibility. I. An overview.* Glenview, IL: Rehabilitation Nursing Foundation of the Association of Rehabilitation Nurses. [Video]

Rancho Los Amigos Medical Center, Continuing Education Center. (May 1, 1987). Intermittent catheterization protocol. In *Nursing rehabilitation: Managing bowel and bladder dysfunction.* Class seminar conducted for nurses at Rancho Los Amigos Medical Center, Downey, CA.

Rehabilitation Nursing Foundation. (1995). *Twenty-one rehabilitation nursing diagnoses: A guide to interventions and outcomes.* Glenview, IL: author.

Saltzstein, R. J., & Romano, J. (1990). The efficacy of colostomy as a bowel management alternative in selected spinal cord injury patients. *Journal of American Paraplegia Society, 13* 9–13.

Staskin, D. R. (1991). Classification of voiding dysfunction. In R. J. Krane & M. B. Sirosky (Eds.), *Clinical neuro-urology* (2nd ed.). Boston: Little, Brown.

Toth, L. (1988). *Alterations in bowel elimination in neuroscience nursing: Phenomena and practice.* Norwalk, CT: Appleton & Lange.

Urinary Incontinence Guideline Panel. (1992). *Urinary incontinence in adults: Clinical practice guidelines.* AHCPR Publication No. 92-0038. Rockville, MD: Agency for Health Care Policy and Research, Public Health Service, U.S. Department of Health and Human Services.

Venn, M. R., Taft, L., Carpentier, B., & Applebaugh, G. (1992). The influence of timing and suppository use on efficiency and effectiveness of bowel training after a stroke. *Rehabilitation Nursing, 17*(3), 116–120.

Voith, A. M. (1986). A conceptual framework for nursing diagnoses: Alterations in urinary elimination. *Rehabilitation Nursing,* 18–20.

Voith, A. M. (1988). Alterations in urinary elimination: Concepts, research and practice. *Rehabilitation Nursing, 13*(3), 122–131.

Wein, A. J. (1990). Pharmacological treatment of incontinence. *Journal of American Geriatrics Society, 38*(3), 317–325.

Wilson, B. A., & Shannon, M. T. (1993). In *Govani & Hayes' Nurses' drug guide 1993.* Norwalk, CT: Appleton & Lange.

Wyman, J. F. (1988). Nursing assessment of the incontinent geriatric outpatient population. *Nursing Clinics of North America, 23,* 169–187.

Zejdlik, C. M. (1983). *Management of spinal cord injury.* Belmont, CA: Wadsworth Health Sciences Division.

CHAPTER 20
Care of the Client with an Amputation

Elizabeth A. Yetzer

Key Terms   *Amputation*
Contracture
Disarticulation
Doffing of the Prosthesis
Donning of the Prosthesis
Edema
Phantom Limb Pain
Phantom Limb Sensation
Prosthesis
Residual Limb/Stump
Socket of the Prosthesis
Stump Shrinker
Limb (Stump) Wrapping

Objectives   1. Identify three major causes of amputation.

2. Describe common feelings about amputation by the client, family, and staff.

3. Identify nursing measures to assist the client and the family with the psychological aspects of amputation.

4. List four educational needs of the client with an amputation, and of the family.

5. Develop (identify) a list of at least three nursing problems and one nursing action/measure for each problem experienced by a client with an amputation.

Introduction   Whether a client's amputation is due to disease, accident, or birth defect, the client requires intensive rehabilitation. The rehabilitation goals are to provide the client with the knowledge, skills, and attitudes necessary for social, physical, and emotional adjustment. The objective is to assist the client to achieve self-care goals and to return to the community. The family and significant others must also be considered and included in the rehabilitation goals.

In this chapter, we discuss the major causes of amputation. Common feelings about amputation, factors that influence those feelings, and measures to assist the client and family with the psychological aspects of amputation are described. The educational needs of the client with an amputation and of the family are identified. An outline of nursing diagnosis, objectives/outcomes, and interventions is developed.

Amputation is defined as the partial or complete surgical removal of a limb as the result of a crushing injury, intolerable pain, gangrene, vascular obstruction, uncontrollable infection, or congenital anomalies. Three major causes of amputation are medical, trauma, and congenital anomalies (Table 1).

Examples of medical causes are diabetes, vascular obstruction, cancer, gangrene, or uncontrollable infection. Seventy-four percent of amputations are due to medical causes. These amputations are usually of the lower extremity.

Accidents or traumatic amputations account for 23 percent of amputations. The majority of these amputations are of the upper extremities.

Congenital anomalies, or birth defects, account for 3 percent of amputations and can be of the upper or the lower extremities.

In 1992, the number of amputations in the United States was estimated at 358,000: 102,000 upper extremity and 256,000 lower extremity. The National Center for Health Statistics estimates that 1 in 200 people in the United States is a lower extremity amputee. There is one upper extremity amputee for every nine lower extremity amputees. Amputation is the eleventh most common procedure performed on the lower extremities. Amputations are increasing in number five times more rapidly in people more than 50 years of age, owing to diabetes and peripheral vascular disease (PVD) (Cutson & Bongiorni, 1996).

Table 1
Major Causes of Amputation

Cause	Examples
Medical	Diabetes, peripheral vascular disease (PVD), cancer, gangrene, and infection
	Usually of lower extremity
	Accounts for 74 percent of amputations
Trauma	Accidents such as crushing injury, burns, frost bite
	Often of upper extremity
	Accounts for 23 percent of amputations
Congenital anomalies or birth defects	Can be upper or lower extremities
	Accounts for 3 percent of amputations

Of the estimated 15 million diabetics, 5 to 15 percent will undergo an amputation in their lifetime. Each year, 54,000 diabetes-related amputations are performed, costing more than $600 million. Amputations can cost between $24,000 and $40,000 each (Diabetes in America, Publication 95-1468, 1995). Amputations can be prevented with good foot care, avoiding injury to the feet, wearing proper shoes, controlling diabetes, and stopping smoking.

Psychological Aspects of Amputation

When you think of the term *amputation,* what do you think about? Is it that amputation is a loss, the removal of a body part, the loss of body image? All of these are negative ideas. Reviewing the causes of amputation, most are due to gangrene or an uncontrolled infection—life-threatening situations. The surgery is to remove a nonfunctioning part and to prepare the residual limb for the use of a prosthesis if possible. If the health care team is to assist the client and the family, the team needs to view amputation as reconstructive surgery, not a mutilating procedure (Tardiff, 1994). Understanding common feelings about amputation, factors that influence these feelings, and measures to assist the client and the family to cope are necessary.

The prospect of an amputation is frightening for both the client and the family. Their concerns include how the amputation will change their lives; the client's ability to walk and to work; the reaction of family and friends to them after amputation; and their own reaction to the changes in self-image.

The client and family will mourn the loss of the body part and the loss of function. No matter how advanced a **prosthesis** (artificial limb) is, it cannot replace the lost body part (Carpenito, 1991). The loss of a body part parallels the death of a loved one (Parks, 1975). But there is no funeral ritual or burial, and mourning is not encouraged (McAteer, 1989).

Grief is a universal reaction to loss. The stages of grief are denial, bargaining, depression, anger, and acceptance (Butler, Turkal, & Seidl, 1992). At first, there may be a denial of the need for amputation. After surgery, the client may refuse to look at the residual limb/stump, that portion of the arm or leg remaining after the amputation. Or the client may deny that the amputation will alter his or her life in any way. The client may bargain, that is, seeking a second opinion about the need for surgery, or attempt any treatment other than amputation. Depression may be demonstrated as anxiety, self-pity, or noncompliance. The client may feel he or she will never be whole again. Anger is expressed at the caregivers, family and friends, and at himself or herself. Often, there are feelings of guilt, "if I had or had not done" what might have resulted in the amputation. Adjustment to the amputation, instead of acceptance, may be a more descriptive term of the last stage of grief. This adjustment often occurs much later after the amputation.

Both the client and the family or significant other will go through the grief process. The stages of grief are not locked into steps. There may be sliding forward and backward between the stages. The client and the family may be at different stages at different times (Butler, Turkal, & Seidl, 1992). The health care team may be dealing with a depressed client and an angry family at the same time. Often, a difficult time is when the client returns home and no longer has the support of the health care team and the protection of the hospital or rehabilitation center. A second difficult time is when the client is being fitted for a prosthesis, an artificial limb, as this forces the client to face the reality of the lost limb. Nursing assessment is used to identify where the client and the family are in the grief process and to identify factors that will influence their reactions to the amputation.

Factors Influencing the Reaction to Amputation

Some of the factors that will influence the client's reaction to amputation include his or her age and developmental stage, the cause of the amputation, the amputation level, the reaction of the family and friends, previous coping mechanisms, a first amputation versus having a second amputation, and other medical problems of the client (Butler, Turkal, & Seidl, 1992).

The age and developmental tasks of the client need to be considered. The child or youth with an amputation will also be dealing with the normal dependency versus independency issues. He or she may adapt easier to the amputation because of limited experience before the amputation. The parents may have more difficulty dealing with the amputation than the child. The adult client is concerned with family responsibilities, work, and marriage. His or her questions will deal with how the amputation will affect these activities and being accepted by others. He or she may have more difficulty adapting to the new body image. Older adults may be retired on a fixed income and adjusting to the physical changes of aging (McCourt, 1993). They often have other health problems that may affect the ability to care for themselves.

The major causes of amputation are disease, trauma, and congenital anomalies. Diseases such as diabetes, PVD, cancer, gangrene, or infection cause the majority of lower extremity amputations. The client often anticipates the need for amputation and may go through some of the grief process even before the surgery. The client with a traumatic amputation may view himself or herself as a victim without a choice. With amputations due to birth defects, the health care team will deal with the parents' as well as the child's feelings about amputation.

The level of amputation may influence the client's reaction. A hand injury or amputation has the impact of a deformity of the face (Mendelson, Burech, Polack, & Kappel, 1986). The reaction depends on what the amputated part means to the client, not just the amount of tissue lost. The loss of a toe or a finger may be more devastating to one client than the loss of an entire limb to another.

The client with an amputation is acutely aware of everyone's reaction to them. If the client feels that the members of the health care team have difficulty caring for the residual limb, how can he or she expect friends or family to deal with the amputation? The client, fearful of rejection, may not want to see friends. The family may avoid or overprotect the client. They may feel anxious or depressed. There might be anger over role reversal if the client is not able to return to previous activities or employment.

All of the health team members need to be aware of the dynamics of family relationships and of the client's and family's previous coping mechanisms for dealing with a crisis. The amputation could be seen as a reason for the client to become dependent.

Because the disease process, such as diabetes or PVD, affects the circulation of both legs, there is always the fear of losing the "good" leg. Within 3 to 5 years of the first amputation due to PVD or diabetes, the client has an 80 percent chance of losing the second leg (Walters, 1992). Sometimes the client and family are more upset by the second amputation because they have been through the "trauma" of one amputation and now know the difficulties. With a second amputation of the lower extremities, the client may not be able to ambulate with a prosthesis, owing to the energy requirements of walking and the stress of other medical problems.

Other medical problems that affect the client's reaction to amputation include cardiac or respiratory disease, blindness, stroke with loss of function of one side of the body and/or short-term memory loss, or spinal cord injury. Each problem is dealt with during rehabilitation to assist the client to reach his or her potential. The health care team plans and implements measures necessary to assist the client and the family in the coping process.

Strategies to Assist the Client and Family

Psychological preparation of the client and the family for a potential amputation should begin as early as possible. The physician should discuss the type of surgery, the benefits of amputation, and a review of the efforts to save the limb. Such preparation pre-operatively often diminishes long-term complications (Butler, Turkal, & Seidl, 1992). There is a need for open communication and realistic encouragement. How the health care team deals with the client before and after surgery affects the client's medical and psychological adjustment (Mendelson, Burech, Polack, & Kappel, 1986). The team must assist the client in learning that the degree of disability depends on his or her ability to accept and adapt to the amputation.

Information must be provided at the appropriate level, at the appropriate time. Most new amputees have knowledge deficits about amputation and how it will affect their lives. Providing information is the key to minimizing the client's and the family's anxiety, enlisting the client's cooperation in the treatment, and expediting the adjustment process (Mendelson, Burech, Polack, & Kappel, 1986).

Be a good listener. Allow time for the client and the family to vent their feelings. They need to feel comfortable about working through their grief. Assure them that grieving is a normal process. Remember that the client and the family may be at different stages of the grief process. Both will need time to come to terms with the loss (Thompson & Haran, 1984).

Suggest that the client and family become involved with a support group to aid in the psychological, social, and physical adjustment to amputation. Some support groups have people who will visit the client before or after surgery. The client has the opportunity to ask questions and to see that there is recovery after amputation. A psychologist may also assist the client and/or family with adjusting to the amputation.

The goal is to assist the client with the physical and psychological adjustments necessary for him or her to return to the family and the community. Using this goal, the health care team can evaluate the client's and the family's progress toward the psychological, physical, and social adjustment to the amputation.

Educational Needs of the Client and Family

The client facing an amputation is dealing not only with the psychological issues, but also with a knowledge deficit of how his or her life will be altered and a lack of skills to deal with the alterations. The health care team will assist the client and the family in learning the knowledge and skills necessary for self-care.

The teaching-learning process, as defined by White (1989), is a "cooperative effort between the teacher and the learner designed to effect change in the learner's knowledge, skills, and attitudes" (p. 64). He states that this process has four steps: assessment, planning, implementation, and evaluation—the same steps as the nursing process. These steps should be used to develop an educational program for the client with an amputation, and the family.

Assessment can begin by using White's (1989) four categories of problems to determine the learning needs to rehabilitation patients: physical functioning, such as transfers, ambulation, and hygiene; social needs, such as financial, living, or structural arrangements; psychological needs; and vocational needs.

During the planning phase, the goals and objectives of an educational program are developed, resources are identified, and a written plan is formulated. Topics the client will need to know include positioning, residual limb care, residual limb wrapping, stump sock care, prosthetic care, transfers, phantom limb sensation or pain, foot care, and emotional adjustment. Behavioral objectives— activities defined in observable and measurable terms—are developed for each topic.

The "five rights" of teaching are used to develop the educational program. Who is the right person to teach the client and/or the family? When is the right time to teach? The right time is when the client is ready to learn, is alert, and does not have other obstructions to learning, such as pain. What is the right information in the right amount to teach? Skills may need to be broken into smaller tasks that are easier to learn. What is the right method of instruction for this client or family? What is their learning style? Is it visual, auditory, or tactile? (McCourt, 1993) (Table 2).

There are many learning resources available. Resources such as booklets, video tapes, and games should be used as the client's reference material and to stimulate questions, not to take the place of teaching. Resources should be reviewed for the reading level of the materials, the size of the print, the use of pictures, and whether they meet the learning style of the client.

Because learning is more effective when the content is relevant to the client's concerns and when the client feels the need to know (White, 1989), the educational needs for the client with an amputation are divided into the pre-operative, postoperative, and rehabilitation phases. The objectives presented in one phase are reviewed in the next phase. The objectives are used to evaluate what the client and family have learned and/or what they still need to know. The client's and family's progress in meeting the objectives must be documented at the end of each teaching session for continuity of care.

Pre-Operative Concerns

The preparation of the client for amputation should include a discussion of the possible level of the amputation. The level of amputation (Figure 1) depends on the circulation of the limb, the disease process involved, other medical problems, and, for the lower limb, whether the client was ambulatory before this hospitalization. The whole person must be evaluated, not only the limb at risk. A noninvasive vascular study is often done to determine the blood flow and the amount of oxygen reaching the tissues (Williamson, 1992). The client may be evaluated for a vascular procedure to improve the blood supply to the limb, therefore, lowering the level of amputation.

Objectives presented pre-operatively are the following:

- Verbalize feelings about amputation. After discussing the psychological aspects and that grief is a normal process for the client and family, they are encouraged to verbalize their feelings about amputation and what the loss means to them.
- Define **phantom limb sensation.** They are able to define phantom limb sensation as a normal sensation that the amputated part is still there. The sensation can be so

Table 2
Five Rights of Teaching

Right person to teach
Right time to teach
Right information
Right amount of information
Right method of instruction

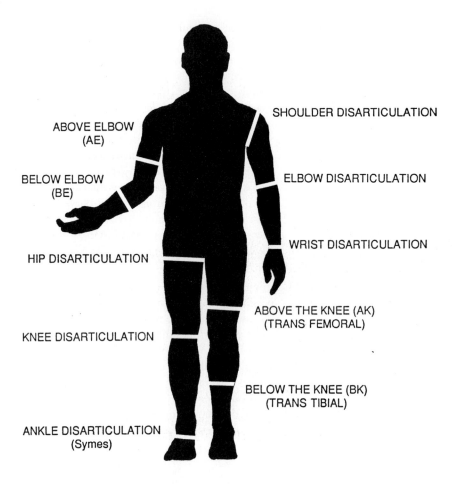

Fig 1. *Different levels of amputation.*

lifelike that the client tries to step on the phantom foot or lift a cup with a phantom hand (Davis, 1993). Unless phantom limb sensation is discussed before surgery, the client may not talk about it for fear of being called crazy.

- Describe the dressings used. The residual limb (stump) dressing may be soft dressings or rigid (cast). The staff will routinely check the dressing frequently after surgery.
- Describe pain control. After surgery, medication will be available. The client needs to inform the staff of the need for medication.
- Identify the goals for rehabilitation. Rehabilitation should begin before the surgery, but often the client may be too ill to participate. The client should be informed that he or she will be evaluated for therapy after the surgery. Therapy will include

such activities as transfer training, ambulation using crutches or walker, evaluation for equipment for home use (such as shower chair or safety rails), driver training, gait training, and learning to walk with the prosthesis if the client is a prosthetic candidate.

- Develop a plan for discharge. Often, the client is ready for discharge from the acute ward about 1 week after surgery. Questions that need to be discussed include the following: If the client is going home, is there wheelchair access? Is there transportation for the client to come to therapy as an outpatient? Is there a need for equipment for the activities of daily living? The client needs to begin therapy before discharge so these questions can also be evaluated by the therapist. Does the client live alone, or is he or she unable to care for himself or herself? Should an extended care or rehabilitation facility be considered? The discharge plan will be reassessed and revised throughout the postoperative and the rehabilitation phases.

Postoperative Concerns

During the postoperative phase, the following objectives are presented and evaluated:

- State the purpose of the residual limb dressing. If a soft dressing is used, it can be changed frequently to inspect the suture line. The Syme's or below-knee residual limb may be casted in surgery. The purpose of the cast is to prevent **edema** (swelling of tissues), prevent knee flexion **contracture** (tightening of muscles around a joint, which restricts range of motion), decrease pain, and provide protection. Because the cast may be in place for 3 to 4 weeks, a window is opened in the distal end to inspect the suture line. After inspection of the surgical area and replacement of the same amount of dressings, the window must be replaced and taped firmly in place to form the complete cast to prevent edema of the end of the residual limb (Figure 2). If the cast slips off, the residual limb should be wrapped with an elastic bandage to prevent edema and the physician should be notified.
- Explain the purpose of proper positioning of the residual limb. Positioning of the residual limb is important to prevent edema and contractures. For the first 24 to 48 hours after surgery, the residual limb is elevated on pillows to prevent edema. After 24 hours, the lower residual limb is positioned flat on the bed or supported straight when the client is in the wheelchair to prevent contractures of the hip and knee.
- Explain the purpose of and demonstrate the prone position. The client with a lower extremity amputation should lie prone for 15 to 20 minutes twice a day to help prevent hip contractures. If hip or knee flexion contractures develop, they may prevent the client from using a prosthesis.

Rehabilitation Concerns

Evaluation for rehabilitation and therapy should begin as soon after surgery as possible. Often, the client is deconditioned because of age, other medical problems, and immobility (Cutson & Bongiorni, 1996). With an amputation, the client must learn transfer techniques from the bed to wheelchair and toilet, and ambulation techniques using crutches, a walker, or a wheelchair.

As the rehabilitation assessment continues, the client with a lower extremity amputation will be evaluated for a prosthesis. Not all clients are candidates for

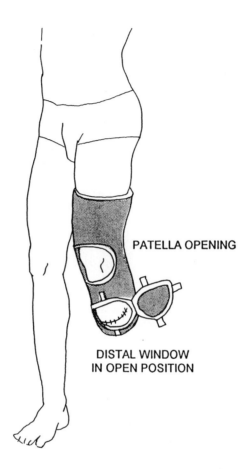

Fig 2. *Below-the-knee stump cast with patella opening and distal window.*

prostheses. The client or family must demonstrate the motivation and the ability to learn the knowledge and skills necessary for self-care. As mentioned previously, it is difficult to fit a lower residual limb for a prosthesis if there are hip or knee flexion contractures. If the client was not ambulatory before amputation due to other medical problems, it is doubtful he or she would be a prosthetic candidate after surgery. Clients with comorbidities, such as cardiopulmonary disease and diabetes, may not have the energy reserves required to use a prosthesis (Table 3). Walters (1992) determined that walking with a below-the-knee prosthesis requires 40 percent more energy, whereas walking with an above-the-knee prosthesis requires 60 percent more energy, as compared with self-propelling a wheelchair, which requires only 12 percent more energy.

Table 3
Criteria for Prosthetic Candidate

Motivation of the client to learn knowledge and skills necessary for self-care
Ability of client and/or family member to learn knowledge and skills for self-care
Absence of hip or knee contractures
Ambulatory status before amputation
Other medical problems such as stroke, blindness, cardiac, respiratory, spinal cord injury

The cost of a prosthesis may be another concern for the client and family. A prosthesis for a below-the-knee amputation begins at $6000; for an above-the-knee amputation, it begins at $10,000. Some insurance plans do not cover the cost of a prosthetic device.

Objectives presented during the rehabilitation phase include the following. Lower extremity amputation care is discussed first, followed by upper extremity amputation care.

- Demonstrate residual limb inspection and care. When the cast and the sutures are removed from the residual limb 3 to 4 weeks after surgery, the client will demonstrate washing the limb with soap and water and drying thoroughly. Inspection of the limb for any open or discolored areas or skin irritation is done daily. A mirror may be needed to view the end or back of the residual limb.
- Demonstrate proper residual **limb (stump) wrapping.** Explain the purpose of limb wrapping. Once the cast and sutures are removed, the residual limb may have edema up to 4 months after surgery. Limb wrapping is begun to prevent edema and to shape the limb for a prosthesis. Using a figure eight, the elastic wrap is applied at the distal end of the limb and continues up to the joint above (Figures 3 and 4). To maintain proper pressure, the wrap is reapplied at least three times a day.

A **stump shrinker,** an elastic sock in the shape of the limb, may be used in place of the elastic wraps. Both the wraps and the shrinker should be washed by hand frequently. They must be thoroughly dry before use.

Clients who are not prosthetic candidates will benefit from therapy to increase their independent function using a wheelchair or assistive devices (Cutson & Bongiorni, 1996). Antitip casters should be applied to the back of the wheelchair to prevent tipping backward when going up an incline (Edelstein, 1992). If the client is a bilateral lower limb amputee, the wheelchair should have an amputee frame. To accommodate the decreased weight from the missing limbs in the front of the wheelchair, the rear axle is set back about 2 inches to adjust the center of gravity (Smeltzer & Bare, 1992).

Stump Wrapping

Below-the-Knee Stump

Wrapping the stump with an ace wrap shapes and shrinks the stump to prepare it for the prosthesis. The ace wrap is to be worn at all times, day and night, except during bathing or when wearing the prosthesis.

The ace wrap will need to be reapplied four to five times during waking hours to maintain an even pressure. The pressure should be greater at the end of the stump. Follow the steps as shown.

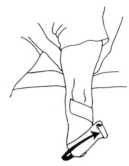

1 To prevent constriction of circulation, all turns must be on the diagonal. Anchor the wrap.

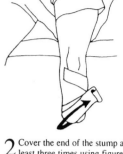

2 Cover the end of the stump at least three times using figure-of-eight turns.

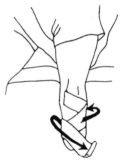

3 Maintain an even tension on the ace wrap. It should be snug, but not tight.

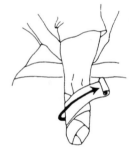

4 Continue up the leg, using figure-of-eight turns. Decrease the tension on the ace wrap as you wrap toward the thigh.

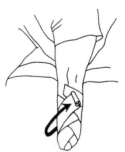

5 Continue wrapping up the leg. The knee can be included in the wrap as a reminder to keep the knee straight.

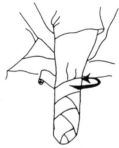

6 If the wrap is extended above the knee, there should be one turn above the knee cap. Do not put excessive pressure on the popliteal area behind the knee as this will decrease the circulation to the leg.

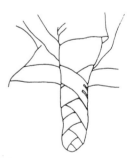

7 Bring the wrap back below the knee, continuing with diagonal turns. Anchor the wrap with tape. Do not use pins as this could injure the skin.

Fig 3. *Stump wrapping: Below-the-knee stump.*

Stump Wrapping

Above-the-Knee Stump

Wrapping the stump with an ace wrap shapes and shrinks the stump to prepare it for the prosthesis. The ace wrap is to be worn at all times, day and night, except during bathing or when wearing the prosthesis.

The ace wrap will need to be reapplied four to five times during waking hours to maintain an even pressure. The pressure should be greater at the end of the stump. Follow the steps as shown.

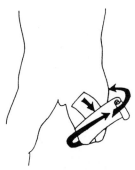

1 To prevent constriction of circulation, all turns must be on the diagonal. Cover the end of the stump well.

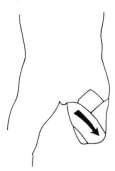

2 Continue figure-of-eight turns to bring the wrap well up into the groin area to prevent adductor muscle from forming roll over bandage.

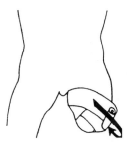

3 Maintain an even tension on the ace wrap. It should be snug, but not tight, on the end of the stump.

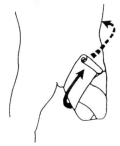

4 The wrap can be finished at this point, or a turn can be taken around the hip to anchor the wrap.

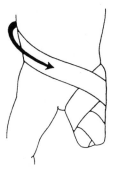

5 Bring the wrap behind the body at the level of the iliac crest. The wrap should not be tight where they cross.

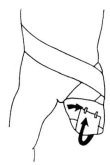

6 Finish the wrap with diagonal turns around the stump. Anchor the wrap with tape. Do not use pins as this could injure the skin.

Fig 4. *Stump wrapping: Above-the-knee stump.*

If the client is a prosthetic candidate, a cast will be made of the residual limb to form the **socket of the prosthesis,** that portion of the prosthesis into which the residual limb is placed. The basic parts of a prosthesis include the socket, a knee joint if the client has a knee disarticulation or above-the-knee amputation, the shank of the prosthesis, and the foot and ankle (Figures 5, 6, and 7).

If the client's weight changes more than 5 pounds, the fit of the socket will be affected and could result in skin breakdown of the residual limb. Owing to the possibility of infection, the prosthesis should not be worn if any open areas on the residual limb are seen (Nevue & Spearbeck, 1994). The client with a lower limb prosthesis should bring a pair of walking shoes when the prosthesis is fitted. The prosthesis is adjusted to the heel height of that shoe. If shoes are changed, the same heel height should be used to maintain alignment of the prosthesis.

- Demonstrate proper cleaning of the socket of the prosthesis. When the prosthesis is removed for the day, the socket should be cleaned with a damp cloth and must thoroughly dry before wearing. Inspection of the prosthesis is done daily, looking for any cracks or rough areas inside the socket and unusual noise or movement in the joints or foot. A new prosthesis should be worn for a short time, removed, and

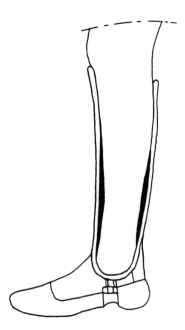

Fig 5. *Syme prosthesis.*

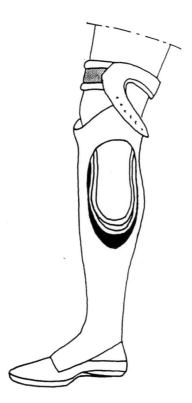

Fig 6. *Below-the-knee amputation prosthesis.*

the residual limb inspected for any skin problems. The wearing time and use of the prosthesis should be increased slowly.

- Describe the purpose of stump socks and their care. Describe when to add or remove stump socks and how to obtain new stump socks. Stump socks of different thicknesses are used to maintain proper fit between the residual limb and the socket of the prosthesis. The usual thicknesses are 1 ply, 3 ply, and 5 ply. The higher the number, the thicker the sock. A combination of socks is used for proper fit. As the socks are usually of wool, the manufacturer's instructions for care should be followed for daily washing. Because the socks must be thoroughly dry before use to prevent stump breakdown, several pair are needed.

  A thin nylon sheath or sock may be used next to the skin to prevent the residual limb from turning within the socket. It also should be washed frequently.

- Demonstrate proper **donning** (putting on) and **doffing** (removing) **of the prosthesis.** In donning the prosthesis, the residual limb, the sheath, stump socks, and the prosthetic socket must be clean and dry. The sheath and stump socks are applied

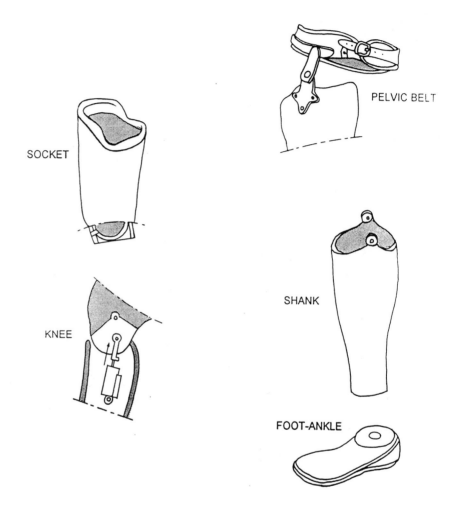

SOCKET

PELVIC BELT

KNEE

SHANK

FOOT-ANKLE

Fig 7. *Above-the-knee amputation prosthesis.*

without wrinkles to prevent skin irritation. If a linear is used inside the socket, it is then applied. The residual limb is then slipped into the socket. The residual limb should not touch the bottom of the socket, as this puts pressure of the skin and could cause skin breakdown. The prosthesis is secured by suction in the socket or by belts around the waist.

- Demonstrate proper foot care. Inspection of the foot for open areas, blisters, or discolorations is done daily. The bottom of the foot is inspected by using a mirror. The foot should be washed and dried well between the toes daily. Toenails are trimmed straight across and not too short to prevent ingrown toe nails. Lotion can be applied to the dry skin on the top and bottom of the foot, but not between the toes, as the moisture may lead to skin breakdown. Shoes need to be wide enough and long enough to prevent pressure on any area of the foot. When buying shoes, the feet should be measured.

The person with an amputation of one foot due to poor circulation is at a 20 to 50 percent risk of losing the other foot due to vascular disease within 3 to 5 years (Cutson & Bongiorni, 1996).

• Describe signs and symptoms of infection and actions to take if noted. The client and the family need to know the signs and symptoms of infection and, if they occur, whom to contact or when to come to the emergency room.

Because the education of the client and family occurs throughout hospitalization, clinic appointments, therapy sessions, and home visits, all of the health care team need to know the educational objectives for each client. Teaching sessions can be individualized or part of a support group presentation. Support group sessions provide a time and place for the client and the family to discuss common concerns and to share information. It provides a safe place for them to vent feelings with others who have had the same experience and to learn they are not the only people facing the stress of coping with an amputation. The ability of the client and family to meet the behavioral objectives for all three phases of care should be documented at the end of each educational session. Those objectives not fully met can then be reviewed at the next session (Table 4). Documentation includes what was taught, to whom, by what method, listing the materials given to the person, how well the behavioral objectives were met, and what further education is needed.

Complications   Beside the problems of flexion contractures of the hip or knee, other complications include residual limb skin breakdown and phantom limb pain. Contractures are preventable with proper positioning of the residual limb and instructing the client in proper positioning and the reason for preventing contractures.

Residual limb skin breakdown may be due to ischemia or infection. Ischemia is due to lack of blood supply to an area. Prevention of edema of the residual limb by proper positioning, avoiding a dependent position of the limb, will assist in increasing circulation to the area. The lower residual limb may require a revascularization procedure, such as angioplasty or bypass, or a surgical revision of the limb. An infection is treated with antibiotics and positioning of the limb. It may require surgery to remove necrotic tissue. Either ischemia or infection will increase the client's hospitalization and prolong rehabilitation.

Phantom limb pain is a painful sensation felt in the missing body part, described as knifelike, burning, or squeezing (Davis, 1993), or resembling pain felt in the limb before amputation (Rounseville, 1992). Up to 85 percent of amputees experience phantom limb pain. It is unpredictable in severity, frequency, duration, and character. There is no cure, but interventions include surgical, physi-

Table 4
Educational Objectives of Client with Amputation

Pre-operative objectives
    Verbalize feelings about amputation
    Define phantom limb sensation
    Describe residual limb dressing used
    Describe pain control measures
    Identify goals of rehabilitation program
    Develop plan for discharge
Postoperative Objectives
    State purpose of residual limb dressing (cast)
    State purpose of proper positioning of residual limb
    State purpose of and demonstrate prone position
    Demonstrate safe transfer techniques
Rehabilitation objectives
    Demonstrate residual limb inspection and care
    State purpose of residual limb wrapping
    Demonstrate residual limb wrapping
    Demonstrate proper care of prosthesis
    Describe the purpose of stump stocks and their care
    Demonstrate proper donning and doffing of prosthesis
    Demonstrate proper foot care
    Describe signs and symptoms of infection and actions if infection noted

cal, medical, and psychological training, and education (Davis, 1993; Maher, Addams, & Shabtaie, 1994; Rounseville, 1992; Williams & Deaton, 1997). Sometimes, a simple exercise of dorsiflexing and plantarflexing the foot up and down on both sides, which contracts and relaxes the muscles, may decrease the painful feeling (Edelstein, 1992).

Upper Extremity Amputation

The major causes for upper extremity amputations are severe trauma (acute injury, electrical burn, frostbite), malignant tumors, infections (fulminating gas gangrene or chronic osteomyelitis), and congenital malformations (Smeltzer & Bare, 1992). Usually, these clients are younger and healthier than the lower extremity amputees.

Psychological reactions to a traumatic upper extremity amputation are often more intense because of the disruption of the ability to do activities of daily living and continue with vocational and recreational activities. Amputations of up per extremities present different problems because of their highly specialized functions (Smeltzer & Bare, 1992).

Occupational therapy is involved immediately postoperatively to begin instruction in self-care skills, such as feeding and grooming. One-handed techniques for shaving, brushing teeth, applying make-up, and using utensils such as a knife-fork or a rocking knife can be learned to increase confidence (Bender, 1974).

Atkins and Meier (1989) stated that it is critical to maintain range of motion in all joints of the upper extremity for the placement and function of the terminal device, the prosthesis. Exercises that maintain or improve the range of motion of the scapular, glenohumeral, elbow, and forearm for pronation and supination are begun early.

Care of the residual limb includes daily washing and patting dry with a towel. This allows the client to become familiar with the body changes. Proper hygiene also provides sensory input. The residual limb should be gently massaged to desensitize and provide sensory input. Desensitization will increase the client's tolerance to pressure placed on the residual limb by the socket (Atkins & Meier, 1989). The upper extremity residual limb also requires stump wrapping (Figures 8 and 9).

If the preferred hand is amputated, training in activities of daily living may require the client to use the remaining hand. Once familiar with the use of the prosthesis, the client may choose to do many activities with the prosthesis (Santschi, 1958). But the prosthesis does have limitations and will never fully duplicate the function of the lost limb. Some clients with upper extremity amputations decide not to wear a prosthesis because they feel it is awkward. If the client uses a prosthesis, it will be used as an assist to the sound limb, to regain lost function (Santschi, 1958) (Figures 10 and 11).

Stump socks may be used for absorption of perspiration, warmth, and padding. Several are needed to facilitate laundering. The prosthesis is usually held in place with a harness. Because the harness should be washed when soiled, two harnesses should be supplied for wearing. A T-shirt worn under the harness absorbs perspiration, serves as padding under the harness, and prevents irritation and pressure in the axilla area (Santschi, 1958).

For the bilateral upper extremity amputee, at least one functional prosthesis is critical. Usually, the longer residual limb is considered the dominant side (Santschi, 1958). Before receiving the prosthesis, the use of a universal cuff with adapted utensil, such as toothbrush or pen, can enhance independence (Atkins & Meier, 1989).

There are a number of textbooks that illustrate specific techniques for using one hand or using the prosthesis for self-care dressing and grooming, food preparation and cooking, household tasks (Bender, 1974), and "clerical activities,"

A. To prevent constriction of circulation, all turns must be diagonal. Anchor the wrap with the first couple of turns.

B. Cover the end of the limb at least three times, using figure-of-eight turns. Maintain an even tension of the wrap. It should be snug, but not tight.

C. Continue up the limb, using figure-of-eight turns; decrease tension when wrapping toward elbow. Avoid pressure on the elbow.

D. Continue wrapping with the diagonal turns until midway above the elbow.

E. Anchor wrap with tape. Do not use pins as they could injure the skin.

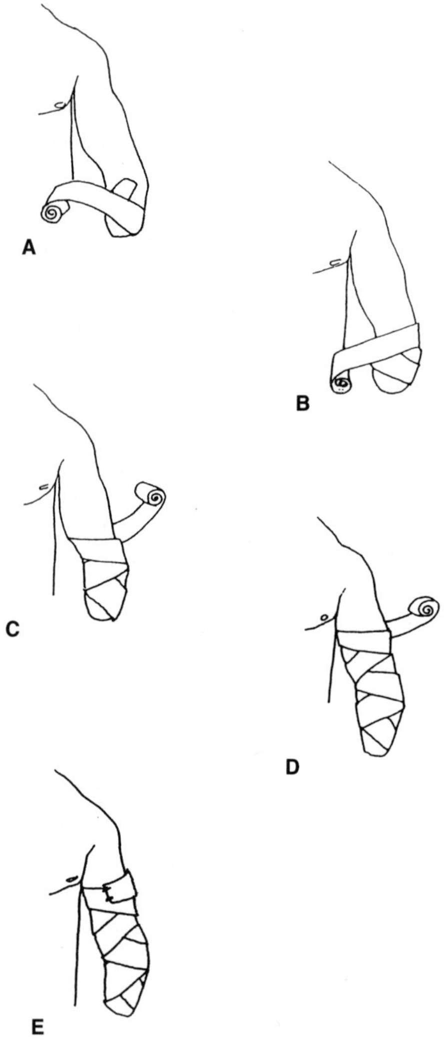

Fig 8. *Stump wrapping: Below the elbow. Wrapping the residual limb with an elastic wrap shapes and shrinks the limb to prepare it for the prosthesis. The wrap is worn at all times, day and night, except during bathing or when wearing the prosthesis. The elastic wrap should be reapplied four or five times a day to maintain an even pressure. The pressure should be greater at the distal end of the limb. Steps A–E are shown.*

A. To prevent constriction of circulation, all turns must be diagonal. Anchor the wrap with the first couple of turns.

B. Cover the end of the limb at least three times, using figure-of-eight turns. Maintain an even tension on the wrap. It should be snug, but not tight.

C. Bring the wrap up to the axilla, avoiding pressure on nerves. The wrap can be finished at this point, and the wrap anchored with tape.

D. If needed, the wrap can go around body through the normal axilla to hold wrap in place. Wrap should not be tight in the axilla. Anchor wrap with tape. Avoid using pins that could injure the skin.

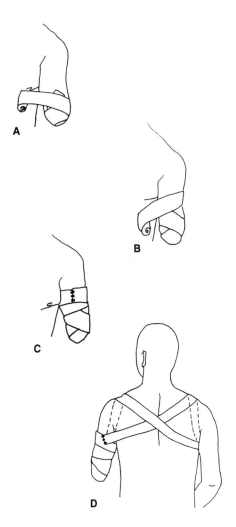

Fig 9. *Stump wrapping: Above the elbow. Wrapping the residual limb with an elastic wrap shapes and shrinks the limb, preparing it for the prosthesis. The elastic wrap is worn at all times, day and night, except during bathing or when wearing the prosthesis. The wrap should be reapplied four or five times a day to maintain an even pressure. The pressure should be greater at the distal end of the limb. Steps A–D are shown.*

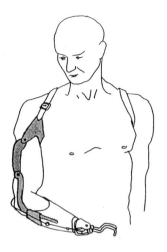
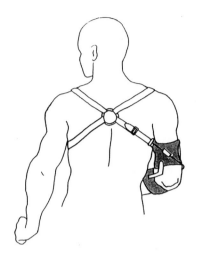

Fig 10. *Below-the-elbow amputation prosthesis.*

such as pencil sharpening, writing, using the telephone, typing, and using scissors (Santschi, 1958). Examples of client and family educational materials are listed at the end of the chapter.

The nurse can assist the rehabilitation process by encouraging the client to use the techniques taught in therapy to foster independence.

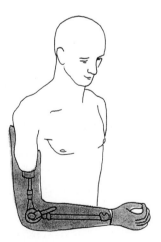

Fig 11. *Above-the-elbow amputation prosthesis.*

Common Nursing Diagnoses, Outcomes, and Interventions

By using the nursing process, several common nursing diagnoses related to the client with an amputation are identified. Six common nursing diagnoses are as follows: body image disturbance, knowledge deficit, self-care deficit, impaired mobility, grieving related to loss of body part, and alteration in comfort owing to phantom pain or operative stump pain. These nursing diagnoses, objectives or outcomes, and the suggested interventions for each diagnosis, are presented. There are other nursing diagnoses that may also be needed for these clients.

Nursing Diagnosis

- Body image disturbance related to loss of body part. Defined by McCourt (1993), *body image* is the conscious and unconscious mental picture a person has of the shape, size, and mass of the body and its parts. Gordon (1993) describes body image disturbance as negative feelings about the characteristics, functions, or limits of one's body or body parts. Clients may not look at or touch the residual limbs. They often have fears of rejection by family and others. There may be feelings of hopelessness, helplessness, or powerlessness or a refusal to acknowledge that the amputation will change the lifestyle (McCourt, 1993). Clients may be unable to participate in their usual lifestyle or vocational and recreational roles owing to the physical limitations imposed by the loss of a limb (Ulrich, Canale, & Wendell, 1986).

Goals/Outcomes

The client and family are able to

- Share feelings about self-concept and acknowledge changes in body image (Nevue & Spearbeck, 1994; Smeltzer & Bare, 1992).
- Express feelings of grief, such as anger, sadness, or loss (McCourt, 1993) and acceptance of an altered self (Tucker, Canobbi, Parquette, & Wells, 1996).
- Participate in social activities without hiding the residual limb (McCourt, 1993).
- Resume role-related responsibilities (Smeltzer & Bare, 1992).
- Maintain relationships with significant others.
- Verbalize a plan for adapting a lifestyle to meet restrictions imposed by the loss of a limb (Ulrich, Canale, & Wendell, 1986).
- Use positive coping skills to deal with the loss of the body part (Tucker, Canobbi, Parquette, & Wells, 1996).

Nursing Interventions

- Encourage both the client and family to express feelings about loss. Note the nonverbal responses (Ulrich, Canale, & Wendell, 1986).
- Provide support by actively listening.
- Support the client and family through the grieving process.
- Assist the family to treat the client in normal manner (McCourt, 1993).
- Assist the client and family to explore sources of support, such as professional and peer groups.

- Encourage the client and family to attend amputee support group (Nevue & Spearbeck, 1994).
- Assist the client and family to identify and use helpful coping techniques.
- With the client's approval, arrange for a visit with an amputee who has successfully adjusted and resumed his or her usual lifestyle (Ulrich, Canale, & Wendell, 1986).

Nursing Diagnosis

- *Knowledge deficit.* Defined by McCourt (1993) as the inability to explain information or demonstrate required skills for disability management or activities of daily living (ADL), the knowledge deficit is usually due to the client having no previous experience with the disability.

Goals/Outcomes

- The client and family are able to verbalize the knowledge or demonstrate the skills needed to meet the behavioral objectives for disability management and activities of daily living (McCourt, 1993).

Examples include demonstrating residual limb care, demonstrating limb wrapping, donning and doffing the prosthesis correctly, verbalizing necessary observations of the residual limb, and demonstrating care of the other foot.

Nursing Interventions

- With the client and the family, develop behavioral objectives for needed instructional experiences (McCourt, 1993) and develop an individualized teaching plan (Nevue & Spearbeck, 1994).
- Tailor the information and the teaching approaches to meet the client's and family's needs.
- Encourage the client and family to ask questions and to participate in daily care (Nevue & Spearbeck, 1994).
- Allow the client and family time for practice and return demonstration (Ulrich, Canale, & Wendell, 1986).
- Document the client and family instruction and their ability to meet the behavioral objectives.

Nursing Diagnosis

- Self-care deficit. Self-care includes such activities as independence in feeding, transfers, toileting, and the ability to dress and bathe. Self-care deficit is the impaired ability to perform activities for oneself (McCourt, 1993). An example would be self-feeding deficit for a client with bilateral upper limb amputations.

Goals/Outcomes

The client and family are able to

- Demonstrate adapted techniques and equipment to meet self-care needs.
- Direct care given by others, if unable to meet own self-care needs (McCourt, 1993).

Nursing Interventions

- Provide an environment in which the client feels safe.
- Teach and assist the client to use adaptive equipment.
- Reinforce safe transfer techniques.
- Reinforce the therapist's instructions for adapted ADL.
- Assist the client to become independent with self-care techniques, providing assistance only as necessary.
- Assist the family to give encouragement and provide only the necessary help until the client is independent (Nevue & Spearbeck, 1994).

Nursing Diagnosis

- Impaired mobility. McCourt (1993) describes physical mobility as having the four aspects of bed mobility, transfers, wheel chair mobility, and ambulation. The client with impaired physical mobility has limitation of ability for independent physical movement within the environment. Ulrich, Canale, and Wendell (1986) suggest that one cause of balance difficulties is associated with the change in the body's center of gravity due to the loss of the lower limb.

Goals/Outcomes

The client and family are able to

- Perform safe transfers.
- Demonstrate safe use of adaptive equipment (Nevue & Spearbeck, 1994).
- Demonstrate positions to avoid joint contractures (Smeltzer & Bare, 1992).

Nursing Interventions

- Teach/supervise the use of safe transfer techniques.
- Reinforce the therapist's instructions in the safe use of adaptive equipment for ambulation, such as walker, cane, crutches, wheelchair, and prosthesis (Nevue & Spearbeck, 1994; Ulrich, Canale, & Wendell, 1986).
- Instruct the client in reasons for prevention of joint contractures and correct positioning, including proning.

Nursing Diagnosis

- Grieving related to loss of body part. Grieving is a normal reaction to loss. Ulrich, Canale, and Wendell (1986) states that grieving is related to the loss of a body part and the resulting changes in body functioning, self-image, and usual lifestyle and roles.

Goals/Outcomes

The client and family are able to

- Express grief and begin to work through their feelings (Smeltzer & Bare, 1992).
- Use available support systems (Ulrich, Canale, & Wendell, 1986).

Nursing Interventions

- Provide support to the client and family by acknowledging the reality of the loss and by active listening (Smeltzer & Bare, 1992).
- Encourage the client and family to express and share their feelings about the loss (Carpenito, 1991).
- Discuss the grieving process, noting that it is an expected response to loss or change.
- Allow time for the client and family to progress through the stages of grief.
- Provide information about support groups and counseling services (Ulrich, Canale, & Wendell, 1986).
- Encourage the client and family to discuss their perception of the short- and long-term effects of the disability.
- Promote grief work by encouragement, acceptance, and open communication with the client and family (Carpenito, 1991).

Nursing Diagnosis

- Alteration in comfort owing to phantom pain or operative stump pain. Residual limb pain in the client with an amputation is commonly caused by the surgical incision, may be an expression of grief and altered body image, may result from postoperative complications of pressure on the bony prominence by the dressing or by a hematoma, or be phantom limb pain. Surgical incision pain usually is time limited and controlled by analgesics. Pain due to the expression of grief and alteration of body image may not be changed by analgesics. Severe pain due to complications must be reported to the surgeon for treatment of its cause (Smeltzer & Bare, 1992). Phantom pain is discussed in a previous section (see Complications). Carpenito (1991) states that phantom sensations are due to severed nerves that continue to send pain impulses and give the sensation of the limb's presence.

Goals/Outcomes

The client and family are able to

- Experience absence of pain as evidenced by appearing relaxed and by verbalizing comfort (Smeltzer & Bare, 1992).
- Participate in self-care and mobility activities without complaints of pain.

- Demonstrate techniques for management of phantom limb sensation and/or pain (Carpenito, 1991).
- Understand the differences between phantom limb sensation and phantom limb pain.

Nursing Interventions

- Assist the client to identify the nature of the discomfort and assess the need for pain medication or other measures to decrease discomfort.
- Administer appropriate pain medication as needed. Assess effectiveness of pain relief measures and document ("Tucker, Canobbi, Parquette, & Wells, 1996).
- Assist the client to find a comfortable position and support the limb during movement.
- Instruct the client in other pain management techniques, such as tapping, massaging, pressure, and contracting, and relaxing muscle groups (Nevue & Spearbeck, 1994).
- Encourage the client to report phantom limb sensation and pain (Ulrich, Canale, & Wendell, 1986).

Other nursing diagnoses may be appropriate for a client depending on age, other medical problems, lifestyle, vocational needs, and concerns. The presented interventions and desired outcomes are examples and suggestions from a variety of sources. The client's needs must be assessed, interventions planned and implemented, and desired outcomes evaluated. This process should be used by the entire health care team for continuity of care for the client and the family.

Summary

This chapter has presented information on the rehabilitation of the client with an amputation. As the general population ages and the complications of diseases such as diabetes and vascular disease are seen, the numbers of clients facing amputation will increase. The client with an amputation will be older with more concomitant and complicating medical problems. The nurse will be a critical member of the health care team during the rehabilitation of these clients. A major function of the nurse will be to assist these clients and their families in dealing with everyday life after an amputation.

References

Atkins, D., & Meier, R. (1989). *Comprehensive management of the upper-limb amputee.* New York: Springer-Verlag.

Bender, L. (1974). *Prostheses and rehabilitation after arm amputation.* New York: Charles C Thomas.

Butler, D., Turkal, N., & Seidl, J. (1992). Amputation: Preoperative psychological preparation. *Journal of American Board of Family Practice, 5*(1), 69–73.

Carpenito, L. (1991). *Nursing care plans and documentation: Nursing diagnosis and collaborative problems.* Philadelphia: J.B. Lippincott.

Cutson, T., & Bongiorni, D. (1996). Rehabilitation of the older lower limb amputee: A brief review. *Journal of the American Geriatrics Society, 44,* 1388–1393.

Davis, R. (1993). Phantom sensations, phantom pain, and stump pain. *Archives of Physical Medicine and Rehabilitation, 74,* 79–91.

Edelstein, J. (1992). Preprosthetic and nonprosthetic management of older patients. *Topics in Geriatric Rehabilitation, 8*(1), 22–29.

Gordon, M. (1993). *Manual of nursing diagnosis: 1993–1994.* St. Louis: Mosby–Year Book.

Maher, A., Addams, S., & Shabtaie, J. (1994). Amputation and replantation. In A. Maher, S. Salmond, & T. Pellino (Eds.), *Orthopaedic nursing* (pp. 762–780). Philadelphia: W.B. Saunders.

McAteer, M. (1989). Some aspects of grief in physiotherapy. *Physiotherapy, 75*(1), 55–58.

McCourt, A. (1993). *The specialty practice of rehabilitation nursing: A core curriculum* (3rd ed.). Rehabilitation Nursing Foundation.

Mendelson, R., Burech, J., Polack, E., & Kappel, D. (1986). The psychological impact of traumatic amputations. *Hand Clinics, 2*(3), 577–582.

National Diabetic Association (1995). Publication 95-1468. Washington, D.C.: Author.

Nevue, V., & Spearbeck, K. (1994). Care of the patient with lower extremity amputation. In P. Maguire (Ed.), *Manual of patient care standards* (pp. 1–7). Gaithersburg, MD: Aspen.

Parks, C. (1975). Psycho-social transitions: Comparison between reactions to loss of a limb and loss of a spouse. *British Journal of Psychiatry, 127,* 204–210.

Rounseville, C. (1992). Phantom limb pain: The ghost that haunts the amputee. *Orthopaedic Nursing, 11*(2), 67–71.

Santschi, W. (1958). *Manual of upper extremity prosthetics* (2nd ed.). Los Angeles: University of California.

Smeltzer, S., & Bare, B. (Eds.). (1992). *Brunner & Suddarth's textbook of medical-surgical nursing* (7th ed.). Philadelphia: J.B. Lippincott.

Tardiff, F. (1994). Playing on the same team: Amputees and nurses. *RN Times, 3,* 10–11.

Thompson, D., & Haran, D. (1984). Living with an amputation: What it means for patients and their helpers. *International Journal of Rehabilitation Research, 7*(3), 283–292.

Tucker, S., Canobbi, M., Parquette, E., & Wells, M. (1996). *Patient care standards: Collaborative practice planning guides* (6th ed.). St. Louis: Mosby.

Ulrich, S., Canale, S., & Wendell, S. (1986). *Nursing care planning guides: A nursing diagnosis approach.* Philadelphia: W.B. Saunders.

Walters, R. (1992). Energy expenditure. In J. Perry (Ed.), *Gait analysis: Normal and pathological function* (pp. 475–479). New York: McGraw-Hill.

White, B. (1989). Teaching-learning process. In S. Dittmar (Ed.), *Rehabilitation nursing: Process and application* (pp. 63–72). St. Louis: Mosby.

Williams, A., & Deaton, S. (1997). Phantom limb pain: Elusive, yet real. *Rehabilitation Nursing, 22*(2), 73–77.

Williamson, V. (1992). Amputation of the lower extremity: An overview. *Orthopaedic Nursing, 11*(2), 55–65.

CHAPTER 21
Burn Injuries and Long-Term Care Concerns

Barbara Kammerer Quayle

Key Terms   *Behavioral and Social Skills Training*
Burn "Survivor" rather than Burn "Victim"
Color Analysis
Corrective Cosmetic Techniques
Donor Site
Facial and Body Disfigurement
First-Degree Burn
Fourth-Degree Burn
Image Enhancement Program
Investment in Rehabilitation
Mesh Graft
Offsetting
Pressure Garments
Second-Degree Burn
Self-Talk
Sheet Graft
Skin Grafts
STEPS to Self-Esteem
Support Group
Third-Degree Burn
Total Body Surface Area (TBSA)

Objectives   1. List three primary causes of burns.

2. Identify the four types of burn according to depth.

3. List five behavioral and social skills that influence the client-professional relationship.

4. Describe the psychological impact of facial/body disfigurement.

5. Identify four behavior/social skills that can be taught to a burn client to help in coping with social encounters.

6. List three body-image issues that burn clients face during rehabilitation.

Introduction   Burn-injured clients present one of the greatest challenges in nursing care. A burn injury is an extremely painful trauma physically, psychologically, and spiritually. Serious burn injuries are sudden, disastrous in magnitude, and require specialized, extensive, and long-term care to assure optimal recovery and rehabilitation. Nurses can assume a significant role in the rehabilitation process.

This chapter introduces strategies to assist rehabilitation nurses to help clients resume their lives after a burn trauma. Physical, psychological, psychosocial, and spiritual concerns receive primary significance. Attention to the social and behavioral skills that enhance the client-professional relationship is stressed. Current image enhancement strategies and behavioral coping skills are explored to enable nurses to help or refer clients. A summary of nursing diagnoses, goals/outcomes, and interventions is presented. Finally, resources for support organizations specific to burn injuries and facial disfigurement are listed to ensure ongoing support.

Burn injuries occur to 2 million people each year because of fire, scalds, electricity, and chemicals. More men than women incur burn injuries owing to their involvement in more dangerous occupations and hobbies. Scald injuries cause the highest incident of burns to children younger than 6. Approximately 4500 people die each year from burns, and 60,000 are hospitalized. Nearly 10,000 children suffer permanent disability. Clients with significant burns to the face, hands, perineum, and extensive body surface areas receive acute care in one of the 135 burn centers throughout the United States. Burn centers are staffed with physicians, nurses, and therapists who are specially trained in burn wound management.

Skin Anatomy   The skin or integumentary system is the largest organ of the body. It acts as a defense against infection and trauma. The skin also regulates body temperature and sensation.

The skin consists of two primary layers: the epidermis and the dermis. The subcutaneous tissue is not regarded as a layer of skin. Muscle and bone lie beneath the subcutaneous tissue.

Burn Injuries   Injuries are categorized according to the depth of the burn. The depth of the burn injury is calculated by the "burning agent, the temperature of the burning agent, the duration of exposure, the conductivity of the tissue, and the thickness of the dermal structures involved" (Trofino & Braun, 1991, p. 24). A **first-degree burn** (or superficial partial thickness burn), such as a mild sunburn, causes damage to the epidermal layer of the skin. First-degree burns create a great deal of pain, are red or pink, dry, and do not blister. They heal within 5 to 10 days.

A **second-degree burn** (or deeper partial thickness burn), according to Trofino and Braun (1991), affects the dermal layer of skin. Second-degree burns are extremely painful, moist, red, and blistered. The blisters prevent excess water loss, dehydration, and death of superficial dermal cells. Some light second-degree burns heal on their own and if deeper require grafting.

The deep second-degree burns or deep partial-thickness burns, Trofino and Braun (1991) state, involve all of the epidermal and dermal layers. They are mottled pink or red to waxy white with blisters and edema. About 1 month is required to heal completely. A great deal of scar formation is produced.

A **third-degree burn** (or full-thickness burn) extends into the subcutaneous tissue and may involve muscle and bone. Third-degree burns cause damage to the vasculature underlying the burned skin. Their color is deep red, black, waxy white, or yellow. They feel hard and dry and are painless unless surrounded by areas of partial-thickness burns. These burns do not heal on their own and require skin grafts.

A **fourth-degree burn** is also full-thickness and involves muscle, fascia, and bone. Fourth-degree burns are black and depressed. If extremely severe, bones and ligaments are exposed. Amputations are required if the damage is too severe and grafting is impossible.

The extent of the burn injury or **total body surface area (TBSA)** is learned by "the Rule of Nine." Each arm is 9 percent, each leg is 18 percent, front and back of the trunk are 18 percent each, the head is 9 percent, and the perineum is 1 percent. From these percentages, along with consideration of age and general health, the required fluid replacement is calculated.

The age of the client may also decide survival of a burn injury. Children younger than 2 and adults older than 60 have the highest mortality rate. The skin in young children is very thin, and skin in the elderly is also thin and loses elasticity. Both groups are at a higher risk for infection because of their lowered immune status.

Individuals have survived second- and third-degree burns that cover as much as 90 percent TBSA. Although survival is important, quality of life is also important, and the standard of rehabilitation care can make the difference for all burn survivors whether the client is a 20 percent or 80 percent TBSA burn injury.

Burn injuries are among the most painful types of trauma. During the acute care period, patients are extremely sick, and pain management by the burn team is critical. From the onset of the injury until the wounds are almost healed, clients experience pain. The physical pain is usually due to continuous pain from damaged tissue and acute pain from chemical or mechanical irritation of damaged tissue during necessary procedures, such as hydrobaths, dressing changes, physical and occupational therapy, or ambulation (Watkins, Cook, Randolph, & Ehleben, 1988).

Treating Burn Victims

Trofino and Braun (1991) stress that a thorough knowledge of the pathophysiology of a burn is necessary to care for burn-injured clients. This understanding guides in planning, implementing, and evaluating care. It also provides the basis for applying the pathologic changes that occur with burn injuries and for assessing and treating systemic manifestations as well. Major burn injuries affect most body systems including cardiovascular, hematologic, pulmonary, and immune systems, as well as fluid and electrolyte function.

Skin Grafts

When physicians decide the client's stability and the conditions are right, **skin grafts** of the deep second- and third-degree burns are begun. Grafting is the method used to gain 100 percent coverage of the injured surfaces. Skin grafts are harvested from healthy, unburned areas in a surgical procedure. The area from which the skin is harvested is termed a **donor site.** This area is very painful due to disruption of the nerve endings and feels like a second-degree burn. The donor site usually heals within 10 days. The same area can be harvested again if necessary.

A successful skin graft depends on an adequate blood supply at the graft site. With optimal conditions, the graft will adhere within 5 days. If it does not adhere, the procedure must be repeated later.

When there is a shortage of skin for *autografts* (grafts of the client's own skin), sheets of available skin are put into a meshing device. This machine cuts the skin, giving it a chicken-wire appearance and increasing the area it can cover. Although it is not as esthetic in appearance as a solid **sheet graft,** it serves a valuable role. The appearance of the skin with a **mesh graft** is uneven as opposed to the smooth surface of a sheet graft. Sheet grafts, if available, are always used for the face.

Once the burned areas have healed, for approximately 1 year the scars mature. During this time, raised scars develop, contractures of the grafted areas occur, and clients suffer from severe itching. The scarring and contractures at graft sites can be controlled by wearing **pressure garments,** and the itching can be relieved by wearing pressure garments and taking antihistamines at night.

Physical, Psychological, Spiritual Care

Understanding the physical, psychological, and spiritual care required by clients demands time and initiative. Recognizing one's own reactions to burn-injured clients is equally important and requires self-examination of one's own body image.

Rehabilitation nurses who openly examine and resolve their own experiences and feelings concerning body-image issues may achieve greater success. They may feel more comfortable speaking candidly about topics concerning body functions, appearance, and sexuality. As caregivers enabling others to adjust and accept a major life change, it is important to realize that our body images are shaped out of every experience we have ever had. According to Macgregor (1979), the way our parents related to and touched our bodies as babies and as growing children, what we learned from our role models about what it is like to live in and value a body, the acceptance and rejection we have felt from peers, every negative and positive piece of feedback we and our bodies have received from people whose opinions count to us, and the ways we have perceived our bodies to fit or not fit the cultural image have all influenced how we perceive our bodies.

It is no accident that some of us handle body issues easily and effortlessly, while others struggle to come to terms with them. One's personal experiences concerning body image affect how comfortably appearance issue discussions with clients proceed.

Hutchinson (1985) believes that to understand how we arrived at our relationship with our bodies, we must understand the culture in which we have developed. We live in a society that places a high premium on physical appearance. A sizeable body of research confirms the benefits of an attractive appearance. Dion, Berschied, and Walster (1972) describe the physical attractiveness stereotype that suggests that attractive people are also considered to possess other positive attributes. People labeled "attractive" are often viewed as more socially acceptable, likely to find better employment, marry earlier and "better," having more successful marriages, and being better parents and spouses.

In our society, a person's attractiveness and physical beauty often receive greater emphasis than qualities of character, intelligence, and competence. Some studies suggest that assumptions relating to intelligence, personality, and success are often made on the basis of on a person's physical appearance.

A client's realization that a burn injury results in permanent facial or body disfigurement often generates feelings of hopelessness and helplessness. Concern with the alteration in appearance frequently gains as much or greater emphasis than functional capability. Nurses play a vital role in helping people to cope during this difficult time of adjustment. Recognizing the early signs of depression and difficulties with acceptance along with knowledge of appropriate interventions to provide support is important.

Most clients and their families have little understanding about burn injuries and the care, recovery, rehabilitation, and required adaptations. Because of the intense daily involvement with the client and family members, nurses may offer not only expert care, but also education and spiritual and psychosocial support. Nursing requires an understanding of treating the whole person—mind, body, and spirit—because all are affected and need to be addressed. During the acute and rehabilitation phases, clients often view their primary care nurses as a strong anchor of security and their greatest allies.

Behavioral and Social Skills in the Treatment of Burn Survivors

Today, health care delivery continually changes. Clients receive discharge programs quicker and sicker. The current and future medical environment requires professionals to act effectively and efficiently. For these reasons, nurses must not only develop excellent clinical skills, but also excellent "people" skills.

The insight that "It takes so little to be above average" synthesizes what it means to be a rehabilitation nurse working with burn-injured clients. Nurses can develop behavioral and social skills that build greater rapport with clients and work toward creating a powerful bond.

Twenty years ago, I sustained burns over 40 percent of my body owing to flame burns resulting from an auto accident. Second- and third-degree burns covered my face, scalp, back, arms, and hands. The depth of burns on my right hand required amputation of my fingers and part of my thumb. Doctors performed many skin grafts during my 2-month hospitalization. During the rehabilitation phase of my recovery, I received numerous grafts and ongoing therapies.

At the time of my injury, I knew nothing about burn injuries. My experience with hospitals was very limited. During the most vulnerable and dependent period in my adult life, I quickly learned which nurses I could count on and who cared. The expression "They'll never care how much you know, until they know how much you care" became very real and very personal.

Communication

Because 7 percent of communication is verbal and 93 percent nonverbal, it is crucial to be aware of the fact that we are always communicating even when we speak few words. Appropriate behavioral and social skills used by nurses during acute and rehabilitation care developed trust, confidence, and rapport. Incorporating these skills into rehabilitation care seems essential and makes a vital difference to the well-being of the client. Some of these skills may sound simple and easy; unfortunately, in the rush and pressure of direct nursing care, they can slip into disuse.

The first skill is to call clients by name. We all like to hear our name and sense the person using it cares. Clients feel somewhat degraded when called "he" or "she," a diagnosis, or a bed number.

Another skill that reaps dividends is to look directly into the eyes of a client. It is eye contact that connects one human being to another, confirms communication, and promotes rapport.

The vital skill of wearing a smile conveys a feeling of friendliness and self-confidence. Clients enjoy being greeted with a smile that says, "I'm glad to see you and care for you." A smile is a great gift and comfort, especially under times of stress.

A nurse's tone of voice can easily reveal either positive or negative feelings to the client. It is important to use a calm, caring, and confident tone of voice when explaining a procedure, asking about comfort level, or answering a question. The energy and warmth in a nurse's voice can influence a patient's response and interactions. With heightened awareness of their environment, clients readily recognize dissatisfaction, insincerity, or moodiness in caregivers. A professional rehabilitation nurse emits comfort, confidence, and care through his or her tone of voice.

Listening to clients with eye contact can help to establish increased harmony between client and nurse. The gift of listening without judgment or comments gives patients a sense of being cared about. Sometimes, patients simply want a sounding board and do not require discussion or even want to hear an opinion. Sometimes, clients may ask questions about their future outcomes that cannot be answered fully. Some information must be given gradually because to tell everything at a single session would overwhelm the client. To be empathetic in our listening and without feeling the need to make everything better is a valuable contribution to the rehabilitation process.

The power of touch establishes rapport and shows care. A high level of comfort and connection can be achieved through touch. Clients frequently associate touch with pain and anxiety during acute and rehabilitation care. Touching patients in a soothing and noninvasive manner feels relaxing and therapeutic. Holding or rubbing a foot, stroking the forehead, or any unburned area offers solace and human connection.

An essential nursing skill in rehabilitation requires the explanation of a procedure before beginning. Skilled nurses familiar with a procedure must remember that although they have experienced it often, it is a first-time experience for the client and the unknown often generates anxiety.

Sitting by the bedside occasionally, rather than standing, brings client and professional to the same communication level. This strategy done for 5 minutes equates to much longer for the client. It exhibits sensitivity and compassion.

As a matter of respect, by the time a client transitions to the rehabilitation phase of his or her recovery, professionals may want to use the term **burn "survivor"** rather than **burn "victim."** It is preferred by most survivors and connotes independence, dignity, and capability. The term *victim* implies helplessness, dependence, and shows a lack respect for an individual who has overcome a tremendous injury and is resuming much of his or her preburn life. It is a term that survivor groups and the Phoenix Society, a national organization for people with burns, continually work toward changing in the media's coverage of burn injuries.

While these skills may appear simple and easy, they are essential gestures and attitudes that say "I care" and simultaneously create a strong relationship between nurse and client. It is important for health care professionals to remember that it is the human being they are caring for and not just the burn injury.

Facial and Body Disfigurement

Most changes in body image, whether caused by trauma, disease, or birth anomaly, create feelings of profound loss and requiretime for adjustment and acceptance. Because of the emphasis placed on physical attractiveness, it is not surprising that an alteration in body image caused by burns creates a tremendous threat.

Nurses play an especially important role for the burn patient who suffers an injury that leaves significant **facial and body disfigurement.** Nurses care for and witness challenging yet successful recoveries during their burn treatment experience. The staff may become desensitized by the disfigured appearance of patients and may overlook the impact of the body transformation on others. For the patient and his or her family, this is not only their first experience, but it is also intensely personal. A patient's mental picture of his or her face and body is how it looked before the burn incident. To see his or her face in a mirror for the first time and begin to adapt to the realization of permanent disfigurement is an important stage of recovery. This assignment challenges a medical team and requires responsible, thoughtful attention before discharge.

The client's first view of his or her altered appearance often evokes feelings and expressions of shock, sadness, anger, and disbelief. An approach that incorporates the skills of nursing, psychology, and family members assists the burn client to experience his or her disfigurement both cognitively and emotionally. Throughout the literature, findings consistently show that severity of disfigurement is not linked to the degree of emotional distress. It is helpful for clients to see photos of others who haveexperienced a facial disfigurement. By viewing reconstructive surgeries, diligent wearing of pressure garments or masks, and appropriate use of image improvement techniques by others, clients and families can probably feel more hopeful and less helpless about the future.

What is remarkable about facial disfigurement and the problem it presents for a burn client stems from the symbolic significance of the face and its enmeshed relationship to the person behind it. Disfigurement is judged by implied public standards of how people should look and what is normal. A person whose facial features deviate from the standard not only receives different treatment, but often becomes the focus of negative judgments and discrimination. A significant change of attitude is difficult because society frequently equates disfigurement with imperfection.

Reactions to facial disfigurement are accurately described by Macgregor (1990), who says that "in their efforts to go about their daily affairs [people with facial disfigurement] are subjected to visual and verbal assaults and a level of familiarity from strangers [such as] naked stares, startled reactions, 'double takes,' whispering, remarks, furtive looks, curiosity, personal questions, advice, manifestations of pity or aversion, laughter, ridicule, and outright avoidance."

Adaptive Stages

While the physical rehabilitation of burn clients is visible and carefully monitored, the psychological rehabilitation ranks equally in importance and also requires accurate and close observation. Watkins, Cook, Randolph, and Ehleben (1988) established a seven stage method of assessing and assisting psychological recovery for burn clients. This method delineates the stages in normal psychological healing and offers interventions to help the client at each stage. The stages usually form a continuum, with each stage overlapping and being replaced by subsequent stages. Some clients go through all of the stages, and others skip one or more. This method can be used in an integrated fashion by all members of the multidisciplinary team to accelerate the client's psychological recovery and to maximize his or her adherence with necessary treatment modalities. Return to maximum independent functioning appears to require a gradual psychological adaptation to losses and changes resulting from injury.

The seven adaptive stages of Watkins, Cook, Randolph, and Ehleben (1988), along with applicable staff interventions to aid the client's conclusion to the particular stage, are presented in Table 1.

Watkins et al. (1988) further stated that each stage consists of a dynamic interaction between cognitive (thinking) and affective(feeling) processes, resulting in the patient displaying stage-specific behavior composed of spontaneous verbalizations, reported emotions, and patterns of interactions with others. Normality or abnormality of a client's behavior postburn can be assessed accurately only within the context of that adaptational stage in which the client is currently engaged. There are two stages in which certain complications can arise and cause particular psychiatric disorders. One occurs in stage 3 and is called *posttraumatic stress disorder,* and the other, called *affective disorder,* may happen in stage 5.

For the purposes of this chapter, let us focus on stage 6: **investment in rehabilitation.** As the client emerges from stage 5, he or she has developed an acceptance of his or her losses and a reality-oriented understanding of at least some disabilities. Entering stage 6, the client focuses on steps that can be taken to allow him or her to resume as much preburn functioning as possible despite disabilities due to accepted losses. Behavior of a client entering stage 6 superficially resembles that displayed at stage 4. He or she begins to show obvious interest in recommended treatments and procedures and increased motivation to become self-sufficient. This stage is marked

Table 1
Seven Adaptive Stages for Psychological Recovery of Burn Patients

Adaptive Stage	Intervention
1. Survival anxiety	1. Orientation
2. The problem of pain	2. Medication
3. The search for meaning	3. Validation
4. Investment in recuperation	4. Education
5. Acceptance of losses	5. Legitimization
6. Investment in rehabilitation	6. Commendation
7. Reintegration of identity	7. Termination

Source: Watkins, Cook, Randolph, and Ehleben (1988).

by interest in or resumption of functions specific to his or her own lifestyle, such as driving and leisure activities, hobbies, and vocational pursuits. Some attempts to resume preburn status may be unsuccessful and make the patient aware of the existence of changes in appearance and/or functional capabilities from his or her preburn norm. The client's own trial-and-error attempts at resuming preburn functioning are the best indicators of ability to return to his or her preburn life and lifestyle. Failure to resume a preburn function often results in hurt, sadness, frustration, anger, anxiety, and a re-entry to stage 5 before he or she can accept the loss and progress toward full psychological recovery.

Eventually, according to Watkins, Cook, Randolph, and Ehleben (1988), the client starts to assess the importance of being able to regain certain preburn skills that are partially or entirely nonessential, because they would now require too much time, effort, energy, money, or pain to regain. Most clients will choose to attempt those rehabilitative procedures and programs that have the best chance for helping them resume the skills they see as paramount for the resumption of a personally valuable and pleasurable life. If a client cannot perform skills in the same manner as he or she did preburn, he or she may use new learning and environmental manipulation to attain the skill; this is called **offsetting.** The client may even use offsetting in supervised rehabilitative programs. This suggests that the client assumes individual responsibility for outcome results. A client enters this stage during acute care and continues through the rehabilitation process to his or her own physical and social environment.

Staff members, in the view of Watkins, Cook, Randolph, and Ehleben (1988), can offer three types of assistance through this stage. First, nurses need to give verbal praise and recognition of the efforts along with encouragement and active listening. Second, nurses can provide reality orienting and educational information regarding the rehabilitation process. As a client continues to progress in gaining preburn function, he or she may also be given additional information on assistive and adaptive devices that may assist in regaining some "nonexpendable" preburn functions.

Finally, nurses can acknowledge the client for taking responsibility for his or her rehabilitation outcome, and respect his or her right to decide which functions to have and which to let go. Also important is acceptance of the client's right to decline further medical or rehabilitative interventions if he or she chooses, and not judging the client negatively for his or her choices.

Pressure Garments

During the long rehabilitation period of a burn injury, clients wear thick, elastic garments called pressure garments over the burned areas. The purpose of the garments is to control the development of scar tissue and attain skin texture that feels and appears smooth, flat, and flexible. This is accomplished by exerting constant pressure against the skin. Pressure garments also help reduce the itching that occurs during the maturation of scar tissue. They are custom made to ensure the correct percentage of pressure and accurate fit. The garments do not constrict movement; however, they are tight and hot to wear during the summer months. Therapists recommend that clients wear the garments 23 hours per day for 1 year to 18 months. The standard color of the garments is tan, although some companies make a variety of colors to suit a variety of individual preferences. These are particularly advantageous for successful compliance by children.

Because pressure garments are visible if worn on the face, arms, and hands, the reactions by the public can be very annoying and make coping difficult. Because of public reactions and the constricted comfort level, compliance can be problematic. Rehabilitation nurses may increase compliance by providing continued reinforcement through literature, videos, and photographs.

Some rehabilitation centers produce custom masks from a clear plastic material. The scar tissue can be seen through the mask and managed easier and more effectively. This type of mask offers social advantages, because it is clear and does not draw as much attention to the wearer.

Clients' Altered Appearance

When a client returns to the community and resumes social, work, school, and recreational activities, he or she may experience distress over the reactions of others to his or her altered appearance. Macgregor (1974) recorded three primary coping strategies used by people with disfigurements. The first was avoidance or withdrawal from social situations. The second involved showing obvious aggression to counter the anticipated negative reactions. Finally, some cope by taking the initiative in their interactions with others. The social skills used appear to influence the impressions that are formed.

Because social skills and image are important issues for clients with disfigurements, it is important that they receive training or "coaching" in these areas. Early in my own rehabilitation progress, I recognized that there was little assistance given to clients about how to go back to the community successfully. How should we react to stares, questions, curiosity, and whispers?

A hospital-based **image enhancement program** provides services to clients in the areas of corrective cosmetic techniques, color analysis, clothing coordination, and **behavioral and social skills training.** These interventions help clients to explore and to expand their image choices. Many people in our society have had little education in this area and are unaware of the harmony and balance that is possible through image enhancement strategies.

During my own burn rehabilitation, I underwent a series of reconstructive surgeries to restore my nostrils and grafts on deep second- and third-degree areas of my face from my forehead to my chin. After an excellent surgical outcome, reinforced by compliant wearing of a pressure garment mask, my skin tones were uneven, I had no eyebrows, and my lip line was not symmetrical. Neither health care professionals from the burn and rehabilitation centers nor the surgeon and his staff could offer much information about what to do next. Through some lengthy research, I found a makeup expert knowledgeable about working with facial disfigurement. This was the beginning of creating yet another new image and transitioning from a burn "injury" to a whole person again. This intervention and others I will identify can bring comfort and confidence to clients during their rehabilitation recovery.

Cosmetics

Corrective cosmetic techniques serve as an adjunct to plastic surgery. People look to the fields of plastic and reconstructive surgery with great hope. This hope is also the great myth. Surgery has limitations and cannot always establish perfect symmetry and create even skin tones. In the words of Partridge (1990), disfigurement is only diminished by surgery, not overcome. Both during and after surgical treatment, corrective cosmetic techniques can produce beneficial psychological results for the patient.

Family and friends may enable or discourage the client's use of corrective cosmetics. People struggle with the imagined and sometimes real opinions of others. Because family and friends may feel uncomfortable with a change in appearance, they may not extend support. Some family and friends react with statements such as, "You don't need makeup, we love you just the way you are" or "Gosh, Mom, why are you wearing that stuff?" Openly discussing and explaining the possible reactions and preparing them can increase their comfort, commitment, and motivation.

Sharing a collection of before-and-after photos and stories of others who have survived burn injuries often encourages clients to do the most with what they have. Seeing others with similar or even worse disfigurements and hearing success stories give a sense of hope.

Using **color analysis** as an enhancement strategy for people with a facial disfigurement produces immediate results. Complementary colors help create a more harmonious appearance and an inner feeling of well-being. Wearing colors close to the face that are not harmonious with skin undertones and hair and eye color emphasizes scars and skin discoloration. Wearing colors in harmony with the skin, hair, and eyes diminishes the intensity of the disfigurement.

When scarring, asymmetry, or skin discoloration is not the primary focus of an observer's attention, one accomplishes communication and daily activities with less difficulty. This reality quickly motivates acceptance of color enhancement knowledge.

STEPS to Self-Esteem

A five-step program I designed called **STEPS to self-esteem** offers skills that provide an easy and effective model for clients with a facial and body disfigurement to follow. Clients' realizations of the powerful role they play in the responses they receive from others can give them new confidence and capability. All of us influence our acceptance or rejection by others. It is important to teach clients techniques they can use to control social encounters. Knowledge of the STEPS and conscious use of them in daily activities aid in developing self-confidence.

The first "S" in STEPS represents **self-talk.** Self-talk is the continual conversation that we have in our minds about ourselves and our circumstances. During each day, we may have up to 50,000 thoughts. This conversation directly affects our actions and feelings and is a powerful force at work in our lives. The words we select become extremely powerful in the meanings, ideas, and emotions they evoke. People need concrete instruction about the power of the mind to aid or hinder their social skills. Introduction of this essential strategy seems critical to community re-entry. When people are in a crisis period, life may look dismal. Coping with the reality of a facial disfigurement requires positive and enabling thoughts and self-talk for optimal results. Self-defeating statements such as, "I can't do it," "I'm too scared," and "It's impossible" render most of us immobilized. Using empowering statements such as, "I can do it," "I'm improving every day," and "Although I'm feeling scared, I trust that things will get better" can produce effective results.

Creating a library of motivational and inspirational books, video and audio tapes, and posters for clients to borrow works toward changing disabling thoughts. When thoughts change, actions have the potential of transforming to more enabling and functional practices.

The "T" in STEPS, *tone of voice,* influences communication results. A warm, enthusiastic, and confident tone of voice reflects an image of being relaxed and at ease with oneself. Understanding this concept and having it modeled clearly illustrate the advantage of incorporating this skill into daily activities. No one responds well to a person who speaks in a weak, timid, or defensive tone. Voice intonation affects the listener's response and judgments about the person making them. If people sense someone is comfortable with himself or herself, they seem to relax and act authentically.

The "E" in STEPS represents *eye contact.* Our eyes are extremely important communication tools. Eyes connect people and can create potentially comfortable and fulfilling interactions. This holds particular importance for a person with a facial disfigurement, whose lack of eye contact may be interpreted negatively. When a person looks away, looks down, or otherwise avoids eye contact, the message communicated is that the person is ill at ease and not comfortable with himself or herself. Working with a client in this area can produce positive results.

The "P" in STEPS, *posture,* also expresses positive or negative self-esteem. Standing or walking with the head and chin up and the rib cage lifted is a communication approach that exhibits composure and self-assurance. Displaying posture with slumped shoulders and the head down may lead others to assume that a person is self-conscious about his or her appearance. When an individual acts ill at ease, others frequently refrain from trying to communicate. Demonstrating the differences in types of posture and the nonverbal messages conveyed can effect a lasting behavior change for some individuals.

The final "S" in STEPS represents *smiling*. A smile can produce immediate results. People who wear a smile have an advantage in forming relationships. A smile often dispels the fears and apprehensions of strangers and, in new situations, breaks barriers or ends prejudicial judgments. It sends messages of being approachable and at ease. A smile also diminishes the visual intensity of scarring and skin discoloration. Energy and warmth radiate from faces wearing smiles. Coaching clients regarding the power of a smile can motivate them to use this step in social situations.

Common Nursing Diagnoses, Goals/Outcomes, and Interventions: Burn Injury

Nursing Diagnosis

- Gas exchange, impaired

Impaired gas exchange may be related to smoke inhalation and damaged tracheal–bronchial tissue.

Goals/Outcomes

- The patient will maintain adequate gas exchange as evidenced by clear lung sounds, respiratory pattern regular and unlabored, Po_2 80 to 100 mm Hg, Pco_2 35 to 45 mm Hg, effective mobilization of secretions.

Nursing Interventions

- Monitor lung sounds—character, rate, and depth of respirations.
- Monitor ability to cough.
- Monitor arterial blood gases (ABGs).
- Encourage patient to cough, deep breathe, and use incentive spirometer every 2 to 4 hours.
- Monitor vital signs.

Collaborative:

- Administer humidified oxygen.
- Administer bronchodilators and antibiotics, as prescribed.
- Obtain sputum cultures.
- Assist in providing/maintaining endotracheal intubation/mechanical ventilation.

Nursing Diagnosis

- Tissue perfusion, alteration in

Alteration in tissue perfusion may be related to the following:

- Decreased circulating blood volume from the fluid shift and tourniquet effect of circumferential burns
- Blood loss with decreased cardiac output and decreased tissue perfusion (associated with problems of lactic acidosis and the potential for renal shutdown)
- Release of myocardial depressant factor

Goals/Outcomes

- The patient will maintain adequate cardiac output and optimal tissue perfusion as evidenced by presence of peripheral pulses and adequate circulation, sensation, and motion (CSM).

Nursing Interventions

- Elevate the burned extremity above the level of the heart.
- Assess peripheral perfusion hourly (pulses, color, swelling, sensation, motion, capillary refill).

Nursing Diagnosis

- Fluid volume deficit, potential

The potential for fluid volume deficit may be related to the following:

- A rapid shift of plasma proteins into the interstitial spaces due to increased capillary permeability and vasodilation, shift of sodium and chloride into the muscle and tissues, and evaporation losses from the wound surface
- Untreated fluid shifts can result in hypovolemic shock
- Metabolic acidosis resulting from decreased circulation and poor peripheral perfusion
- Decreased fluid intake.

Goals/Outcomes

- The patient will maintain adequate fluid and electrolyte balance.
- Tissue perfusion will be maintained and hypovolemia prevented.

Nursing Interventions
Independent:

- Obtain admission weight and monitor weight daily.
- Record all input and output (I&O), hourly. Record hourly specific gravity.
- Report urine output of less than 3 milliliters per hour.
- Monitor the patentcy of the urinary catheter.
- Monitor electrolytes, complete blood count (CBC).
- Monitor dressings and burn sites to assess for bleeding.
- Monitor intravenous (IV) patentcy.

Collaborative:

- Administer IV fluids and electrolyte replacements as prescribed.
- Elevate the head of the bed as prescribed.
- Assist in the placement of hemodynamic monitoring lines (central venous pressure [CVP], pulmonary artery catheter).
- Administer blood and blood products as prescribed.
- Administer fluid challenges/mannitol for myoglobinuria.

Nursing Diagnosis

- Fluid volume excess, potential

The potential for fluid volume excess may be related to the following:

- Iatrogenic causes of overhydration during fluid resuscitation
- Surgical stress response
- Excess fluid and/or sodium intake

Goals/Outcomes

- The patient will maintain optimum fluid and electrolyte balance.
- Tissue perfusion will be maintained and hypervolemia prevented.

Nursing Interventions

Independent:

- Obtain admission weight and monitor daily at the same time of day with the same amount of clothing.
- Record I&O hourly in the critical period. Record hourly specific gravity.
- Monitor vital signs and hemodynamic parameters at least hourly, and report abnormal results. Titrate fluid replacement according to hemodynamic pressures.
- Monitor electrolytes, CBC, and other diagnostic tests, and report abnormal results.
- Monitor for physical assessment changes at least every 4 hours.
- Monitor for breath sounds and heart sounds. Monitor for fluid overload, edema, especially in dependent body areas. Assess for neck vein distention. Monitor peripheral pulses. Monitor mental status.
- Limit the amount of time in the Hubbard tank to no more than 20 minutes.

Collaborative:

- Assist in the placement of hemodynamic monitoring lines (CVP, pulmonary artery catheter).
- Elevate the head of the bed, as prescribed.
- Administer IV fluids and electrolyte replacements as prescribed.
- Restrict sodium and fluid intake, as necessary.
- Administer diuretic and/or mannitol as needed.

Nursing Diagnosis

- Pain

Pain may be related to the following:

- Exposure to nerve ending in partial thickness burns
- Donor site procurement

Goals/Outcomes

- The patient's pain is minimized and controlled.

Nursing Interventions

Independent:

- Assess and record the nature and location, quality, intensity, and duration of pain.
- Assess the level of pain through client verbalization, facial expression, and body positioning. Rate the pain or have the patient rate the pain on a visual analog scale.
- Accept individual responses to pain.
- Observe for physiologic responses to pain, such as increases in blood pressure, pulse, and respiratory rate; increased restlessness and irritability; increased muscle tension; facial grimaces; and guarding.
- Offer pain medication a half hour before pain-provoking treatments.
- Evaluate effectiveness of analgesics.
- Offer diversional activities: music, radio, television, books, games.
- Properly position the patient. Elevate his or her extremities above the level of the heart.
- Use relaxation techniques to increase comfort.
- Explain procedures and their importance (e.g., range of motion [ROM], tubbings, dressing changes).
- Perform dressing changes efficiently. Have supplies ready.
- Attempt to allay fear and anxiety by allowing time to verbalize concerns.
- Maintain comfortable environment (30 to 33°C, bed cradle, quiet environment).

Collaborative:

- Administer analgesics and sedatives, as prescribed.
- Administer IV morphine sulfate during the critical period. Other medications such as methadone or fentanyl may also be used.
- Cover the wound with biologic dressings and grafts.
- Instruct patients in the use of self-administered analgesics.

Nursing Diagnosis

- Infection, potential for

Potential for infection may be related to the following:

- Loss of skin integrity.
- Decreased resistance to infection; in addition, multiple dressing changes and tubbings increase fluid loss and provide increased opportunity for contamination.

Goals/Outcomes
- The patient will not develop wound infection and sepsis.

Nursing Interventions
Independent:

- Shave hair at least 1 inch around the burn area (excluding eyebrows).
- Maintain strict isolation during tubbing and dressing changes.
- Monitor vital signs at least hourly in the critical period.
- Monitor white blood cell (WBC) count.
- Monitor wound cultures.
- Monitor wound changes in drainage: odor, redness, tenderness, swelling, and amount of drainage.
- Monitor indwelling catheters—IV, Foley, and other invasive lines.
- Date and time insertions, line changes, and so on.
- Maintain strict aseptic technique during wound management.
- Monitor the effect of topical agents.
- Implement isolation techniques.
- Instruct visitors in appropriate burn unit protocols.

Collaborative:

- Administer antibiotics and topical agents as prescribed.
- Collect wound cultures as ordered.
- Administer antibiotics by subeschar clysis.

Rehabilitation nurses play an important role in motivating and supporting facially disfigured clients. Their sensitivity and ability to model and teach image enhancement techniques and the STEPS to self-esteem make the quality of life more successful and satisfying. Experiencing ongoing assistance through follow-up sessions, motivational books and tapes, and support groups provides encouragement during the journey to accepting and loving themselves.

A burn **support group** formed for the ongoing support of burn "survivors" and their families and friends can be highly beneficial. Burn clients feel comfort and strength knowing they are not the only ones. Seeing others who have "made it" provides motivation and inspiration. This is an area often neglected in rehabilitation of burns, and it is extremely important to the outcome.

Development of a school re-entry program on a local level is an extemely important rehabilitation technique. To go to the school before a child returns, or even after he or she has started, has an impact on the entire student body. This intervention not only provides education but also reduces misconceptions and myths that surround burn injuries. Students have an opportunity to ask questions, learn appropriate responses, and begin to be more comfortable around the burned child.

It is also vital for the rehabilitation team to meet with the child and his or her family to discuss school re-entry and teach coping skills. Children can learn through role playing with parents, nurses, and therapists how to answer questions, react calmly, and deal with stares and comments. Teaching parents and children to react with love and warmth rather than anger and hostility can create a smoother and more successful re-entry into the community and school.

Several national organizations focus on support. The Phoenix Society is an organization devoted exclusively to the support of burn survivors. They publish a quarterly newsletter called *The Icarus File* and have area coordinators in every state who offer support where there may be none otherwise. Another organization, About Face, has regional chapters throughout the United States. About Face is dedicated to serving all people with a facial difference. It has literature available on many types of facial differences and a highly developed program for school re-entry. An organization called Let's Face It offers support for all disfigurements and a thorough resource book.

Norman Bernstein (1976), a noted psychiatrist with years of experience with burn-injured clients, states,

> The enormity of facial disfigurement shifts and alters the overall personality pattern and methods of adaptation. The people who work with these patients need to make large shifts in their own perceptions in order to put together the special patterns of professional and humane intervention that will yield the most gratifying lives for these patients. The approach needs to have an experimental and venturesome quality; the goals must be long-term and not require perfect results or continually smooth relations with grateful subjects.
>
> Societal attitudes about deviance and people who look damaged can be modified only a little, but determined professionalism coupled with humane feeling can yield great increments in improved living for many people who would otherwise be lost to society and whose lives would be largely lost to them.

These thoughts of Dr. Bernstein summarize the mission of rehabilitation nurses dedicated to the quality of care and optimal recovery of people with burn injuries.

References

Bernstein, N. (1976). *Emotional care of the facially burned and disfigured.* Boston: Little, Brown.

Hutchinson, M. (1985). *Transforming body image.* Freedom, CT: Crossing Press.

Macgregor, F. (1974). *Transformation and identity: The face and plastic surgery.* New York: Quadrangle/New York Times Books.

Macgregor, F. (1979). *After plastic surgery: Adaptation and Adjustment.* New York: Praeger.

Macgregor, F. (1990). Facial disfigurement: Problems and management of social interaction and implications for mental health. *Aesthetic Plastic Surgery, 14*(4), 249–257.

Partridge, J. (1990). *Changing faces: The challenge of facial disfigurement.* London: Penguin Books.

Trofino, R. B., & Braun, A. E. (1991). *Nursing care of the burn injured patient.* Salem, MA: F.A. Davis.

Watkins, P. N., Cook, E. L., Randolph, M., & Ehleben, C. (1988). Psychological stages in adaptation following burn injury: A method for facilitating psychological recovery of burn victims. *Journal of Burn Care and Rehabilitation, 94,* 376–384.

Suggested Readings

Blakeney, P., Herndon, D., Desai, M., Beard, S., & Wales-Seale, P. (1988). Long-term psychosocial adjustment following burn injury. *Journal of Burn Care and Rehabilitation, 9*(6), 661–665.

Dion, K., Berschied, E., & Walster, E. (1972). What is beautiful is good. *Journal of Personality and Social Psychology, 24,* 285–290.

CHAPTER 22

Cardiac Rehabilitation
Anita Rosebrough

Key Terms   *Acute Myocardial Infarction (AMI)*
Angina Pectoris
Atherosclerosis
Cardiac Rehabilitation
Cardiovascular Disease
Coronary Heart Disease
Coronary Stent
Percutaneous Translumenal Coronary Angioplasty
Thrombolytic Therapy
Unstable Angina

Objectives   1. Discuss the etiology of coronary artery disease.

2. Describe the learning needs of a cardiac rehabilitation client.

3. Identify and describe the risk factors associated with the development of coronary artery disease.

4. Describe the atherosclerotic process.

5. Identify the symptoms commonly associated with coronary artery disease.

6. Describe angina pectoris, unstable angina, and myocardial infarction.

7. Identify and describe common treatment strategies designed to establish reperfusion to the myocardium.

8. Identify and state the action of common classifications of drugs used to treat heart disease.

9. Identify and describe the components of a comprehensive cardiac rehabilitation program.

10. Describe phase I cardiac rehabilitation.

11. Describe phase II cardiac rehabilitation.

12. Describe phase III cardiac rehabilitation.

13. Describe the role of exercise in cardiac rehabilitation.

14. Describe common lifestyle changes recommended for clients in cardiac rehabilitation.

15. Discuss the outcomes of cardiac rehabilitation programs.

Introduction

Cardiovascular disease (CVD) is the leading cause of mortality and morbidity, and accounts for about 50 percent of all deaths in this country (Agency for Health Care Policy and Research [AHCPR], 1996). According to the American Heart Association (AHA) about 250,000 people per year die within 1 hour of developing symptoms and before they can access the health care system. About 13.5 million people have **coronary heart disease.** During 1996, 1.5 million people had heart attacks, and 500,000 of those died. Those individuals who recover may experience damage to the heart that limits their activities. The estimated annual cost of providing medical treatment for cardiovascular disease is $85 billion.

Etiology

Coronary heart disease is most frequently caused by **atherosclerosis,** or narrowing of the coronary arteries. Atherosclerosis is a progressive disease that is characterized by the build-up of plaque in large, medium-sized, and coronary arteries. Atheromas form in areas of vessel bifurcation with high turbulent blood flow (Misinski, 1990). The exact etiology of atherosclerotic plaque formation is unknown. Researchers believe that the process begins when the endothelium is damaged. The damage can be caused by elevated levels of cholesterol and triglycerides, hypertension, and cigarette smoking. Over time, fats, cholesterol, fibrin, platelets, cellular debris, and calcium are deposited in the damaged areas. The arterial walls thicken and narrow. As the diameter of the artery decreases, blood flow decreases, thus decreasing myocardial oxygen supply. Partial or total blockage of a coronary artery can cause ischemia, angina pectoris, unstable angina, acute myocardial infarction (AMI), and sudden cardiac death (AHA, 1996a). Several factors are known to contribute to the development of atherosclerotic plaque formation and cardiovascular disease.

Risk Factors Associated with the Development of Heart Disease

Research has demonstrated that several risk factors play a major role in the development of cardiovascular disease. These factors are categorized as those over which the individual has no control and those that can be changed or modified. The nonmodifiable risk factors are heredity, ethnicity, sex, and age. There is a tendency for heart disease and atherosclerosis to run in families. The children or siblings of individuals with cardiovascular disease are more likely to develop it themselves.

African-Americans are at increased risk of heart attack owing to their increased incidence of hypertension. The death rate from CVD for African-American males is 47 percent higher than for Caucasian males. Asian/Pacific Islanders are at increased risk for cardiovascular disease due to obesity, smoking, elevated serum cholesterol levels, and hypertension (AHA, 1996c).

Men have heart attacks earlier in life than women, and have them more frequently. Women with AMI are twice as likely to die within the first few weeks post-AMI than men. Morbidity following AMI is higher for women than for men (Hamilton & Seidman, 1993) CHD is the major cause of death for post-menopausal women (Margolis & Goldschmidt-Clermont, 1996).

The incidence of heart disease and the death rate from heart disease increase steadily with age. Symptomatic coronary artery disease appears predominantly in individuals over the age of 40. More than 55 percent of heart attack victims are over the age of 65 (AHA, 1996).

The modifiable risk factors are cigarette smoking, hypertension, elevated cholesterol levels, and sedentary lifestyle. Smokers have twice the risk of heart attack and are more likely to die from a heart attack than are nonsmokers. The American Heart Association (AHA, 1996) approximates that one-fifth of all deaths from cardiovascular disease are directly related to smoking. Consistent exposure to second-hand smoke increases the risk of heart attack, and approximately 40,000 nonsmokers exposed to second-hand smoke die from CVD yearly. Women who smoke and use oral contraceptives are 40 percent more likely to have a heart attack. According to data from the Centers for Disease Control (CDC, 1996), the number one cause of death in chronic illness is cigarette smoking.

Approximately 50 million Americans are hypertensive. Hypertension increases the workload of the heart, and causes the left ventricle of the heart to enlarge and weaken. This increases oxygen demand. Blood pressure increases with age. Men have a higher risk of hypertension until age 55. After age 65, women are more prone to develop high blood pressure. Hypertension accelerates the atherosclerotic process (Margolis & Goldschmidt-Clermont, 1996).

A serum cholesterol level above 240 milligrams per deciliter doubles the risk of heart attack. Twenty percent of American adults have blood cholesterol levels above 240 milligrams per deciliter. This doubles the risk of developing cardiovascular disease. This risk factor is the most influential in the development and progression of coronary artery disease (Fletcher, 1992). The AHA (1996) recommends that cholesterol intake be limited to 300 milligrams per day, and total fat intake should be less than 30 percent of total calories.

Lack of exercise and a sedentary lifestyle increase the risk of heart attack. Inactivity leads to excess weight and elevated serum cholesterol levels, which increase the risk of heart disease. Approximately 60 percent of American adults do not engage in daily activity, and 25 percent do not engage in any physical activity at all (CDC, 1996).

Several contributing factors are associated with increased risk of CVD, but their significance and prevalence are yet to be determined. They include diabetes, obesity, and stress. Diabetes increases the risk of developing cardiovascular disease. More than 80 percent of individuals with diabetes die from some form of heart disease. Elevated serum cholesterol and triglyceride levels, hypertension, and obesity are more common in diabetics than in nondiabetics. Even individuals with good glucose control are at increased risk for CHD. To lower their risk of heart attack, it is essential that diabetics control other modifiable risk factors such as smoking (Margolis & Goldschmidt-Clermont, 1996).

Individuals more than 30 percent above their ideal body weight are more prone to develop heart disease even in the absence of other risk factors. Excess weight increases the workload of the heart, influences blood pressure and serum cholesterol levels, and contributes to the development of diabetes. All of these factors increase the risk of cardiovascular disease (AHA, 1996).

Excessive stress over long periods of time increases the risk of heart disease. The normal physiological response to stress releases adrenaline and other hormones that increase the heart rate and blood pressure. This increase in vital signs increases the workload of the heart and increases the demand for oxygen by the myocardium (AHA, 1996).

Symptoms of Coronary Heart Disease Angina Pectoris

Coronary heart disease can lead to angina, unstable angina, acute myocardial infarction, and sudden cardiac death. **Angina pectoris** refers to acute intermittent pain in the chest. The pain is caused by transient myocardial ischemia. Angina occurs when there is an imbalance between myocardial oxygen supply and myocardial oxygen demand. The onset of angina is frequently associated with atherosclerosis in the coronary arteries. Symptoms of angina do not appear until the lumen of a coronary artery is 75 percent occluded by atherosclerotic plaque formation. Pain is the predominant symptom of angina. It may be described as pressure, tightness, burning, heaviness, aching, constricting, squeezing, or viselike. It is most commonly felt beneath the sternum, but may radiate to the jaw, left arm, or other sites.

Angina is a subjective symptom, and the pain of angina can range from mild to sharp. It is usually sudden and of short duration. The intensity of pain increases gradually, plateaus, and gradually decreases with rest. A typical attack lasts 3 to 5 minutes. Most attacks subside in 3 to 15 minutes. If ischemic chest pain persists for more than 20 minutes, ischemic necrosis results. The pain of angina is usually precipitated by physical exertion, emotional stress, temperature extremes, or other factors that increase the workload of the heart. Angina is relieved by rest and/or the administration of nitroglycerin. It is also referred to as *stable angina* because a known amount of activity triggers an episode, and the intensity and duration of pain are usually the same with each episode.

Unstable Angina

Unstable angina is due to the rapid narrowing of coronary arteries by a blood clot at a site of atherosclerotic plaque formation, or may be due to spasm of a coronary artery. Unstable angina occurs at rest, lasts longer than 20 minutes, causes activity limitations, is different in pattern from stable angina, and is caused by smaller amounts of physical activity. Many consider it to be a "preheart attack" condition. The risk of acute myocardial infarction and sudden cardiac death significantly increases during an episode of unstable angina (Margolis & Goldschmidt-Clermont, 1996).

Myocardial Infarction

Acute myocardial infarction (AMI) refers to the destruction of myocardial cells owing to an interruption in the blood supply to the myocardium. Symptoms associated with AMI include chest pain, weakness, dysrhythmias, electrographic changes, elevated serum enzyme levels, and signs of inflammation. Pain is the most significant symptom. Unlike the pain of angina, it is not relieved by rest or the use of nitroglycerin. The pain is more prolonged and more severe. Many clients with an AMI have a history of angina, and may experience more frequent episodes before the heart attack.

Complications of an acute myocardial infarction include sudden cardiac death. Sudden cardiac death refers to death that occurs within the first hour of cardiac symptom onset, and is due to a malfunction of the heart's electrical system. It accounts for approximately 50 percent of deaths related to acute myocardial infarctions. Sudden cardiac death is often due to bradyarrhythmia, ventricular tachycardia, ventricular fibrillation, reinfarction, or progressive cardiac failure (NIH, 1993).

Routine Medical Management

Treatment of myocardial infarction falls into two broad categories: strategies designed to re-establish blood flow and increase oxygen and nutrients, such as thrombolysis, angioplasty, and coronary bypass surgery; and strategies that reduce the demand for oxygen and nutrients, such as β-adrenergic blockers, calcium channel blockers, and nitrates (Scavone, Turissini, & Salem, 1992).

Coronary artery disease can be treated surgically with coronary artery bypass graft surgery (CABG), percutaneous translumenal coronary angioplasty (PTCA), and angioplasty with insertion of coronary stents. Nonsurgical interventions include thrombolytic therapy, lipid-lowering drugs, and anti-anginals.

The first procedure developed to correct arterial stenosis was coronary artery bypass graft surgery. This procedure is performed on clients with significant narrowing or blockages of the coronary arteries. The procedure involves opening the chest to gain access to the heart and coronary arteries. The occluded area is identified, excised, and replaced with a donor artery usually from the saphenous system in the lower extremities, or the left internal mammary artery (MedicineNet, 1995).

Percutaneous Translumenal Coronary Angioplasty

Percutaneous translumenal coronary angioplasty is an effective method of revascularization in some individuals with coronary artery disease, and angina. It is used to dilate narrowed coronary arteries via the insertion of a balloon-tipped catheter. Once the catheter reaches the area of occlusion, the balloon is inflated several times and the area of occlusion is widened. The plaque is not removed.

The procedure is performed in a cardiac catheterization laboratory and is done without general anesthesia (Margolis & Goldschmidt-Clermont, 1996).

Angioplasty with Insertion of Coronary Stents

A **coronary stent** is a permanent implant into a coronary artery or vein. Stents have an open lattice work, wire mesh design, and are made of stainless steel. The stent is expanded against the inner wall of a coronary artery in an area where atherosclerotic plaque build-up is reducing coronary blood flow. The stent insertion procedure is similar to that of percutaneous translumenal coronary angioplasty. Stents require balloon inflation to expand, and to embed the stent into the arterial wall. To prevent or reduce the possibility of thrombus formation over the stent, anticoagulants and platelet inhibitors are prescribed (AHA, 1996).

Thrombolytic Therapy

Intravenous **thrombolytic therapy** as a means of establishing reperfusion to the damaged myocardium is considered a safe and highly effective method of reperfusing occluded coronary arteries by dissolving the clot responsible for causing the heart attack. The AHA (1996) recommends that for maximal benefit thrombolytic therapy should be initiated within 30 to 60 minutes of the client's arrival in the emergency department. However, studies show that clients continue to benefit from thrombolysis as much as 12 hours after the onset of symptoms. Clients presenting in the emergency department with chest pain are evaluated to establish evidence of an acute MI and to determine candidacy for thrombolysis. The criteria include recent onset of chest pain lasting 20 to 30 minutes, chest pain unrelieved by nitroglycerin, ST-segment elevation of at least 1 millimeter in two leads of a 12-lead electrocardiogram. The two most commonly used thrombolytic agents are streptokinase (SK) and tissue plasminogen activator (t-PA) (Slovis & Weaver, 1995). Intravenous heparin and aspirin are administered after thrombolysis to reduce the risk of clot formation.

Pharmacological Treatment

Anti-Anginals

The pharmacological treatment of angina pectoris is directed at increasing the oxygen supply to the heart and decreasing the oxygen demand of the heart. Anti-anginal medications such as nitrates, β blockers, and calcium channel blockers are often effective in controlling anginal symptoms. The nitrates cause generalized vasodilation, which increases the blood flow to the heart. Generalized vasodilation leads to peripheral pooling of blood in the lower extremities, which in turn decreases the total volume that the heart has to circulate. This decreases myocardial oxygen demand. Nitrates are given to treat episodes of angina, and can be taken prophylactically before engaging in activities that increase myocardial oxygen demand.

β blockers decrease myocardial contractility and heart rate, thus decreasing the workload of the heart and myocardial oxygen demand. Calcium channel blockers inhibit the movement of calcium ions across the cell membrane, and dilate the coronary arteries. This decreases myocardial contractility and myocardial oxygen demand. Some patients require treatment with a combination of these drugs before effective relief of angina is achieved.

Anticoagulants

Anticoagulant therapy is frequently used prophylactically in patients with known atherosclerosis or to prevent a second heart attack. Aspirin, warfarin, and ticlopidine are commonly prescribed agents.

Lipid-Lowering Drugs

Individuals with elevated serum cholesterol and triglyceride levels not responding to low-fat diets may be treated with lipid-lowering drugs. Four types of lipid-lowering agents are available. These include reductase inhibitors such as lovastatin and pravastatin; ion-exchange resins such as cholestyramine and colestipol; nicotinic acid such as niacin; and fibrates such as gemfibrozil and clofibrate. These drugs slow the progression of atherosclerotic plaques, promote plaque regression, and prevent the formation of new plaques (Margolis & Goldschmidt-Clermont, 1996).

Components of a Cardiac Rehabilitation Program

An important cornerstone of the management of heart disease is a comprehensive multidisciplinary cardiac rehabilitation program. **Cardiac rehabilitation** is a multidimensional process through which individuals are assisted to return to an optimal level of physical, psychosocial, emotional, spiritual, and economic functioning. Cardiac rehabilitation should include a medical evaluation, prescribed and monitored exercise, risk factor reduction, education, and counseling (AHA, 1996). The client with heart disease plays a pivotal role in the cardiac rehabilitation process. The client must be an active participant in the acquisition of knowledge, skills, and behaviors to optimize adherence and decrease the risk of future cardiac events. Clients must learn to manage their illness, and prevent or retard the progression of the atherosclerotic process.

Cardiac rehabilitation programs are effective in reducing rehospitalizations, decreasing the need for cardiac drugs, decreasing cardiac symptoms, instilling confidence to resume normal activities of daily living, increasing the quality of life, and increasing return-to-work rates (AHA, 1996). The cardiac rehabilitation process begins during the acute hospitalization recovery phase following an acute cardiac event. It continues with referral to an outpatient program after discharge (AHA, 1996).

Phase I: Inpatient Cardiac Rehabilitation

The first phase of a cardiac rehabilitation program is designed for the client who has recently sustained a major cardiac event, such as a myocardial infarction or coronary artery bypass surgery. It begins during hospitalization when the client is medically stable. The major focus of this phase is early structured, progressive ambulation, and basic teaching related to the pathophysiology of heart disease. The goal of phase I cardiac rehabilitation is to prepare the individual for independence in performing activities of daily living after discharge.

Activity is resumed slowly. Supervised activities may progress from sitting up in bed, to sitting up in a chair, to performing range-of-motion exercises while sitting, to taking short walks. The client's heart rate, respirations, blood pressure, and electrocardiogram are closely monitored during activities. Clients are usually encouraged to perform self-care tasks such as brushing their teeth and combing their hair within 1 to 2 days after an acute myocardial event.

Exercise training is an important component of cardiac rehabilitation. Exercise training is provided to increase functional capacity by increasing endurance, strength, and flexibility. It is important that risk factors leading to the development or progression of CHD be identified and controlled. Incremental physical activity is correlated with increased survival rates, improved functional capacity, return to work, and management of cardiac risk factors (AHA, 1996). Other benefits of regular physical activity include a decreased pulse rate, decreased blood pressure, improved lipid profile, improved sense of psychological well-being, and improved self-care capacity. Exercise frequency, time, and intensity are individualized to client condition and response (Fletcher, 1992; Pashkow, 1993).

Exercise training for individuals with coronary artery disease is important because of the many beneficial physiological changes produced by regular exercise. Exercise decreases cardiac ischemia both at rest and during submaximal exercise, and slows the progression of coronary artery disease, increases the capacity to engage in physical work, decreases heart rate, increases cardiac output, lowers systolic blood pressure, lowers circulating catecholamine levels, reduces anxiety and depression, and increases self-confidence (Fletcher, 1992). The AHCPR (1996) recommends exercise training for individuals who have experienced angina pectoris, a myocardial infarction, CABG, or PTCA.

Client teaching begins during phase I and continues as part of the phase II outpatient program. The client is taught the physiological aspects of coronary heart disease, signs and symptoms of cardiac disease, medication management, dietary restrictions or modifications, and activity guidelines, and risk factor modification such as weight loss and smoking cessation is introduced.

The survivor of an acute cardiac event should be provided psychological counseling related to the emotional stress such an event produces. The client and family members often need assistance in coping with such issues as fear of death, fear of having another heart attack, fear of returning to work, and fear related to resuming normal sexual activity.

Phase II: Outpatient Cardiac Rehabilitation

Phase II begins 1 to 3 weeks after the client is discharged from the acute care setting, and the duration varies depending on client need, from 4 to 6 weeks to 6 months. The hallmark of outpatient cardiac rehabilitation is structured and supervised exercise. Clients free from cardiac symptoms are the best candidates for this type of program. An exercise test is administered by a trained professional before discharge from the acute care setting to establish the individual's functional capacity and response to exercise. The AHA (1996) recommends the use of dynamic exercise testing on a stationary cycle or a treadmill for 6 to 12 minutes.

Phase II exercise training programs are based on the principles of frequency, intensity, and time. Most programs offer three sessions per week for approximately 12 weeks. Exercise intensity is based on a percentage of the maximal heart rate obtained during the exercise test. Sessions are designed to provide safe exercise without causing excessive fatigue. Sessions vary from 30 to 90 minutes in length, at an intensity of 70 to 85 percent of the baseline exercise test heart rate. The client's heart rate and blood pressure are monitored before, during, and after exercise. In some programs, clients are placed on cardiac monitors while exercising (Fletcher, 1992; Pashkow, 1993). The goal of this phase is to gradually work the client up to a standard aerobic workout, which includes 5 to 10 minutes of warm-up and stretching; 20 to 40 minutes of an aerobic activity such as walking, jogging, or swimming; and 5 minutes of cool-down and stretching.

During phase II group education and counseling sessions are provided. These sessions are open to the client and family. The focus of teaching sessions is the long-term management of cardiovascular disease, and risk factor modifications. The emphasis is on the long-term maintenance of healthy lifestyle habits. Participation in a structured program provides continual reinforcement and encouragement to improve and maintain lifestyle habits, and increases a client's adherence rate.

Phase III: Maintenance Program

Phase III is a community-based or home-based maintenance exercise program. Risk factor and lifestyle modifications are continued during this phase. Some programs include abbreviated nutritional counseling, stress management, and smoking awareness counseling sessions. Phase III programs are also beneficial for clients who are at increased risk for developing cardiovascular disease but have not experienced a cardiac event.

Teaching and Counseling for Risk Factor Modification

Risk factor modification can prevent, delay the development of, or prevent existing CHD from becoming worse (Margolis & Goldschmidt-Clermont, 1996). Nutritional counseling with a focus on lipid management should be provided by a registered health care professional. Special considerations should be given to obese individuals, hypertensive individuals, and diabetics. Research has shown that lowering serum cholesterol levels has a positive effect on cardiovascular mortality and morbidity. Lowering cholesterol levels in symptomatic individuals slows the progression of the atherosclerotic process (Gattiker, Goins, & Dennis, 1992). Aggressive dietary management plus the addition of lipid-lowering pharmacological agents may be needed to achieve the most beneficial results. Controlling serum lipid levels is crucial to the success of cardiac rehabilitation and to preventing future cardiac events (Fletcher, 1992).

Management of elevated serum lipid levels includes dietary changes, weight loss, exercise, fiber supplements, and lipid-lowering drugs. These strategies are used singly or in combination, depending on the severity of the lipid abnormality. The American Heart Association cholesterol-lowering dietary guidelines are recommended. Regular physical exercise results in weight loss and a reduction in total body fat, which in turn decreases total cholesterol levels. Adding water-soluble dietary fiber, such as pectin, gum, and mucilage, can lower serum cholesterol levels by approximately 6 to 20 percent (Bell, Hectorn, Reynolds, & Hunninghake, 1990).

Research demonstrates that dietary changes such as limiting fat consumption, combined with moderate levels of physical activity, are successful in reducing total body weight and lowering serum cholesterol levels. Stopping the progression of the atherosclerotic process requires an energy expenditure of approximately 1600 calories per week. Reversing the atherosclerotic process requires an energy expenditure of approximately 2200 calories, or 5 to 6 hours of exercise per week (Hambrecht, Niebauer, Marburger, Grunze, Kalberger, Hauer, Schlierf, Kubler, & Schuler, 1993).

Smoking Cessation   Cardiac rehabilitation programs should include a structured approach to smoking cessation. Individuals who stop smoking benefit from reduced risk of reinfarction, sudden death, and decreased total mortality. After smoking cessation, the risk of MI is lowered to that of nonsmokers within 3 years (Gattiker, Goins, & Dennis, 1992). Referrals to smoking clinics, nicotine gum or patches, or support groups are helpful. Smoking cessation post-MI lowers the risk of reinfarction, sudden death, and mortality rate.

Moderate to severe depression, anxiety, cessation of sexual activity, social isolation, and family problems are common after MI. Depression and anxiety often contribute to failure to return to normal sexual activity, failure to adhere to or participate in a cardiac rehabilitation program, and can lead to social isolation. Psychological and psychosocial impairments can limit the recovery process. Everyone entering a cardiac rehabilitation program should be assessed and referrals to psychiatrists, psychologists, social workers, or mental health workers should be made as needed. Teaching sessions on stress management, and group sessions focusing on psychosocial issues, are also beneficial (Fletcher, 1992).

Hypertension is often associated with coronary artery disease and other cardiac problems and should be addressed in cardiac rehabilitation programs. An individual's blood pressure should be monitored and recorded during cardiac reha-bilitation sessions. Dietary guidelines for weight reduction and controlling or lowering sodium intake are important components of lowering blood pressure (Fletcher, 1992).

Adherence

The AHCPR (1996) states that adherence to a comprehensive cardiac rehabilita-tion program may improve client outcomes. Clients need to be active partners in health care decisions that affect them and their families. Increased client involve-ment in decision-making increases satisfaction and improves adherence. Several strategies for success are recommended. These include clear communication be-tween the client, family, and health care provider about cardiovascular disease and its treatment; emotional support and alleviation of fears and anxieties; under-standable and sensible explanations about the program that are compatible with the client's values, preferences, and needs; recognizing the client's social and cul-tural needs; and continuity of care between transitions. Other factors that influ-ence adherence to a cardiac rehabilitation program include complexity, duration, convenience, location, time of day, cost, and client personal and demographic characteristics.

The American Heart Association has identified several factors leading to pro-gram noncompliance. These factors include lack of individual attention, inconve-nient location, inconvenient schedule, poor program leadership, lack of positive feedback, cigarette smoking, history of two previous MIs, sedentary occupation, sedentary lifestyle, and blue-collar employment.

Outcomes of Cardiac Rehabilitation Programs

The AHCPR recognizes the following as positive outcomes of a multidimensional cardiac rehabilitation program. Prescribed exercise training improves exercise toler-ance without cardiovascular complications or other adverse side effects. Exercise maintenance is required to sustain improvement in exercise tolerance. The great-est benefit occurs with exercise three times per week for 12 weeks or more at an intensity of 70 to 85 percent of baseline maximal heart rate. Exercise training de-creases cardiac symptoms of angina and anginal pain. A multidisciplinary ap-proach including exercise training, counseling, behavioral interventions, and cli-ent education decreases dietary fat and weight, decreases serum cholesterol levels, low-density lipoprotein (LDL) cholesterol, and serum triglycerides levels. Compre-hensive cardiac rehabilitation programs report success rates of 16 to 26 percent in smoking cessation efforts. Smoking cessation decreases coronary risk, and im-proves psychosocial well-being and quality of life. Improvements in overall qual-ity of life are indicated by increased functional independence, prevention of pre-mature disability, and postponement or lessening of the need for custodial care. After completion of a cardiac rehabilitation program clients report fewer symp-toms, and return to work and leisure time activities. After cardiac rehabilitation clients report a decrease in emotional stress, and a decrease in type A behaviors. A 25 percent reduction in mortality rates is reported at 3-year follow-up (AHCPR, 1996).

Teaching/Learning Needs

- Basic anatomy and physiology of the heart
- Coronary artery disease
- Atherosclerosis
- Risk factors of coronary artery disease
- Myocardial infarctions
- Why heart attacks occur
- Emotional reactions to heart attack and cardiac disease
- Safe recovery from heart attack
- Risk factor modification strategies
- Nutrition and dietary modifications
- Medications
- Relaxation techniques
- Self-monitoring of pulse and blood pressure
- Safe and effective exercise activity
- Sexual activity
- Stress management
- Community resources
- Return to work
- Signs and symptoms of complications
- What is normal and what to expect after a cardiac event
- Self-care

Nursing Diagnoses

- Activity intolerance
- Altered nutrition
- Altered role performance
- Altered sexual functioning
- Altered tissue perfusion
- Anxiety
- Depression
- Fear
- Grieving
- Ineffective individual coping
- Knowledge deficit
- Management of therapeutic regimen
- Self-concept disturbance
- Self-esteem disturbance

Summary

Cardiac rehabilitation makes a significant difference in perceived quality of life. Participants enjoy and value the experience. Cardiac rehabilitation programs are a safe and cost-effective way of modifying coronary risk factors and providing client education. Cardiac rehabilitation is an important part of the continuum of treatment for heart disease.

References

Agency for Health Care Policy and Research. (1996). *Cardiac rehabilitation.* Clinical Practice Guideline, Number 17 (on-line). Available http://text/nim.nih.gov/ahcpr.

American Heart Association (AHA). (1996a). Biostatistical fact sheets information (on-line). Available http://www.amhrt.org/biostat/html.

American Heart Association (AHA). (1996b). Cardiovascular disease statistics (on-line). Available http://www.amhrt.org/heartg/ac9.html.

American Heart Association (AHA). (1996c). Risk factors for heart disease (on-line). Available http://www.reg.uci.edu/UCI/CARDIOLOGY/PREVENTIVE/FACTS/risk.html.

Bell, L. P., Hectorn, K. J., Reynolds, H., & Hunninghake, D. B. (1990). Cholesterol-lowering effects of soluble-fiber cereals as part of a prudent diet for patients with mild to moderate hypercholesterolemia. *American Journal of Clinical Nursing, 53,* 1020–1026.

Fletcher, G. F. (1992). Current status of cardiac rehabilitation. *Current Problems in Cardiology, 17*(3) 147–203.

Gattiker, H., Goins, P., & Dennis, C. (1992). Cardiac rehabilitation: Current status and future directions. *Western Journal of Medicine, 156*(2), 183–188.

Hambrecht, R., Niebauer, J., Marburger, C., Grunze, M., Kalberger, B., Hauer, K., Schlierf, G., Kubler, W., & Schuler, G. (1993). Various intensities of leisure time physical activity in patients with coronary artery disease: Effects on cardiorespiratory fitness and progression of coronary atherosclerosis lesions. *Journal of the American College of Cardiology, 22*(2), 468–477.

Hamilton, G. A., & Seidman, R. N. (1993). A comparison of the recovery period for women and men after an acute myocardial infarction. *Heart and Lung, 22*(4), 308–315.

Margolis, S., & Goldschmidt-Clermont, P. J. (1996). *Coronary heart disease.* Baltimore, MD: The Johns Hopkins Medical Institutions.

MedicineNet. (1995). Coronary artery bypass graft (CABG) surgery (on-line). Available http://www.medicinenet.com/mainmenu/encyclop/article/Art_C/cagb.html.

Misinski, M. (1990). Pathophysiology of acute myocardial infarction: A rationale for thrombolytic therapy. *Heart and Lung, 17*(6), 743–749.

National Institutes of Health. (1993). Rapid identification and treatment of patients with acute myocardial infarction. NIH Publication No. 93-3278. Bethesda, MD: U.S. Department of Health and Human Services, Public Health Service, National Institutes of Health, National Heart, Lung, and Blood Institute.

Pashkow, F. J. (1993). Issues in contemporary cardiac rehabilitation: A historical perspective. *Jouranl of the American College of Cardiology, 21*(3), 822–834.

Scavone, J. M., Turissini, C. J., & Salem, D. N. (1992). *Overview of thrombolytic therapy for acute myocardial infarction* (pp. 4–16). Medford, MA: Tufts University School of Medicine.

Slovis, C. M., & Weaver, W. D. (1995). *State-of-the-art management of acute myocardial infarction in the emergency department.* Monograph of The American College of Emergency Physicians. Califon, NJ: Gardiner-Caldwell Syner-Med.

Suggested Readings

Ades, P. A., Huang, D., & Weaver, S. O. (1992). Cardiac rehabilitation participation predicts lower rehospitalization costs. *American Heart Journal, 123*(4), 916–921.

Ades, P. A., Waldmann, M. L., Polk, D. M., & Coflesky, J. T. (1992). Referral patterns and exercise response in the rehabilitation of female coronary patients aged >62 years. *American Journal of Cardiology, 69,* 1422–1425.

Allen, J. K., Becker, D. M., & Swank, R. T. (1990). Factors related to functional status after coronary artery bypass surgery. *Heart and Lung, 19*(4), 337–343.

Allen, J. K., & Redman, B. K. (1996). Cardiac rehabilitation in the elderly: Improving effectiveness. *Rehabilitation Nursing, 21*(4), 182–186.

American Heart Association Cardiac Care Committee and Subcommittees. (1992). Guidelines for cardiopulmonary resuscitation and emergency cardiac care. *Journal of the American Medical Association, 268*(16), 2171–2298.

Ashton, K. C., & Saccucci, M. S. (1996). A follow-up study of ethnic and gender differences in cardiac rehabilitation. *Rehabilitation Nursing, 21*(4), 187–191.

Balady, G. J., Fletcher, B J., Froelicher, E. S., Hartley, L. H., Krauss, R. M., Oberman, A., Pollock, M. L., & Taylor, C. B. (1994). Cardiac rehabilitation programs: A statement for healthcare professionals from the American Heart Association. *Circulation, 90*(3), 1602–1610.

Bennett, P., & Carroll, D. (1995). Cognitive-behavioural interventions in cardiac rehabilitation. *Journal of Psychosomatic Research, 38*(3), 169–182.

Bennett, S. J. (1992). Perceived threats of individuals recovering from myocardial infarction. *Heart and Lung, 21*(4), 322–326.

Blumenthal, J. A., & Emery, C. F. (1988). Rehabilitation of patients following myocardial infarction. *Journal of Consulting and Clinical Psychology, 56*(3), 374–381.

Blumenthal, J. A., Rejeski, W. J., Walsh-Riddle, M., Emery, C. F., Miller, H., Roark, S., Ribisl, P. M., Morris, P. B., Brubaker, P., & Williams, R. S. (1988). *American Journal of Cardiology, 61,* 26–30.

Bondestam, E., Breikss, A., & Hartford, M. (1995). Effects of early rehabilitation on consumption of medical care during the first year after acute myocardial infarction in patients >65 years of age. *American Journal of Cardiology, 75,* 767–771.

Brown, G., Albers, J. J., Fisher, L. D., Schaefer, S. M., Lin, J., Kaplan, C., Zhao, X., Bisson, B. D., Fitzpatrick, V. F., & Dodge, H. T. (1990). Regression of coronary artery diseases a result of intensive lipid-lowering therapy in men with high levels of apolipoprotein B. *New England Journal of Medicine, 323*(19), 1289–1297.

Cannistra, L B., Balady, G. J., O'Malley, C. J., Weiner, D. A., & Ryan, T. J. (1992). Comparison of the clinical profile and outcome of women and men in cardiac rehabilitation. *American Journal of Cardiology, 69,* 1274–1279.

Centers for Disease Control and Prevention. (1996). Physical activity and health: A report of the surgeon general (on-line). Available http://www.cdc.gov/nccdphp/sgr/sgr.html.

Conn, V. S., Taylor, S. G., & Abele, P. B. (1991). Myocardial infarction survivors: Age and gender differences in physical health, psychological state and regimen adherence. *Jouranl of Advanced Nursing, 16,* 1026–1034.

Coronary Drug Project Research Group. (1980). Influence of adherence to treatment and response of cholesterol on mortality in the coronary drug project. *New England Journal of Medicine, 303*(18), 1038–1041.

Dattilo, A. M., & Kris-Etherton, P. M. (1992). Effects of weight reduction on blood lipids and lipoproteins: A meta-analysis. *American Journal of Clinical Nursing, 56,* 320–328.

DeBusk, R. F., Miller, N. H., Superko, H. R., Dennis, C. A., Thomas, R. J., Lew, H. T., Berger, W. E., III, Heller, R. S., Rompg, J., Gee, D., Kraemer, H. C., Bandura, A., Ghandour, G., Clark, M., Shah, R., Fisher, L., & Taylor, C. B. (1994). A case-management system for coronary risk factor modification after acute myocardial infarction. *Annals of Internal Medicine, 120*(9), 721–729.

DeLunas, L. R. (1996). Beyond type A: Hostility and coronary heart disease—implications for research and practice. *Rehabilitation Nursing, 21*(4), 196–201.

Denollet, J. (1993). Sensitivity of outcome assessment in cardiac rehabilitation. *Journal of Consulting and Clinical Psychology, 61*(4), 686–695.

Doctor's Guide to the Internet. (1996). Cardiac rehabilitation beneficial but under used (on-line). Available http://www.pslgroup.com/dg95101b.html.

Doctor's Guide to the Internet. (1996). FDA clears Prinvil to save lives when initiated 24 hours after heart attack (on-line). Available http://www.pslgroup.com/dg951129d.html.

Doctor's Guide to the Internet. (1996). Heart attack treatment varies regionally according to NEJM paper (on line). Available http://www.pslgroup.com/dg950831.html.

Doctor's Guide to the Internet. (1996). Landmark study: Pravastatin reduces risk of heart attack and saves lives (on-line). Available http://www.pslgroup.com/dg9511a.html.

Doctor's Guide to the Internet. (1996). Statement from Merck & Co., Inc. on results from WOS trial (on-line). Available http://www.pslgroup.com/dg951116f.html.

Doctor's Guide to the Internet. (1996). Zestril cleared for treating heart attack patients (on-line). Available http://www.pslgroup.com/dg951129e.html.

Faigenbaum, A. D., Skrinar, G. S., Cesare, W. G., Kraemer, W. J., & Thomas, H. E. (1990). Physiologic and symptomatic responses of cardiac patients with resistance exercise. *Archives of Physical Medicine Rehabilitation, 71,* 395–398.

Featherstone, J. F., Holly, R. G., & Amsterdam, E. A. (1993). Physiologic responses to weight lifting in coronary artery disease. *American Journal of Cardiology, 71,* 287–292.

Fletcher, B. J., Dunbar, S. B., Feiner, J. M., Jensen, B. E., Almon, L., Cotsonis, G., & Fletcher, G. F. (1994). Exercise testing and training in physically disabled men with clinical evidence of coronary artery disease. *American Journal of Cardiology, 73,* 170–174.

Fletcher, G. F., Blair, S. .N, Blumenthal, J., Caspersen, C., Chaitmen, B., Epstein, S., Falls, H., Froelicher, E. S. S., Froelicher, V. F., & Pina, I. L. (1992). Statement on exercise: Benefits and recommendations for physical activity programs for all Americans. A statement from the American Heart Association. *Circulation, 86*(1), 340–343.

Fletcher, G. F., Froelicher, V. V., Hartley, L. H., Haskell, W. L., & Pollock, M. L. (1990). Exercise standards: A statement for health professionals from the American Heart Association. *Circulation, 82*(6), 2286–2322.

Fleury, J. D. (1991). Wellness motivation in cardiac rehabilitation. *Heart and Lung, 1*(20), 3–8.

Fleury, J. D. (1993). An exploration of the role of aocial networks in cardiovascular risk reduction. *Heart and Lung, 22*(2), 134–144.

Frasure-Smith, N., Lesperance, F., & Talajic, M. (1995). Depression and 18-month prognosis after myocardial infarction. *Circulation, 91*(4), 999–1005.

Froelicher, E. S., Kee, L. L., Newton, K. M., Lindskog, B., & Livingston, M. (1994). Return to work, sexual activity, and other activities after acute myocardial infarction. *Heart and Lung, 23*(5), 423–434.

Fuster, V., Badimon, L., Badimon, J. J., & Chesebro, J. H. (1992). The pathogenesis of coronary artery disease and the acute coronary syndromes. *New England Journal of Medicine, 326,* 310–317.

Gibler, W. B., Braunwald, E., & Topol, E. J. (1995). *Thrombolytic therapy for acute myocardial infarction: Evolving concepts in patient selection.* Cincinnati, OH: University of Cincinnati College of Medicine.

Gould, K. L. (1994). Reversal of coronary atherosclerosis: Clinical promise as the basis for noninvasive management of coronary artery disease. *Circulation, 90*(3), 558–571.

Gulanick, M. (1991). Is phase 2 cardiac rehabilitation necessary for early recovery of patients with cardiac disease? A randomized, controlled study. *Heart and Lung, 20*(1), 9–15.

Hanisch, P. (1993). Informational needs and preferred time to receive information for phase II cardiac rehabilitation patients: What CE instructors need to know. *Journal of Continuing Education in Nursing, 24*(2), 82–89.

Harlan, W. R., Sandler, S. S., Lee, K. L., Lam, L. C., & Mark, D. B. (1995). Importance of baseline functional and socioeconomic factors for participation in cardiac rehabilitation. *American Journal of Cardiology, 76,* 36–39.

Haskell, S. F., Alderman, E. L., Fair, J. M., Williams, P. T., Johnstone, I. M., Champage, M. A., Krauss, R. M., & Farquahar, J. W. (1994). Effects of intensive multiple risk factor reduction on coronary atherosclerosis and clinical cardiac events in men and women with coronary artery disease. *Circulation, 89*(3), 975–990.

Heath, G. W., Ehsani, A., Hagberg, J. M., Hinderliter, J. M., & Goldberg, A. P. (1983). Exercise training improves lipoprotein lipid profiles in patients with coronary artery disease. *American Heart Journal, 105*(6), 889–894.

Hedback, B. E. L., Perk, J., Engvall, J., & Areskog, N. H. (1990). Cardiac rehabilitation after coronary artery bypass grafting: Effects on exercise performance and risk factors. *Archives of Physical Medicine Rehabilitation, 71,* 1069–1072.

Hellman, E. A., & Williams, M. A. (1994). Outpatient cardiac rehabilitation in elderly patients. *Heart and Lung, 23*(6), 506–512.

Horwitz, R. I., & Horwitz S. M. (1993). Adherence to treatment and health outcomes. *Archives of Internal Medicine, 153,* 1863–1868.

Horwitz, R. I., Viscoli, C. M., Berkman, L., Donaldson, R. M., Horwitz, S. M., Murray, C. J., Ransohoff, D. F., & Sindelar, J. (1990). Treatment adherence and risk of death after a myocardial infarction. *Lancet, 336,* 542–545.

Hsia, J., Hamilton, W. P., Kleiman, N., Roberts, R., Chaitman, B. R., & Ross, A. M. (1990). A comparison between heparin and low-dose aspirin as adjunctive therapy with tissue plasminogen activator for acute myocardial infarction. *New England Journal of Medicine, 323*(21), 1433–1437.

Johnson, C., & Greenland, P. (1990). Effects of exercise, dietary cholesterol, and dietary fat on blood lipids. *Archives of Internal Medicine, 159,* 137–141.

Johnson, J. L., & Morse, J. M. (1990). Regaining control: The process of adjustment after myocardial infarction. *Heart and Lung, 19*(2), 126–135.

Kugler, J., Dimsdale, J. E., Hartley, L. H., & Sherwood, J. (1990). Hospital supervised vs home exercise in cardiac rehabilitation: Effects on aerobic fitness, anxiety, and depression. *Archives of Physical Medicine Rehabilitation, 71,* 322–325.

LaRosa, J. H., Becjer, D. M., & Fitzgerald, S. (1990). Elevated blood cholesterol: A risk factor for coronary heart disease. *AAOHN Journal, 38*(5), 211–215.

Lavie, C. J., & Milani, R. V. (1994). Effects of cardiac rehabilitation and exercise training on low-density lipoprotein cholesterol in patients with hypertriglyceridemia and coronary artery disease. *American Journal of Cardiology, 74,* 1192–1195.

Lavie, C. J., & Milani, R. V. (1995). Effects of cardiac rehabilitation programs on exercise capacity, coronary risk factors, behavioral characteristics, and quality of life in a large elderly cohort. *American Journal of Cardiology, 76,* 177–179.

Lavie, C. J., Milani, R. V., & Littman, A. B. (1993). Benefits of cardiac rehabilitation and exercise training in secondary coronary prevention in the elderly. *Journal of the American College of Cardiology, 22*(3), 678–683.

Levin, L. A., Perk, J., & Hedback, B. (1991). Cardiac rehabilitation—a cost analysis. *Journal of Internal Medicine, 230,* 427–434.

Newman, M. A., & Moch, S. D. (1991). Life patterns of persons with coronary heart disease. *Nursing Science Quarterly, 4*(4), 161–167.

Oldridge, N., Guyatt, G., Jones, N., Crowe, J., Singer, J., Feeny, D., McKelvie, R., Runions, J., Streiner, D., & Torrance, G. (1991). Effects on quality of life with comprehensive rehabilitation after acute myocardial infarction. *American Journal of Cardiology, 67,* 1084–1089.

Orinsh, D., Brown, S. E., Scherwitz, L. W., Billings, J. H., Armstrong, W. T., Ports, T. A., McLanahan, S. M., Kirkeeide, R. L., Brand, R. J., & Gould, K. L (1990). Can lifestyle changes reverse coronary heart disease? *Lancet, 336,* 129–133.

Pepine, C. J. (1996). Percutaneous transluminal coronary angioplasty (on-line). Available http://www.sma.org/dialmon/percutan.html.

RITA Trial Participants. (1993). Coronary angioplasty versus coronary artery bypass surgery: The Randomized Intervention Treatment of Angina (RITA) trial. *Lancet, 341*(8845), 573–580.

Rosal, M. C., Downing, J., Littman, A. B., & Ahern, D. K. (1994). Sexual functioning post-myocardial infarction: Effects of beta-blockers, psychological status and safety information. *Journal of Psychosomatic Research, 38*(7), 655–667.

Suter, P. M., Suter, W. N., Perkins, M. K., Bona, S. L., & Kendrick, P. K. (1996). Cardiac rehabilitation survey: Maintenance of lifestyle changes and perception of program value. *Rehabilitation Nursing, 21*(4), 192–195.

Taylor, C. B., Houston-Miller, N., Killen, J. D., & DeBusk, R. F. (1990). Smoking cessation after acute myocardial infarction: Effects of a nurse-managed intervention. *Annals of Internal Medicine, 113*(2), 118–123.

Thomas, J. J. (1995). Reducing anxiety during phase I cardiac rehabilitation. *Journal of Psychosomatic Research, 39*(3), 295–304.

Thompson, D. R. (1995). Cardiac rehabilitation: How can it be improved? *Journal of Psychosomatic Medicine, 39*(5), 519–523.

Warner, J. G., Brubaker, P. H., Zhu, Y., Morgan, T. M., Ribisl, P. M., Miller, H. S., & Herrington, D. M. (1995). Long-term (5-year) changes in HDL cholesterol in cardiac rehabilitation patients. Do sex differences exist? *Circulation, 92*(4), 773–777.

CHAPTER 23
Degenerative Joint Disease: Rheumatoid Arthritis and Osteoarthritis

Anita Rosebrough

Key Terms
Anti-Inflammatory Agents
Bony Ankylosis
Disease-Modifying Antirheumatic Drugs (DMARDs)
Fibrous Ankylosis
Osteoarthritis (OA)
Osteophyte
Pannus Formation
Rheumatoid Arthritis (RA)
Rheumatoid Factor
Rheumatoid Nodules
Synovitis

Objectives
1. Identify and describe three characteristics of osteoarthritis and rheumatoid arthritis.

2. Describe the pathophysiology associated with osteoarthritis and rheumatoid arthritis.

3. Identify and describe the causal theories behind osteoarthritis and rheumatoid arthritis.

4. Identify nursing interventions for nursing problems related to the arthritic client.

5. Describe joint protection guidelines.

6. Identify and describe common pharmacological agents used to treat osteoarthritis and rheumatoid arthritis.

7. Describe and review the benefits of thermal treatments.

8. Review the importance of proper positioning and body mechanics for clients with osteoarthritis and rheumatoid arthritis.

Introduction
The term *arthritis* refers to more than 100 different diseases affecting the joints and connective tissue throughout the body. Arthritis is a chronic, progressive condition. The disease process itself varies from person to person. Approximately 40

million Americans have some form of arthritis. Anyone can develop arthritis. However, almost two-thirds of arthritis sufferers are women. Arthritis is the number one cause of physical limitations in Americans. Arthritis limits activities of daily living such as bathing, dressing, and mobility. The estimated cost of providing health care combined with income lost because of arthritis is approximately $95 billion per year. Arthritis is the leading cause of employee absenteeism and the second leading reason for receiving disability benefits. The two most common types of arthritis are osteoarthritis and rheumatoid arthritis. Osteoarthritis is the most prevalent form of arthritis in the United States.

Osteoarthritis
Etiology

Osteoarthritis (OA) is a disease of unknown origin that attacks the large weight-bearing joints such as the hips, knees, and ankles. Research suggests that there may be a hereditary tendency to pass on defective cartilage or the way joints fit together, or that the abnormal release of cartilage-destroying enzymes is responsible for the development of OA.

Although the exact etiology of OA remains unknown, several factors are associated with the development of the disease. Excessive weight stresses the large weight-bearing joints, particularly the knees. Weight loss benefits those who already have OA and reduces joint stress. For women, losing as little as 10 pounds can decrease the risk of developing osteoarthritis. Injury from accidents such strains, sprains, fractures, and dislocations, or repeated use, such as jogging, increase the risk of developing OA. Joint inflammation, joint instability, and congenital or acquired skeletal deformities contribute to the development of OA. Complications from other forms of arthritis can eventually lead to osteoarthritis. For example, rheumatoid arthritis can lead to the development of osteoarthritis.

Osteoarthritis occurs in both men and women over the age of 40. Females tend to be more severely effected than males. It usually does not develop in women until after menopause. Almost everyone over the age of 70 has osteoarthritis in at least one joint. An estimated 17 million people per year seek medical treatment for osteoarthritis. Approximately 37 million Americans experience limitations in movement or activity due to osteoarthritis (Arthritis Foundation, 1995).

A diagnosis of osteoarthritis is made on the basis of a thorough physical examination, history of symptoms, and radiological evidence. Approximately one-third of individuals with radiological evidence of osteoarthritis are asymptomatic. The radiographic changes in early osteoarthritis are minimal. Typical radiographic changes include **osteophyte** formation, sclerosis of the subchondral plates, and the presence of subchondral cysts. Laboratory tests are within normal limits. A blood test to detect the breakdown of joint cartilage may be available in the near future (Oddis, 1996).

Pathophysiology

Osteoarthritis is a localized noninflammatory process. Symptoms of osteoarthritis usually come on slowly and are limited to the involved joints. Common symptoms include joint pain, stiffness, or swelling lasting more than 2 weeks. The primary defect in osteoarthritis is the loss of articular cartilage. The cartilage becomes thin and may be absent from the bone in some areas, leaving the underlying bone unprotected. Bone grating against bone can lead to ulceration of the subchondral plates. Other joint changes that can occur with osteoarthritis include sclerosis of the subchondral bone, development of bone cysts, and osteophytes.

Joint pain is the predominant symptom of osteoarthritis and the reason most people seek medical help. Weight bearing and use of the joint aggravate the pain. Resting the joint relieves the pain. Stiffness occurs after periods of inactivity, but dissipates within a few minutes of beginning joint motion. Joint motion may be accompanied by sounds of crepitus, creaking, or grating. Degeneration of the large weight-bearing joints is the most debilitating form of osteoarthritis.

Routine Medical Management

Treatment of osteoarthritis includes both pharmacological and nonpharmacological interventions. Nonpharmacological treatments include thermal treatments, therapeutic exercises, and joint protection guidelines.

The use of thermal treatments, i.e., the application of hot or cold packs, provides temporary relief of pain and stiffness. Heat relaxes aching and stiff muscles, relieves joint pain and stiffness, and increases circulation to the area. Cold reduces edema through vasoconstriction, and has a local analgesic effect. Ice numbs the area by blocking nerve impulses, thus decreasing the sensation of pain.

Therapeutic exercise is beneficial for many individuals with osteoarthritis and should include a warm-up period with range-of-motion exercises and muscle-strengthening exercises, a period of aerobic activity (such as walking or swimming), and a cool-down period. Exercise reduces the symptoms of OA and promotes a generalized sense of well-being. Moderate and low-impact exercise relieves pain, maintains muscle strength, and maintains or increases joint flexibility.

Protecting involved joints means avoiding the mechanical stress encountered in activities of daily living. Alternating light and heavy tasks, changing position frequently, and using good body mechanics reduce stress on painful joints and allow weakened muscles to rest. The use of splints; orthotics; and assistive devices such as canes, raised chairs, grip and reaching aids, grab bars, and shower seats is an effective way of protecting damaged joints. Making environmental adjustments or changes such as reducing chair height, reducing the use of stairs, and using shoe orthotics has a protective effect (Oddis, 1996). Joint protection guidelines and assistive devices such as canes and walkers should be recommended on an individualized basis. Maintaining body weight at the recommended weight per height level reduces joint stress and pain.

The primary goal of pharmacological treatment for osteoarthritis is pain control in order to maintain joint mobility and functional independence. Nonprescription medications such as acetaminophen, aspirin, and ibuprofen provide temporary pain relief. Aspirin in small doses is one of the most common treatment modalities for OA. Nonsteroidal anti-inflammatory drugs (NSAIDs) given in low to moderate doses provide relief of chronic pain and inflammation.

Investigational treatments for osteoarthritis include tissue transplants and cytokine-modulating drugs. Viscosupplementation is a relatively new treatment for osteoarthritis of the knee that involves injecting a clear, gel-like substance into the joint. The gel helps the joint fluid to regain its elasticity and ability to lubricate the cartilage, thus reducing friction and pain and increasing mobility (Blackburn, 1996).

Surgical options for OA include arthroscopic surgery, repair of joint deformities, joint fusion, or joint replacement. Surgery reduces pain and increases joint mobility and function.

Nursing interventions for clients with osteoarthritis should be designed to decrease pain, increase or maintain joint mobility, decrease joint deformities, and encourage independent functioning. A major effort should be directed at teaching the client and family about the disease and its potential physical impairments.

Rheumatoid Arthritis

Rheumatoid arthritis (RA) is a chronic, progressive, inflammatory disease of diarthrodial joints that is accompanied by systemic manifestations. RA causes chronic inflammation of the joints, the tissues surrounding joints, and other organs of the body. It affects 3 percent of the adult population in the United States. The female-to-male ratio is 3 : 1. The average age of onset is 35 years. RA has the potential to cause substantial disability and permanent functional impairment. The extent of damage and disease progression varies widely.

Etiology

The exact etiology of rheumatoid arthritis is unknown. The disease probably occurs in a genetically susceptible host. Most people with RA have a genetic marker called HLA-DR4 (human leukocyte antigen). Not everyone with the genetic marker develops the disease and some people without a genetic marker develop rheumatoid arthritis. Researchers believe infectious or environmental factors trigger an autoimmune response resulting in inflammation (Arthritis Foundation, 1995).

The diagnosis of rheumatoid arthritis is often difficult to make. RA is based on pattern of symptoms, medical history, physical examination, radiographic findings, and laboratory tests to measure the presence of rheumatoid factors and anti-nuclear antibodies. Approximately 80 percent of individuals with rheumatoid arthritis have rheumatoid factors in their blood and/or synovium (Arthritis Foundation, 1995).

The symptoms of rheumatoid arthritis vary from person to person. In some individuals, the disease is relatively mild with periods of exacerbation, or joint inflammation, and periods of remission. In other individuals the disease is continuously active and progresses steadily over time. When the disease is active common signs and symptoms include joint pain, morning stiffness, stiffness after periods of inactivity, generalized weakness, fatigue, fever, weight loss, and polyarthritis. When body tissues are inflamed, the disease is active. When tissue inflammation subsides, RA is in remission. Remission can occur spontaneously or because of treatment. During periods of remission symptoms disappear. Symptoms return when the disease becomes active again. Remission can last for weeks, months, or years. Remission is achieved in approximately 20 percent of individuals with RA. Twenty-five percent achieve remission with mild residual effects. Forty-five percent have persistent disease, 20 percent are unable to return to work, and 10 percent become severely disabled (Arthritis Foundation, 1995).

The pathological changes of rheumatoid arthritis begin with inflammation of the synovial membrane. The inflammation may spread to the articular cartilage, the fibrous joint capsule, the ligaments, and the tendons. The cells in the edematous and inflamed synovial membrane start multiplying. The synovium becomes thick and fibrous, resulting in **pannus formation.** The pannus tissue adheres to and erodes the articular cartilage. Pannus is probably the most destructive force to joint and soft tissue structures (Figures 1 and 2). The presence of pannus between the joint margins results in decreased joint mobility, which eventually leads to the development of **fibrous ankylosis** and **bony ankylosis.** The structural changes associated with RA cause pain, joint deformity, and loss of joint function (Figure 3).

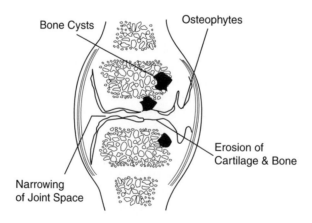

Fig 1. *Joint changes in osteoarthritis.*

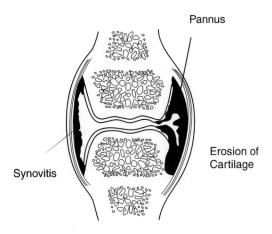

Fig 2. *Joint changes in rheumatoid arthritis.*

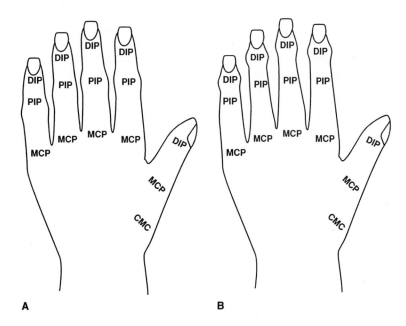

Fig 3. A. *Joint involvement in rheumatoid arthritis.* **B.** *Joint involvement in osteoarthritis. DIP, distal interphalangeal joint; PIP, proximal interphalangeal joint; MCP, metacarpophalangeal joint; CMC, carpometacarpal joint.*

Rheumatoid arthritis can affect any synovial joints. However, it has a great affinity for the small joints of the hand, wrist, and foot. (RA usually does not affect the distal interphalangeal joints.) In many individuals, joint involvement in the extremities is symmetrical.

The onset of rheumatoid arthritis is variable and insidious. It begins with general systemic signs and symptoms of inflammation such as fever, malaise, anorexia, muscle aches, weakness, weight loss, generalized aching, and stiffness. Localized manifestations appear gradually over a period of weeks or months. The symptoms often begin in the hands, particularly in the proximal interphalangeal joints, and the metacarpal phalangeal joints. The joints become painful, tender, and stiff. Pain early in the disease process is caused by pressure from swelling. Later it is caused by sclerosis of the bone and new bone formation. The systemic manifestations associated with RA include skin rash, lymph node enlargement, anemia, cardiac dysfunction, and rheumatoid nodules. **Rheumatoid nodules** occur in approximately 20 percent of RA cases. They are frequently found in subcutaneous tissue covering the extensor surfaces of the elbows and fingers. The nodules may be freely moveable or fixed to tendons and bones. Rheumatoid nodules can be life-threatening if they invade the structures of the heart or lungs. Rheumatoid nodules can cause the enlargement of the spleen, glaucoma, and necrotizing vasculitis.

Routine Medical Management

There is no known cure for rheumatoid arthritis. Conventional treatment of rheumatoid arthritis is conservative and includes both pharmacological and nonpharmacological interventions. The goals of treatment are to prevent disease progression, relieve pain and inflammation, restore or maintain function, prevent joint deformity, and maintain quality of life. Successful treatment requires early diagnosis and aggressive treatment to prevent functional impairment and irreversible joint damage.

The pharmacological treatment of RA is designed to induce disease remission and includes **anti-inflammatory agents** such as aspirin, nonsteroidal anti-inflammatory drugs (NSAIDs), and corticosteroids, **disease-modifying antirheumatic drugs (DMARDs),** and experimental agents. This first line of defense in RA includes the use of salicylates and NSAIDs in moderate to high doses, NSAIDs, rest, and physical therapy.

Nonsteroidal anti-inflammatory drugs are prescribed to reduce joint pain and swelling, and improve function. In most patients, pharmacological treatment of RA is initiated with NSAIDs. NSAIDs provide relieve from symptoms but do nothing to alter the ultimate outcome of the disease process. Nevertheless, they are effective in providing symptomatic relief. Gastrointestinal (GI) irritation is a common side effect of these drugs and the client should be taught strategies for minimizing GI irritation, such as taking with food. If or when pain becomes more severe owing to disease progression, then other pharmacological agents are added (Blackburn, 1996).

Corticosteroids are used to treat extreme inflammation and the systemic effects of RA. Low-dose corticosteroids can provide rapid relieve from pain (Blackburn, 1996). The goal of corticosteroid therapy is to find the lowest effective dose while minimizing the many side effects associated with steroid use. NSAIDs and steroids are effective in alleviating symptoms, but joint damage may continue to progress (Arthritis Society, 1996).

Diseases-modifying antirheumatic drugs (DMARDs) are frequently used to treat RA clients whose disease remains active in spite of treatment with anti-inflammatory drugs. DMARDs have the potential to prevent joint damage and preserve joint integrity and function. The most commonly used DMARDs are antimalarial drugs (hydroxychloroquine), gold salts, and methotrexate. DMARDs are prescribed when inflammation continues for more than 6 weeks or when several joints are affected simultaneously. DMARDs target the immune cells responsible for the inflammation. They do nothing to reverse permanent joint damage. DMARDs have several common characteristics. They are slow acting, with a delayed response of 1– 6 months. They are all toxic agents that require close monitoring.

Antimalarial agents such as hydroxychloroquine are used primarily to treat mild cases of RA. The primary mechanism of action of hydroxychloroquine involves an alteration in intracellular pH, which in turn alters cellular immune functions. The dose ranges from 400 to 600 milligrams per day. There is a risk of irreversible retinopathy with this medication. Regular ophthalmological examinations are strongly recommended.

Parenteral gold salts, or chrysotherapy, is effective for approximately two-thirds of RA clients. It is given in weekly injections for a period of 20 weeks. For many individuals, no improvement in symptoms is noted for 12 to 16 weeks. A complete blood count and urinalysis must be done before each injection to monitor for renal toxicity. Gold salts are also available in an oral form. The oral form has a lower rate of renal toxicity and appears to be less effective than parenteral gold. Methotrexate therapy is associated with a variety of side effects such as gastrointestinal toxicity, hepatotoxicity, and pulmonary complications (Blackburn, 1996).

Several new experimental agents such as Tenidap, intercellular adhesion molecule 1 (ICAM-1), and tumor necrosis factor α (TNF-α), as well as gene therapy, hold great promise for the future of RA therapy. These drugs alter the macrophages, cytokines, and inflammatory cells responsible for joint deterioration in RA. As triggering agents for some forms of arthritis are identified it may become possible to develop vaccines for disease prevention. Vaccines for Lyme disease are already being tested. Advances in arthritis research provide great hope for the future (Arthritis Foundation, 1996).

Individuals with severe damage to the large weight-bearing joints such as the hips or knees can benefit from joint replacement surgery or surgical correction of joint deformities. The most common surgical treatment is joint replacement or *arthroplasty*. The goal of arthroplasty is to provide a pain-free, stable, fully functioning joint. The joints most commonly replaced are the hips and knees. Shoulder, toe, and finger joint replacements are becoming more common.

Deficits and Limitations

Osteoarthritis and rheumatoid arthritis are chronic, progressive conditions that exact both physical and psychological tolls. Pain is the predominant limitation associated with arthritis. Clients with rheumatoid arthritis report that pain is present 70 percent of the time and that pain disrupts sleep about 40 percent of the time (Conwal Incorporated, 1993). Poor pain management and pain control contribute to decreased quality of life and disability. Pain and impaired mobility can interfere even with simple activities of daily living such as dressing, bathing, or walking. The psychological pain associated with arthritis leads to increased stress, fatigue, anger, depression, and strained interpersonal relationships (Arthritis Foundation, 1995). Pain management includes the use of analgesics, rest, therapeutic exercise, joint protection guidelines, and the application of heat and cold.

The management of stress and fatigue includes a regular exercise program, relaxation techniques, learning to say no, balancing rest and activity, maintaining proper body alignment, using good body mechanics, and adequate rest. A daily exercise program is an important component of arthritis treatment. The benefits of a regular exercise program include increased muscle strength, increased joint flexibility, increased range of motion, increased endurance, improved cardiovascular functioning, decreased fatigue and stress, decreased pain, fewer doctor visits, and improved quality of life. Benefits are also achieved through participation in recreational activities such as walking or swimming. Therapeutic exercise programs should be recommended by a trained medical professional.

A balanced diet and weight control can assist with pain management in arthritis. Maintaining an ideal body weight decreases pressure on the large weight-bearing joints. A healthy and nutritious diet should be encouraged. Pain, fatigue, and disease exacerbation decrease appetite, resulting in weight loss. To meet caloric needs, a diet high in protein, vitamins, and minerals is recommended. Alcohol intake should be limited for individuals taking aspirin and NSAIDs, and avoided altogether by those on methotrexate. The Arthritis Foundation recommends the following dietary guidelines: eating a variety of foods; limiting the intake of fat, cholesterol, salt, sugar, and alcohol; and increasing the intake of vegetables, fruits, and grains (Arthritis Foundation, 1996).

Individuals with RA need to maintain a balance between rest and activity. Exercise should be adjusted to the disease course. A task timer can be used to carefully time activities that cause pain. The timer can be set for periods of 20 to 30 minutes. When the timer goes off, the activity is stopped and the client rests for an equal amount of time. When joints are warm, swollen, and painful fatigue and morning stiffness are increased. During these times, activity should be reduced. Light, gentle range-of-motion exercise to maintain joint mobility is recommended. When the individual is not experiencing swelling, pain, or fatigue the exercise program should be expanded. Any physical exercise should be combined with joint protection guidelines. The emphasis should be on strengthening muscles, maintaining flexibility, and minimizing wear and tear on the joints and connective tissues.

People with RA generally need more rest. They should get adequate rest at night, and a nap during the day is beneficial. Relaxation training such as progressive muscle relaxation, biofeedback, and guided imagery is effective in reducing muscle tension, decreasing cognitive concerns such as worry and fear, and promoting rest.

Rheumatoid arthritis is unpredictable and is often characterized by chronic pain, emotional stress, and depression. These make it difficult to cope with the disease process. It is important that individuals and their families learn as much as they can about the disease process and its effects on everyday life. Counseling can assist in the development of positive coping skills and the services offered by local support groups may be beneficial. The Arthritis Foundation offers a variety of services including support groups, home study courses, exercise classes, and educational brochures. Depression is a significant problem in arthritis suffers. Medications are available to treat depression.

The progression of rheumatoid arthritis leads to loss of functional independence and disability. Approximately 50 percent of individuals with RA are unemployed within 10 years of disease onset (Blackburn, 1996). Vocational rehabilitation referrals should be made early in the disease process. Successful vocational rehabilitation focuses on remaining abilities, maintenance of personal independence, and the removal of environmental barriers.

Sexual dysfunction in individuals with RA is likely to occur. Problems related to sexual functioning can be due to role changes, physical changes, or psychological changes. (See Chapter 29 on altered sexual functioning for nursing interventions related to these issues.)

The individual with arthritis must learn to make lifestyle modifications designed to protect the joints and to simplify everyday tasks. Many options are available to assist in this process. The following are some tips for simplifying tasks:

- Use assistive devices such as reach extenders, canes, and long-handled brushes to make tasks easier and reduce reaching and bending. These items can be personalized by painting them or adding decorative items such as flowers or stickers.
- Ask for help with activities that stress the joints or cause pain.

- Learn to say no. Saying no is never easy. Rules for saying no include admitting limitations, explaining your answer, saying no gently and lovingly, being honest with children, and cherishing the yeses.
- Wear rubber gloves to improve grip.
- Use long-handled tongs to pick up items.
- Wind rubber bands around door knobs to make grasping easier.
- Purchase lamps that come on when touched lightly.
- Use long-handled utensils such as ice teaspoons for eating.
- Purchase a self-inking address stamp.
- Always follow joint protection guidelines:
  Respond to pain by decreasing or stopping activity.
  Use good body mechanics.
  Change position frequently.
  Alternate tasks and activities.

Nursing interventions for individuals with arthritis should promote a sense of empowerment and control of their condition. The client must become an active partner in the management of his or her condition. One technique for achieving this is a comprehensive educational program.

Teaching/Learning Needs

A planned program of client education should be designed to improve client knowledge regarding their disease and disability, enhance pain management skills by increasing knowledge regarding medication regimen, improve functional living skills, provide joint protection guidelines, and promote adherence.

Nursing Interventions

Nursing interventions should be designed to assist the client in managing the disease independently. And to:

- Decrease pain
- Decrease inflammation
- Increase joint mobility and strength
- Prevent deformities
- Promote independent functioning
- Decrease weight bearing
- Assist in finding new and creative ways of coping with physical limitations
- Encourage sharing frustrations, feelings, and successes with family and friends
- Encourage honest and open communication
- Assist in setting flexible and realistic goals
- Learn to say no without guilt

Common Nursing Diagnoses

- Sleep pattern disturbance
- Impaired physical mobility
- Alteration in comfort: Pain
- Depression

- Altered sexual functioning
- Altered nutrition
- Adherence
- Anxiety
- Health maintenance management
- Ineffective coping
- Guilt
- Knowledge deficit
- Low self-esteem
- Hopelessness
- Powerlessness
- Stress
- Diminished quality of family life
- Diminished professional satisfaction

Summary

Life for individuals with degenerative joint disease is difficult and unpredictable. Pain, stiffness, or deformities may occur at any time and afflict any part of the body. Symptoms range from mild to severe. There are many social and psychological implications associated with arthritis. Individuals with arthritis experience a higher divorce rate; have more difficulty remaining gainfully employed; 60 percent suffer major family, marital, and sexual changes; and 42 percent suffer major depressive disorders (Conwal Incorporated, 1993).

References

Arthritis Foundation. (1995). Arthritis research fact sheet; Living with arthritis fact sheet; Exercise and arthritis fact sheet; Diet and arthritis fact sheet; Topical pain relievers; New dosage form of NSAID available for osteoarthritis and rheumatoid arthritis; Normal intestinal bacteria may trigger certain types of arthritis; New pathway found for some types of arthritis; New method to replace cartilage/bone; Microdose therapy (very low-dose prednisone); Guidelines for the medical management of osteoarthritis of the hip and knee; Glucosamine sulfate treatment; New NSAID, Daypro (Oxaprozin), approved for osteoarthritis and rheumatoid arthritis; News alert: cartilage growth factor (TGFB) in osteoarthritis (on-line). Available http://www.arthritis.org/connectios.

Arthritis Foundation. (1996). Arthritis research highlighted; Arthritis Foundation pain relievers; Targeting the debilitating effects of arthritis (on-line). Available http://www.arthritis. org/connections/qanda/pimemos/pimemo.96.03.shtml.

Blackburn, W. D. (1996). Management of osteoarthritis and rheumatoid arthritis: Prospects and possibilities. *The American Journal of Medicine, 100*(Suppl. 2A), 2A-25S–2A-29S.

Conwal Incorporated. (1993). Arthritis: An overview of research findings (on-line). Available gopher://val-dor.cc.buffalo.edu:70/00/.naric/.briefs/.arthritis.

Oddis, C. V. (1996). New perspectives on osteoarthritis. *The American Journal of Medicine, 100*(Suppl. 2A), 2A-10S–2A-15S.

Suggested Readings

American College of Rheumatology Ad Hoc Committee on Clinical Guidelines. (1996a). Guidelines for the management of rheumatoid arthritis. *Arthritis & Rheumatism, 39*(5), 713–722.

American College of Rheumatology Ad Hoc Committee on Clinical Guidelines. (1996b). Guidelines for monitoring drug therapy in rheumatoid arthritis. *Arthritis & Rheumatism, 39*(5), 723–731.

The Arthritis Society. (1996). Types of arthritis (on-line). Available: http://www.ca:80/types/osteo. html#general.

Fifield, J., Reisine, S., Sheehan, T., & McQuillan, J. (1996). Gender, paid work, and symptoms of emotional distress in rheumatoid arthritis patients. *Arthritis & Rheumatism, 39*(3), 427–435.

Hochberg, M. C., Altman, R. D., Brandt, K. D., Clark, B. M., Dieppe, P. A., Griffen, M. R., Moskowitz, R. W., & Schnitzer, T. J. (1995). Guidelines for the medical management of osteoarthritis. II. Osteoarthritis of the knee. *Arthritis & Rheumatism, 38*(11), 1541–1546.

Pope, R. M. (1996). Rheumatoid arthritis: Pathogenesis and early recognition. *American Journal of Medicine, 100*(Suppl. 2A), 2A-3S–2A-7S.

Rehabilitation Institute of Chicago. (1996). *Rehabilitation of persons with rheumatoid arthritis.* Gaithersburg, MD: Aspen.

Reisine, S., McQuillan, J., & Fifield, J. (1995). Predictors of work disability in rheumatoid arthritis patients. *Arthritis & Rheumatism, 39*(11), 1630–1637.

Stratton, K. V., Maisiak, R., Wrigley, J. M., White M. B., Johnson, P., & Fine, P. R. (1996). Barriers to return to work among persons unemployed due to arthritis and musculoskeletal disorders. *Arthritis & Rheumatism, 39*(1), 101–109.

CHAPTER 24

Chronic Neurological Disorders: Multiple Sclerosis, Parkinson's Disease, Myasthenia Gravis, and Guillain-Barré Syndrome

Anita Rosebrough

Key Terms *Akinesia*
Antibodies
Ataxic Gait
Autoimmune Disorder
Axons
Benign Multiple Sclerosis
Bradykinesia
Central Nervous System (CNS)
Cerebrospinal Fluid
Chronic Progressive Multiple Sclerosis
Chronic Relapsing Multiple Sclerosis
Demyelination
Dopamine
Myelin Sheath
Optic Neuritis
Plaques
Plasmapheresis
Postural Instability
Ptosis
Relapsing-Remitting Multiple Sclerosis
Rigidity
Substantia Nigra
Tremor

Objectives 1. Describe the pathophysiology associated with multiple sclerosis.

2. Discuss the theories of multiple sclerosis etiology.

3. Describe factors associated with exacerbation of multiple sclerosis.

4. Describe symptoms frequently associated with multiple sclerosis.

5. Describe the types or patterns of the multiple sclerosis disease process.

6. Discuss the current medical and nursing management options for multiple sclerosis.

7. Compare and contrast alterations in thought processes related to chronic neurological diseases.

8. Describe the pathophysiology associated with Parkinson's disease.

9. Discuss the etiology of parkinsonism.

10. Describe the common manifestations of Parkinson's disease.

11. Describe the action of levodopa in the treatment of Parkinson's disease.

12. Discuss the current pharmacological and surgical treatment options for Parkinson's disease.

13. Describe four common impairments associated with Parkinson's disease and their appropriate nursing interventions.

14. Describe the prognosis of multiple sclerosis, Parkinson's disease, myasthenia gravis, and Guillain-Barré syndrome.

15. Identify assessment findings associated with multiple sclerosis, Parkinson's disease, myasthenia gravis, and Guillain-Barré syndrome.

16. Identify and describe the pathophysiology associated with myasthenia gravis and Guillain-Barré syndrome.

17. Identify possible causes of Guillain-Barré syndrome.

18. Identify and describe the clinical manifestations of Guillain-Barré syndrome and myasthenia gravis.

19. Describe the prognosis of Guillain-Barré syndrome.

Multiple Sclerosis
Introduction

Multiple sclerosis (MS) is a chronic, progressive, degenerative disease of the **central nervous system (CNS)** affecting the **myelin sheath.** The **axons** and cell bodies are unaffected by the disease process. **Demyelination,** an inflammatory process, destroys the myelin sheath in scattered areas along the conduction pathways of the nerves. MS is a disease of the white matter and affects the brainstem, cerebrum, cerebellum, optic nerve, and spinal cord. The peripheral nerves are spared. Myelin, a fatty substance coating nerve fibers, promotes the rapid and efficient transmission of nerve impulses. As the myelin is destroyed, it is replaced by scar tissue or sclerotic **plaques.** The plaques disrupt and slow the transmission of neural impulses to the brain, and produce symptoms specific to the involved areas.

Multiple sclerosis is a common disorder and a leading cause of neurological disability during early adulthood. There are approximately 300,000–500,000 cases of multiple sclerosis in the United States. About 8000 new cases are diagnosed each year. The average age of onset is 20 to 40 years, and can vary from 10 to 59 years. However, the incidence of MS in children is very low. Multiple sclerosis affects women twice as often as it affects men. There is a higher incidence of MS in Caucasians than in African-Americans and Asians. Life expectancy after diagnosis is approximately 25 years (National Institutes of Health [NIH], 1996; Rudick, 1990).

Etiology

The exact cause of multiple sclerosis is unknown. However, several causative theories exist. Multiple sclerosis cannot be inherited or genetically transmitted. However, a person is at 15 times the risk of developing the disease if a family member has been diagnosed with MS. Environment influences the incidence of MS worldwide. MS is more prevalent between 40 to 60 degrees north latitude. The incidence of MS in colder, northern climates is 30 to 80 per 100,000 whereas in more tropical climates the incidence is 1 per 100,000. Another theory suggests that the destruction of the myelin sheath is due to an abnormal immune response. Viral **antibodies** are thought to trigger a delayed autoimmune response that causes the body's T cells to attack its own myelin sheaths. Many viruses have been implicated as the causative agent of multiple sclerosis. However, no definitive evidence exists to link one specific virus with the demyelinating autoimmune reaction of MS. It is also suggested that a specific, slow-acting MS virus exists. At this time no such virus has been identified. The exact cause of MS remains unknown. There is no known cure or preventive treatment (NIH, 1996; Rudick, 1990).

The course of the disease is unpredictable and can be crippling. Typically it is characterized by periods of exacerbation and remission, especially during the early stages. The majority of individuals have recognizable but vague and transitory symptoms. Neurological deficits vary widely from individual to individual and are related to the location and the severity of nerve involvement. Deficits are more pronounced during the period of exacerbation and may disappear completely during remission. Early in the disease process, the remission of symptoms is due to partial healing of the myelin sheath. Eventually, scar tissue replaces the myelin sheath and symptoms become permanent. Some individuals experience only minor neurological deficits, whereas for others the disease progresses rapidly to total disability and dependence. Several common patterns of disease progression have been identified.

Benign Multiple Sclerosis

- Incidence: 20 percent.
- The individual with **benign multiple sclerosis** experiences one or two episodes of neurological dysfunction and recovery is complete or nearly complete. This form does not progress or worsen over time. There is minimal to no disability after 10 to 15 years. Symptoms at onset tend to be less severe.

Relapsing-Remitting Multiple Sclerosis

- Incidence: 25 percent.
- **Relapsing-remitting multiple sclerosis** is characterized by more frequent periods of exacerbation, during which the person experiences new neurological deficits or old deficits become more severe. The exacerbations can last from several days to several months. The exacerbation is followed by a period of remission, during which partial healing takes place. During the remission phase the person may experience recovery from the neurological deficits. Remissions can last from months to years.

Chronic Relapsing Multiple Sclerosis

- Incidence: 40 percent.
- **Chronic relapsing multiple sclerosis** usually starts as relapsing-remitting MS and later develops into progressive disability. Remissions after each exacerbation are fewer and incomplete. There is a cumulative effect, with more neurological deficits following each episode. Disability ranges from moderate to severe.

Chronic Progressive Multiple Sclerosis

- Incidence: 15 percent.
- **Chronic progressive multiple sclerosis** is characterized by the absence of clearly identifiable periods of exacerbation. Instead, there is a slow and steady progression of symptoms over a period of months or years, without remissions.

Symptoms   Several factors are frequently associated with the onset of symptoms, and the periods of exacerbation, of multiple sclerosis. These factors include infection, trauma, fatigue, exposure to temperature extremes, pregnancy, physical stress, and/or psychological stress. Exacerbations are more common during the early stages of the disease process. Mild upper respiratory infections of viral origin are thought to be responsible for the majority of exacerbations in relapsing-remitting MS (Panitch, 1994).

There is no typical profile of an individual with MS. Multiple sclerosis is a variable condition and symptoms depend on the areas of the CNS effected. Each person has a unique set of symptoms that vary over time. Symptoms may be mild or severe, of short or long duration. They may appear alone or in combination. There are symptoms that are common to many people. However, no one will experience all of them. Early in the disease process symptoms are often vague and transitory, and vary widely. The first symptom is often blurred or double vision. Many individuals experience numbness and muscle weakness in an extremity, and problems with coordination or balance. Symptoms may be severe enough to impair mobility. Fatigue, tremors, dizziness, and speech impediments are other common initial complaints. As the disease progresses, bowel, bladder, and sexual dysfunction may occur. Depression is a common reaction and some clients experience memory impairment (NIH, 1996). The following list includes frequently experienced symptoms or neurological deficits.

Impaired Vision
- Diplopia
- Blurred vision
- Nystagmus
- Optic neuritis
- Loss of vision or blindness

Altered Sensation
- Paresthesia (numbness, tingling, or burning)
- Pain (moderate to severe)
- Impairment in ability to sense pain, temperature, touch, vibration, and position

Impaired Verbal Communication
- Slurred speech
- Changes in speech rhythm (words may be clipped or broken; scanning speech, staccato speech)
- Slowing of words
- Dysarthria

Alteration in Elimination
- Change in urinary retention, frequency, or urgency
- Incomplete emptying of the bladder
- Incontinence
- Constipation

Impaired Physical Mobility
- Muscle weakness in the lower extremities
- Spasticity
- Muscle spasms
- Loss of balance
- **Ataxic gait**
- Loss of balance
- Incoordination

- Tremor (greater with fine movement)
- Fatigue
- Vertigo

Altered Sexual Functioning
- Impotence
- Loss of sensation
- Diminished arousal
- Orgasmic dysfunction
- Ejaculatory dysfunction
- Decreased libido

Altered Thought Processes
- Short-term memory problems
- Lack of concentration
- Lack of judgment
- Impaired ability to reason
- Emotional lability (Britell, 1995a; Hanak, 1992; Hickey, 1992)

Diagnosing Multiple Sclerosis

Owing to the vague and transitory nature of symptoms during the early stages of MS, a medical diagnosis may be difficult to make, and may take an extended period of time. There are no specific tests for MS and the ones that are used are not 100 percent conclusive. The evaluation process should include a complete medical history, and a complete neurological examination. The history includes a record of signs and symptoms, their onset and pattern. Evidence of central nervous system demyelination is often found during the clinical examination. However, a neurological examination cannot determine the exact cause of the neurological deficits. Diagnostic studies are used to determine the presence of multiple sclerosis and to rule out other possible causes. Frequently ordered diagnostic tests include magnetic resonance imaging (MRI), lumbar puncture, and evoked potential studies.

Magnetic resonance imaging scans take very detailed pictures of the brain and spinal cord. The scans show the number, size, and distribution of sclerotic plaques in the brain and spinal cord. Scan results are abnormal in 70 to 90 percent of MS clients. MRI is superior to other tests. It can even show asymptomatic lesions. However, not all lesions are detected by the scanner and other illnesses can produce similar results. It is critical that scan findings be correlated with clinical findings. A lumbar puncture is performed to evaluate the **cerebrospinal fluid (CSF)** for the presence of blood, bacteria, malignant cells, glucose, protein, color, chloride, lactic dehydrogenase, serology, oligoclonal gammaglobulin bands, glutamine, and antibodies. CSF findings suggestive of MS include the presence of protein, IgG, and oligoclonal bands (National Multiple Sclerosis Society, 1996; Giang et al., 1994).

The demyelination process causes slowing of the conduction of nerve impulses. Evoked potential testing measures the time it takes for the brain to receive and interpret messages. Normal reaction time is instantaneous, and with demyelination delays occur. Evoked potential testing includes the visual evoked response (VER), auditory brainstem evoked potentials (ABEPs), and the somatosensory evoked response (SER). The VER machine records the length of time it takes for an impulse to travel from the eye to the occipital area of the brain. This test is abnormal in 85 to 90 percent of clients with definite MS. The ABEP test is used to test for lesions in the auditory pathways. It is abnormal in 67 percent of clients with definite MS. The SER test measures the length of time it takes for a small electrical current to travel to the cerebral cortex. Results are abnormal in 77 percent of clients with definite MS (National Multiple Sclerosis Society, 1996-Giang et al., 1994).

The diagnosis of MS is difficult to make. Test results often are unclear. The transitory and vague nature of the initial symptoms can be confusing. The diagnosis is often a shock to the client and the family. With treatment and symptom management most people with MS lead active and productive lives.

Routine Medical Management

At this time there is no known cure or preventive treatment for multiple sclerosis. Treatment modalities include the use of anti-inflammatory agents, symptom management, and/or investigational pharmacological agents. During periods of acute exacerbation steroids with anti-inflammatory properties are given to reduce both the duration and the severity of the exacerbation. Steroids are associated with many side effects and are not intended for long-term use. Drugs commonly used include adrenocorticotropic hormone (ACTH), prednisone, prednisolone, methylprednisolone, betamethasone, and dexamethasone. Their exact mechanism of action in multiple sclerosis is unknown. Over time, clients may become resistant to steroid therapy. Current investigational treatments are designed to limit the inflammatory process and to repair damaged myelin. Clinical trials are in progress for the use of azathioprine, cyclosporine, cyclophosphamide, mitoxantrone, Copolymer 1, interferons, methotrexate, plasma exchange, and myelin transplantation (Compston, 1994; Mitchell, 1993; van Oosten, Truyen, Barkhof, & Polman, 1995).

Symptom Management

Altered Urinary Elimination The demyelination process of MS affects the motor and sensory pathways of the bladder. Approximately 75 percent of individuals with MS experience neurogenic bladders. Up to 90 percent experience urinary dysfunction at some time during the course of their illness. Urinary symptoms vary and can change over time. The majority of symptoms experienced are related to either a small bladder capacity or to an irritable bladder with high postvoiding residuals. Normal micturition requires that the detrusor muscle of the bladder contract at the same time that the sphincters relax. Relaxation of the sphincters opens the outlet, and contraction of the detrusor muscle expels the urine from the bladder. If the detrusor is unable to inhibit contractions until a reasonable amount of urine has accumulated, the client experiences frequency, urgency, and/or incontinence. If the force of the detrusor muscle contraction is weakened, urinary retention occurs. Simultaneous contraction of the bladder and contraction of the urinary sphincters cause urinary retention. Some MS clients experience a combination of symptoms. However, urinary urgency, urinary frequency, and urinary hesitancy are the most common problems (Mitchell, 1993; Rudick, 1990; Schapiro, 1994; Britell, 1995a; van Oosten, Truyen, Barkhof, & Polman, 1995).

Urinary symptoms are inconvenient and disrupt all aspects of life, particularly social activities and employment. Urinary dysfunction increases the mortality and morbidity of multiple sclerosis. With proper identification of the underlying pathology, most symptoms can be managed effectively, and complications can be prevented. The goals of treatment are to maintain continence, prevent infection, and maintain normal kidney function.

Treatment modalities vary depending on the underlying cause of the symptoms. Urinary urgency and frequency can be effectively treated with anticholinergic drugs such as probantheline or oxybutynin. Urinary hesitancy or retention is frequently managed with a clean intermittent self-catheterization program. Most individuals are capable of performing self-catheterization, and thus, of maintaining independence. Clients experiencing a combination of symptoms usually require both anticholinergic drugs and intermittent catheterization. Other treatment options are a timed voiding schedule, Credé maneuver, controlling fluid intake, external collection devices, and absorbent pads. Long-term surgical options include bladder augmentation, artificial sphincter, and suprapubic cystostomy (Bemelmans, Hommes, van Kerrebroeck, Lemmens, Doesburg, & Debruyne, 1991; Betts, D'Mellow, & Fowler, 1993; Britell, 1995a; Holland, 1994; Rudick, 1990).

Nursing Interventions
- Administer medications as ordered.
- Teach about medication regimen.
- Teach about urological problems.
- Teach preventive measures.
- Teach management of urological interventions.
- Teach self-catheterization.
- Teach to maintain adequate hydration.
- Teach to schedule fluid intake and voiding times.
- Teach strategies to prevent urinary tract infections.

Altered Bowel Elimination

The most common bowel problem with multiple sclerosis is constipation. Constipation is characterized by difficult or incomplete emptying. Occasionally incontinence is associated with constipation or fecal impaction. Prevention is the best intervention. Regular evacuation of a soft stool is facilitated by a high-fiber diet, adequate fluid intake, physical activity, and regularly scheduled evacuations.

Nursing Interventions

- Teach diet management of bowel program.
- Teach preventive measures.
- Teach to maintain adequate fluid intake.
- Assist the client to identify the best time for day for regular evacuations.
- Teach the client to massage lower abdomen gently.
- Emphasize the need for regular exercise.

Impaired Vision

Visual problems are common manifestations of multiple sclerosis because the optic nerve and the oculomotor tracts are often affected. In fact, more than one-third of MS clients report experiencing ocular symptoms (McDonald & Barnes, 1992). **Optic neuritis,** an inflammation of the optic nerve, is a common early symptom. It results in blurring, variable loss of vision, and loss of visual acuity or blindness. Optic neuritis is usually self-limiting with good recovery of vision. Diplopia and nystagmus are also common. Diplopia, double vision, occurs when eye movement is poorly coordinated owing to weakness of the eye muscles. It usually resolves without treatment. An eye patch may be beneficial to the client with diplopia. Nystagmus is uncontrollable horizontal or vertical movement of the eye. It can be mild or severe enough to impair vision. If blindness occurs the client benefits from a referral to a local society for the blind. Currently, no specific pharmacological treatment exists for visual problems. The use of steroids is under investigation for optic neuritis (Hickey, 1986; Martin, Holt, & Hicks, 1981; McDonald & Barnes, 1992; National Multiple Sclerosis Society, 1996).

Nursing Interventions

- Assist the client in learning to compensate for visual deficits.
- Teach scanning techniques.
- Maintain a safe environment.
- Monitor for environmental hazards.

Impaired Mobility: Spasticity

Spasticity is increased voluntary muscle tone and is stimulated by movement. It can cause stiffness, difficulty in moving, pain, contractures, and deformities. Cold temperatures aggravate spasticity. Standard treatment modalities include physical therapy and skeletal muscle relaxants such as Lioresal/baclofen, Valium/diazepam, Klonopin/clonazepam, and Zanaflex/tizanidine hydrochloride (National Multiple Sclerosis Society, 1996).

Nursing Interventions

- Administer medications as ordered.
- Teach the client management of medication regimen.
- Teach preventive measures.
- Teach side effects of medications.
- Perform passive range-of-motion exercises.
- Position in normal alignment to prevent contractures.
- Teach the use of assistive aids such as canes and walkers.
- Teach safety precautions.
- Encourage the use of adaptive equipment.

Fatigue

Fatigue has a major impact on all activities of daily living for individuals with MS. The exact pathophysiology behind the fatigue is unclear. Almost everyone with multiple sclerosis experiences fatigue to some degree. Pharmacological treatment with amantadine is beneficial for some clients (van Oosten, Truyen, Barkhof, & Polman, 1995).

Nursing Interventions

- Teach energy conservation techniques.
- Teach to alternate activities and rest.
- Teach the client to recognize signals indicating endurance limitations.
- Encourage expression of feelings regarding fatigue.
- Refer to community resources as appropriate (Meals on Wheels, and so on).

Heat Sensitivity

Temperature variations, either hot or cold, have a negative effect on symptoms of multiple sclerosis. Many MS clients experience a temporary worsening of neurological deficits owing to overheating. When a demyelinated nerve fiber becomes hot, its ability to conduct electrical impulses becomes more impaired. Increased temperatures do not cause demyelination or scarring, and the neurological deficits quickly return to their prior state when the temperature returns to normal (Uhthoffs sign). MS clients should avoid sunbathing, taking hot baths or hot showers, and exposure to temperature extremes (National Multiple Sclerosis Society, 1996).

Nursing Interventions

- Teach impact of exposure to temperature extremes.
- Teach to check water temperatures.

Altered Sensation

Pain in multiple sclerosis takes many forms and is not uncommon. Stabbing, electric, shocklike pains can occur. Acute burning, or "pins and needles" in the extremities, can also occur. Untreated spasticity can lead to tightness, aching, and pain in the muscles. Acute pain such as trigeminal neuralgia can occur early in the disease and may be the initial presenting symptom. Pharmacological treatment of trigeminal neuralgia includes daily doses of carbamazepine (National Multiple Sclerosis Society, 1996; van Oosten, Truyen, Barkhof, & Polman, 1995). Individuals with multiple sclerosis may also experience a decrease in or loss of sensation.

Nursing Interventions
- Teach nonpharmacological pain management techniques.
- Teach relaxation therapy.
- Teach good skin care.
- Teach client to check temperature of bath water.
- Teach client to avoid temperature extremes.
- Teach pressure release techniques.

Altered Sexual Functioning

Both physiological and psychogenic sexual dysfunction is common with multiple sclerosis. Anywhere from 20 to 91 percent of MS clients indicated that they had to modify sexual activities to accommodate problems associated with their disease. Normal sexual functioning depends on an intact neurological system. Motor and sensory deficits can lead to problems with the physical activity of sexual intercourse. Physiological problems encountered include fatigue, decreased libido, impotence, ejaculatory dysfunction, decreased lubrication, and orgasmic dysfunction. The neurological deficits associated with multiple sclerosis affect body image and self-esteem, and change the clients perception of relationships. Everyone has the need to feel that they are appealing to others, and that they have value as a person. Sexual dysfunction of a psychogenic nature relates to issues of body image, sexual identity, role performance, and self-esteem (Britell, 1995b; Rudick, 1990; Schapiro, 1994).

Many options are available to the client and the sexual partner. However, options need to be discussed on an individual basis. Options should be comfortable to both partners. Because fatigue is a primary concern, timing and positioning changes can be implemented. Supplemental hormone therapy can assist with decreased libido. Erectile dysfunction can be managed with penile implants, papaverine injections, or vacuum devices. Lubricants and vibrators are available to enhance sensation (Korejwo, 1994; Schapiro, 1994). The rehabilitation nurse should conduct a thorough assessment and discuss alternative means of expressing sexuality. The permission limited information/specific information intensive therapy (PLISSIT) model of altered sexual function should be followed and referrals for intensive counseling should be made as needed.

Nursing Interventions
- Maintain privacy.
- Assist the client in maintaining sexual identity.
- Acknowledge feelings and concerns.
- Allow the client to express feelings and concerns.
- Refer for counseling as needed.
- Assess stage of grieving process.
- Identify barriers to normal sexual functioning.
- Assist the client and partner to identify acceptable alternatives.

Altered Thought Processes

Neuropsychological tests demonstrate that 43 to 65 percent of MS clients experience cognitive impairments that are associated with subcortical brain pathology (Britell, 1996). Cognitive functions commonly affected by MS include complex attention, information processing, learning, recent memory, concept formation, problem-solving, and executive functions. Cognitive impairments cause problems at home and at work. They affect a person's ability to perform activities of daily living, lead to decreased social interaction, and to loss of employment (Britell, 1996; Kujala, Portin, & Ruutiainen, 1994; Rao, Leo, Ellington, Nauertz, Bernardin, & Unverzagt, 1991; Rudick, 1990).

Nursing Interventions
- Teach compensatory mechanisms.
- Teach use of memory aids.
- Teach to minimize deficits.
- Teach effect of MS on cognitive processes.

Individuals with multiple sclerosis experience a wide variety of progressive problems. Many of the symptoms and problems take years or decades to develop. The long-term management of individuals with MS presents a challenge to the interdisciplinary rehabilitation team. With appropriate management the client with MS can achieve and maintain an optimal level of independence.

Parkinson's Disease
Introduction

Parkinsonism was first described in 1817 by Dr. James Parkinson as paralysis agitans. Today, it is more commonly referred to as Parkinson's disease (PD). PD is a chronic progressive, degenerative disorder of the CNS. Parkinson's disease is one of the most common neurological disorders causing progressive disability in middle to late adulthood.

Roughly 500,000 to 1 million Americans have Parkinson's disease, and 40,000 new cases are diagnosed each year. PD affects the 40- to 90-year age groups, and the average age of onset is 57 years. A small percentage (5 to 10 percent) of individuals develop symptoms of Parkinson's disease before the age of 40. The disease is slightly more common in men than in women, and is four times more common in whites than in darkly pigmented individuals. The life expectancy of an individual with PD is reduced owning to complications associated with physical immobility (National Institute of Neurological Disorders and Stroke [NINDS], 1996; Wilson, 1995).

Parkinson's disease occurs when the neurons located in the **substantia nigra** of the midbrain degenerate or become impaired. As a result, the neurotransmitter **dopamine** that is produced by the substantia nigra is depleted. Symptoms of PD do not appear until the dopamine supply is reduced by 80 percent. In the normal brain, dopamine, an inhibitory neurotransmitter, and acetylcholine, an excitatory neurotransmitter, are in balance. Together, they control normal motor function. Normal motor functioning is initiated by the release of dopamine from the substantia nigra. Dopamine transmits messages to the corpus striatum. Loss of dopamine causes the striatum to fire out of control, and control of movement is lost. The dopamine deficiency produces the classic symptoms of tremor, bradykinesia, rigidity, and postural instability associated with Parkinson's disease (Hanak, 1992; Johnson, 1994).

Etiology   Either primary or secondary Parkinson's disease can occur. Secondary Parkinson's disease is associated with specific factors such as trauma, infection, tumors, toxins, atherosclerosis, and drugs. Primary PD is idiopathic in nature.

The exact cause of cell death in idiopathic Parkinson's disease is unknown. A number of theories are currently under investigation. One theory suggests that toxins are responsible for the degeneration of the substantia nigra. There are a number of toxins, such as methylphenyltetrahydropyridine (MPTP), and neuroleptic drugs that are known to cause parkinsonian symptoms in humans. No specific toxin is linked to the development of Parkinson's disease. Environmental factors are also implicated. Parkinson's disease is more prevalent in rural areas where people are exposed to well water and pesticides. Increased levels of serum iron in the substantia nigra and the striatum may play a role in exacerbating neuronal degeneration. Elemental iron is known to increase free radical formation in the CNS. A relatively new theory suggests that there may be a genetic link to PD. About 15 to 20 percent of individuals with Parkinson's disease have a close relative with the illness. Last, the presence of excessive free radicals and consequent oxidative damage to the cells is blamed for the destruction of the substantia nigra. Although many theories exist, none has been definitively proven to cause Parkinson's disease. Some researchers believe that a combination of genetic and environmental factors causes the degeneration of the substantia nigra (American

Academy of Neurology [AAN], 1994; Johnson, 1994; McDermott et al., 1995; NINDS, 1996; Silverstein, 1996).

Diagnosis　There are no specific diagnostic tests for Parkinson's disease. A diagnosis is usually made after a thorough neurological examination establishes the presence of parkinsonian-type symptoms, and other diseases resembling Parkinson's disease have been ruled out.

Symptoms　Early symptoms of Parkinson's disease are subtle, and often are attributed to the normal aging process. As the disease progresses, the classic symptoms of PD become more pronounced. The primary features of Parkinson's disease are tremor, bradykinesia, rigidity, and postural instability. The symptoms and rate of disease progression vary from person to person. Some individuals become severely disabled and others suffer only minor symptoms.

Tremor

Tremor is the most common symptom associated with Parkinson's disease. It is an involuntary rhythmic movement that affects the head, hands, extremities, or the entire body. The tremor is most pronounced and noticeable in the hands. Hand tremors frequently involve a back-and-forth motion of the thumb and index finger, producing a "pill-rolling" motion. Stress exacerbates the tremor. The tremor stops during sleep, and decreases with intentional movements. Tremor is the least disabling of all PD symptoms; but it is the most noticeable and the most troublesome.

Rigidity

Rigidity is another symptom of Parkinson's disease, caused by tense, contracted muscles. Both the flexor and the extensor muscles are involved. The rigidity may initially be localized, but eventually it becomes a diffuse problem. When tremor and rigidity combine, a "cogwheeling" effect occurs, and movements are short and jerky. Rigidity also contributes to the postural changes and the postural instability associated with PD. Rigidity of the intercostal muscles and decreased chest expansion can lead to alterations in respiratory functioning. Rigidity leads to severe motor impairment that interferes with the client's ability to engage in activities of daily living.

Akinesia/Bradykinesia

Akinesia and **bradykinesia** refer to a generalized inability to move, and to a slowness of movement. It is the most disabling characteristic of PD. Bradykinesia affects all motor functions, including the ability to blink the eyes, change facial expressions, eat, chew, and walk. Facial expressions remain fixed and masklike.

Simple activities of daily living may take hours to perform. The individual may sit motionless for long periods of time as if frozen in place. The person with Parkinson's disease becomes unable to perform more than one motor activity at a time. When asked to perform two motor activities they will "freeze," and be unable to perform either activity.

Postural Instability

One of the most recognizable features of PD is **postural instability.** Individuals with PD develop a stooped posture with head bowed down and knees flexed. The arms are flexed, and fail to swing when walking. The person walks in a shuffling, small-stepped, toe-first manner. The gait is unsteady and unbalanced (see Figure 1). These individuals are prone to falls, and are at high risk for injury.

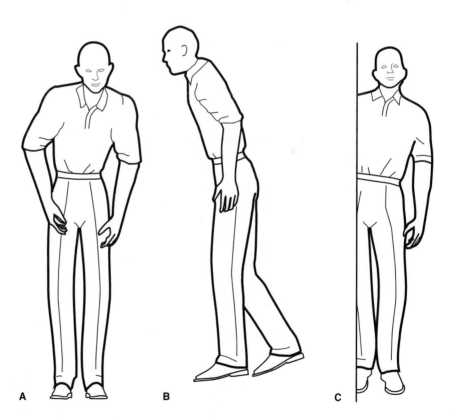

A   B   C

Fig 1. *Postural instability associated with Parkinson's disease.*

Sleep Pattern Disturbance

Many individuals with Parkinson's disease experience sleep disruptions. The exact causes of the sleep disturbances are unclear but appear to be linked to the loss of dopamine. A variety of sleep disturbances occur, including difficulty falling asleep, waking frequently during the night, waking very early in the morning, vivid dreams and nightmares, leg cramps and restlessness, difficulty with bed mobility, and nocturia. Factors such as depression, anxiety, shortness of breath, medications, or other sensory complaints contribute to nonrestful sleep patterns. Loss of nighttime sleep leads to daytime drowsiness and fatigue.

Nursing Interventions
- Teach to avoid dietary stimulants in the evening.
- Teach relaxation techniques.
- Teach to avoid excessive daytime napping.
- Teach to establish a regular sleep/wake schedule.
- Encourage regular physical exercise.
- Avoid loud noises.
- Avoid excessively warm nighttime temperatures.
- Encourage the client to drink a warm glass of milk, or to eat a light snack at bedtime.
- Discuss the medication regimen with the physician.

Altered Bowel Elimination

Individuals with Parkinson's disease experience decreased gastric motility, and decreased transit time. As a result, constipation is a common problem. It is important that a normal pattern of elimination be maintained. This can be achieved by establishing a regular bowel program. A good bowel program should include dietary fiber, adequate fluid intake, and a regular exercise program.

Altered Urinary Elimination

Most parkinsonians develop a hyperactive detrusor muscle. Consequently, urinary urgency, frequency, and nocturia are common problems.

Altered Sexual Functioning

The most common sexual problem for men with PD lies in achieving or sustaining an erection. Little is known about the sexual functioning of women with PD. Sexual dysfunction is a major side effect of many of the pharmacological agents used to treat Parkinson's disease. Depression also plays an important role in sexual dysfunction and should not be overlooked as an influencing factor. Clients experiencing sexual dysfunctioning should be referred for counseling by a licensed therapist.

Impaired Swallowing

Individuals with Parkinson's disease often experience dysphagia during the latter stages of the disease process. Frequently experienced swallowing problems include poor tongue control, difficulty moving the food bolus to the pharynx, difficulty chewing, aspiration of food, and reflux of food. For many it is more difficult to swallow solid foods than liquids. It is not unusual for the person with Parkinson's to lose 20 to 30 pounds of weight. A dietitian and speech therapist should be consulted to maintain adequate nutrition. Clients should be taught to plan meals during the peak times of levodopa therapy. The motor disturbances leading to dysphagia in PD can also lead to dysarthria. Dysarthria is a common speech problem that may improve with levodopa therapy.

Medical Management

There is no known cure for Parkinson's disease, and medical management is symptomatic. About three-quarters of clients with PD experience symptoms severe enough to warrant pharmacological treatment within 2 years of onset of their illness. Medical treatment does not halt the progression of the disease process. The pharmacological agents are used in an attempt to restore or replenish the dopamine levels in the CNS. Ongoing adjustments in medication dosages are required as the disease progresses. With proper treatment and symptom management it is possible for clients with PD to lead normal and productive lives.

Antiparkinson medications function in one of three ways: to replenish the supply of dopamine, to reverse the process in the brain regulating the amount of dopamine available, or to supply substitutes that are similar to dopamine. Medications commonly used include dopamine precursors, dopamine agonists, antiviral agents, monoamine oxidase type B (MAO-B) inhibitors, and anticholinergic drugs. These drugs may be used alone or in combination (McDermott et al., 1995; Silverstein, 1996).

Levodopa (L-Dopa, Dopar, Larodopa). The cornerstone of treatment for Parkinson's disease since the 1960s has been levodopa, a precursor of dopamine. Levodopa is used by the body to make dopamine and to replenish the diminishing supply in the brain. It delays the onset of debilitating symptoms, and extends the productive life of individuals with Parkinson's disease. However, it does not stop the progress of the disease. Not all symptoms respond to levodopa therapy. The dosage of the drug may need to be increased gradually to achieve maximum benefit.

Levodopa has many side effects. The most common side effects are nausea, vomiting, hypotension, involuntary movements (dyskinesias), and restlessness. The dyskinesias may be mild or severe. Drug dosages need to be titrated to achieve maximum benefit and minimum side effects. Clients are usually given levodopa and carbidopa (Sinemet) in combination. Carbidopa prevents the conversion of levodopa to dopamine until it reaches the brain. It decreases the amount of levodopa needed, and decreases the number and severity of levodopa side effects. As more of the dopamine-producing cells degenerate, higher doses of Sinemet are needed. Sinemet in high doses causes dyskinesia (Bernstein, 1995; NINDS, 1996).

Dopamine agonists mimic the effect of dopamine, and stimulate dopamine receptors. Currently, there are two dopamine agonists on the market Parlodel (bromocriptine) and Permax (pergolide). These drugs act directly on the receptor sites and are long-lasting. They can be taken less frequently, and allow for a decrease in levodopa/carbidopa dosages (Bernstein, 1995).

Amantadine (Symmetrel) is an antiviral drug that reduces the symptoms of Parkinson's disease in the early stages of the disease process. However, its effectiveness wears off after several months. Amantadine causes more dopamine to be released, and may block the action of acetylcholine (NINDS, 1996).

Another commonly used drug is selegiline (deprenyl, or Eldepryl), an MAO-B enzyme inhibitor. By preventing the breakdown of dopamine, the dopamine is available for a longer period of time. This drug can delay the need for levodopa therapy for 1 year or more. Selegiline inhibits the metabolism of dopamine in the brain (Bernstein, 1995; NINDS, 1996). When Sinemet and selegiline are given in combination, lower doses of Sinemet are needed, thus decreasing the dyskinesias associated with high doses of Sinemet.

Anticholinergic medications were used to treat Parkinson's disease before the introduction of levodopa. They control tremor and rigidity in some individuals. They act by blocking acetylcholine in the brain, and are used in the early stages of PD (NINDS, 1996). Currently used anticholinergics are trihexyphenidyl hydrochloride (Artane), benztropine mesylate (Cogentin), and diphenhydramine hydrochloride (Benadryl). Side effects of these drugs include dry mouth, urinary retention, and constipation (Mishra, 1996).

Nursing Interventions

- Teach management of medication regimen.
- Teach side effects of medications.
- Teach to read food and drug labels to monitor for vitamin B_6.
- Monitor for side effects.

Surgical Options Since the introduction of levodopa during the 1960s surgery for Parkinson's disease has been limited to rare and severe cases. However, some of the older surgical procedures are making a comeback. Two surgical procedures are being evaluated: ablative surgeries and cell transplantation. The ablative surgeries cryothalamotomy and pallidotomy involve inserting a supercooled probe into the thalamus. High-resolution MRI is used to pinpoint the exact location of the cells causing the tremor. The cryoprobe is inserted and the targeted cells are identified. The probe is cooled in 10-degree increments and the cells are destroyed. Thalamotomy is effective for severe tremor, and pallidotomy is performed for bradykinesia. Ablative surgeries were used during the 1960s. Fetal cell transplantation is a more recent and experimental phenomenon. Both procedures decrease the symptoms of PD, but clients must continue to take antiparkinsonian medications (Fazzini, 1995; NINDS, 1996).

Activities of Daily Living

Because Parkinson's disease leads to slowness and awkwardness in movement, freezing in midmotion, and unstable postures, many accommodations need to be made in the home and in the schedule of activities of daily living to promote independent functioning. Fall prevention is a high priority. Environmental clutter (scatter rugs and bric-à-brac) and hazards (doorsills and stairs) should be removed. Safety devices such as grab bars and railings should be installed. Toilet seats will need to be raised and grab bars installed next to the toilet.

The person with Parkinson's disease cannot perform more than one motor activity at a time. This coupled with bradykinesia leads to slowness in performing all tasks. It may take three to five times as long to complete ordinary tasks, such as brushing teeth or combing hair. Dressing is problematic, and clothing may need to be altered to facilitate independence in this area.

The individual with Parkinson's disease slowly loses the ability to engage in self-care activities. The client should be encouraged to do as much as possible without assistance for as long as possible, and to maintain a healthy and active lifestyle. A regular exercise program is important to prevent stiffness, and maintain joint range of motion. Participation in hobbies and community programs provides a sense of accomplishment and self-worth.

Summary

Parkinson's disease affects every dimension of life. Pharmacological management of symptoms often improves the quality of life for the person with PD. Unfortunately, medication side effects can also be disabling. An interdisciplinary team process must be used to assist clients in achieving maximum independent functioning.

Myasthenia Gravis
Introduction

The term *myasthenia gravis* (MG) is derived from the Greek and Latin words for grave muscle weakness. MG is a chronic, progressive neuromuscular disease manifested by weakness of the voluntary (striated) muscles. Muscles innervated by the cranial nerves and proximal muscles are more affected than distal muscles. It can affect any voluntary muscles but is more common in the extraocular muscles, facial muscles, and muscles used for chewing, swallowing, and speaking. **Ptosis** and ocular palsies are often the initial presenting symptoms. Muscle weakness associated with MG increases with activity and improves with rest. It can affect a single muscle or a group of muscles. In some individuals it is limited to ocular and eyelid muscles, producing ptosis and double vision. Others experience dysphagia, dystonia, and/or respiratory problems. MG is potentially life-threatening when respiratory functioning is impaired. Muscles in the neck and the extremities can also be affected. Extremity weakness can result in self-care deficits. Symptoms vary widely. The classic manifestations of MG are muscle weakness and fatigability. Weakness associated with MG is proximal and fluctuates. The weakness occurs after repeated use of a muscle. Clients may complain of generalized weakness, drooling, difficulty in swallowing, choking, or blurred vision.

MG is progressive during the first 5 to 7 years after onset of initial symptoms. After that the disease remains relatively stable. However, severity of muscle weakness fluctuates from day to day and from hour to hour.

MG occurs in all races, in both sexes, and can affect an individual at any age. It is seen more frequently in young adult females and older males. The incidence for women peaks around 30 years of age. The onset for men is 60 to 70 years of age. The female-to-male ratio is 6:4. The rate of occurrence of myasthenia gravis is 25 to 125 cases per million people (Irvives, 1997).

Etiology and Pathophysiology

Myasthenia gravis is an **autoimmune disorder.** Antibodies destroy postsynaptic acetylcholine receptor sites at the neuromuscular junction, blocking the transmission of nerve impulses. Acetylcholine production is normal but the number or receptor sites and their efficiency are reduced (Kshatri, 1996).

The onset of MG may be gradual or sudden. Initial symptoms include ptosis or diplopia (50 percent), dyphagia or dysarthria (30 percent), and/or extremity weakness (20 percent) (Wiederholt, 1995). The hallmarks of MG are muscle weakness and fatigability. Sensation, reflexes, and coordination remain intact. MG is characterized by periods of exacerbation and remission. Several factors are known to temporarily worsen myasthenic muscle weakness. These things include infections, fever, temperature extremes, pregnancy, thyroid activity, surgery, diuretics, overexertion, and emotional stress. MG in some cases is associated with tumors of the thymus gland, thyrotoxicosis, rheumatoid arthritis, systemic lupus erythematosus, and other immune system disorders.

MG remains localized to the extraocular and eyelid muscles in approximately 15 percent of cases. Generalized weakness occurs in approximately 85 percent of individuals with MG (Drachman, 1994).

Diagnosis

The diagnosis of MG is based on four basic elements. These include clinical presentation and history of symptoms, edrophonium test, electromyography, and anti-acetylcholine receptor antibody test. The edrophonium (Tensilon) test is performed by administering the drug intravenously, and monitoring the client for improvement in the function of a specific muscle group such as the eyelid. Edrophonium inhibits acetylcholinesterase, thus prolonging the life of acetylcholine.

Individuals with MG exhibit increased muscle strength with the administration of edrophonium. The drug takes effect in approximately 30 seconds, has a duration of 5 minutes, and is specific for MG. Occasionally an individual with MG will have a negative test (Irvives, 1997).

Electromyography is part of the routine evaluation for MG. A decrease occurs in the evoked action potential in a muscle affected by MG during repetitive stimulation. This can occur in other disorders of the neuromuscular junction (Irvives, 1997).

Serum antibody testing is more specific for MG. Approximately 85 percent of individuals with MG have detectable levels of acetylcholine receptor antibodies. Occasionally, all tests are negative even in the presence of obvious muscle weakness. Positive clinical findings by an experienced neurologist take precedence over negative diagnostic studies.

Routine Medical Management

There is no known cure for MG; however, treatment can lead to prolonged periods of symptom-free remission. Short-term treatment of MG consists of strategies designed to prolong the life of acetylcholine (Kshatri, 1996) and plasmapheresis. Drugs blocking the breakdown of acetylcholine include neostigmine, pyridostigmine, and ambenonium chloride. These drugs are not a cure for MG. They provide temporary relief of symptoms of MG and improve client functioning. The dosage and administration schedule vary depending on muscle involvement and severity of symptoms.

Therapeutic **plasmapheresis** or therapeutic plasma exchange removes toxic elements, metabolic substances, antibodies, and other constituents implicated in disease from the blood. Its ability to remove antibodies and other immunologically active substances from the blood has led to its therapeutic use in neurological conditions in which autoimmunity plays a role. Plasmapheresis is a short-term alternative treatment used to strengthen individuals before to thymectomy and during the postoperative period. It is also useful in decreasing symptoms before the initiation of immunosuppressive drug therapy and during an acute respiratory crisis. The beneficial effects of plasmapheresis last for several weeks (Kshatri, 1996).

Administration of intravenous human immune globulin (IVIG) boosts the client's immune system with pooled gammaglobulin antibodies from many donors. The effects last several weeks. IVIG can be used to prevent/treat a myasthenic crisis, which may be life threatening. It appears to work by binding to the receptor antibodies or to the leukocytes that destroy the receptors. There are fewer side effects with IVIG than with plasmapheresis.

Short-term treatments do not completely relieve the symptoms of MG and sometimes make them worse. Approximately 20 percent of MG clients go into a spontaneous remission lasting 1 year or longer.

Long-term treatment strategies include thymectomy and immunosuppressive drugs. The mainstay of therapy in younger individuals is thymectomy. Removal of the thymus gland decreases symptoms; for some, symptoms disappears completely. Thymectomy reduces the dosage of immunosuppressive drugs needed to induce remission. Immunosuppressive drug therapy to induce remission includes azathioprine, cyclophosphamide, cyclosporine, and prednisone. How these drugs work to induce remission in MG is unclear and there are many side effects associated with their use.

Myasthenia gravis can result in disruptions in activities of daily living. Symptoms vary from person to person, and differences in symptoms can be quite severe. Some of the problems frequently encountered include impaired vision, distorted facial appearance, impaired mobility, impaired verbal communication, impaired swallowing, activity intolerance, and knowledge deficit. The following nursing interventions are specific to the client with MG.

Nursing Interventions for Clients with Myasthenia Gravis

Activity Intolerance

Teach the client to alternate activity (play and work) with rest periods. This enables continuation of activities. Exercise is recommended to prevent muscle atrophy. Teach the client to exercise at his or her own pace and never to the point of fatigue. Exercise should be nonstrenuous and low-output, such as stretching and walking in a climate-controlled environment. Encourage the client to eat regular and well-balanced meals. Encourage the client to get adequate sleep. Plenty of rest and a well-balanced diet may help reverse muscle weakness. Teach the client to exercise and perform strenuous activities only at peak drug times. Teach energy conservation strategies such as sitting rather than standing: for example, sitting to shave, brush teeth, comb hair, and so on.

Impaired Vision

Eye patching is recommended for diplopia. Teach the client to patch alternate eyes to avoid eye strain. Teach the client to rest the eyes by closing them for 15 to 30 minutes. Teach the client to use eye crutches to relieve droopy eyelids. Temporary eye crutches can be made with stretchy adhesive tape. Teach the client to use sunglasses or tinted glasses to protect the eyes from bright light. If reading is problematic, books on tape maybe a viable alternative.

Risk for Injury

Teach the client to avoid hot baths, showers, sunbathing, and hot tubs. Teach the client to avoid or decrease stress to reduce the risk of symptom exacerbation. Teach the client relaxation techniques. Encourage the client to join a myasthenia support group to share experiences and problems.

Knowledge Deficit: Medication Management

Teach the action, onset, duration, and side effects of medications used to treat myasthenia gravis. Instruct the client to keep a dose of medication at the bedside to take on waking. Teach the client to avoid over-the-counter medications (some drugs can aggravate myasthenia gravis). Teach clients that if weakness is experienced within 30 to 60 minutes of taking MG medications, call 911. Instruct the client to have extra doses of medications available at all times.

Impaired Swallowing

Teach the client to take MG drugs 30 minutes before meals. This improves the ability to chew and swallow. Teach the client to avoid hot foods as they weaken muscles.

Other client recommendations include wearing a medical alert bracelet, avoiding alcoholic beverages, avoiding cigarette smoke, avoiding exposure to infections, and avoiding exposure to aerosol pesticides. These factors aggravate symptoms of MG.

There is still much to be learned about the diagnosis and treatment of myasthenia gravis. The client with generalized myasthenia gravis can experience weakness of respiratory muscles leading to apnea and respiratory arrest. The client with a compromised respiratory system is said to be in a *myasthenic crisis.* This is a neurologic emergency requiring hospitalization in an intensive care unit. The clinical picture of an acute myasthenic crisis must be distinguished from other neuromuscular disorders such as Guillain-Barré syndrome.

Guillain-Barré Syndrome
Introduction

Guillain-Barré syndrome (GBS) is a rare autoimmune disorder of the peripheral nervous system resulting in generalized and symmetrical weakness involving the extremities and the trunk, loss of sensation, pain, and paralysis. The incidence of GBS is 1.7 in 100,000 per year (Hickey, 1992). It can affect anyone at any age. However, it is more common between the age of 30 to 50 years. Both sexes are equally affected. It is a leading cause of neuromuscular paralysis. Weakness develops rapidly. Approximately 30 percent of individuals with GBS require hospitalization in medical intensive care units. The mortality rate during the acute phase is 2 to 3 percent, and 75 percent recover completely within 6 months to 1 year after onset of symptoms (Bolton, 1995).

Etiology

The exact etiology of Guillain-Barré syndrome is unknown. Approximately 50 to 60 percent of individuals with GBS experience a sore throat, intestinal influenza, or stress syndrome 1–3 weeks before the unset of symptoms (Wiederholt, 1995). The most common viral infections associated with GBS are cytomegalovirus and Epstein-Barr virus. Other risk factors include recent immunization, recent surgery, Hodgkins disease, and lupus erythematosus. The first symptoms include tingling and numbness in the fingers and toes. This is followed by progressive weakness in the arms and legs. In mild cases of GBS the weakness does not progress beyond this point. These individuals have moderately impaired mobility necessitating the use of a walker, crutches, or cane. In other cases, the weakness continues to progress to complete paralysis of the arms and legs. In approximately 25 percent of cases, the paralysis progresses to the chest muscles, requiring mechanical ventilation. If the neck and facial muscles are involved, dysphagia occurs and a gastrostomy tube is needed.

Pathophysiology

GBS is an acute inflammatory demyelinating polyneuropathy probably triggered by an autoimmune response. Demyelination occurs in the cranial and spinal nerves. The demyelination process begins distally and ascends symmetrically (Hickey, 1992).

Diagnosis

Diagnosing GBS is difficult because the symptoms can easily be confused with other illnesses. Positive outcomes for GBS clients are dependent on early diagnosis and treatment. A diagnosis of GBS is based on clinical presentation. A thorough history reveals a recent viral infection with acute onset of symptoms. The flu symptoms are followed by rapid development of weakness and paralysis involving the proximal and distal limbs with an absence of muscle atrophy. Two tests, lumbar puncture and EMG, are used to confirm the diagnosis. The cerebrospinal fluid reveals an elevated total protein with a normal cell count. Electrophysiological testing indicates an absence or a slowing of motor and sensory nerve conduction (Wiederholt, 1995).

Routine Medical Management

The treatment of Guillain-Barré syndrome during the acute phase usually requires admission to the medical intensive care unit to monitor disease progression and to prevent complications. In many cases GBS resolves spontaneously. Several factors can assist in or hasten the recovery process. Medical treatment involves the use of steroids, plasmapheresis, respiratory support, and support therapy. Steroids are given in high doses for their anti-inflammatory properties.

Plasmapheresis is beneficial for clients with severe weakness due to GBS. It reduces the duration of the disease process if initiated within 2 weeks of symptom onset. Four to six treatments are usually needed to achieve maximum benefit. Plasmapheresis decreases the duration of muscle weakness, and thus ultimately reduces hospital length of stay and time spent on mechanical ventilation. There are many risks associated with therapeutic plasma exchange (TPE), therefore hospitalization is recommended. Its use should be reserved for situations in which maximum benefit can be expected. Similar results are now being obtained with immunoglobulin therapy.

Supportive therapy is the mainstay of treatment for individuals with GBS. The major focus is on excellent nursing and respiratory care to prevent the complication frequently associated with Guillain-Barré syndrome. Approximately 50 percent of clients with Guillain-Barré syndrome recover completely. Some individuals are left with residual deficits such a numbness or weakness. A small percentage are unable to return to their previous occupations. Following the acute phase of GBS, individuals with residual neurological deficits have many functional benefits to gain from participation in a comprehensive rehabilitation program.

Summary

The symptoms and responses associated with chronic neurological disorders vary from person to person. The following are possible nursing diagnoses for these individuals. Nursing care plans must be individualized and appropriate to client needs.

Common Nursing Diagnoses for Clients with Chronic Neurological Disorders

Activity Intolerance
Alteration in Comfort
Alteration in Nutrition
Alteration in Respiratory Function
Alteration in Skin Integrity
Altered Bowel Elimination: Constipation
Altered Family Processes
Altered Role Performance
Altered Sexual Functioning
Altered Urinary Elimination
Body Image Disturbance
Caregiver Role Strain
Disuse Syndrome
Fatigue
Fear
Grieving
Impaired Cognition
Impaired Physical Mobility
Impaired Sensation
Impaired Swallowing
Impaired Verbal Communication
Impaired Vision
Ineffective Airway Clearance
Ineffective Breathing Pattern
Ineffective Individual Coping
Ineffective Family Coping
Knowledge Deficit

Powerlessness
Risk for Injury
Risk for Social Isolation
Self-Care Deficit
Sleep Pattern Disturbance
Spiritual Distress

Discharge Planning   Most individuals with multiple sclerosis, parkinsonism, myasthenia gravis, and Guillain-Barré syndrome are capable of some level of independent functioning and remain in the community. Health care services are accessed during periods of exacerbation of neurological symptoms. At these times it is important that referrals to support groups and other community resources be initiated to ensure continuity of care.

References   American Academy of Neurology. (1994). An algorithm for managing Parkinson's disease. A supplement of the American Academy of Neurology—Part 2 (on-line). Available http://neuro-chief-e.mgh.harvar...onsweb/Main/Drugs/MainPark2.html.

Bemelmans, B. L. H., Hommes, O. R., van Kerrebroeck, P. E. V., Lemmens, W. A. J. G., Doesburg, W. H., & Debruyne, F. M. J. (1991). Evidence of early lower urinary tract dysfunction in clinically silent multiple sclerosis. *The Journal of Urology, 145,* 1219–1224.

Bernstein, K. (1995). The basics of drug therapy in Parkinson's disease (on-line). Available http://neuro-chief-e.mgh.harvar...sonsweb/ Main/Drugs/agonist.html.

Betts, C. D., D'Mellow, M. T., & Fowler, C. J. (1993). Urinary symptoms and the neurological features of bladder dysfunction in multiple sclerosis. *Journal of Neurology, Neurosurgery, and Psychiatry, 56,* 245–250.

Bolton, C. F. (1995). The changing concepts of Guillain-Barré syndrome. *The New England Journal of Medicine, 333*(21), 1415–1417.

Britell, C. W. (1995a). The multiple sclerosis problem list (on-line). Available http://colossus.infosci.org/MS-Internat/problist.html.

Britell, C. W. (1995b). Sexual dysfunction in MS (on-line). Available http://colossus.infosci.org/MS-Internat/sex.html.

Britell, C. W. (1996). Cognitive and perceptual problems in MS (on-line). Available http://weber.u.washington.edu/~britell/coginfo.html.

Compston, A. (1994). Future prospects of the management of multiple sclerosis. *Annals of Neurology, 36,* S146–S150.

Drachman, D. B. (1994). Medical progress: Myasthenia gravis. *New England Journal of Medicine, 330*(25), 1797–1810.

Fazzini, E. (1995). A comparison of neurosurgical procedures in the treatment of Parkinson's disease (on-line). Available http://neuro-chief-e.mgh.harvar...eb/Main/Surgery/APDANssp95.html.

Giang, D. W., Grow, V. M., Mooney, C., Mushlin, A., Goodman, A. D., Mattson, D. H., Schiffer, R. B., & the Rochester-Toronto Magnetic Resonance Study Group. (1994). Clinical diagnosis of multiple sclerosis: The impact of magnetic resonance imaging and ancillary testing. *Archives of Neurology, 51,* 61–66.

Hanak, M. (1992). *Rehabilitation nursing for the neurological patient* (pp. 197–210). New York: Springer.

Hickey, J. V. (1986). *The clinical practice of neurological and neurosurgical nursing* (2nd ed.). Philadelphia, PA: J.B. Lippincott.

Hickey, J. V. (1992). *The clinical practice of neurological and neurosurgical nursing* (3rd ed.). Philadelphia, PA: J.B. Lippincott.

Holland, N. (1994). Bladder management in multiple sclerosis (on-line). Available http://www.infosci.org/IFMSS/SEPT94/bladmgmt.html.

Irvives. (1997). Myasthenic crisis: Diagnosis and management (on-line). Available http://www.geocities.com/HotSprings/4357/myasthenis.html.

Johnson, C. W. (1994). Parkinson's disease (on-line). Available http://www.personal.engin.umich.edu/~jxm/parkinson.html.

Korejwo, R. L. (1994). Sexual dysfunction in MS (on-line). Available http://colossus.infosci.org/MS~Internat/sex.html.

Kshatri, A. (1996). Management of a patient with myasthenia gravis (on-line). Available http://www.anes.hmc.psu.edu/CaseCo...gust95caseFolder/August95Case.html.

Kujala, P., Portin, R., & Ruutiainen, J. (1994). Automatic and controlled information processing in multiple sclerosis. *Brain, 117,* 1115–1126.

Martin, N., Holt, N. B., and Hicks, D. (1981). *Comprehensive rehabilitation nursing.* New York: McGraw-Hill.

McDermott, M. P., Jankovic, J., Carter, J., Fahn, S., Gauthier, S., Goetz, C. G., Golbe, L. I., Koller, W., Lang, A. E., Olanow, C. W., Shoulson, I., Stern, M. B., Tanner, C. M., Weiner, W. J., & the Parkinson Study Group. (1995). Factors predictive of the need for levodopa therapy in early, untreated Parkinson's disease. *Archives of Neurology, 52,* 565–570.

McDonald, W. I., & Barnes, D. (1992). The ocular manifestations of multiple sclerosis: Abnormalities of the afferent visual system. *Journal of Neurology, Neurosurgery, and Psychiatry, 55,* 747–752.

Mitchell, G. (1993). Update on multiple sclerosis. *Contemporary Clinical Neurology, 77*(1), 231–249.

National Institute of Neurological Disorders and Stroke (NINDS). (1996). Parkinson's disease: Hope through research (on-line). Available http://www.nih.gov/ninds/healinfo/disorder/parkinso/pdhtr.htm#whogets.

National Institutes of Health (NIH). (1996). Multiple sclerosis-research highlights (on-line). Available http://www.nih.gov/ninds/healin....der/ms/mspecial.html#coordinated.

National Multiple Sclerosis Society. (1996). Multiple Sclerosis Information (on-line). Available http://www.nmss.org/Msinfo.

Panitch, H. S. (1994). Influence of infection on exacerbations of multiple sclerosis. *Annals of Neurology, 36,* S25–S28.

Rao, S. M., Leo, G. J., Ellington, L., Nauertz, T., Bernardin, L., & Unverzagt, G. (1991). Cognitive dysfunction in multiple sclerosis. II. Impact on employment and social functioning. *Neurology, 41,* 692–696.

Rudick, R. A. (1990). Helping patients live with multiple sclerosis. What primary care physicians can do. *Postgraduate Medicine, 88*(2), 197–207.

Schapiro, R. T. (1994). Symptom management in multiple sclerosis. *Annals of Neurology, 36,* S123–129.

Silverstein, P. M. (1996). Moderate Parkinson's disease. *Postgraduate Medicine, 99*(1), 52–68.

van Oosten, B. W., Truyen, L., Barkhof, F., & Polman, C. H. (1995). Multiple sclerosis therapy. *Drugs, 49*(2), 200–212.

Wiederholt, W. C. (1995). *Neurology for the nonneurologists* (3rd ed.). Philadelphia, PA: W.B. Saunders.

Wilson, L. (1995). Focus on . . . Parkinson's disease (on-line). Available http://pharminfo.com/pubs/msb/pd__focus.html.

Suggested Readings

American Academy of Neurology. (1994). Neuroprotective strategies for Parkinson's disease: MAO-B inhibition, vitamin E, and beyond (on-line). Available http://synapse.uah.ualberta.ca/aan/001u001a.html.

American Academy of Neurology. (1996a). Multiple sclerosis (MS) (on-line). Available Microsoft Internet Explorer.

American Academy of Neurology. (1996b). Practice parameters: Selection of patients with multiple sclerosis for treatment with Betaseron (on-line). Available Microsoft Internet Explorer.

American Parkinson Disease Association. (1994). Deprenyl—A 1994 update (on-line). Available http://neuro-chief-e.mgh.harvar.../Drugs/deprenyl.html#deprenylup.

Anouti, A., & Koller, W. C. (1995). Tremor disorders: Diagnosis and management. *Western Journal of Medicine, 162,* 510–513.

Bernstein, K. (1995a). The agonist & the ecstasy: A primer on PD (on-line). Available htt-://neuro-chief-e.mgh.harvar...sonsweb/Main/Drugs/agonist.html.

Bernstein, K. (1995b). Sleep and Parkinson's disease (on-line). Available http://neuro-chief-e.mgh.harvar...nsweb/Main/Coping/SleepPDU.html.

Bonander, A. (1995). Problem drugs in PD (on-line). Available http://neuro-chief-e.mgh.harvar...ons web/Main/Drugs/BadDrugs.html.

Breeze, R. E., Wells, T. H., & Freed, C. R. (1995). Implantation of fetal tissue for the management of Parkinson's disease: A technical note. *Neurosurgery, 36*(5), 1044–1048.

Britell, C. W. (1996). Exercise in multiple sclerosis (on-line). Available http://weber.u.washington.edu/~britell/exercise.html.

Caparros-Lefebvre, D., Pecheux, N., Petit, V., Duhamel, A., & Petit, H. (1995). Which factors predict cognitive decline in Parkinson's disease? *Journal of Neurology, Neurosurgery, and Psychiatry, 58,* 51–55.

Cullen, K. A. (1995). Sleep problems and Parkinson's disease (on-line). Available http://neuro-chief-e.mgh.harvar.../Main/Coping/Sleep1.html.

Cunnington, R., Iansek, R., Bradshaw, J. L,. & Phillips, J. G. (1995). Movement-related potentials in Parkinson's disease. Presence and predictability of temporal spatial cues. *Brain, 118,* 935–950.

Date, I., Asari, S., & Ohmoto, T. (1995). Two-year follow-up study of a patient with Parkinson's disease and severe motor fluctuations treated by co-grafts of adrenal medulla and peripheral nerve into bilateral caudate nuclei: Case report. *Neurosurgery, 37*(3), 515–519.

Decker, T. W., & Decker, B. B. (1994). Effects of multiple sclerosis on physical and psychosocial functioning. *Perceptual and Motor skills, 79,* 753–754.

Doble, S. E., Fisk, J. D., Fisher, A. G., Ritvo, P. G., & Murray, T. J. (1994). Functional competence of community-dwelling persons with multiple sclerosis using the assessment of motor and process skills. *Archives of Physical Medicine Rehabilitation, 75,* 843–851.

Durif, F., Vidailhet, M., Bonnet, A. M., Blin, J., & Agid, Y. (1995). Levodopa-induced dyskinesias are improved by fluoxetine. *Neurology, 45,* 1855–1858.

Duvoisin, R., & Sage, J. (1995). Parkinson's disease: A guide for patient and family (on-line). Available http://neuro-chief-e.mgh.harvar.../parkinsonsweb/Main/Chap14.html.

Feldman, R. G., Mosbach, P., Thomas, C., & Perry, L. M. (1995). Psychosocial factors in the treatment of Parkinson's disease: A contextual approach (on-line). Available http://neuro-chief-e.mgh.harvar...nsonsweb/Main/Psychosocial.html.

Fitzsimmons, B., & Bunting, L. K. (1996). Parkinson's disease: Quality of life issues (on-line). Available http://www.Cnsonline.org/www/archive/parkins/park-07.txt.

Freed, C. R. (1990). Transplantation of human fetal dopamine cells for Parkinson's disease—results at fifteen months. *Parkinson Report, XI*(III), 8.

Freeman, T. B., Olanow, C. W., Hauser, R. A., Nauert, M., Smith, D. A., Borlongan, C. V., Sanberg, P. R., Holt, D. A., Kordower, J. H., Vingerhoers, F. J. G., Snow, B. J., Calne, D., & Gauger, L. L. (1995). Bilateral fetal nigral transplantation into the postcommissural putamen in Parkinson's disease. *Annals of Neurology, 38,* 379–388.

Friedman, Y. (1996). Parkinson's disease: A teaching presentation (on-line). Available http://www.grfn.org/~morph/present/park2__1.html.

Gehlsen, G., Beekman, K., Assmann, N., Winant, D., Seidle, M., & Carter, A. (1986). Gait characteristics in multiple sclerosis: Progressive changes and effects of exercise parameters. *Archives of Physical Medicine Rehabilitation, 67,* 536–539.

Gilchrist, A. C., & Creed, F. H. (1994). Depression, cognitive impairment and social stress in multiple sclerosis. *Journal of Psychosomatic Research, 38*(3), 193–201.

Guillain-Barré Syndrome Support Group. (1997). The Guillain-Barré syndrome (GBS). A quick guide (on-line). Available http://Glaxocentre.merseyside.org/gbs.html.

Harden, D. G., & Grace, A. A. (1995). Activation of dopamine cell firing by repeated L-DOPA administration to dopamine-depleted rats: Its potential role in mediating the therapeutic response to L-DOPA treatment. *Journal of Neuroscience, 15*(9), 6157–6166.

Harris, J. (1996). Staging of Parkinson's disease (on-line). Available http://www.kumc.edu/instruction...dietetics/jharris/ldstages.html.

Honig, L. S., Wasserstein, P. H., & Adornato, B. T. (1991). Tonic spasms in multiple sclerosis. Anatomic basis and treatment. *Western Journal of Medicine, 154*(6), 723–725.

Howard, R. S., Wiles, C. M., Hirsch, N. P., Loh, L., Spencer, G. T., & Newsom-Davis, J. (1992). Respiratory involvement in multiple sclerosis. *Brain, 115,* 479–494.

Jacobs, D. M., Marder, K., Cote, L. J., Sano, M., Stern, Y., & Mayeux, R. (1995). Neuropsychological characteristics of preclinical dementia in Parkinson's disease. *Neurology, 45,* 1691–1696.

Jacobs, M. B., & Heller, S. J. (1994). A clinical review of Parkinson's disease. *Hospital Physician, 30*(3), 30–34.

Jankovic, J., Cardoso, F., Grossman, R. G., & Hamilton, W.J. (1995). Outcome after sterotactic thalamotomy for parkinsonian, essential, and other types of tremor. *Neurosurgery, 37*(4), 680–687.

Johnston, B. T., Li, Q., Castell, J. A., & Castell, D. O. (1995). Swallowing and esophageal function in Parkinson's disease. *American Journal of Gastroenterology, 90*(10), 1741–1746.

Keesey, J. C., & Sonshine, R. (1995). A practical guide to myasthenia gravis (on-line). Available http://www.med.unc.edu/mgf-prac.

Kidd, D., Thorpe, J. W., Kendall, B. E., Barker, G. J., Miller, D. H., McDonald, W. I., & Thompson, A. J. (1996). MRI dynamics of brain and spinal cord in progressive multiple sclerosis. *Journal of Neurology, Neurosurgery, and Psychiatry, 60,* 15–19.

Koller, W., Silver, D., & Lieberman, A. (1995). An algorithm for managing Parkinson's disease. A supplement of the American Academy of Neurology—Part 1 (on-Line). Available http://neurochief-e.mgh.harvar...onsweb/Main/Drugs/ManPark1.html

Kurtzke, J. F. (1994). Clinical definition for multiple sclerosis treatment trials. *Annals of Neurology, 36,* S73–S79.

Levin, B. E., & Weiner, W. J. (1990). Psychological aspects of Parkinson's disease. *Parkinson Report, XI*(III), 5–7.

Lieberman, A. (1993). New drug treatments on Parkinson's disease APDA Newsletter, Winter 1993–1994 (on-line). Available http://www.med.upenn.edu/~mednews/june94/7258__10.html.

Marder, K., Tang, M., Cote, L., Stern, Y., & Mayeux, R. (1995). The frequency and associated risk factors for dementia in patients with Parkinson's disease. *Archives of Neurology, 52,* 695–701.

McKhann, G. M. (1988). Plasmapheresis and Guillain-Barré syndrome: Analysis of prognostic factors and the effect of plasmapheresis. *Annals of Neurology, 23*(4), 347–353.

Menza, M. A., & Rosen, R. C. (1995). Sleep in Parkinson's disease. *Psychosomatics, 36*(3), 262–266.

National Institute of Neurological Disorders and Stroke. (1997). Guillain-Barré syndrome fact sheet (on-line). Available http://www.ninds.nih.gov/healinfo/disorder/guillain/guillain.html.

National Institutes of Health (NIH). (1994). Hope through research (on-line). Available http://neuro-chief-e.mgh.harvar...web/Main/IntroPD/NIHPub139.html.

Nirenberg, M. J., Vaughan, R. A., Uhl, G. R., Kuhar, M. J., & Pickel, V. M. (1995). The dopamine transporter is localized to dendritic and axonal plasma membranes of nigrostriatal dopaminergic neurons. *Journal of Neuroscience, 16*(2), 436–447.

Norris, S.A. (1994). Parkinson's disease—A summary (on-line). Available http://www.personal.engin.umich.edu/~jxm/parkguide.html.

Noseworthy, J. H. (1994). Clinical scoring methods for multiple sclerosis. *Annals of Neurology, 36,* S80–S85.

O'Connor, P., Detsky, A. S., Tansey, C., Kucharczyk, W., & the Rochester–Toronto MRI Study Group. (1994). Effect of diagnostic testing for multiple sclerosis on patient health perceptions. *Archives of Neurology, 51,* 46–51.

Offenbacher, H., Fazekas, F., Schmidt, R., Freidl, W., Flooh, E., Payer, F., & Lechner, H. (1993). Assessment of MRI criteria for a diagnosis of MS. *Neurology, 43,* 905–909.

Paty, D. W., Li, D. K. B., the UBC MS/MRI Study Group, & the IFNB Multiple Sclerosis Study Group. (1993). Interferon beta-1b is effective in relapsing-remitting multiple sclerosis. II. MRI analysis results of a multicenter, randomized, double-blind, placebo-controlled trial. *Neurology, 43,* 662–667.

Rao, S. M., Huber, S. J., & Bornstein, R. A. (1992). Emotional changes with multiple sclerosis and Parkinson's disease. *Journal of Consulting and Clinical Psychology, 60*(3), 369–378.

Research Society for Parkinson's Disease and Movement Disorders, Inc. (1996). Surgery for Parkinson's disease—Stereotactic cryosurgical pallidotomy/thalamotomy (on-line). Available http://www.caprica.com/~parkinsons/.

Sengstock, G. J., Olanow, C. W., Dunn, A. J., Barone, S., & Arendash, G. W. (1994). Progressive changes in striatal dopaminergic markers, nigral volume, and rotational behavior following iron infusion into the rat substantia nigra. *Experimental Neurology, 130,* 82–94.

Scheinberg, L. C. (1994). Managing individuals with multiple sclerosis: Therapeutic strategies. *Annals of Neurology, 36,* S122.

Schwab, R. S., & Doshay, L. J. (1996). The Parkinson patient at home (on-line). Available http://www.cnsonline.org/www/archive/parkins/park-02.txt.

Singaram, C., Ashraf, W., Gaumnitz, E. A., Torbey, C., sengupta, A., Pfeiffer, R., & Quigley, E. M. M. (1995). Dopaminergic defect of enteric nervous system in Parkinson's disease patients with chronic constipation. *Lancet, 346,* 861–864.

Singer, C. (1990). Sexual dysfunction in Parkinson's disease. *Parkinson Report, XI*(III), 3–5.

Spieker, S., Jentgens, C., Boose, A., & Dichgans, J. (1995). Reliability, specificity and sensitivity of long-term tremor recordings. *Electroencephalography and Clinical Neurophysiology, 97,* 326–331.

Swirsky-Sacchetti, T., Field, H. L., Mitchell, D. R., Seward, J., Lublin, F. D., Knobler, R. L., & Gonzalez, C. F. (1992). The sensitivity of the Mini-Mental State Exam in the white matter dementia of multiple sclerosis. *Journal of Clinical Psychology, 48*(6), 779–786.

Tartaglino, L. M., Friedman, D. P., Flanders, A. E., Lublin, F. D., Knobler, R. L., & Liem, M. (1995). Multiple sclerosis in the spinal cord: MR appearance and correlation with clinical parameters. *Radiology, 195,* 725–732.

Weiner, H. L., Mackin, G. A., Orav, E. J., Hafler, D. A., Dawson, D. M., LaPierre, Y., Herndon, R., Lehrich, J. R., Hauser, S. I., Turel, A., Fisher, M., Birnbaum, G., McArthur, J., Butler, R., Moore, M., Sigsbee, B., Safran, A., & the Northeast Cooperative Multiple Sclerosis Treatment

Group. (1993). Intermittent cyclophosphamide pulse therapy in progressive multiple sclerosis: Final report of the Northeast Cooperative Multiple Sclerosis Treatment Group. *Neurology, 43,* 910–918.

Weiner, W. J. (1990). Parkinson's disease and walking. *Parkinson Report, XI*(III), 1–3.

Weinshenker, B. G. (1994). Natural history of multiple sclerosis. *Annals of Neurology, 36,* S6–S11.

Whittaker, D. (1996). Life with myasthenia (on-line). Available http://pages.prodigy.com/lifewithmg/body.html.

Wolters, E. Ch., Tissingh, G., Bergmans, P. L. M., & Kuiper, M. A. (1993). Dopamine agonists in Parkinson's disease. *Neurology, 45,* S28–S34.

FUNCTIONAL LIVING SKILLS FOR SELF-CARE

CHAPTER 25
Self-Care Techniques

Susan Arakaki, Honor Duderstadt Galloway, and *Robin Johnson Zableckis*

Key Terms   *Adaptive Equipment*
Bathing Techniques
Doffing
Donning
Dressing
Hygiene and Grooming
Toileting

Objectives   1. Demonstrate an increased awareness of clients' problems with self-care.

2. Recognize the different methods and equipment used to teach self-care for different diagnoses.

3. Demonstrate the ability to support team self-care goals and specific training programs.

4. Be aware of the occupational therapist's role in self-care programs.

Introduction   Self-care tasks such as dressing, bathing, and toileting are such automatic parts of our daily lives that it is difficult to realize how complex these tasks can become in the presence of disability. When faced with disability simple tasks may suddenly become difficult if not impossible. A person may need to ask for help with tasks as basic as brushing teeth. As self-care tasks are very private activities, it can be difficult to ask for assistance. While someone is acutely ill, these tasks are frequently performed for them. As improvement is seen there is often a preference for more control and increased ability to perform these activities. The transition to become more independent is often gradual and learned through a systematized, efficient method to prevent the frustration often associated with trial and error, or possible failure. Initially, these tasks may take longer but as clients become more proficient, it will decrease the burden of care for the staff.

In rehabilitation settings, all clients are assessed by the occupational therapist when they have difficulty performing their daily occupations, which includes self-care. The occupational therapist's role is to assess and determine the extent of the client's self-care deficits and functional goals, and to establish a treatment plan along with the client's family to remediate these barriers. This will help determine the skills clients lack for completing self-care. After the initial assessment and training the occupational therapist can collaborate with nursing staff to foster carryover of newly learned tasks.

Nurses play a vital role by recognizing clients' self-care difficulties and initiating consultations with occupational therapy. Nurses also play an important role in helping clients learn how to direct others to assist them with completion of their self-care tasks. In some cases directing care may be only a temporary need, but for others this skill may result in helping clients prepare to supervise attendants that they will need after discharge. Nurses can help introduce clients to attendant management by educating and encouraging them to direct their own care.

Clients who have a recent onset of disability or limitations frequently are not at a point where they feel ready to begin daily self-care. Being faced with such basic tasks is often a painful reminder of how limited they now are. They may prefer to wait until they are better to begin caring for themselves. It may be difficult for these clients to recognize that by performing these activities they are slowly improving to the extent that their disability allows. Health care provider recognition that the initial goals of the client may differ from the goals of the rehabilitation team is important. For example, brushing their own teeth may not be of value to clients, but they may feel a strong need to feed themselves. In the process of learning to feed themselves, they are gaining the skills necessary to brush their teeth, which may increase in importance to the clients over time.

A wide variety of effective approaches to learning self-care skills exists. The diagnoses of arthritis, spinal cord injury, traumatic brain injury (TBI), and cerebrovascular accident (CVA) are indicative of the need for different approaches to self-care training. This chapter describes common approaches to self-care training for clients with these diagnoses. Precautions pertaining to these diagnoses will also be addressed. Many of these techniques can be applied to clients with other diagnoses, with modifications made for any significant differences in impairment. The occupational therapist will help identify the best approach.

Cerebrovascular Accident and Traumatic Brain Injury

Following a CVA clients may be limited in activities by a variety of secondary diagnoses, which include hypertension and cardiac issues. Blood pressure can be significantly increased at rest and increased further with any task performance. In addition, it is important to keep in mind that the amount of effort required for any upper extremity task can raise blood pressure to unsafe levels during self-care. Thus, it is essential to monitor the client's blood pressure before and after self-care tasks to determine whether or not it is safe to perform the tasks at that time.

In the same manner, cardiac problems such as tachycardia, bradycardia, or preventricular contractions (PVCs) may indicate a need to monitor levels of task performance. Electrocardiograph (EKG) monitoring during the performance of a new task such as self-care, transfers, or walking has been found effective. If an abnormal reading is noted, self-care tasks should be discontinued until evaluated and cleared by a physician.

Clients who have sustained a TBI may have associated fractures that might interfere with the ability to perform self-care tasks. For example, clients may require adaptive equipment to dress themselves when a knee is immobilized in extension, or may need to dress in bed if weight-bearing status is restricted. When clients require complex splinting or casting to protect a fractured extremity physician clearance is needed to initiate self-care training.

In addition to medical issues, clients who have sustained a significant CVA or TBI may present with *hemiplegia* (weakness of one side of the body), decreased sensation, decreased cognition, visual impairments, and visual perceptual impairments. These deficits, either singularly or in combination, can interfere with a client's ability to achieve independence in self-care and frequently necessitate an individualized training program designed by an occupational therapist. For example, clients who demonstrate cognitive or visual perceptual deficits may have a difficult time learning new methods or learning to use new equipment; thus, these clients may be issued adaptive equipment less frequently than clients with other disabilities. For training to be effective with the use of adaptive equipment or special methods for performing self-care, it is important that learning be reinforced outside the training session by all staff and family members. Clients with cognitive deficits may initially require frequent cueing from staff to perform self-care. Cueing is decreased as client cognitive levels improve.

Hygiene and Grooming

Hygiene and grooming include washing, brushing hair and teeth, shaving, and applying make-up.

Hemiplegia

Washing the Face and Hands. Washing the face is generally not a problem for clients who have hemiplegia. When washing their hands, clients may need assistance to access the sink with the affected arm but should always be encouraged to incorporate this side in the task.

Brushing Hair. Clients who have long hair or complicated hairstyles may have difficulty with this task unless the hair is altered to a more manageable style.

Brushing Teeth. To brush teeth, clients place the toothbrush with the bristles positioned upward on the edge of the sink. Clients then open the toothpaste, using thumb and forefinger to twist off the cap. Clients then apply toothpaste to the toothbrush and proceed to brush their teeth. Alternatively, clients with minimal grasp in the affected hand should be encouraged to hold the toothbrush in the affected hand to apply the toothpaste. For clients who have dentures special brushes with suction cups are available to allow a one-handed method for cleaning.

Shaving the Face. Clients should be encouraged to begin shaving, using an electric razor for safety. If clients use manual razors, they should be encouraged to apply the shaving cream to the affected hand, and then use the unaffected hand to apply the shaving cream to the face. Clients can then shave as usual with close supervision for the sake of safety.

Applying Make-Up. Make-up is applied as usual although clients may need problem-solving help in opening containers. This may require occupational therapy intervention to determine the easiest method.

Cognitive Impairment

Clients who have cognitive impairments may require close supervision, appropriate cueing, and a daily routine to achieve increased independence with hygiene and grooming tasks. They may be impulsive and lack judgement, thus making it unsafe to use a manual razor. Clients who display decreased initiation or distractibility may require cueing to begin and follow through with a task. For example, clients may have difficulty proceeding with a task while the television is on or when there are visitors in the room. These clients may not notice that the water has been left running when they are finished at the sink. Some clients may simply not recognize the need to perform daily hygiene and grooming tasks and require tactful reminders from staff or family. Some clients may tend to perseverate on a task, such as shaving one area of their faces or combing one portion of their hair, and require verbal or physical prompting to move on and complete the task. It is important that the whole team work together to develop and maintain a regular daily routine of self-care tasks with cognitively impaired clients.

Visual Perceptual Impairment

Impairments in vision or visual perception may take a variety of forms, all of which can interfere with hygiene and grooming tasks. Clients may present with decreased ability to recognize one side of the body or locate items on the affected side. Clients may need prompting to attend to the affected side while performing all hygiene and grooming tasks. They should perform these tasks at the sink or in a setting as appropriate as possible to increase their familiarity with the task. They may need prompting to be aware of items placed on the affected side. This does not mean that items should be placed only on the unaffected side. Clients will develop increased awareness of that side if frequently encouraged to attend to the neglected side. It is important that items such as the call light and drinking water be placed on the unaffected side, for the sake of client safety. Clients may have difficulty finding one object in a crowded drawer and may need to limit the number of objects placed in the drawer. Drawers may need to be kept uncluttered, with only a few regularly used items, or staff may need to help clients locate objects. These clients may also benefit from having a variety of different-colored utensils (such as a red hairbrush, a blue toothbrush, and a yellow razor).

Dressing Each client's approach to **dressing**—that is, the **donning** and **doffing** of clothes—must be individualized.

Hemiplegia

When initiating dressing with a client with hemiplegia, the safest method is to start with the client dressing in bed, especially when limited supervision is available. As the client becomes stronger, and staff become more familiar and comfortable with the client's mobility, the occupational therapist may recommend that the client progress to dressing in the wheelchair or at the edge of the bed. The occupational therapist will advise the team on the amount of assistance the client requires to complete the task safely. Staff should encourage the client to do as much as possible without help but to be prepared to assist with any step at which the client appears to be having difficulty or becoming frustrated. It will take the client longer to dress than expected and extended time is necessary during training. The occupational therapist will recommend individualized approaches, often based on the following principles.

Upper Body Dressing. To don a shirt, clients

1. Position the shirt with the front facing lap and the back facing upward.
2. Insert the hemiplegic arm into the correct sleeve (Figure 1).
3. Push the sleeve up above the elbow on the hemiplegic arm.
4. Insert the unaffected arm into the opposite sleeve.
5. Pull the shirt over the head (Figure 2).
6. Adjust the shirt in the back and front as needed.

Donning a brassiere is often a very difficult task for clients and may not be a goal, depending on their preferences; if they do choose to wear a brassiere, clients

1. Hook the brassiere.
2. Lay the brassiere on the lap with the cups facing downward and hooks upward.
3. Insert the hemiplegic arm through bottom of the brassiere and the correct strap.
4. Pull the brassiere up and over the affected shoulder.
5. Insert the unaffected arm through the bottom and the correct strap.
6. Pull the brassiere over the head.
7. Adjust the back and cups as needed.

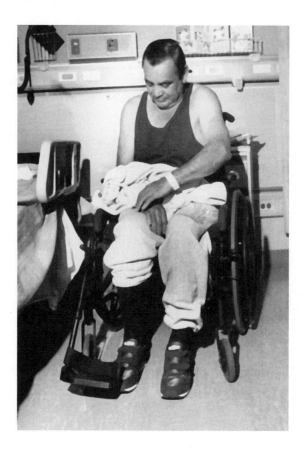

Fig 1. *Inserting the hemiplegic arm into a sleeve.*

Lower Body Dressing. To don pants in bed, clients

1. Position the pants with the front facing upward, waistband at thighs, and pant legs as close to their feet as possible.
2. Cross the hemiplegic leg until the foot can be inserted into the pant leg. (Clients may use the unaffected arm or leg to assist with bending the affected leg.)
3. Insert the hemiplegic leg into the pant leg (Figure 3).
4. Pull the pants toward their hips until the waistband is at the knee.
5. Insert the unaffected leg into opposite pant leg.
6. Pull the pants toward their hips as far as possible.
7. Bend their knees with feet flat on the bed, lift their hips to pull the pants over their hips (clients with one weak leg often need help stabilizing this leg to assist

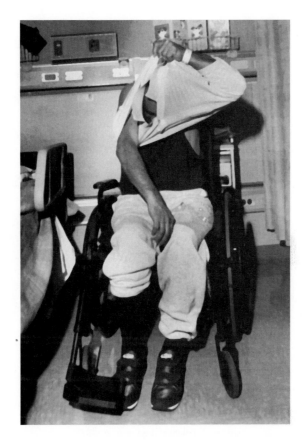

Fig 2. *Using the unaffected arm to pull the shirt over the head.*

with bridging their hips) (see Figure 4, p. 485). *Note:* Some clients cannot bridge their hips owing to weakness, pain, or contractures. They should be taught to roll from side to side to pull their pants up.

To don pants while in a wheelchair, clients

1. Cross the affected leg over the unaffected leg.
2. Insert the affected leg into the pant leg (Figure 5, p. 486).
3. Pull the pant leg until the foot is exposed and the waistband is at the knees.
4. Insert the unaffected leg into the appropriate pant leg and pull over the foot.
5. Pull the pants as high as possible while remaining seated in the wheelchair by shifting body weight from side to side.

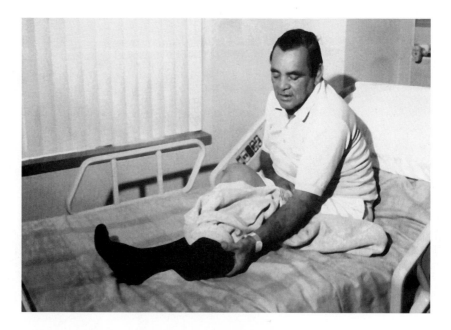

Fig 3. *Crossing the hemiplegic leg over the unaffected leg and inserting the foot into the pant leg.*

6. Stand to pull their pants over their hips (clients may need assistance to stand and should be encouraged to use the unaffected hand to manage clothing while staff assists with balance (Figure 6, p. 487).

The following method of donning socks can be used in bed or at the wheelchair level. This method can also be used for donning pressure hose, although clients often need additional assistance, depending on the tightness. To don socks, clients

1. Cross the affected leg over the unaffected leg. (In bed, clients may need to bend the unaffected knee to hold the affected leg in place.)
2. Hook the elastic edge of the sock over their toes; or insert their fingertips inside the elastic edge, spreading their fingers to pull the sock over their toes.
3. Pull the sock up, using the unaffected hand.

The following method of donning shoes can be used in bed or at the wheelchair level. Velcro closures are recommended, as these are easier to manage than learning one-handed shoe tying and safer for ambulation than slip-on shoes. To don shoes, clients

1. Cross one leg over the other. (In bed, clients may need to bend the unaffected leg slightly to hold the affected leg in place.)

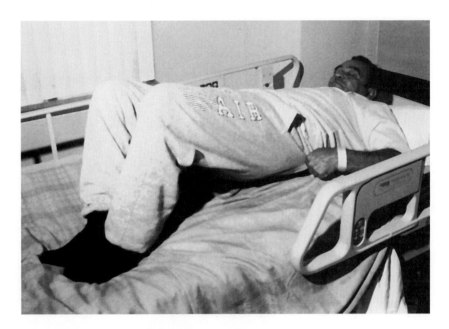

Fig 4. *Bridging hips to pull pants over hips.*

2. Loosen their shoelaces and place the shoe on the foot.
3. Place the foot on the floor and adjust the shoe to assure that it is on completely. (Owing to lower extremity weakness clients may need to use the unaffected arm to push the hemiplegic leg into the shoe.)
4. May be unable to tie their shoes unless taught a one-handed method by the occupational therapist.

Donning an ankle-foot orthosis (AFO) is more easily done with clients seated in a chair, wheelchair, or on the edge of a bed. A variety of AFOs may be issued to clients. Clients should be encouraged from the start to participate in donning the AFO. The client's ability to don the AFO independently will be greatly influenced by the amount of muscle tone present in the hemiplegic leg. This may not be a realistic goal for all clients.

> *If the AFO inserts into the shoe.* Clients should begin with the AFO in the shoe. After the laces have been loosened as much as possible, clients should insert the foot into the shoe and slide the heel into the AFO. Initially this is often difficult, as the AFO can move within the shoe and become dislodged. Clients then fasten the shoe (either with ties or Velcro straps) and the AFO strap. This frequently requires patience and practice to achieve independence.

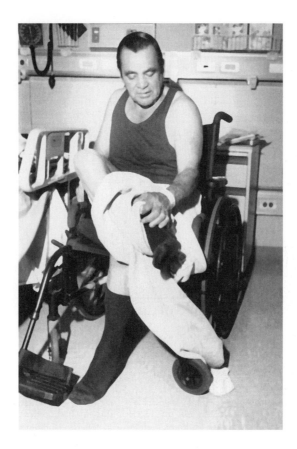

Fig 5. *Inserting the hemiplegic foot into the pant leg.*

If the AFO is attached to the shoe. The laces (or Velcro) should be loosened as much as possible. With the shoe resting on the floor clients can manipulate the foot into the shoe. Alternatively, clients can cross the affected leg over the unaffected leg and, holding the AFO by the leg strap, maneuver the shoe onto their foot. Clients can then place the foot on the floor and press into the heel (using either muscle strength in the leg, or the hand to push the knee), to position the heel into the shoe. Clients then secure the calf strap and fasten the shoes (i.e., tie or close the Velcro straps).

Cognitive Impairment

Clients who display cognitive deficits without physical limitations may not require a specialized dressing technique, as dressig is often a very automatic task. An assessment by an occupational therapist may be necessary when clients require

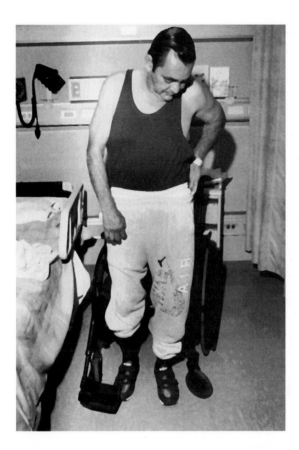

Fig 6. *Standing to pull pants over the hips.*

close supervision for safety, or display decreased initiation or decreased ability to organize tasks. Staff may note unsafe, impulsive movements in clients whose mobility is impaired, requiring close supervision and the use of bed rails when clients are left alone.

Clients who have hemiplegia along with cognitive deficits will need to learn the dressing techniques previously described. Cognitive deficits can greatly interfere with the ability of clients to learn new methods. Thus, these clients will often need more repetition and consistency to learn new techniques. Clients who are impulsive may need to be encouraged to slow down in order to process new techniques. They may need to have tasks broken down into simple steps. For example, clients may be trained to pull a shirt over the head after both sleeves have been placed on their arms by staff, or the training technique used may have staff place the affected arm into the sleeve and ask the client to pull the sleeve up over his or her elbow.

Visual Perceptual Impairment

Following a CVA or TBI, clients may experience alterations in their visual perception. For example, objects may seem closer or further away than they really are. Clients may have difficulty observing items placed on the affected side (more frequently on the left), or they may have difficulty distinguishing one object from another in a drawer, or finding a white sock on white sheets. Clients with perceptual deficits may have difficulty knowing if they are sitting upright or if they are leaning to one side. These factors may lead to the need for close supervision during the training process to increase independence in dressing.

To achieve effective learning these tasks may need to be broken down into steps that diminish the effects of the impairment. For example, an initial step may be to find the opening of the sleeve or pant leg with assistance from staff, before dressing. With the presence of visual deficits or unilateral neglect, items may need to be placed toward the unaffected side. White clothing may need to be placed on a colored backdrop to make it easier to find. Clients may need prompting to recognize that they are leaning to one side or the other and help to correct themselves.

Toileting

To achieve independence in **toileting,** clients often need an individualized assessment.

Hemiplegia

Clients with hemiplegia should begin using the toilet rather than a urinal, bedpan, or incontinence pad as soon as they begin to develop continence and can transfer onto the toilet safely. Clothing management at the toilet is safer and easier if closures such as buttons or zippers are unfastened while clients are seated in the wheelchair. Clients may need staff assistance to transfer onto the toilet. While clients stand to transfer onto the toilet, staff may need to help with stabilization for balance, while clients lower their clothing. It is important to keep in mind that clients will need the unaffected hand to manage clothing and thus the hand will not be available to hold onto grab bars for balance. Clients may need assistance to clean themselves following toileting if they present with impaired balance, poor body-handling skills, or decreased safety judgment. When possible, clients should close fasteners while seated, following the transfer to the wheelchair (although this is frequently more difficult than closing fasteners while standing). If closing fasteners while standing is necessary, owing to body type or the fit of the clothing, clients may need additional stabilization from staff while standing.

Cognitive Impairment

Clients with only cognitive impairment(s) are more likely to display issues related to decreased continence rather than toileting. Occasionally, clients who are at a fairly low cognitive level may not recognize the correct location for toileting and may require close supervision and prompting to use the toilet or urinal. If cognition is decreased in combination with limited motor skills, clients may display poor safety judgment and impulsivity, and attempt unsafe toilet transfers without notifying staff, thus risking falls.

Bathing Techniques

This section, on **bathing techniques,** focuses on full showers rather than bed baths. If clients receive bed baths, they should be encouraged to perform as much of the washing as possible with minimal assistance.

Hemiplegia

It is recommended that clients with hemiplegia initially bathe on a tub bench or bath chair rather than stand or sit on the bottom of the tub, as this allows for greater independence and safety. In addition, clients may achieve greater independence by using a hand-held shower hose to reach all parts of the body. Clients may need assistance with transfers and with bathing, according to occupational and physical therapy recommendations. Clients should be encouraged to wash as much of the body as possible without risking falls. The occupational therapist may issue a long-handled bath brush to allow clients easier access to their feet, back, and under the unaffected arm. Some clients find it easier to lay the bath brush or washcloth on one knee to apply soap, whereas others find it easier to apply the soap directly to the body.

Clients who are cleared by occupational or physical therapy to stand in order to wash their buttocks may need to use grab bars to gain balance before washing. Clients who are not safe when standing may need to be prompted to shift their weight from one side to the other in order to wash their buttocks. Clients who are unsafe with shifting their weight may need assistance with bathing.

To apply shampoo or conditioner, it is recommended that clients place the shampoo into the palm of the affected hand and apply the shampoo using the unaffected hand. Some clients prefer to apply the shampoo directly to the head. This method makes it difficult for clients to ascertain how much shampoo is being used and often results in too much or too little being applied. Clients can then use a hand-held shower hose to rinse their hair.

Cognitive Impairment

Impaired cognition may interfere with the ability of clients to recognize the degree of safety in a given situation, and could result in clients acting impulsively and risking falls. Thus, it is important to supervise clients with cognitive deficits while they are bathing. These clients may also lack the ability to attend to details and may neglect to wash thoroughly, thus requiring prompting to complete the process. Clients may lack insight into the need to bathe and may require tactful, sometimes direct, reminders. Lack of initiation or perseveration may require that clients be cued to continue to the next step in the task.

Visual Perceptual Impairment

Visual perceptual deficits such as unilateral neglect may require that staff prompt the client to wash the affected side as well as the unaffected side. Clients may display poor awareness of where the body is in space and may have a difficult time maintaining balance on a tub bench or bath chair. When necessary, the occupational or physical therapist may apply a chest strap to help increase client awareness of where the center of gravity is to assist with safety.

Spinal Cord Injury

Initially following a spinal cord injury, clients may be restricted from performing self-care tasks owing to spinal instability. Therefore, before beginning training, it is important to obtain orthopedic clearance from the physician.

This section describes special techniques and adaptive equipment used to perform self-care tasks by clients with *complete* spinal cord injuries. These guidelines assume that clients do not have interfering problems such as contractures, spasticity, pain, and pressure ulcers. They also presume that clients have sufficient strength, endurance, body-handling skills, and motivation to accomplish specific self-care tasks. Clients with incomplete injuries exhibit varying degrees of motor recovery; therefore, their functional goals are addressed individually.

Summarized in Table 1 are key muscles of the upper extremities, potential self-care goal(s), and commonly used adaptive equipment by levels of complete spinal cord injury. These potential goals of self-care are not always achieved or desirable to clients. The determination of equipment and self-care goals requires assessment by an occupational therapist who tests for presence of specific muscles, range of motion (ROM) limitations, abnormal muscle tone, sensory deficits, and other biopsychosocial areas that influence self-care goal setting.

At all levels of spinal cord injury, self-care tasks can be time consuming and physically demanding. For example, lower body dressing and bathing for the C6–7 tetraplegics can initially take 1 to 1.5 hours to complete. Clients may ultimately choose to direct their time and energy toward other activities and hire an attendant to assist with self-care. However, while participating in rehabilitation programs, clients are encouraged to engage in their self-care not only to gain independence, but also to improve their ROM, strength, and endurance.

Levels C1 Through C4

Clients with spinal injuries at levels C1–4 are dependent in self-care. Therefore, the goal of rehabilitation is to be able to give verbal instructions to their caregiv-

Table 1
Level of Spinal Cord Injury, Self-Care Goals, and Adaptive Equipment

Level of Injury	Key Muscles	Potential Self-Care Goals	Equipment
C4	Diaphragm Upper trapezius	Dependent with all self-care	Not applicable
C5	Deltoids Biceps	Dependent to assisted with hygiene and grooming	Hand orthosis Suction soap holder Universal cuff Wash mitt
		Dependent with remaining self-care	Not applicable
C6	Clavicular pectoralis Extensor carpi Radialis longus Serratus anterior	Independent with hygiene and grooming	Hand orthosis Universal cuff Built-up handle Phone holder Wash mitt Nail clippers
		Independent with upper body dressing. Assisted to independent with lower body dressing	Zipper pull Button hook Elastic shoelaces Push cuffs Dressing stick Dressing loops and straps Leg straps Long-handled shoe horn
		Assisted to independent with bathing	Chain loops Finger brushes Long-handled sponge
		Assisted to independent with toileting	Suppository inserter Digital stimulator Velcro leg bag straps Labia spreader
C7	Triceps	Similar to level C6	Similar to level C6
C8	Flexor digitorum profundus	Independent with all self-care tasks	Similar to level C6
T1-below	Thumb and finger intrinsics	Independent with all self-care tasks	None indicated

ers. This provides clients with an opportunity to gain control in managing their lives. Clients will have preferences for how tasks are to be approached and when they are to be completed. Thus, they must learn to communicate instructions effectively regarding their care to caregivers. This will ensure that tasks are completed in the most accustomed manner. Practice and feedback are essential for learning. Clients need to direct their self-care in hospital units with support and encouragement from nursing personnel. Nurses can enhance client learning by performing the tasks as directed and by providing verbal feedback about the clarity of the instructions.

Level C5   Clients with level C5 spinal injuries can perform simple hygiene and grooming tasks with adaptive equipment and assistance with set-up. They are generally dependent with the remaining self-care tasks.

Hygiene and Grooming
To wash the face, clients

1. Are assisted with donning a hand orthosis to stabilize the wrist.
2. Are assisted with placing a washcloth in their hands. A wash mitt with a Velcro strap is recommended.
3. Are assisted with turning the faucet on and off. Clients may be independent, contingent on the type and accessibility of the faucet handle.
4. Wet the wash mitt and blot excess water onto a dry towel.
5. Apply soap to the wash mitt by moving it across a bar of soap. Soap can be stabilized on a suction soap holder.
6. Wash the face. Head and neck movements may be necessary to reach the other side of the face.
7. Place the wash mitt under running water to rinse off the soap and blot excess water onto dry towel. Clients rinse the face with the wash mitt.
8. May be able to remove the wash mitt independently by using their teeth to loosen the Velcro strap.
9. Can use a second wash mitt to dry the face.

Clients at this level of injury are unable to cross midline. Therefore, it is important to keep the bar of soap, extra dry towel, and running water on the same side as the arm that is being used.

To brush teeth, clients

1. Are assisted with donning an orthosis to stabilize the wrist.
2. Are assisted with donning a universal cuff over the orthosis. If the orthosis has a built-in utensil holder, a universal cuff will not be required.
3. Are assisted with placing the toothbrush into the utensil holder or universal cuff (Figure 7).
4. Are assisted with applying toothpaste to the toothbrush.

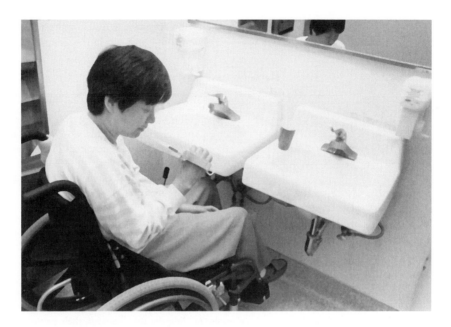

Fig 7. *Using a utensil cuff to hold a toothbrush.*

5. Brush one side of the mouth, then use their teeth to change the direction of the bristles. Clients proceed to brush the other side.
6. Rinse the mouth by sipping water through a straw and emptying the contents into a cup. Clients are assisted with setting up the cups.

To shave the face, clients

1. Are assisted with donning an orthosis to stabilize the wrist.
2. Are assisted with donning a universal cuff over the orthosis. If the orthosis has a built-in utensil holder, a universal cuff will not be required.
3. Are assisted with placing a razor into the utensil holder or universal cuff. If an electric razor is preferred, an adapted handle may enable clients to hold the razor. For client safety, it is recommended that they begin training with an electric razor.
4. Will need assistance with dispensing and placing shaving cream into their hands. Clients then apply the shaving cream to the face and shave. Head and neck movements may be necessary to reach the other side of the face.

Levels C6 and C7

Clients at the C6–7 level of spinal injury can achieve independence with hygiene and grooming and may eventually become independent with the remaining self-care tasks. However, in the initial months postinjury, they often require assistance with dressing, toileting, and bathing. Clients may need to use adaptive equipment if they do not have a functional tenodesis grasp. (*Definition:* With active wrist extension, fingers passively flex creating a grasping motion.)

Hygiene and Grooming

To wash the face, clients

1. Don and doff a wash mitt by using their teeth or the thumb of the opposite hand to loosen and tighten the Velcro strap. If a standard washcloth is preferred, clients can hold the washcloth using tenodesis or between their palms.
2. Turn the faucet on.
3. Wet the wash mitt and blot excess water onto a dry towel; or the other hand can be used to apply pressure.

Clients may be able to pick up a bar of soap using tenodesis. If this is difficult, soap can be stabilized on a suction soap holder or liquid soap dispensers can be used. Clients then proceed to wash the face.

To brush their teeth, clients

1. Remove the cap of the toothpaste tube, using tenodesis or their teeth. Rubber bands can be placed around the cap to provide friction. Clients squeeze out toothpaste by holding the tube between their palms. Toothpaste can be applied to the toothbrush or directly into the mouth. Use of toothpaste in tubes with flip-top caps or in pump dispensers may simplify this task.
2. Hold the toothbrush, using tenodesis or between their palms. Brushing their teeth requires adequate pressure, therefore some clients may prefer using a universal cuff or built-up handle to improve their grip.
3. Can hold a cup of water, using tenodesis or between their palms, to rinse the mouth.

To shave the face, clients

1. Apply shaving cream to the face. An adapted lever may be needed to apply the necessary pressure to dispense shaving cream.
2. Commence shaving. The razor can be held, using tenodesis or between the palms. As with brushing teeth, shaving also requires adequate pressure. Therefore, some clients may prefer using a universal cuff or built-up handle to improve their grip.

Shaving Legs and Underarms. Clients may choose to shave their legs in bed or in the bathroom if there is adequate room to prop their legs up on a toilet seat or on the edge of a tub. If a safety razor is used for shaving, the length of the handle may need modification. If the clients are having difficulty gripping the razor, built-up handles can be attached. Although electric razors are cumbersome, they are recommended over safety razors because when the client has impaired or absent sensation they offer extra protection when shaving legs and underarms. Clients should inspect their legs for cuts after shaving.

Brushing Hair. A hairbrush can be held using tenodesis. If the tenodesis grasp is inadequate, an adapted phone holder or built-up handle can be attached to improve the grip (Figure 8).

Applying Deodorant. Tenodesis can be used to hold a roll-on or stick deodorant. If the tenodesis grasp is inadequate, adapted handles can be attached with Velcro straps to the deodorant. If an aerosol can is preferred, an adapted lever arm can be attached to the nozzle of the can.

Applying Make-Up. Make-up can be applied with minimal equipment and adaptations if the tenodesis grasp is functional. A hand orthosis can be used to as-

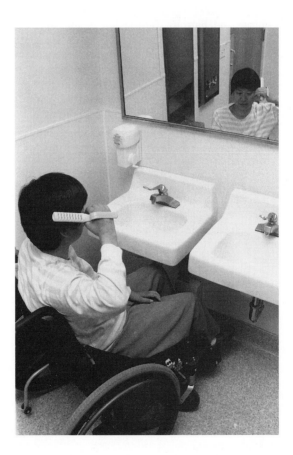

Fig 8. *Using a phone holder to hold a hairbrush.*

sist with the fine motor skills involved in the application of make-up. This is dependent on the needs of the clients and their personal preferences. Clasps on plastic compacts can be filed down, making them easier to open. In addition, Velcro finger loops can be fabricated and attached to the top of the compact. If tubes, applicators, and brushes are difficult to manipulate, Velcro can be applied to the surface to stabilize grasp or pinch. Custom-made containers to hold tubes upright allows easier access to make-up.

Nail Care. Nails can be trimmed with an adapted nail clipper. To file nails, an emery board can be laced through the fingers or taped to a table.

Dressing

The amount of effort needed for upper and lower body dressing can be reduced by choosing garments that are loose-fitting, with minimal numbers of zippers and buttons. Button hooks and zipper pulls can be used to facilitate fastening garments (Figure 9). Buttons and zippers can be converted into Velcro closures.

Upper Body Dressing. Upper body dressing can be completed in bed or in the wheelchair. It is recommended that clients begin in the wheelchair for trunk support.

Two common methods for donning a shirt are the *over-the-head* and the *around-the-back* methods.

To don a shirt over the head, clients

1. Position the shirt on their lap, front face down with the collar close to the knees. When donning an open-front shirt, fasten all but the top three buttons before positioning on the lap.
2. Insert their arms through the bottom of the shirt and into the sleeves one at a time. If a cuff gets caught around the hand, they can use their teeth or the friction of the hand against their lap to pull up the sleeve.
3. Raise their arms to don the shirt over the head and pull down the back of the shirt. A dressing stick may be helpful if clients are having difficulty reaching for the garment.

To don a shirt around the back, clients

1. Position the shirt on their lap, front face up with the collar close to the knees.
2. Insert one arm into the sleeve and pull the collar over the shoulder.
3. Push the shirt around the back.
4. Insert their other arm into the sleeve.
5. Fasten the closures, using tenodesis or adaptive equipment.

To don a brassiere, clients

1. Fasten the closure.
2. Position the fastened brassiere on the lap, cups face down.

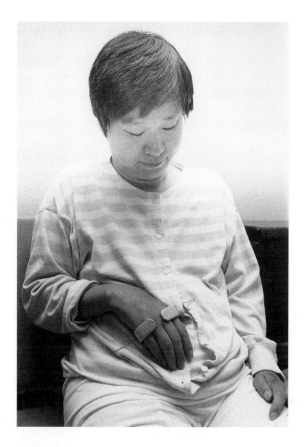

Fig 9. *Using a button hook to fasten a garment.*

3. Insert their arms through the bottom of the fastened brassiere and through the straps past the elbows.
4. Place the brassiere over their head and pull down.

Brassieres with either front or back closure can be converted into front Velcro closures with adapted thumb loops. They are fastened by placing the left thumb through the left loop and the right thumb through the right loop. The ends are pulled together simultaneously to overlap.

ABDOMINAL BINDER Abdominal binders are for clients who have decreased trunk innervation. The binders assist with respiration and blood pressure. Abdominal binders can be modified by attaching thumb loops to the Velcro straps. Binders can be donned in the supine or sitting position.

Lower Body Dressing. Lower body dressing demands greater exertion, body-handling skills, and endurance than upper body dressing. Throughout dressing training, it is important to be aware of the clients' lower extremity ROM. Hamstring ROM (hip flexion with knee fully extended) of 110 degrees is necessary, specifically when the client leans forward to dress in long sitting. (*Definition:* Sitting with hips flexed and knees extended.) Clients are at risk of overstretching their back extensors if hamstring ROM is limited. This can have serious implications for future sitting posture and trunk balance. Thus, when hamstring ROM is limited, clients need to position their legs in external rotation for dressing.

Training initially begins in a hospital bed with the head of the bed raised to support the trunk. As clients become skilled in maintaining trunk balance while unsupported, they will gradually progress to dressing on a flat bed.

A preliminary step to dressing training is for the clients to learn how to use their upper extremities to position their legs. If this is difficult, another way to manage their legs is to use a leg strap (Figure 10).

Methods for lower body dressing are broken down into three parts: pants over feet, pants over legs, and pants over hips.

Three common methods for donning pants over feet are as follows: legs crossed at ankles, legs crossed at knees, and hips and knees flexed.

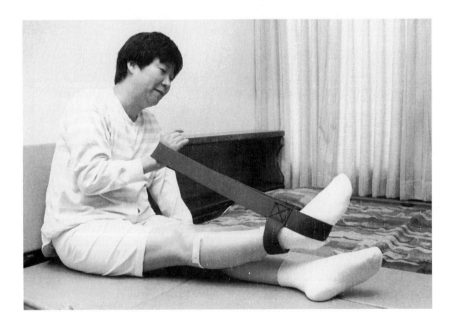

Fig 10. *Using a leg strap to position the leg for dressing.*

To don pants with legs crossed at the ankles, clients

1. Assume the long sitting position.
2. Position the pants distal to the foot opposite the leg to be maneuvered.
3. Lean forward and place a wrist under the ankle to lift the foot. *Note:* Heels often dig into the bed when clients lean forward in long sitting. This makes lifting the foot a difficult task. Therefore, clients may need to lean onto the elbow to un-weight the heel (Figure 11).
4. Place the foot over the opposite ankle.
5. Don the pant leg over the foot.
6. Repeat the process for the other leg.

To don pants with legs crossed at the knees, clients

1. Assume the long sitting position.
2. Position the pants distal to the knee opposite the leg to be maneuvered.
3. Place a wrist under the knee to bring it into flexion.
4. Place the other wrist under the ankle to life the foot.
5. Place the foot over the opposite knee (Figure 12, p. 500).
6. Don the pant leg over the foot.
7. Repeat the process for the other leg.

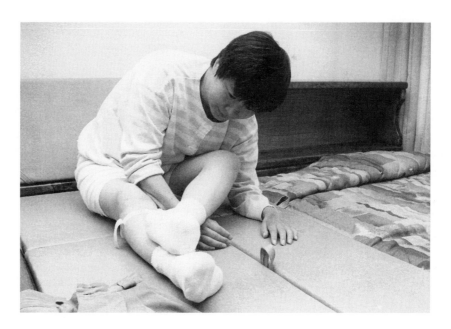

Fig 11. *Crossing the leg at the ankle.*

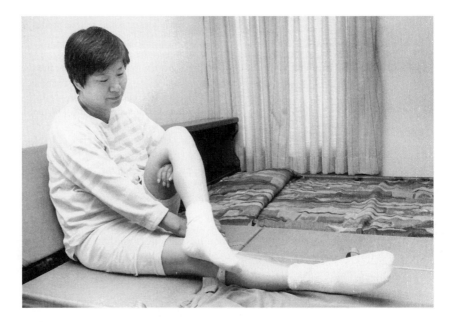

Fig 12. *Crossing the leg at the knee.*

To don pants with hips and knees flexed, clients

1. Assume the long sitting position.
2. Position the pants distal to the knee on the side of the leg to be maneuvered.
3. Place a wrist under the knee to bring it into flexion (Figure 13, p. 501).
4. Insert the foot into the pant leg.
5. Push down on the knee to slide the foot into the pant leg.
6. Repeat the process for the other leg.

To don pants over the legs, clients

1. Pull their pants up over their legs, using various hand placements such as hand-over-hand, double-hand-over, and holding the material between their palms. Clients can also use push cuffs or moisten their palms for friction (Figure 14, p. 502). When pulling pants up over the legs, it is important for clients to use head and shoulder movements to shift weight forward and backward. When the trunk is shifted backward, the legs become slightly unweighted. This makes it easier to pull pants up over the legs.
2. Place a forearm under the crotch of the pants to pull up the inseam (Figure 15, p. 503).
3. Pull the pants up toward the hips as far as possible.

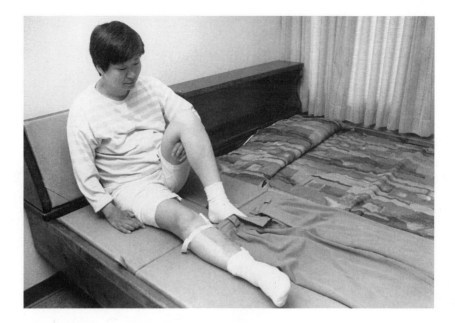

Fig 13. *Flexing the leg to insert into the pant leg.*

To don pants over the hips, clients

1. Assume a supine position.
2. Roll to a side-lying position. Initially, clients may need assistance with this task. The goal is for clients to achieve side lying independently, using the momentum of their head, neck, and arms without the use of the bed rails. If this is difficult, chain loops can be attached to the sides of the bed to assist the clients with rolling.
3. Place one hand inside the pants, starting from the front and moving toward the back.
4. Pull the pants up as much as possible.
5. Roll onto their back while maintaining placement of the hand. This helps keep the pants from sliding back down below the hips.
6. Continue rolling from one side to the other until the pants are over the hips.

If clients are having difficulty manipulating pants over the feet, legs, or hips, adapted dressing loops or straps can be used to assist further with donning pants.

To doff pants, clients

1. Assume a supine position.
2. Roll from side to side to remove the pants from the hips. Clients can also remove pants while sitting by shifting their weight from side to side.

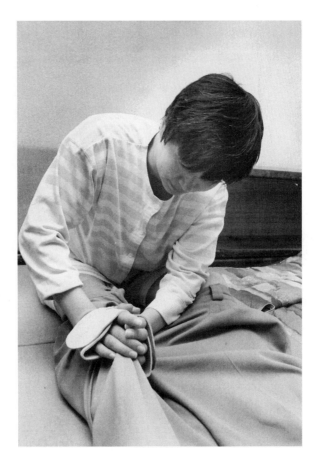

Fig 14. *Using push cuffs to pull pants up.*

3. Assume the long sitting position.
4. Place the palm of one hand on the crotch of the pants and push the pants down toward the feet.
5. Bring one knee into flexion and remove their foot from the pant leg. If clients have difficulty managing their legs, an adapted dressing stick may be helpful for removing pants.
6. Repeat the process for the other leg.

Toileting

An occupational therapist's primary responsibility is to determine if clients have the motor skills necessary for bowel and bladder management, and to provide them with adapted equipment and train them in its use.

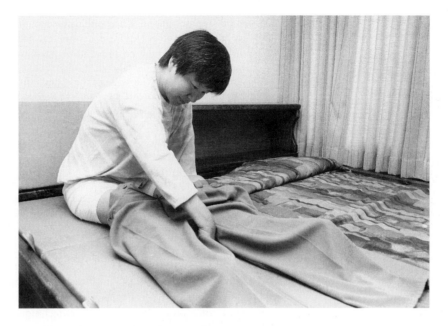

Fig 15. *Pulling up pants by placing a forearm in the crotch of the pants.*

Once proper equipment has been issued and training has been completed, the occupational therapist and nurse can work collaboratively on the clients' bowel and bladder training.

Client participation in bathing following discharge is dependent on having the appropriate equipment and an accessible environment. It is essential to be aware of the layout of the client's bathroom at home so that training can be set up to simulate their home environment.

To bathe, clients

1. Transfer onto a tub bench, using the upper extremities or using a transfer board. It is helpful to position the tub bench level with the wheelchair to facilitate the transfer. A towel or powder may be placed on the transfer board to reduce friction on bare skin.
2. Turn on the faucet. It is recommended to start with cold water and gradually add hot water. Clients should test the water temperature on a part of the body with normal sensation.
3. Wash hair using their fingers or the heels of their hands. If unable to attain adequate pressure, finger brushes are useful for scrubbing the scalp. Shampoo in squeeze bottles or dispensers that mount to the wall are recommended to reduce the chance of spillage.
4. Wash the face, arms, trunk, and buttocks with a standard washcloth or wash mitt. If clients have difficulty handling a bar of soap, liquid soap dispensers or a soap-

on-a-rope are options. When bathing, one arm is generally used to maintain balance while the other arm is free to wash the body. A chest strap and seat belt can be attached to the tub bench for stability and safety. No special methods are needed for washing the face, arms, and trunk.

5. Shift weight to one side and use the opposite hand to wash the buttocks. There are bath benches designed with a cut-out around the buttocks area. If this type of tub bench is used, clients can lean forward to reach the buttocks area.
6. Can use a long-handled sponge to wash the back. A phone holder can be attached to the handle of the sponge if their tenodesis grasp is inadequate.
7. Lean forward until the chest rests on the knees to wash their legs. Legs can also be crossed for washing.
8. Dry their hair, face, arms, legs, and trunk while on the tub bench. To dry the back and buttocks, towels can be placed on the wheelchair. If the towel is difficult to manage, loops can be sewn on both ends. Clients may prefer to wear a terry-cloth robe.

Level C8

Clients at the C8 level of spinal injury can perform self-care independently. They have approximately 50 percent of normal grip strength and may need adaptive equipment because they do not have full function of their hands. Trunk stability, however, is still compromised. Therefore, techniques and adaptive equipment for dressing, bathing, and toileting used by clients with C6 and C7 tetrapelgia are applicable.

Level T1 and Below

Clients at the T1 level of spinal injury (or below) can perform self-care independently. They have full function of upper extremities and generally do not need adaptive equipment. Trunk stability, however, is still compromised. Therefore, dressing and bathing techniques used by clients with C6 and C7 tetraplegia are also applicable to the paraplegic population.

In addition to dressing in bed, clients with paraplegia should also be trained to dress in the wheelchair, as there may be occasions when a bed is not available.

To dress in the wheelchair, clients

1. Cross the leg at the knee or ankle level.
2. Don pants, socks, and shoes over the foot.
3. Repeat the process for the other leg.
4. Pull the pants up toward the hips as high as possible. Clients may shift weight from side to side to help pull pants up over their hips.

Arthritis

Arthritis frequently occurs in middle age, and may occur simultaneously with other diseases secondary to or independent of the arthritis. A condition often accompanied by painful or swollen joints, the term *arthritis* literally means inflammation of the joint. There are more than 100 different rheumatic conditions or diseases, most with an inflammatory process in one or more joints. The two most common rheumatic diseases are rheumatoid arthritis (RA) and osteoarthritis (OA), also known as degenerative joint disease. The focus of this section is on RA and OA, and on the functional implications for clients impacted by these diseases. The interventions listed, however, are appropriate for most joint diseases. Before beginning a rehabilitation program, clients should be cleared by a physician, for there may be other concerns (such as cardiac or pulmonary disease, postoperative restrictions, myocardial infarctions, cancer, or peripheral nerve involvement).

Decreased endurance, joint limitations, pain, or weakness may interfere with the ability to perform basic hygiene and grooming tasks. Use of compensatory techniques or adaptive equipment may be critical to enable clients to continue to perform these personal tasks independently. In some cases a specific piece of adaptive equipment, or training the client in compensatory techniques, may be all that is needed. Other cases, however, may be extremely complex and require the skilled analysis of a multitude of factors. The occupational therapist can collaborate with the client to establish the importance of specific activities as well as the manner in which they are performed. Often, the methods by which tasks are completed may be as important to the client as the task results.

Joint Limitations

Joint limitations are frequently interfering factors in the functional abilities of clients with arthritis. For example, limitations in the shoulder joint may make it difficult for clients to reach the top of the head or feet. Clients may experience frustration when faced with this type of limitation in their daily routines. When limitations are present at the elbow clients may not be able to reach the face, axilla, or perineal areas for hygiene purposes. If joint limitation is present on one side only, clients may be able to use the opposite arm to compensate. If pronation or supination is affected, clients will have difficulty in rotating the palm down toward the tabletop to pick up small items, or in rotating the palm back up toward the ceiling when attempting to wash the face or axilla.

Distal joints of the hands and feet are often affected. There may be involvement of multiple small joints of the hands, affecting the ability to form a fist for grasping items. There may also be difficulty with managing sink/tub faucets, or with the fine motor skills required to open toiletry items (toothpaste, bottle caps, make-up compacts). For these limitations, adaptive equipment may make the difference between dependence and independence. Orthoses may be required when there is a limited ability to open the hand for functional and hygiene purposes. Clients may also require extended devices if ROM limitations are present in the hips or knees, limiting the ability to access the feet. The degree of ROM limitations, the presence of limitations at other joints, and the task-specific demands should be evaluated in order to grasp the entirety of functional limitations. A thorough assessment by an occupational therapist to determine specific techniques and equipment is crucial to achieve optimum function.

Pain
To perform self-care with joint limitations due to pain, compensatory techniques or adaptive equipment may be used. Clients may experience pain in single or multiple joints; the pain may be insidious or rapid in onset, and may be localized to a specific joint or present as generalized total body pain. Clients may complain of a constant dull, aching pain, or acute, debilitating pain that can limit or prevent function. Clients should be encouraged to be aware of and to respect pain. Acute, severe pain may be an indicator of increased disease activity or of worsening joint deformity and should be monitored closely. Its frequency and duration should be reported to the physician, as well to as the rehabilitation team. Nurses should communicate with the occupational and physical therapists if pain is limiting function. The interventions for pain are essentially the same as those for weakness and decreased ROM or endurance (see Tables 2 through 5 [and Figures 16 through 22, pp. 515–521] on self-care tasks for specific interventions). The increased effort required to work through pain in order to complete activities may leave clients exhausted and discouraged.

Clients need to understand that swollen or painful joints should be rested, and stress on the joints minimized. Along with medical management, pain can be relieved or reduced with lightweight adaptive equipment (see Tables 2 through 5 for solutions). It is also important to allow increased time for activities; clients may be unable to complete an entire task at one sitting. Activities should be paced with frequent rest breaks, and performed while sitting instead of standing whenever possible. Tasks may also be planned around the painful periods, or started after the morning medicines have begun to take effect. For some clients, a warm bath or shower in the morning can ease the general aches and pains, making morning tasks easier. Some clients perform part of their daily exercises while seated in a warm shower. Others wake up to take medicines one-half to 1 hour before getting out of bed. Staff should encourage clients to keep an activity log documenting the time and frequency when pain occurs, and of activities performed. A pattern of activity may emerge with subsequent periods of pain up to 1 or 2 days later. Pain that presents after a period in which the client felt good, and participated in more activity than usual, suggests overuse on the "good," or less painful, days. When this pattern (typical of RA) is noted, it is important to educate clients in energy conservation techniques, and the need to space their activities with frequent rest periods, or to spread them over several days. When hand pain is present, handles should be built up on items such as a toothbrush or comb to decrease the joint stress during grasping activities and to assist with reducing pain. The occupational therapist may issue orthoses to enable functional use, and to provide stability and pain relief.

Special Considerations for Rheumatoid Arthritis
Rheumatoid arthritis is a systemic disease that affects the entire body. Symptoms include joint and muscle pain, limited ROM, swelling (inflammation and synovitis), weakness, decreased endurance, morning stiffness, and fatigue. RA is typi-

Table 2
Hygiene and Grooming: Deficits and Solutions

Deficit	Hygiene and Grooming Problem	Solution
Limited shoulder flexion (0–45 degrees)	Managing hair (brush, comb, style and fasten) Washing face	May be able to use compensatory techniques, such as bringing head down to hands, or switch to other hand (if unaffected)
Limited shoulder flexion with (neck) limitations	Managing hair (brush, comb, fasten)	Same as above; also may use extended devices (brush or comb).
		May need devices with adjustable angle to effectively reach both sides and back of head. Hair dryer and mirrors can be attached to walls or counters on extended holders (see Figure 16)
		Wear hair in shorter, easy-to-manage style (if acceptable solution to client). If hair is kept long, may require assistance to style and manage fasteners other than simple headband
	Accessing face to: wash, brush teeth, place or remove dentures, apply make-up, shave	Extended sponges, washcloths, toothbrush, make-up applicators, and razors; may be able to use lightweight electric razor as it extends reach an inch or two
Limited ability to bend elbow	May be unable to access head, face, or axilla areas for hygiene, shaving, or applying deodorant	Extended sponge or cloth, razor, or depilatory creams/lotions; extended toothbrush, hairbrush, or comb; adjustable angle on handles is best
		May be able to use electric toothbrush, or switch to other side if unaffected (or less affected)
Decreased ability to rotate palm up to ceiling (supination)	Turning palm up to make contact with opposite side of face or head for applying make-up, shaving, or brushing hair	Angled hairbrush or comb; shorter length hair would be easier to manage
	May be unable to wash armpit	Compensatory techniques; may require adaptive device if limitation is severe
Difficulty rotating palm up and down (supination and pronation)	Manipulating toothbrush; flossing teeth	Compensatory techniques and/or adaptive device
	Picking up supplies from counter	Compensatory techniques
	Wringing out washcloth	May be able to press between palms, or against sink; may also use small sponge, which is lighter weight and can be managed with one hand
	Opening containers	If no young children around, and in absence of any other safety concerns, client may be able to leave lids loosened or off, or shop with easy access in mind when making selections of products

(Continued)

Table 2
Hygiene and Grooming: Deficits and Solutions (*Continued*)

Deficit	Hygiene and Grooming Problem	Solution
Limited hand closure or grasp	Washing face, oral care, brushing/ styling hair, and manipulating hair fasteners	Compensatory techniques, specific needs for adaptive devices need to be assessed individually with OT
	May have difficulty holding and squeezing out washcloth to wash face	May use lightweight sponge, or terrycloth wash mitt with Velcro strap around wrist (eliminates need to grasp cloth)
	May have difficulty manipulating objects in environment for:	
	Cleaning dentures	May use suction denture or fingernail brush; allows bimanual grasp of dentures
	Holding toothbrush, make-up brushes and pencils, razor	Built-up handles, adapted handles or devices, or Velcro straps; universal cuffs on items
	Holding soap	Use pump lotion soaps, soap-on-a-rope (can get expensive unless someone makes for client), or place soap in a nylon mesh bag and hang on a hook in shower or bath
	Opening containers (toothpaste, lotions, creams, bottles, etc.)	May use pump-style or flip-top toothpaste, toothpaste "key," pump lotions and creams; leave tops on bottles loosened. (*Caution:* This may not be safe if young children or cognitively impaired individuals have access to items)
	Managing finger- and toenails	Adaptive devices such as extended or suction-based clippers to allow use with gross grasp. (*Caution:* Need to be evaluated for safety with use, and not indicated for clients with diabetes or impaired circulation)
	Managing faucets	May use extended level faucets, or extended devices to turn faucets, or shower hose with easy on/off trigger if showering to avoid adjusting faucets during bath
Decreased ability to use thumb	Difficulty using pinch to grasp objects	Universal cuff or d-ring straps on items, small pliers, or jar opener may help to compensate for lack of closure; pump toothpaste, lotion, cream. *Note:* Clients need individual assessment to adequately assess unqiue needs when unable to grasp items
Pain	Pain when attempting to perform activities	Use joint protection techniques: Transfer stress to larger joints whenever possible, avoid positions of deformity or stressing joints by placing them in positions of deformity (example: pushing wheelchair forces fingers into ulnar deviation and

Table 2
Hygiene and Grooming: Deficits and Solutions (Continued)

Deficit	Hygiene and Grooming Problem	Solution
		should be avoided, especially for clients with RA); the OT will communicate with the nurse and client which activities may cause further deformity for individual clients
		Respect pain—it serves as a warning sign to decrease activities
		Learn to distinguish "good" pain from "bad" pain (acute inflammatory pain)
Upper extremity pain	Pain in shoulders, elbows, wrists, or hands when attempting activities	Built-up handles on toothbrush, brushes, razors, etc., may help to decrease stress on joints, which may decrease pain
	Pain at rest or with use	Orthosis may provide pain relief at hand, wrist, and elbow; may require different orthosis for night and day (to allow increased function during day)
	Pain with holding cane or walker (often issued when lower extremity pain is present)	Discuss alternative types of devices with therapist (canes and walkers can be fitted with forearm troughs to decrease stress on wrists and hands)
Lower extremity pain	Standing, ambulating; hip/knee flexion may be limited by pain	Sit whenever possible to perform hygiene and grooming tasks; physical therapist can help assess cause of pain
Decreased endurance	Unable to complete task	Use energy conservation techniques: Allow time needed to complete task. Pace activities by breaking down into several smaller tasks. Example: Assemble items (rest), wash face/hands (rest), apply make-up or shave (rest)
		Plan activities: space those with higher energy cost over the week; sit to complete activities whenever possible; keep high stool in bathroom to allow access to sink and mirror; keep supplies accessible to areas where they will be needed and used to eliminate extra trips
Weakness*	Lacks strength required to accomplish specific tasks, interferes with function or energy†	Report to OT, who will initiate strengthening and endurance program if medically cleared and appropriate for client†

* See preceding entries on decreased endurance; many functional problems are the same.
† See preceding entries on decreased endurance.
Abbreviations: OT, occupational therapist; RA, rheumatoid arthritis.

Table 3
Dressing: Deficits and Solutions

Deficit/Limitation	Dressing Problem	Solution(s)
Limited shoulder flexion	Difficulty reaching head and/or feet	May be able to use compensatory techniques or extended equipment
Limited shoulder flexion on one side only (0–45 degrees)	Donning and doffing pullover shirt	Can use hemidressing techniques, modified to individual needs*
Limited flexion of bilateral shoulders		Thread bilateral sleeves onto arms, push up over elbows, then thread head through neck hole (can also use dressing stick to gather back of shirt and push over head, if severe loss in ROM; refer to OT for full evaluation)
	Doffing upper body clothing	May be more difficult depending on type of clothing—consider loose clothing without fasteners (pullover shirt). Doff in reverse, gather back of shirt behind neck, remove head first, then arms. Or, pull arms out, then push up over head with hands or dressing stick
	Donning and doffing buttonfront shirt	Thread both arms through first, at waist level, use dressing stick to push up over shoulders, then button. If loose fitting, can button, then don over head like a pullover. To doff: Unbutton, then push over shoulders, then over arms (may need dressing stick) (see Figure 17)
	Back closures	Not recommended, but will be evaluated with therapist if important to client; may require assistance with this type clothing
Difficulty bending elbow (flexion)†	Managing fasteners on clothing; buttons, zippers, ties	Button hooks or zipper pulls, Velcro tabs to replace buttons, hooks, and snaps; may need equipment extended significantly (see Figure 18)
	Donning and fastening bras, pulling clothing up over shoulders (especially if both elbows are involved)	May be able to fasten with compensatory techniques, such as fastening at low waist, then slide straps up over shoulders with dressing stick; front hook bras (or fasten in front, then slide to back); may try sports bra, or camisole in lieu or bra if acceptable to client; use pullover blouses to avoid fasteners. Therapist can problem solve individually and share solution with client's nurse
	Pulling pants on; difficulty with closures, belts	Avoid closures by using elastic waist pants; or Velcro closures; may be able to use button hook, depending on amount of elbow limitation—see occupational therapist for individualized problem-solving

Table 3
Dressing: Deficits and Solutions (*Continued*)

Deficit/Limitation	Dressing Problem	Solution(s)
Difficulty straightening elbow (extension)	Accessing lower body to don pants, socks, shoes	Will require extended equipment such as sock cone, dressing stick, and reacher, and training in safe use of equipment
	Men's neckties	Consider placing on a hook that can be clipped on to a shirt (pretied); may also fasten with compensatory techniques onto equipment—can problem-solve individually with therapist
	Managing shoe fasteners	Can use Velcro loops, dressing stick, and reacher, slip-on type shoes, or shoes with elastic shoe laces; shoes should be sturdy and comfortable with sufficient room in toe box in presence of toe deformities
Decreased wrist ROM; may also have instability or pain	May interfere with strength or manipulation of clothing or fasteners—will vary greatly depending on the extent of the limitation	See therapist for individual assessment; may be able to use compensatory techniques or may require assistive devices or orthoses
Decreased hand function[‡]	Managing fasteners; buttons, grasping tools, items	Avoid fasteners whenever possible, with pullover shirts and blouses, elastic-waist pants; try Velcro tabs (in place of buttons or hooks); button hook; zipper pull; loops on clothing such as pants, underwear, etc., can be pulled up using larger forearm muscles instead of wrists and hands
		May precipitate change in dominance to complete tasks, or begin to complete bimanually or with built-up handles; button hook with zipper pull may be helpful
Decreased ROM at hips; or status post total hip arthroplasty (or other hip surgery or orthopedic condition that limits or restricts hip range)	Unable or restricted from specific hip movements, such as hip flexion. (*Note:* Specific restrictions will vary depending on surgery performed)	This is critical if client is required to maintain postoperative precautions, usually temporary (3 months on average); will require extended equipment such as reacher, dressing stick, sock cone, and extended bath sponge in order to complete lower body dressing independently (see Figures 19–22)
Limited knee ROM	Unable to reach feet to pull on pants, or don socks and shoes	If limitation is due to stiff knee, may be able to complete dressing with compensatory techniques; may require adaptive devices such as dressing stick and sock cone
Limited knee ROM and post total knee replacement	Post total knee replacement	Avoid use of any extended equipment as this is counterproductive and does *not* encourage knee flexion, which clients are working hard to achieve with physical therapy; however, there are occasionally

Table 3
Dressing: Deficits and Solutions (*Continued*)

Deficit/Limitation	Dressing Problem	Solution(s)
		specific instances where equipment may need to be issued in spite of knee replacement when other significant range limitations are present, or if client is to be discharged home alone and independence is critical
Pain	Limited ability to use available strength or motion	Compensatory techniques, adaptive equipment such as dressing stick, built-up handles, button hook/zipper pull, universal cuffs, lightweight items, elastic shoe laces, Velcro tabs, extended levers/knobs, joint protection techniques, energy conservation methods, and client education
Decreased endurance	Lacks sufficient endurance or stamina to complete dressing tasks	Energy conservation techniques§
Weakness	Lacks sufficient strength to complete dressing tasks; may be total body weakness or weakness at specific joints	Energy conservation techniques, compensatory techniques, strengthening program tailored for individual needs if appropriate and with physician approval; no resistive or repetitive strengthening if joint involvement present or if active disease present

* See text on dressing with CVA.

† *Note:* Client may need to be seen by an occupational therapist to initiate a splinting program to slow progression of deformity and further functional loss unless the joint is already ankylosed (spontaneously fused).

‡ Functional deficits may vary greatly, therefore requiring individualized assessment by an occupational therapist.

§ See text on decreased endurance in hygiene and grooming.

Abbreviations: ROM, range of motion; OT, occupational therapist.

cally characterized by periods of exacerbations, with hot, swollen, painful joints, and periods of remissions. Clients often refer to these periods as "bad days" and "good days," although a good day may be better only in comparison with a bad day. It is during the periods of exacerbation when most of the joint damage occurs. With each exacerbation the supporting structures are further weakened, causing damage to the joint. Further damage can occur when clients attempt to perform daily tasks that place stress on the weakened joints. After initial damage occurs the affected joints may become misaligned, with the result that mechanical forces become progressively more destructive and further limit function.

Table 4
Bathing: Deficits and Solutions

Deficit	Bathing Problem	Solution
Decreased mobility (upper and lower extremity)	Donning and doffing clothing, drying off	May try terrycloth robe (lightweight); can don/doff in bedroom sitting on bed*
Decreased ROM, strength, and/ or endurance of lower extremities	Reaching forward to faucets unsafe or difficult, may be restricted after hip replacement	Use shower hose (some have automatic on/off switches, decreasing the need to repeatedly manipulate faucets to adjust water; also increases safety during the task); use transfer bench or bath chair
Decreased upper extremity ROM	Difficulty reaching head, face, back, lower legs, or feet; buttocks or perineal areas	Extended equipment such as shampoo brush, bath sponge (with built-up handles as needed) or long string washcloth; seat with cut-out for easier perineal access
	Difficulty grasping washcloth, bottles, bar of soap	Use sponge, wash mitt, lightweight net ball or scrunchie in place of heavy wet washcloth; soap-on-a-rope, pump soap, bar of soap placed in cut-off length of stocking or net bag hung on a hook in place of grasping slippery bar of soap[†]
Fatigue, decreased endurance	Difficulty managing heavy towels	Don lightweight terrycloth robe or air dry (may get cold, or be impractical if not living alone); sit down to dry; use several smaller hand towels
	Unable to stand long enough to perform task; exhausted at end of bath	Use energy conservation and work simplification techniques[‡]

* See dressing solutions in Table 3.
[†] See also solutions for hygiene and grooming in Table 2.
[‡] See text on decreased endurance in hygiene and grooming.

The primary objective of the occupational therapist is to assess the areas of difficulty, provide and train clients in the use of orthoses, and issue adaptive equipment when appropriate. The occupational therapist will also educate clients in energy conservation, and train them in joint protection techniques, including alternative methods for self-care to minimize joint stress and pain. Frequently, clients may have end-stage disease that has "burned out," or is no longer active. These clients may not have pain, but may have severe deformities, unstable joints, or fixed contractures that significantly limit function.

Staff should educate clients on the disease process, and on the importance of medications in controlling symptoms and preventing or minimizing progression

Table 5
Toileting: Deficits and Solutions

Deficit	Toileting Problem	Solution(s)
Decreased ROM at shoulders, elbows, or wrists	May not be able to reach perineum for hygiene purposes	Compensatory techniques if range limitations are mild; if severe may require adaptive devices such as a toilet aid. The occupational therapist will help determine which type will be most appropriate and useful
Decreased hand function	May have difficulty adjusting clothing	*
	May have significant difficulty grasping and manipulating toilet paper	May need adaptive device; individual needs and deficits should be assessed by the occupational therapist, and communicated with the nurses
Decreased upper extremity and hand function	May be unable to access perineum for effective hygiene	If unable to use adaptive devices: Toilets are now available that automatically spray-clean and dry the perineum area (can be quite costly); there are also less expensive bidets and similar-type devices that may enable independence without use of hands
	May have difficulty adjusting clothing	Velcro clothing; may wear dresses (in home); may choose not to wear underclothing if in home alone, or if urinary urgency present*
Limited mobility due to weakness or joint limitations at hips and/or knee; or due to pain at hips and/or knees	May have significant difficulty sitting and standing from toilet; may be painful to sit down or stand up	Raised toilet seat and/or bars around toilet are helpful; should be seen by physical and occupational therapists to explore individual equipment needs. May also require devices to reduce the number of times required to transfer: female urinals, or a funnel-type device with tubing that allows females to urinate from seated or standing position; male urinals
Limited abduction	Unable to access perineum for hygiene	Individual needs should be explored; may need adaptive devices such as toilet aid, split toilet seat, or orthopedic evaluation if limitation is severe
Difficulty managing bowel or bladder appliances		If client has colostomy bag, or other special needs, the occupational therapist and nurse can collaborate to problem-solve ways in which client may be able to assume management of own devices

* See dressing solutions in Table 3.

of deformities. Well-informed clients can take a more active role in developing their own program, thus increasing their ability to care for themselves.

Special Considerations for Osteoarthritis

Osteoarthritis, also called degenerative joint disease, is a disease that may affect single or multiple joints of the hands, spine, knees, hips, or large toe metatarsal phalan-

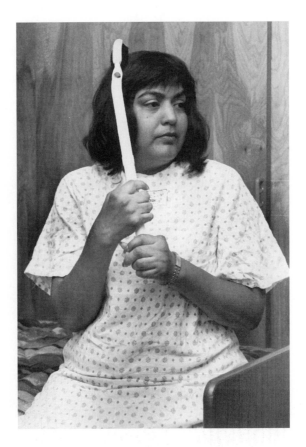

Fig 16. *Using an extended brush to brush hair.*

geal joints. Involvement may not be symmetrical (as is typical of RA). Symptoms typical of OA include joint pain (often affected by the weather), stiffness after static positioning of longer than 15 to 30 minutes, crepitation with movement, limited ROM, enlarged joints or deformities, and weakness from disuse atrophy. Hand deformities are usually due to a severe build-up of bony formation around the joints, which may limit the ability to make a fist or grasp items small in diameter; however, there may not be significant interference with client function. Clients most often seen in the rehabilitation setting are those with significant orthopedic needs involving mobility, such as hip or knee replacements.

Therapeutic interventions include devices such as orthoses to stabilize joints and improve function, training with adaptive equipment, and instruction in tech-

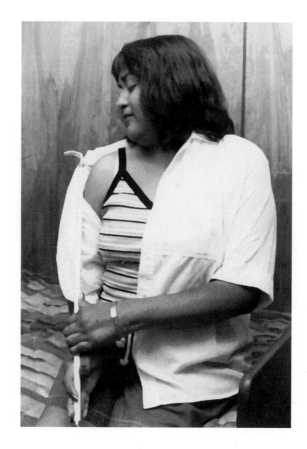

Fig 17. *Using a dressing stick to doff a shirt.*

niques to protect the joints. Therapists may also teach methods for decreasing stiffness, pain, and inflammation.

Problems and Solutions

For each self-care problem, related impairments (deficits) are listed in Tables 2 through 5, along with a range of solutions offered to accomplish the task. In addition, descriptions are provided of many pieces of **adaptive equipment** that may be beneficial to clients. Because there are many varied patterns of joint involvement, each case must be considered individually.

Whereas adaptive equipment may be critical in regaining or maintaining function for one client, it may be inappropriate for another. For this reason, therapists should collaborate with clients as early as possible. By working closely together, the therapist can identify the appropriate equipment for the client's unique functional needs (see Tables 2 through 5 for equipment commonly issued

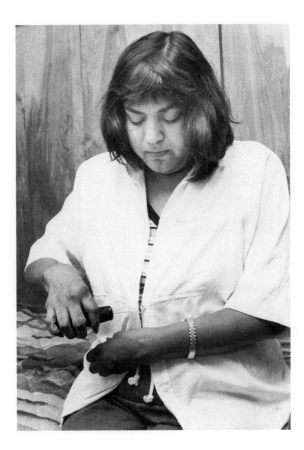

Fig 18. *Using an adapted button hook to fasten a garment.*

to clients with joint disease). The equipment helps compensate for losses in ROM, muscle strength, decreased endurance, joint stability, manual dexterity, or mobility, and assists with decreasing pain, improving functional capability, extending reach, maintaining and preserving joint integrity, and decreasing stress on joints.

Alternative methods such as compensatory techniques, joint protection, or energy conservation techniques may also be used (see Tables 2 through 5 for brief descriptions).

Environmental modifications may be required in addition to adaptive equipment in order to provide safe surroundings and to optimize functional access. In the rehabilitation setting, modifications may include rearranging the client's room to simulate his or her home environment, or suggesting modifications of the home environment. The therapists should perform a thorough clinical and

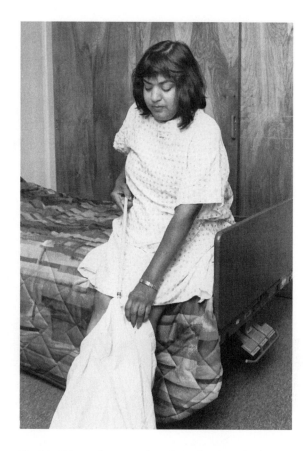

Fig 19. *Using a dressing stick to don a skirt over the feet.*

performance-based assessment, and discuss client interests and values before initiating a treatment plan. To optimize client participation and follow-through, clients must have an active role in planning their own programs.

Clients and their families should be actively involved in the rehabilitation program whenever possible, as a transitional step toward discharge from hospital care. This will provide practical experiences to all involved during the rehabilitation program, with the goal being to achieve and maintain maximum function.

Conclusion This chapter has described self-care techniques for clients who have experienced cerebral vascular accidents, traumatic brain injuries, spinal cord injuries, and arthritis. All clients are unique; therefore, these techniques may need to be varied according to individual needs. Following the occupational therapist's assessment,

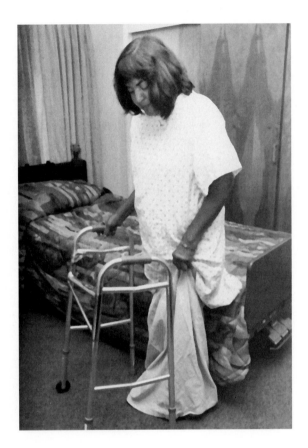

Fig 20. *Using a walker to stand and pull a skirt up over the hips.*

self-care goals and intervention programs are determined with the clients. As soon as clients are ready to function outside of the training program, they are expected to establish daily routines in rehabilitation units in order to promote greater independence on discharge. Because nurses see clients over a 24-hour period, they have multiple opportunities to observe and support performances of self-care tasks under varied conditions to establish a routine. When clients continue to have self-care performance difficulties after participation in a training program, nurse feedback to therapists is vital to make modifications needed to assure a successful rehabilitation outcome. It is beneficial to be familiar with common self-care techniques and equipment clients use, as this will facilitate carryover of self-care training programs. Clients who will not be independent in all phases of self-care will need to be able to direct others in their care. By providing opportu-

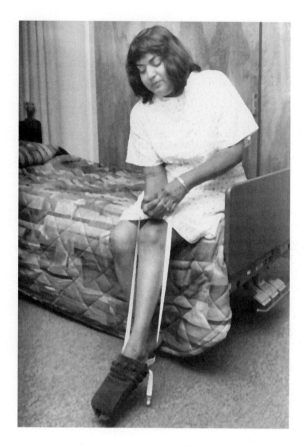

Fig 21. *Using a sock cone to don socks.*

nities for clients to direct staff in helping to complete self-care tasks, and by providing feedback, nurses can enhance the communication skills needed. Thus, clients who are not physically able to care for themselves can achieve greater control in their lives.

Nursing Diagnosis

- Self-care deficit: Hygiene and grooming related to musculoskeletal impairment; cognitive or perceptual impairment

Goals/Outcomes

- The client will perform hygiene and grooming activities at the optimal level of independence.

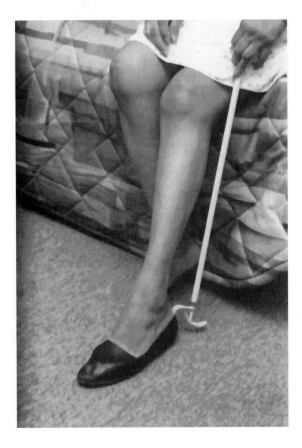

Fig 22. *Using a dressing stick to don slip-on shoes.*

- The client will demonstrate the ability to direct hygiene and grooming techniques correctly to the caregiver.
- The client will demonstrate the correct use of adaptive equipment for hygiene and grooming activities.

Nursing Interventions

- Instruct and assist the client as necessary with hygiene and grooming activities that are safe and appropriate.
- Reinforce the use of adaptive equipment and special techniques for hygiene and grooming.
- Provide ample time and an appropriate setting (at the sink versus in bed) for hygiene and grooming.
- Provide easy access to items necessary for hygiene and grooming.

- Encourage and assist the client with developing and managing a hygiene and grooming routine that is individually appropriate, consistent, and realistic.

Nursing Diagnosis

- Self-care deficit: Dressing related to musculoskeletal impairment; cognitive or perceptual impairment

Goals/Outcomes

- The client will perform dressing activities at the optimal level of independence.
- The client will demonstrate the ability to direct dressing techniques correctly to the caregiver.
- The client will demonstrate the correct use of adaptive equipment for dressing activities.

Nursing Interventions

- Instruct and assist the client as necessary with dressing activities that are safe and appropriate.
- Instruct the client on the use of adaptive equipment for dressing as necessary (such as a dressing stick and button hook).
- Instruct the client to dress the most limited side of the body first.
- Provide ample time and privacy (as appropriate) for the client to dress.
- Provide easy access to clothes.
- Encourage the client to wear loose, easy-to-manage clothing.

Nursing Diagnosis

- Self-care deficit: Toileting related to musculoskeletal impairment; cognitive or perceptual impairment

Goals/Outcomes

- The client will perform self-toileting activities at an optimal level of independence.
- The client will demonstrate safe toileting practices, including transferring.
- The client will demonstrate the ability to direct toileting techniques to caregivers correctly.

Nursing Interventions

- Instruct and assist the client as necessary with transferring, clothing management, and perineal hygiene.
- Instruct the client in safety issues such as safe lighting, and keeping hygiene items within easy reach.
- Provide privacy when safe, and ample time for elimination.
- Reinforce the use of special equipment, such as a raised toilet seat.
- Instruct and assist the client in developing and managing a toileting routine that is individually appropriate, consistent, and realistic.

Nursing Diagnosis
- Self-care deficit: Bathing related to musculoskeletal impairment; cognitive or perceptual impairment

Goals/Outcomes
- The client will perform bathing activities at an optimal level of independence.
- The client will demonstrate safe bathing practices.
- The client will demonstrate the ability to direct bathing techniques correctly to caregivers.

Nursing Interventions
- Instruct and assist the client as necessary with a bathing routine that is safe and appropriate for the client.
- Instruct the client in all safety issues involved with bathing such as water temperature, use of grab bars, wet floors, and transfer techniques.
- Instruct and assist the client with the use of appropriate adaptive equipment, such as a long-handled sponge brush and tub bench.
- Provide necessary equipment within safe reach.
- Maintain privacy during the bathing routine when safe.

Suggested Readings

Axtell, L. A., & Yasuda, L. Y. (1993). Assistive devices and home modifications in geriatric rehabilitation. *Geriatric Rehabilitation, 9,* 803–821.

Daniel, M. S., & Strickland, R. L. (1992). *Occupational therapy protocol management in adult physical dysfunction.* Gaithersburg, MD: Aspen.

Intagliata, S. (1986). *Spinal cord injury: A guide to functional outcomes in occupational therapy.* Rehabilitation Institute of Chicago procedure manual. Chicago: Rehabilitation Institute of Chicago.

Lehmkuhl, L. D., & Smith, L. K. (1983). *Clinical kinesiology.* (rev. ed.). Philadelphia: F.A. Davis.

Mann, W. C., Hurren, D., & Tomita, M. (1995). Assistive devices used by home-based elderly persons with arthritis. *The American Journal of Occupational Therapy, 49,* 810–820.

Melvin, J. L. (1989). *Rheumatic disease in the adult and child: Occupational therapy and rehabilitation* (3rd ed.). Philadelphia: F.A. Davis.

Noaker, J. A. (1996). Enhancing functional ability: Alternatives, techniques, assistive devices, and environmental modification. In: S. T. Wagner et al. (eds., pp. 89–93), *Clinical care in the rheumatic diseases.* Atlanta, GA: American College of Rheumatology.

Orr, P. M., & Bratton, G. N. (1992). The effect of an inpatient arthritis rehabilitation program on self-assessed functional ability. *Rehabilitation Nursing, 17,* 306–310.

Riggs, G. K., & Gall, E. P. (eds.). (1984). *Rheumatic diseases: Rehabilitation and management.* Stoneham, MA: Butterworths.

Shlotzhauer, T. L., & McGuire, J. L. (1993). *Living with rheumatoid arthritis.* Baltimore, MD: The Johns Hopkins University Press.

Trombly, C. (ed.). (1995). *Occupational therapy for physical dysfunction.* Baltimore, MD: Williams & Wilkins.

Wilson, D. J., McKenzie, M. W., Barber, L. M., & Watson, K. L. (1984). *Spinal cord injury: A treatment guide for occupational therapists.* Thorofare, NJ: Slack.

CHAPTER 26
Physical Management of the Neurologically Involved Client: Techniques for Bed Mobility and Transfers

Kathryn A. S. Kumagai

Key Terms
Bed Mobility
Bed Positioning
Modified Depression Transfer
Normal Movement
Pressure Release
Prone
Rolling
Scooting
Side-Lying
Sitting to Standing Transfer
Sliding Board Transfer
Standing Pivot Transfer
Supine
Supine to Sitting
Transfers
Wheelchair Positioning

Objectives

1. Identify components of normal movement for bed mobility, and transfers.

2. Describe the etiology, pathophysiology and clinical manifestation associated with stroke, amyotrophic lateral sclerosis, Guillain-Barré syndrome, multiple sclerosis, Parkinson's disease, traumatic brain injury, and traumatic spinal cord injury.

3. Describe the components of abnormal movement of the hemiplegic client.

4. Describe the appropriate bed mobility, bed positioning, and transfer techniques for the client with hemiplegia and spinal cord injury.

5. Describe the role of the nurse in assisting the neurologically involved client with bed positioning and transfer techniques.

Introduction
Restoring function and improving the quality of life for the neurologically involved client are the primary goals of the rehabilitation team. Members of the rehabilitation team, which includes the physician, nurse, physical therapist, occupational therapist, speech therapist, social worker, psychologist, and the client,

along with his or her family members, must all work together to create a therapeutic environment where essential functional skills can be acquired. Although each team member will focus on different aspects of the rehabilitation process, the team must have one comprehensive plan of care, with each team member reinforcing continually, throughout the day, the essential skills necessary for the client to return to an independent level of function. For example, a client states that his primary goal is to get on and off the toilet by himself because that will allow him to return to living alone. After carefully assessing this activity, the team decides that using a modified depression transfer is the safest and most effective way for this particular client to accomplish his goal. From that point on all team members must incorporate this skill or components of this skill into their therapy sessions when appropriate. If some team members follow the plan of care and others do not, the amount of time in which the client can practice this skill is drastically reduced. At the time of discharge, the client may not be familiar enough with the techniques for performing this activity to use them at home; this means that he cannot independently get himself on and off the toilet and therefore will not be able to return to living alone.

Now consider the same client, but for whom all members implement the plan of care. In addition to working on this skill in physical therapy and occupational therapy there are numerous opportunities to work on the same activity throughout the day: for example, every time the nurse assists the client in and out of bed or on and off the toilet, and every time the speech therapist and psychologist assist the client into a chair in their office during their sessions. At the end of the hospital stay, the client will have practiced the same skill throughout the day, every day, in a variety of different settings. Therefore, the client not only will be able to assist with his own care while he is in the hospital, but he will also have a much greater opportunity to master the skills needed to be as independent as possible at home and in the community once he is discharged.

Nurses spend more time with the client on a day-to-day basis than any other team member and, therefore, play a crucial role in the rehabilitation process. In this chapter, we look at strategies for bed positioning, bed mobility, and transfers that will not only assist the nursing staff in managing the client, but will emphasize the basic components of movement necessary for all functional activities.

Normal Movement

Restoring function means more than just teaching a client to perform an activity that he or she can no longer perform. How the client completes the activity must also be addressed. Even a nonmedical practitioner can recognize that the way a neurologically involved person moves differs from that of an uninvolved person performing the same activity. The neurologically involved person will look asymmetrical, will move much slower, and will not be able to alter the activity that he or she is performing to adjust to different settings or changes in the environ-

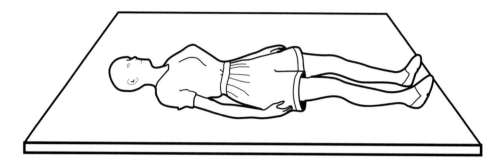

Fig 1. *Normal Movement: Supine to sit. Moving from a supine to a sitting position; starting position.*

ment. The client will also expend a greater amount of effort to accomplish the same activity. To truly restore function, the client must be able to move symmetrically, and efficiently, in a variety of different settings, transitioning easily from one activity to another. This will not be possible unless the movement patterns that the client uses allow for this. To identify the movement patterns that must be incorporated into each activity, it is best to review **normal movement.**

Let's look at the normal sequence of movement that a person goes through each morning when getting out of bed. Remember that even though the components of movement may be discussed separately, they all occur simultaneously to create one fluid motion from beginning to end. This person starts in a supine position and gets up on the right side of the bed (Figure 1). To move from a supine to a sitting position, the person turns the head to the side as it lifts off the pillow (Figure 2). The abdominals contract as

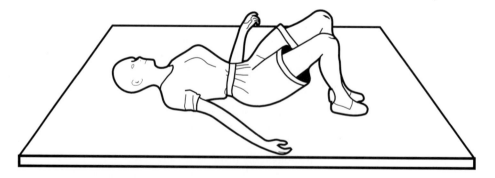

Fig 2. *The movement from supine to sit is started as the knees and hips flex and the head lifts slightly off the pillow.*

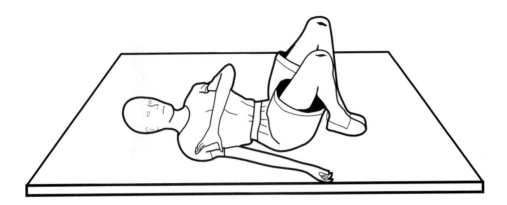

Fig 3. *The left scapula follows the head as it continues to lift off the pillow. The left upper extremity reaches across the body as the person starts to roll to the right.*

the trunk becomes dynamic and prepares for movement. The left scapula protracts and the left shoulder lifts off the bed as the person starts to roll to the right (Figure 3). At the same time legs will flex at the hips and knees and start to move forward off the edge of the bed (Figure 4). As the legs lower to the floor the trunk continues to lift off the bed until it has achieved an erect position and the feet are flat on the floor (Figures 5–7). Keep in mind that during this time the body is making fine postural adjustments and balancing at each point along the way to create one smooth motion.

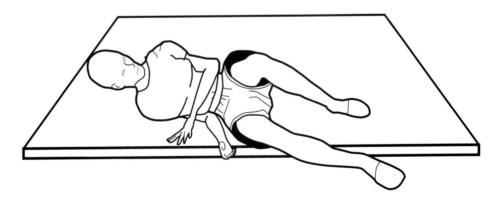

Fig 4. *The legs have already begun to reach for the floor before the person has rolled onto the right side.*

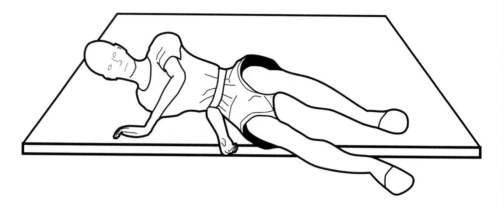

Fig 5. *The body lifts away from the surface as the legs continue to reach for the floor.*

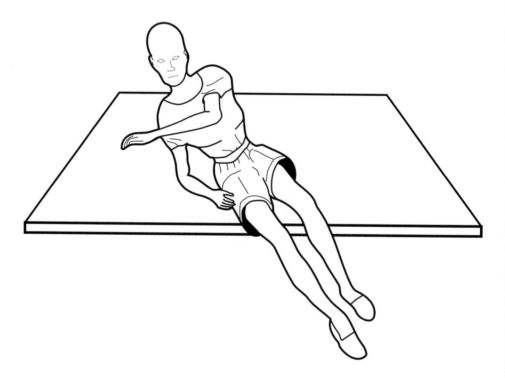

Fig 6. *The right arm assists the body to an erect position. Note the trunk remains dynamic throughout the entire motion, making fine postural adjustments as needed.*

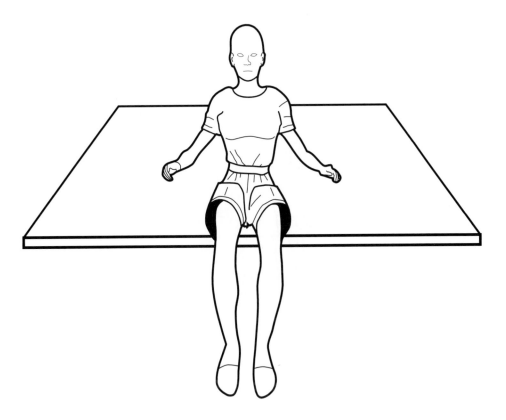

Fig 7. *Sitting erect.*

Once sitting up at the edge of the bed, a variety of different movement options becomes available (Figure 8). The person can reach over to pick up a robe at the bottom of the bed, lean forward to adjust a slipper (Figures 9 and 10), stand up to get dressed, or reach up to stretch (Figures 11–13). One activity is done just as easily as the other is. For any movement to occur, the body must be positioned where the trunk can become dynamic, creating a stable foundation for the extremities to move from. Both feet are flat on the floor and in line with the hip joints. To prepare for movement, the pelvis moves anteriorly to a neutral position, the hips flex, and the trunk becomes dynamic and moves into an erect position until the shoulders are over the hips.

To move into a bedside chair or to stand up, the person would have to scoot to the edge of the bed. Scooting is initiated by a lateral weight shift of the lower trunk. If the right side is going to be moved forward first, then the weight shift occurs to the left as the right side of the pelvis lifts. Simultaneously, the right

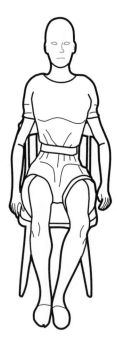

Fig 8. *Normal sitting position. Note that both feet are flat on the floor in line with the hips. Trunk and pelvis are in neutral position and prepared for movement.*

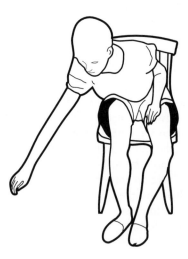

Fig 9. *The client is able to reach over with either hand easily without compromising balance.*

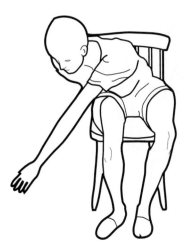

Fig 10. *The client is able to reach over with either hand without compromising balance.*

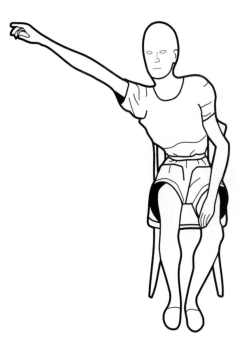

Fig 11. *The client is able to reach overhead easily with either upper extremity. The trunk remains dynamic in all positions.*

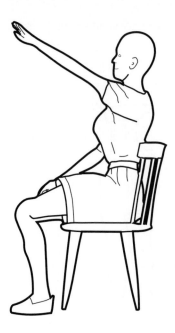

Fig 12. *Side view of overhead reaching. Note the feet are flat on the floor to create a stable base. The pelvis and trunk are in a neutral position, creating a stable foundation for the extremities to move on.*

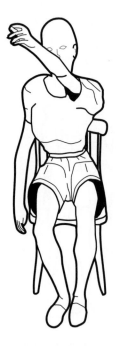

Fig 13. *Overhead reaching.*

side of the trunk shortens and the left side elongates while the head and shoulders stay level. The entire time, the trunk is dynamic and maintains an upright stable position with the weight centered on the left side of the pelvis. The right side can now be moved forward, advancing the body toward the edge of the bed. The pelvis lowers on the right side as the trunk dynamically returns to a neutral position to allow controlled reseating of the pelvis in a neutral position. The process is repeated on the left until the person is sitting with two-thirds of both femurs forward off the edge of the bed. The body is now positioned to move away from the surface.

To move from a sitting to a standing position, the feet must first slide backward until the forefeet are just under the knees (attempting to stand with both feet out in front of the body is very difficult) (Figure 14). Next, the trunk remains dynamic in an erect position as the hips flex forward, transferring the weight off the pelvis and onto the feet (Figures 15 and 16). As weight comes off of the ischial tuberosities, the lower extremities must become dynamic and accept more and more of the weight until all of the weight is centered over the feet (Fig-

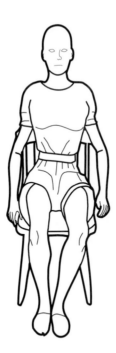

Fig 14. *Moving sit to stand. The pelvis and trunk are in a neutral position, and both feet are flat on the floor and slide back under the knees. They remain in line with the hips. The trunk remains dynamic as the lower extremities prepare to accept the weight.*

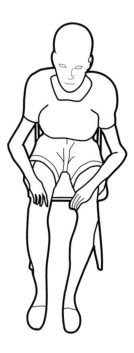

Fig 15. *The trunk remains erect as the hips flex forward, activating the legs. As the weight comes off the ischial tuberosities, it is transferred onto the dynamic lower extremities, lifting the pelvis off the seat.*

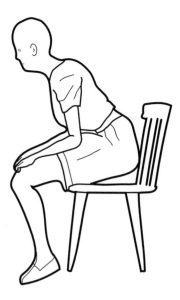

Fig 16. *Side view. Note the feet are behind the knees. The trunk remains erect as the hips flex forward.*

ure 17). At this point, the pelvis slowly lifts off of the bed. The person can now pivot over the feet into a bedside chair or gradually unfold the hips, knees, and trunk until the shoulders are directly over the hips in a fully upright standing position (Figure 18). Note that this occurs in one smooth motion that can be stopped anywhere along the way without total collapse of the body back onto the bed.

Conditions Creating Movement Dysfunction
Stroke

We now look at several conditions that can impair normal movement and the basic treatment strategies that can be used to optimize function. The first is a cerebro vascular accident (CVA), more commonly known as a *stroke*. There are two types of CVA: infarction or hemorrhagic. An infarction-type CVA is the most common and accounts for approximately 70 to 75 percent of all CVAs.

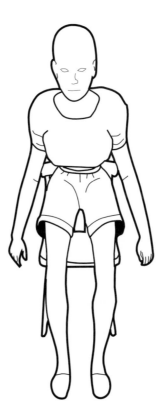

Fig 17. *As the body moves away from the surface, the trunk and legs slowly unfold, moving the person toward an erect standing position. Note the controlled movement that occurs throughout the entire motion.*

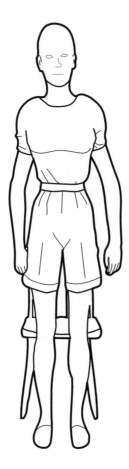

Fig 18. *Erect standing posture.*

There are also two types of infarction CVA: thrombotic and embolitic. A thrombotic infarction can occur when arteriosclerotic changes gradually narrow blood vessels, decreasing blood flow to the brain. This condition together with hypertension can further reduce blood flow, creating permanent or temporary ischemia. If the restriction of blood flow occurs gradually enough, the body may establish collateral circulation before complete occlusion of the blood vessel occurs. If blood flow is reduced rapidly, the result is usually loss of brain tissue supplied by those vessels. The second type of infarction CVA, and far more devastating than the thrombotic infarction, is the embolitic infarction. This condition occurs suddenly, when an embolus obstructs a blood vessel, and results in immediate loss of blood supply to that area of the brain. Because there is no time for collateral circulation to develop, the potential for preservation of brain tissue is much less than with a thrombotic infarction.

The second type of CVA is the hemorrhagic CVA, in which a leakage in a blood vessel occurs. The blood that would normally be carried to the brain is lost into the surrounding brain tissues. Not only is there potential damage from loss of blood to the area, but as the blood accumulates in the brain tissues it forms a mass that becomes a space-occupying lesion compressing the surrounding tissue, thus creating further damage.

Although the location and severity of the CVA will determine the resulting neurological deficits, the most common movement dysfunction associated with CVA is unilateral sensory, motor, and cognitive impairment on the side opposite to the lesion, called *hemiplegia*. A CVA is a devastating condition that essentially leaves the client with only half of the body functioning properly. Typically what is seen is decreased motor control, and flaccidity followed by hypertonicity, in which normal movement is unregulated and occurs in set patterns. Balance and coordination deficits are seen along with other problems, including visual-perceptual impairment and behavioral-intellectual deficits such as poor safety judgment, impulsivity, denial, lability, and irritability. Recovery time can be very lengthy and frustrating for the client. In most instances, the goal of rehabilitation is to re-integrate the involved trunk and extremities back into all functional activities. By doing this, the remaining function in the involved side will be used while facilitating new movement patterns, thus improving the quality of the client's movement with all functional activities. If left without any intervention, the client will compensate for the involved extremities with the uninvolved extremities, creating abnormal movement patterns.

Movement Dysfunction of the Hemiplegic Client

As a result of the hemiplegia, several alterations in a client's movement will be present. Let's look at the same sequence of movement as discussed earlier, that is, moving from a supine to a sitting position. For example, suppose that a male client has suffered a left CVA, which would result in right-sided hemiplegia. As the client is lying supine in bed, the normal pattern would be to lift the head and left shoulder as the client begins to sit up. In this hemiplegic client, because he has difficulty controlling his trunk and head, he performs the opposite pattern: extending his head and trunk and using his left lower extremity to push over onto the right. Once on his side he uses his left leg to kick his right leg off the mat, and uses his left arm to push himself up to a sitting position. Because his trunk is not dynamic, he is now slouched in a posterior pelvic tilt with a flexed trunk (Figures 19 and 20). The client is weight bearing asymmetrically, that is, on one side of the pelvis more than the other (Figures 21 and 22). Because his balance is impaired, no postural adjustments are made, and the client must use his left upper extremity to support his trunk. At this point, no options for move-

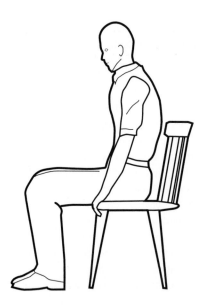

Fig 19. *Slumped sitting posture of the hemiplegic client. Note the posterior pelvic tilt and flexed posture of the trunk.*

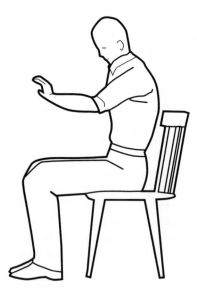

Fig 20. *Hemiplegic client attempting to reach up while maintaining a slumped posture. Note the severely compromised motion of the upper extremity if the trunk and pelvis do not move into a neutral position.*

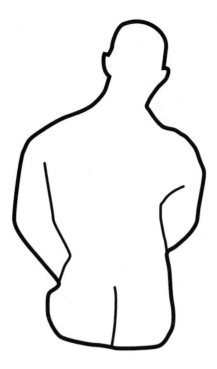

Fig 21. *Asymmetrical weight bearing in sitting.*

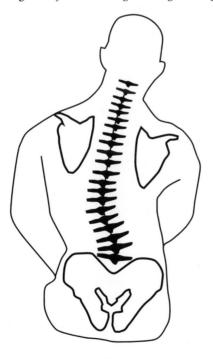

Fig 22.

ment are available. Potential for all upper extremity function is eliminated because his left arm is being used for support to remain upright.

If asked to move forward to the edge of the bed, the client will typically maintain the posterior pelvic position and flexed trunk and will slide his pelvis forward, keeping his weight posterior on the ischial tuberosities. His pelvis and scapula remain retracted, and his left arm will then be used to re-erect himself, pulling his upper trunk over his lower trunk. His trunk and right lower extremity do not become active and provide little support. As the client transitions from sitting to standing, all of the client's weight is still centered over the uninvolved lower extremity.

To maximize use of the involved extremities and to improve the quality of movement, it is critical to restore as many components of normal movement as possible, even if this requires breaking down the activity to allow the client to incorporate each component separately. It is obviously much quicker to do the movement for the client or to allow abnormal compensatory movements to occur, but it will be detrimental to the recovery process of the client if the extra time and effort are not taken to ensure that appropriate movement patterns are used. Even if the client cannot actively complete the entire motion, it is imperative that the nurse assist with the proper movements and allow the client to experience what normal movement is. Only then will the client be familiar enough with the patterns to begin to use them independently.

Treatment

The following treatment strategies are directed toward the adult hemiplegic client, but can be used for clients with various diagnoses including brain injury, multiple sclerosis, amyotrophic lateral sclerosis, Guillain-Barré syndrome, and Parkinson's disease. The approach used for clients with spinal cord injury differs slightly from the following techniques, and is discussed later in the chapter.

Bed Positioning

Our clients spend a considerable amount of time in bed, resting and sleeping. The time that a client spends in bed should be used to reinforce therapeutic procedures as well as to provide comfort, allowing the client to achieve a normal sleep schedule. The goals of **bed positioning** are to

1. Provide comfort at rest and while sleeping
2. Reinforce appropriate movement patterns
3. Prevent decubitus ulcers
4. Inhibit abnormal tone and abnormal movement patterns
5. Encourage awareness of the affected side

The environment that the client is placed in should also be therapeutic both in the hospital and at home. If possible, the objects and pictures in the room that the client would find simulating should be placed on the client's involved side to encourage the client to look toward the involved side. This is especially important if the client is suffering from a condition known as *neglect*, wherein awareness of the involved side of the body is decreased. It can be so severe that the client does not see objects on the involved side or recognize the involved extremities as a part of his or her own body. The family and caregivers should also address the client on the involved side, to further encourage awareness of the involved side. The positions reviewed in this section include

1. Supine
2. Side-lying on the involved side
3. Side-lying on the uninvolved side
4. Prone

Supine

In the **supine** position, the bed should be positioned flat unless the client is in danger of aspiration (see Chapter 18 on dysphagia). When swallowing problems or respiratory problems are present, the head of the bed should be elevated slightly. The areas that should be closely watched for excessive pressure that may lead to sores include the back of the head, the spinous processes of the spine, the spine of the scapula, the sacrum and gluteal area, the elbows, and especially the heels. Any area that is in direct contact with the bed (especially areas that are not visible) may be a potential site for skin breakdown, particularly if the client has impaired sensation. Any areas of tenderness, localized redness, and warmth should be noted immediately.

One pillow should be placed under the head. Some clients, who demonstrate an increased thoracic kyphosis with a forward head, may need one or two additional pillows to support the head comfortably. Often the client's head will be turned away from the involved side. A small towel roll should be placed behind the pillow or behind the uninvolved side of the client's head to gently reposition the head in a neutral position. If the towel is under the pillow it is less likely to fall out of place. Care should be taken not to use too much force to turn the client's head. It should be turned as far as is comfortable. The goal is to restore neutral alignment, not to overcorrect the problem.

The scapula on the involved side will likely be in a retracted position. The nurse should reach under the client's involved scapula and gently protract it forward into a neutral position. A small washcloth may be placed under the shoulder to support the shoulder complex, especially with clients who have forward shoulders (Figure 23).

The involved shoulder should be placed in a slightly abducted position away from the body with a pillow. Clients who demonstrate flaccid upper extremities are in danger of subluxating or dislocating the glenohumeral joint, because there is no muscular support to protect the shoulder. The clients with potential for

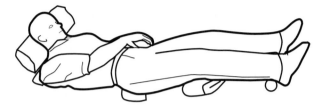

Fig 23. *Positioning supine. The scapula and pelvis must be protracted to a neutral position. A small towel roll can be placed under the scapula and pelvis to maintain the position. Be careful not to overconect. A small towel roll can be added along the lateral aspect of the thigh to prevent excessive external rotation of the femur. A small towel roll can be used to avoid heel contact with the bed. The lower extremities should remain extended. The towels should not cause the knee to bend.*

shoulder subluxation should be handled with great care. Other clients may present with hypertonic upper extremities, in which the involved upper extremity demonstrates increased resistance to passive movement. Active movement will often occur in a set pattern called a *synergy,* in which mass flexion, mass extension, or a combination of the two occurs. These clients are in danger of losing mobility in all joints of the upper extremity in the direction opposite of their synergy pattern. For example, if a client is able to move only in mass flexion, mobility into extension will be quickly lost if great efforts are not taken to stretch and position the extremity out of the flexed posture. The shoulder should be placed in as much external rotation as possible, but not past neutral. If the extremity is flaccid, great care should be taken to avoid excess rotation of the shoulder (Figure 24).

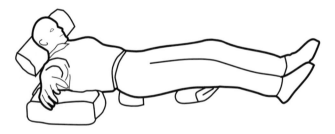

Fig 24. *Positioning supine. The upper extremity should be slightly abducted and placed comfortably on a pillow. If swelling is present in the hand, the extremity should be elevated slightly and placed in a neutral position.*

The elbow, wrist, and hand may be slightly elevated on a pillow if swelling is present. The elbow should be placed in as much extension as possible if a flexor synergy is present. If an extensor synergy is present, slight flexion should be maintained to keep the arm out of the synergy pattern. The wrist should be supported in a neutral position with a towel roll. Occasionally a splint or cone may be used to keep the fingers in a neutral alignment. If a device is used, it should be made of a hard material because soft materials such as washcloths may stimulate the palm of the hand, causing the client to clench the fist closed even harder. The skin of the hand and forearm that are in contact with the device must also be inspected at set intervals to check for high-pressure areas that may lead to sores if not relieved.

The trunk and pelvis should be placed in a neutral position. There should not be a curvature of the spine one way or the other. If it was necessary to elevate the head of the bed, a small, folded towel can be placed under the lumbar spine to keep the back in extension, because elevating the head of the bed has a tendency to make the client slouch. The pelvis will often be retracted on the involved side. The nurse should reach under the pelvis and gently guide it into a neutral position. A small towel roll should be placed under the pelvis to keep it from falling back into retraction. Remember not to overcorrect. If one side of the pelvis is visibly higher than the other, the towel roll may be too big (Figure 23).

Just as the upper extremities can demonstrate synergy patterns, the lower extremities may also move in mass flexion or mass extension. If increased extension is noted, a pillow should be placed under the knees and positioned in flexion out of the synergy pattern (Figure 25). The feet should be placed flat on the bed so that the entire plantar surface is in full contact with the bed to maintain weight bearing through the heels. If a flexor synergy is present or if the client is developing a knee flexion contracture, the lower extremity should be positioned in full extension flat on the bed. If the leg tends to roll outward a small towel roll may be placed under the outside of the thigh to reposition the thigh in neutral align-

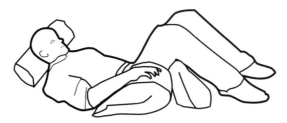

Fig 25. *Positioning supine with excessive lower extremity extensor tone. The scapula is protracted with the upper extremity supported in slight abduction. The trunk and pelvis are in neutral position, with the lower extremities flexed over a pillow.*

ment. Remember, if the towel roll is too big it may lift the thigh enough to flex the knee (Figure 24).

A small towel can be placed under the Achilles tendon to avoid excessive heel contact with the bed. A footboard should not be used to attempt to maintain dorsiflexion. If a footboard is used, the client will usually end up moving away from the board so that only the forefoot is in contact with the board. Stimulating this part of the foot will only encourage further plantar flexion of the ankle.

Side-Lying on the Involved Side

Side-lying a client on his or her involved side is very important for increasing awareness on that side and to begin early weight bearing. The bed should be in a flat position with the client lying on the hemiplegic side. Be sure to watch for potential skin breakdown at the side of the head and ear on the involved side, the spine of the scapula and shoulder, the iliac crest of the pelvis, the greater trochanter of the femur, the head of the fibula, and the lateral malleoli.

The head should be supported with one pillow. If the client has broad shoulders, additional pillows may be added until the neck is in neutral alignment. Be careful not to add so many pillows that the neck in bent away from the bed.

If it is uncomfortable for the client to lie directly on the involved shoulder, a pillow can be placed directly behind the trunk to allow the client to semirecline back onto the pillow. The caregiver should reach under the scapula and guide it into a protracted position. The shoulder should be abducted and externally rotated. If swelling is present in the wrist and hand or if an extensor synergy is present, then the hand and forearm should be elevated on a pillow. If full elbow extension is desired, the upper extremity should be positioned flat against the bed. The wrist should be supported with a towel roll in a neutral position. Necessary splints and hand devices may also be used in this position.

The trunk is usually in an elongated position with full weight bearing on the entire involved side. The semireclined position will also promote protraction in the pelvis; however, if the pelvis is still retracted the nurse may need to reach under the pelvis and pull it into further protraction to reach a neutral position. The client should not be allowed to roll forward because this will put excessive pressure on the shoulder, unweight the involved side, and promote retraction of the pelvis and scapula. The uninvolved upper extremity can be positioned comfortably over a pillow or wherever the client prefers.

The lower extremity should be placed in slight flexion at the hip and knee. Maintaining full extension of the lower extremity at the knee and hip can be difficult in this position. The uninvolved lower extremity can be flexed at the hip and knee to 90 degrees and adducted until it rests on the bed. This will also promote slight rotation of the trunk. If the client desires, the uninvolved leg can be placed on a pillow for comfort (Figure 26).

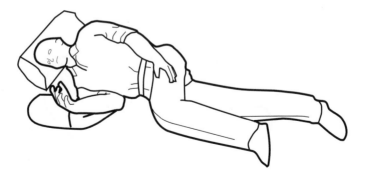

Fig 26. *Side-lying on the involved side. The client should lie on the involved side. If it is too painful for the client to be directly on the involved shoulder, a pillow should be placed lengthwise along the client's back. The client should recline back into the pillow to avoid full weight bearing on the painful shoulder. The involved upper extremity should be positioned comfortably on the bed, or on a pillow if swelling is present.*

Side-Lying on the Uninvolved Side

Positioning a client on the uninvolved side allows for full view of the extremities with impaired sensation, and therefore pressure sores are less likely to develop unless prolonged immobility on the uninvolved side leads to problems. The bed should be flat, with the client lying on the uninvolved side. The head should be supported with one pillow, with the neck in a neutral position. Again, if the client has broad shoulders, additional pillows may be added.

The scapula should be protracted with the upper extremity positioned in flexion and neutral rotation at the shoulder (Figure 27). The arm should be placed comfortably on a pillow to avoid positioning the arm in excessive adduction; however, if the pillow is too high, the upper extremity may be elevated to the point at which the scapula falls back into retraction. The wrist and hand should be supported in neutral with a towel roll. If swelling is not present early weight-bearing may be started by placing the palm of the hand in a weight-bearing position on the bed. Allow the fingers to flex comfortably; do not force the fingers flat against the bed.

The trunk and pelvis should be in a neutral position. A small towel roll may be placed under the uninvolved side of the trunk to prevent excessive shortening on the involved side of the trunk. The towel roll should fit just in between the iliac crest and the scapula. The pelvis should be protracted forward to a neutral position.

The involved lower extremity should be in slight flexion at the hip and knee, positioned on top of several pillows to avoid excessive adduction and internal ro-

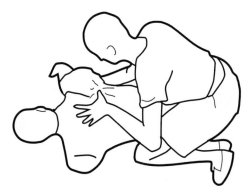

Fig 27. *Side-lying on the uninvolved side. The involved scapula should be protracted, with the shoulder placed in flexion and neutral rotation.*

tation. Avoid elevating the leg so high that the pelvis falls back into retraction. The ankle will tend to fall into inversion and should be supported in neutral with towel rolls. The uninvolved lower extremity can rest in extension flat against the bed (Figure 28).

Prone   The **prone** position is avoided if the client's respiratory status is compromised in any way, or if insufficient mobility in the extremities, trunk, or neck prevents the

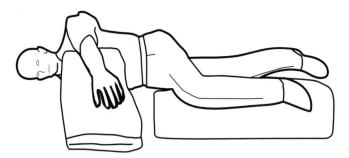

Fig 28. *Side-lying on the uninvolved side. The upper extremity should be supported on a pillow. An additional towel roll may be added under the wrist avoiding the palmar surface of the hand to maintain a neutral position. If excessive shortening on the involved side of the trunk occurs, a towel roll can be added under the trunk to maintain neutral alignment. The lower extremity should be supported in a neutral position on pillows. A towel roll may be needed to support the ankle.*

client from assuming the prone position. The majority of clients who present with hemiplegia as a result of a CVA are often elderly and are unable to tolerate this position for the preceding reasons. Other clients who do not have respiratory compromise and have adequate range of motion should be encouraged to lie prone. Lying prone will stretch the hip flexors, especially for those clients who sit in a wheelchair for the majority of the day, and it facilitates trunk extension and weight bearing through the upper extremities.

The client can be positioned with a pillow under the chest for comfort and to avoid excessive hyperextension of the neck. A small towel roll can be used to support the forehead, or the client can turn his or her head to the side. The upper extremities can be positioned either flexed above the head or resting comfortably down at the client's sides. A small towel roll should be placed under the ankles to avoid excessive plantar flexion of the ankles.

All bed positions should be used at least once in order to ensure that adequate pressure relief is provided for all areas of the body. This is critical in the prevention of pressure sores for the client who is too physically dependent to move on his or her own. A program should be established and posted above the bed with diagrams or pictures so all team members responsible for positioning the client will have access to the program. Each position should be used if possible, alternating every 2 hours throughout the night. The variety of positions will also provide different sensory experiences, and several components of the client's rehabilitation can be reinforced with each position.

Bed Mobility

Before attempting to move the client in bed, the nurse must remember several things to ensure personal safety. To avoid a serious back injury, strict body mechanics must be observed at all times.

1. The nurse should always elevate the bed to avoid stooping over to assist the client. Keep the person or object you are lifting close to you. Never reach across the bed to lift.
2. The nurse should always remember to keep the back straight and to tighten the abdominals before attempting to lift anything, including equipment.
3. All lifting must be done with the legs, not the back.
4. Remember that back braces may add additional support, but in no way substitute for your body's own internal support.
5. Regular exercise will keep the muscles of the abdomen strong and able to support the spine with most activities.
6. If you feel that you are unable to assist a client safely, get help from another rehabilitation team member.

When assisting a client with any functional activity, it is important to remember to allow the client to do as much of the activity as he or she can before assisting. This may take extra time, but the client will not improve if the nurse is always completing the activity for the client. Our role is to guide the client through the motion, providing externally what the client's nervous system is no longer able to do internally. The components of **bed mobility** reviewed in this section include

1. Moving in bed upward and laterally
2. Rolling to the involved side and uninvolved side
3. Moving from a supine to a sitting position, and vice versa

Moving in Bed

The head and foot of the bed should be lowered until the bed is flat, otherwise the client will be fighting to move uphill. The lower body will be moved first, then the upper body. Start by flexing the lower extremities up so that both feet can be positioned flat on the bed as close to the client's body as possible (Figure 29). Remember to allow the client to do as much as possible. The client may need assistance in initiating the movement, especially if an extensor synergy pattern is present, but will complete the motion once out of pattern. The nurse may need to hold the involved lower extremity in place by placing a hand over the dorsum of the client's foot. The client will then perform a bridge high enough to clear the buttocks from the bed. The nurse may need to assist the motion by giving a cue under the buttocks, over the gluteus maximus muscle of the involved side. At the same time, the client moves his or her buttocks up toward the shoulders. The nurse can also assist this motion by guiding the pelvis upward (Figure 30). Next, the upper body will be moved by asking the client to tuck the chin, lifting as much as possible of the neck and shoulders off the bed (Figure 31). If

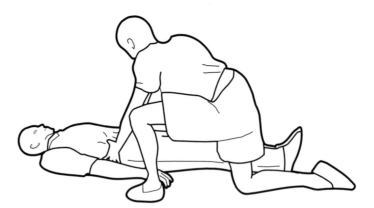

Fig 29. *Moving in bed. The nurse can stand beside the client's bed or kneel next to the client. The nurse assists the clients involved lower extremity into a flexed position. The client flexes the uninvolved extremity.*

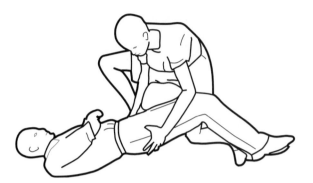

Fig 30. *The client performs a bridge and, at the same time, moves the buttocks up in bed. The nurse assists by helping the client to lift the pelvis. The buttocks are slowly lowered back onto the bed.*

assistance is needed, the nurse should reach behind the scapula and assist the client in coming up off the bed. This will elongate the trunk and allow the client to move up the bed in an inchworm fashion (Figure 32). Never assist the client by grabbing behind the neck or by the arms; this could cause serious injury to the client. This sequence should be repeated until the client is positioned appropriately in the bed. If the client is physically dependent or extremely obese, a

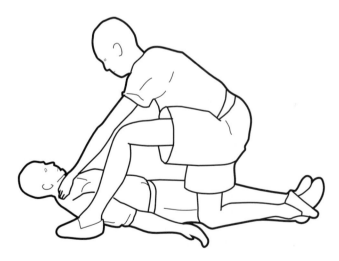

Fig 31. *The client should be asked to tuck their chin and lift the shoulders off the bed.*

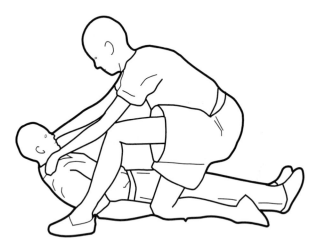

Fig 32. *The client should lift off the bed, elongating the trunk and allowing the client to move up in bed. The nurse can assist by reaching behind the client's scapula. The nurse should never pull on the client's neck or arms to lift the client forward off the bed.*

draw sheet can be used to move the pelvis. The same movements can also be used to move the client sideways in bed, except that the client will be moving laterally instead of upward in the bed. Having the client practice bridging and half-bridging with the involved lower extremity in a weight-bearing position will facilitate this process (Figure 33).

Rolling to the Involved Side

Before **rolling,** the client should be in a supine position with the bed flat. All pillows or bedding that may impede movement should be moved out of the way. The nurse will stand on the side that the client is rolling to (in this case, the involved side). The client should scoot toward the edge of the bed, leaving enough room to roll over safely into a side-lying position. Make sure that the scapula that the client is lying on is in a protracted position before starting the movement. Start by having the client turn his or her head and look toward the involved side. If the client is unable to rotate the head in that direction, the nurse can gently turn the client's head toward the involved side. Also, if the client's head is bent toward the involved side, another pillow may be added to lift the head away from the bed. This will also promote the desired movement pattern. The client will start to turn his or her head and lift away from the pillow. The nurse should assist this motion by giving downward pressure on the uninvolved shoulder. Never pull the client over by the arm or the neck. Continue to assist

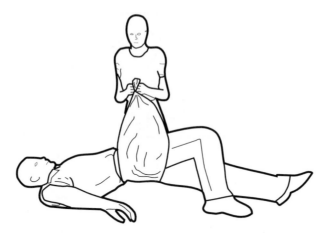

Fig 33. *Practicing half bridge in the physically dependent client in preparation for bed mobility. If the client is too physically dependent to move, a draw sheet under the client's buttocks can be used to assist the client.*

the client over on his or her side, allowing the lower trunk to follow the upper trunk. The uninvolved leg should slightly flex up and follow the lower trunk until a side-lying position is reached (Figure 34). If the client is to remain on this side, add appropriate support as needed.

Rolling to the Uninvolved Side

The client should be supine with the bed flat. Start by protracting the scapula of the involved side. The upper extremity should be placed in front of the trunk with the palm of the hand weight bearing on the bed (Figure 35). The involved lower extremity should be flexed up so that the entire plantar surface of the foot is weight bearing on the bed (Figure 36). The nurse may need to hold the lower extremity in place or trap the foot of the involved lower extremity under the leg of the uninvolved lower extremity. If the nurse is unable to control the lower extremity and assist the roll, the involved lower extremity should be allowed to fall toward the direction the client is rolling to, never out to the side. Have the client initiate the movement by turning his or her head toward the side they are rolling to. The nurse should assist the client by reaching over the involved scapula, giving downward pressure toward the hip to facilitate the head lift. The upper trunk should be guided over, followed by the lower trunk. The leg should follow over and rest gently on a pillow. If the client is to remain this position, place the appropriate pillows for support (Figure 37).

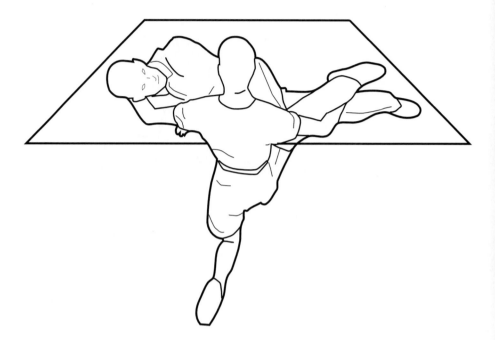

Fig 34. *Rolling to the involved side. The involved scapula should be protracted before starting the motion. To initiate the movement, the nurse should help the client turn and lift the head off the pillow. If the client is unable to support their weight on the involved shoulder, the nurse can reach behind the client's back to support the shoulder and scapula. Never hold onto the client's head or neck. The nurse can also reach under the uninvolved extremity to reposition the involved lower extremity.*

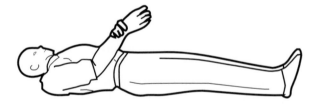

Fig 35. *Rolling to the uninvolved side. The nurse should prepare the client by protracting the scapula and pelvis. If necessary, the client should assist their own upper extremity if possible by guiding it toward the side they are rolling to.*

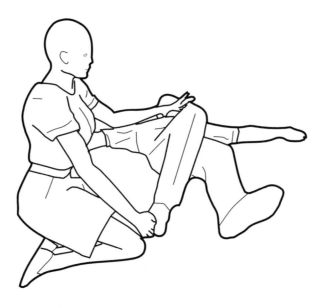

Fig 36. *The lower extremity should be flexed up so that the entire plantar surface of the foot is weight bearing on the bed.*

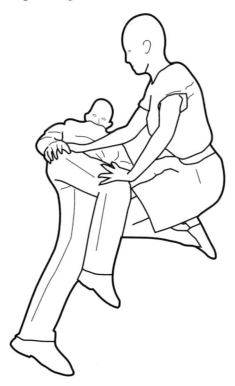

Fig 37. *If the client is able to move the upper body, the nurse can also assist the roll from the pelvis and involved lower extremity. The leg should be guided over and positioned on a pillow if the client remains in sidelying position.*

Supine to Sitting and Vice Versa: Through the Involved Side

To move from **supine to sitting** through the involved side, the sequence of steps is the same as when rolling onto the involved side. Before the movement is started, the nurse should position the client's hand so that the palm of the uninvolved extremity is fully weight bearing either on the bed or on the therapist's thigh. The client will use this upper extremity to push up into sitting. Start by having the client look to the involved side. As the head lifts off the bed, the nurse assists at the shoulder; however, instead of guiding the client onto his or her side, the client should be guided forward and up diagonally toward a sitting position (Figure 38). As the upper body leaves the bed, the uninvolved upper extremity can assist in erecting the trunk up by pushing up from the bed or the therapist's thigh. At the same time, the lower extremities are flexed up and guided toward the edge of the bed. Discourage the client from hooking the in-

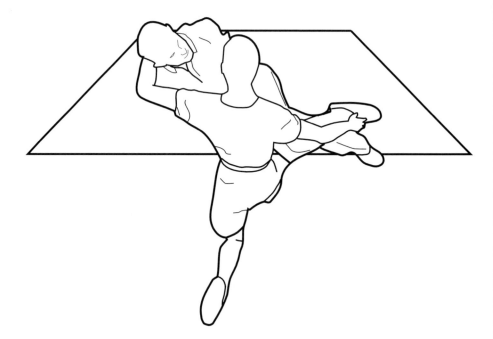

Fig 38. *Supine to sit from the involved side. The nurse should assist the client in initiating the movement as in Fig 34. The client's uninvolved hand should be positioned fully weight bearing to allow the client to use the arm for support. In one fluid motion, the nurse assists the client in moving away from the pillow diagonally up to a sitting position. Remember to support the client under the scapula, not the head or neck.*

volved extremity with the uninvolved extremity; instead, guide the legs together or place the legs side by side and allow the uninvolved leg to guide the involved leg (Figure 39). Once sitting, cue the client to assume an erect sitting posture (Figures 40 and 41).

If the client is unable to perform this sequence in one fluid motion, each step can be performed separately. First, perform the steps for rolling to guide the client onto the involved side, with extra pillows under the head to promote the lift off the bed. Next, guide the lower extremities forward, to the edge of the bed. Remember to allow the client to do as much as possible without hooking the legs together. Make sure to position the uninvolved hand where the client can push up into sitting. Initiate the lift off the bed by giving downward pressure into the uninvolved shoulder. The nurse's other hand is also free to give additional cues by giving pressure through the uninvolved pelvis or on the underside of the client's trunk or scapula. If the client can weight bear on the involved upper extremity, guide the client up onto the elbow, allowing him or her to remain

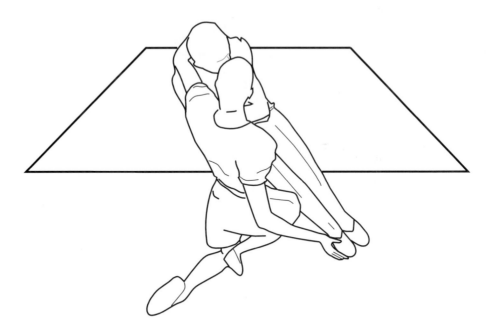

Fig 39. *The client should be encouraged to support as much body weight on the involved extremity as possible, pushing up from the bed. Both legs should be lowered off the mat together, using the uninvolved extremity as a guide for the involved extremity. The client should be discouraged from hooking their legs together.*

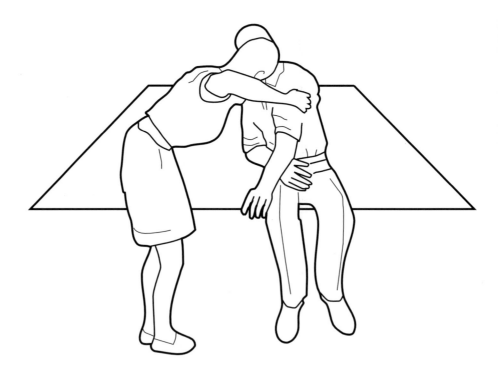

Fig 40. *The client should be assisted to a sitting position and cued to assume an erect posture to prepare for the next activity.*

propped while the legs are assisted off the bed. If the client cannot weight bear on the elbow, then the legs must be taken off the edge of the bed first before the transition into sitting is initiated. Finally, guide the client from the elbow into a full sitting position. The client can assist by fully extending the arm. Breaking up the movement sequence will allow the client to perform as many components as possible, but remember that this type of segmented movement is not normal. The final goal is to progress to such a point that the client performs the movement components in one fluid motion.

To transition from sitting to the supine position through the involved side, the same sequence of steps is performed but in reverse. Start with the client sitting at the edge of the bed. First, position the involved upper extremity so that it is weight bearing on the bed or on the nurse's thigh. The uninvolved upper extremity will reach across the body to the bed. If the involved lower extremity is flaccid, the uninvolved leg can be crossed over the involved leg to assist with the lift onto the bed. If possible, avoid hooking the involved leg with the uninvolved leg. Slowly allow the client to lower him- or herself down toward the bed. Clients can lower themselves onto their elbow first, and then down to their side. Be sure to support the client through the whole motion at the shoulder or under the trunk if needed. Never force a client to weight bear on a flaccid or hypotonic shoulder because there is no muscular support to stabilize the joint. Assist the client in lifting the legs up onto the bed. Finally, help the client roll back into the supine position.

Supine to Sitting and Vice Versa: Through the Uninvolved Side

Clients will usually prefer to come to a sitting position from the uninvolved side. This is because it is much easier to push up with the uninvolved upper extremity. Be sure to encourage performing the sequence from both sides and do not

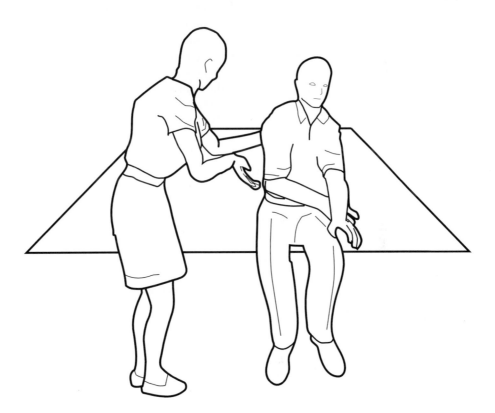

Fig 41. *Once the client is sitting, the nurse must be sure to keep one hand on the client's trunk. Note how the nurse stands close to the involved side in case the client loses balance. Once sitting, never leave a client with balance deficits unattended.*

get in the habit of always allowing the client to perform the easier movement. The initial steps of the sequence will be the same as for rolling onto the uninvolved side (Figure 35 and 36). Instruct the client to turn the head to the uninvolved side. As the head turns and lifts up off the bed, assist the client up to sitting position. Make sure to keep the scapula of the involved upper extremity protracted with the arm placed across the body, so that the involved hand can weight bear and assist with the motion. Encourage the client to use the involved upper extremity as much as possible, as the tendency will be for the client to do the entire motion with the uninvolved arm. Assistance should be given at the involved scapula and at the pelvis or the underside of the trunk if needed. The involved lower extremity should be placed on top of the uninvolved lower extremity and guided off the side of the bed. Again, avoid hooking the involved leg. If the client is having difficulty performing the activity, each component can be broken down into individual steps.

To lower back down to a supine position, the scapula of the involved upper extremity should be protracted with the arm placed on the bed or on the nurse's thigh to assist with the motion. Encourage as much weight bearing through the involved upper extremity as possible, and do not allow the scapula to retract. As the client lowers the trunk down to the bed, the uninvolved lower extremity can assist the involved lower extremity up onto the bed. Assist the client at the involved scapula, pelvis, or underside of the trunk. Assist the legs up onto the bed if needed.

Transfers Once the client is sitting up in bed, there are several methods that can be used to transfer the client into a wheelchair, bedside chair, or to a standing position. In this section several types of **transfers** are reviewed, along with the prepatory activities preceding the transfer. They include

1. Scooting to the edge of the bed
2. Modified depression transfers
3. Sliding board transfers
4. Sitting to standing transfers
5. Standing pivot transfers
6. Sitting from a standing position
7. Scooting back in the chair

Before the client can be transferred to another surface, the nurse must be sure that the client is in the proper starting position. The client must be sitting in an upright position with the head in midline, trunk and pelvis in a neutral position, both shoulders directly over the hips, with both feet in full contact with the floor. The client's knees and feet are in direct line with the hips, weight bearing equally on both ischial tuberosities (Figure 42). The client must also be sitting at the edge of the bed. If the client is not close enough to the edge or is not

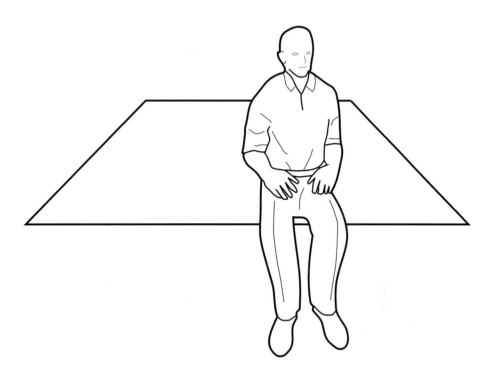

Fig 42. *Ideal sitting alignment for the hemiplegic client prior to initiating a transfer. Note the head is in midline with the trunk. The trunk and pelvis are in neutral position, with equal weight bearing on the ischial tuberosities. Both feet are in full contact with the floor and in line with the hips. Also note that the knees are slightly lower than the hips. This makes it easier to transfer the weight lower onto the lower extremities.*

sitting erect, the transfer will be very difficult for both the client and the nurse. Furthermore, the appropriate movement patterns will not be promoted and the client may be forced to use compensatory movements to complete the activity.

Scooting

To move the client to the edge of the bed, the nurse must first encourage the proper upright position as described above. Do not allow the client to attempt **scooting** forward if he or she is sitting in a slouched position. This will only encourage the client to use abnormal movement patterns. Typically, the client will extend backward, sliding the entire pelvis forward, then using the upper extremity, pull the trunk back over the pelvis. To ensure that this does not happen, apply light pressure at the lumbar spine and tell the client to "sit up straight" to encourage the client to move the pelvis anteriorly and to extend the trunk (Figures 43–45). To move the uninvolved side forward, the client must first shift weight to the involved side. Cue the uninvolved side of the pelvis to lift as the weight is shifted onto the involved side of the pelvis. This can be done by reaching under the hip or by guiding the side of the trunk.

Do not allow the client to lean in order to unweight the pelvis. The shoulders should stay level while the client is scooting (Figure 46). The goal is to achieve controlled shortening of the uninvolved side and controlled lengthening of the involved side of the trunk. Once unweighted, the uninvolved leg is advanced forward. The nurse can assist in pulling the leg forward if necessary. The pelvis is gently lowered back down to neutral and the process is repeated with the other side (Figure 47). The client will now lift the involved side of the pelvis while shifting weight onto the uninvolved ischial tuberosity (Figure 48). The involved lower extremity is now advanced forward. This is repeated until the client

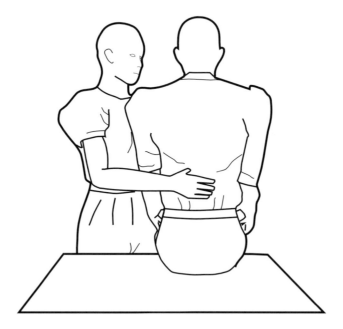

Fig 43. *Encouraging a neutral pelvis and trunk. Before the client can scoot forward, the correct upright posture must be assumed. Because the hemiplegic client usually maintains a slumped posture, the nurse should apply light pressure at the lumbar spine, telling the client to "sit up straight."*

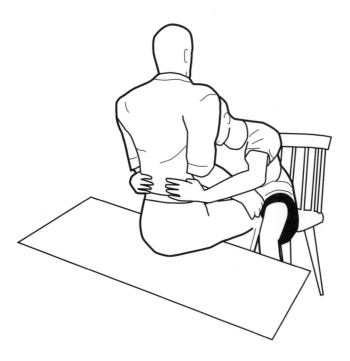

Fig 44. *If the client is too physically dependent to assume a neutral position independently, the nurse can give additional assistance by sitting in front of the client and using both hands to assist the lumbar spine while using the top of the head to give light pressure at client's sternum.*

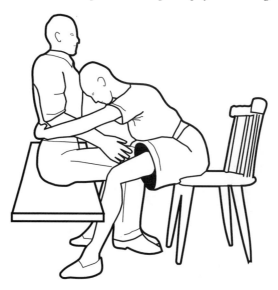

Fig 45. *Note that the nurse is extremely careful not to press on the client's throat or abdomen. Only light pressure is applied with the nurse's head to facilitate the trunk to a neutral position. If the nurse feels too much pressure is being applied, the head should not be used to support the client's trunk.*

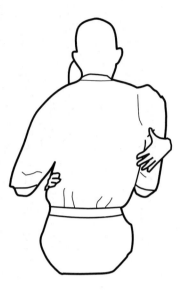

Fig 46. *Scooting to the edge of the mat. First, the client must shift their weight laterally. If the client is going to scoot the left hip forward, the left ischial tuberosity must be unweighted. The nurse sits in front of the client and cues the weight shift by giving upward pressure on the lengthening side of the trunk and lateral pressure at the pelvis on the shortening side of the trunk. Note the shoulders stay level. Do not allow the client to lean.*

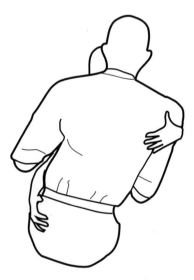

Fig 47. *Once the client has fully unweighted the left ischial tuberosity, the nurse can reach down to the pelvis and cue the left side to move forward. Note that the nurse maintains the support at the trunk on the right side. Once the left side of the pelvis is moved forward, it is gently lowered back down and reseated on the bed.*

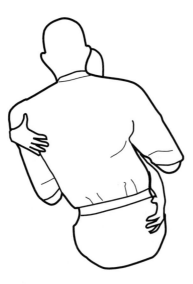

Fig 48. *Once the client is back in a neutral sitting posture, the same procedure is repeated on the opposite side. This process is repeated until the client is sitting at the edge of the bed.*

is sitting at the edge of the bed so that two-thirds of both femurs are unsupported by the bed.

Modified Depression Transfers

To ensure that a **modified depression transfer** is done efficiently and safely, special attention must be give to the set-up of the transfer. The wheelchair should be placed at a 20- to 30-degree angle to the bed. Both brakes should be securely locked to prevent the chair from rolling out from under the client. Both armrests and footrests should be removed or positioned out of the client's way. The height of the bed should be adjusted so that it is even with the height of the seat of the wheelchair. To make the transfer slightly easier, the bed height can be adjusted so that it is slightly higher than the seat height (Figure 49). The client should also be encouraged to transfer in both directions. The client will usually find it easier to transfer to the uninvolved side; however, transferring in only one direction is not practical. Transferring to the involved side will encourage further awareness of that side and weight bearing on the involved extremities.

The client should start in the proper upright position with both feet in full contact with the floor (Figure 50). Clients who are very short may need their feet positioned on a stool or block. The client's feet should be tucked under the cli-

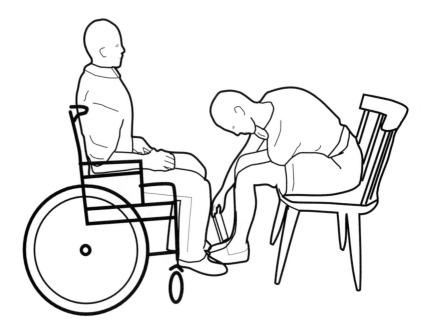

Fig 49. *Modified depression transfers. The nurse must sit in front of the client. The nurse removes the footrest and armrest on the side that the client is transferring to. Remember to place the wheelchair at a 20-30 degree angle to the bed. If possible, the surface that the client is transferring to should be slightly lower than the surface they are sitting on.*

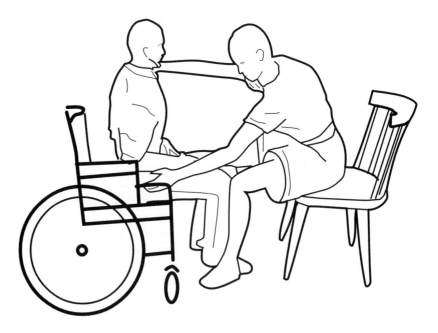

Fig 50. *The client should be scooted to the edge of the wheelchair as in Figs 46 and 47. The nurse can assist the client in advancing the lower extremity. One hand should remain on the client's trunk to help the client maintain balance.*

ent so that the forefeet are under the knees. The feet should also be turned very slightly so that both heels are facing the wheelchair. This will ensure that the client's legs do not cross during the transfer. The nurse is positioned in front of the client, and is either standing or sitting on a chair. If the client is much shorter than the nurse it is best to sit, to avoid stooping over to assist the client. The upper extremities can be placed either on the client's own knees, on the surface that the client is sitting on, or on the nurse's knee to encourage weight bearing through the arm (Figure 51). The nurse may need to support the hand if the extremity is flaccid. The nurse should not allow the client to pull him- or herself up by grabbing onto the wheelchair or around the nurse's neck. The nurse can support the client by reaching around the sides of the trunk and placing both hands at the low back, under the ischial tuberosities, or on the scapula. Wherever the client is lacking the most control is where the nurse should support the client.

To initiate the transfer, the client should maintain neutral alignment of the trunk and pelvis as the trunk flexes forward at the hips, transferring the weight

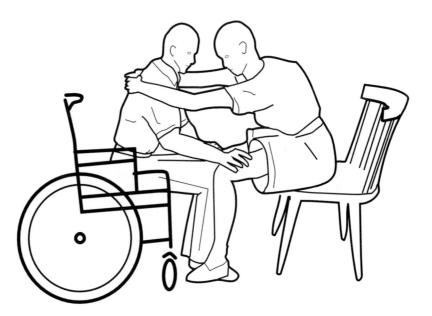

Fig 51. *The client should have both feet in full contact with the floor and tucked under the knees. The feet should be turned so that both heels are facing the direction that the client is transferring to. The upper extremities are placed on a weight bearing surface. The client should not be allowed to pull the body up by grabbing onto the nurse. The nurse should support the client by reaching around to the scapula, low back, or pelvis, wherever the client needs the most support.*

from the ischial tuberosities to the feet. Both of the client's upper extremities should be used to maintain symmetry and to stabilize the trunk. If the involved lower extremity is hypotonic or flaccid and cannot support the body weight of the client, the leg can be supported by sandwiching the leg between the nurse's legs, or by crossing the nurse's leg in front of the client's tibia to prevent the client's leg from buckling and to facilitate weight bearing through the extremity. The nurse should never attempt to "block" the knee (Figure 52). This will prevent the normal forward progression of the femur as the client transfers. To unweight the client's pelvis, the nurse should slowly rock backward as if about to sit down, bringing the client forward in a teeter-totter fashion. The nurse should never attempt to lift the client straight up from the chair. Telling the client to rock back and forth to gain momentum for the transfer should be strongly discouraged. Instead, the client should be encouraged to shift weight gradually onto the lower extremities. This should be done until the nurse is confident that the

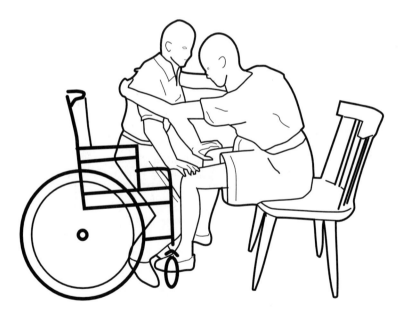

Fig 52. *The client should maintain neutral alignment of the trunk and pelvis as the hips flex forward, transferring the client's weight from the ischial tuberosities onto the lower extremities. As the pelvis is unweighted, the client should pivot over the feet and move laterally toward the bed. The client is then slowly reseated onto the bed. If the client's hemiplegic lower extremity is unable to support the weight, the client's leg can be sandwiched between the nurse's for support. The nurse should be careful not to "block" the client's knee.*

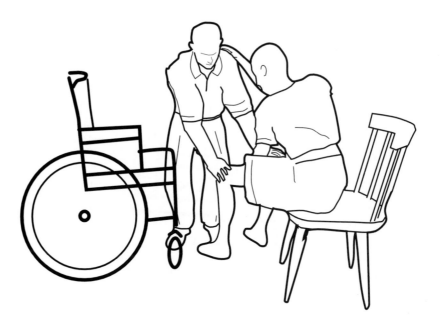

Fig 53. *Note that the client is discouraged from standing all the way up. The nurse must keep at least one hand on the client's trunk at all times. Note that the client does not pull the body over onto the bed, but gently pivots over the feet and gently lowers onto the bed.*

client is accepting weight symmetrically through both legs. As the client lifts off the bed, the client should maintain a flexed position with the shoulders over the feet and pivot slightly, moving the pelvis laterally and gently lowering onto the seat of the wheelchair (Figure 53). If the client is unable to transfer the entire distance from the bed to the wheelchair in one motion, the transfer can be repeated several times, with the client moving closer to the wheelchair with each scoot. After the client is seated safely in the wheelchair, the proper upright position should be assumed.

Sliding Board Transfers

If the client requires considerable physical assistance or if the wheelchair cannot be placed close to the surface the client is transferring to, a **sliding board transfer** may be attempted, in which a sliding board is used to create a bridge between the two surfaces (Figure 54). The client should first scoot to the edge of the surface before the board is placed. One end of the board should be under the client's thigh and angled toward the opposite hip. The other end should be securely resting on the surface the client is transferring to. If the board is posi-

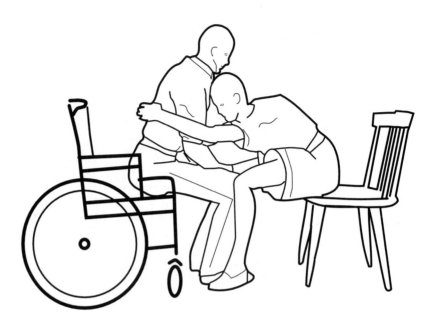

Fig 54. *Sliding board transfers. If the client requires heavy physical assistance, the nurse can use a sliding board to bridge the gap between the two surfaces for additional support. Note that the nurse moves closer to the client, uses the head or shoulder to support the client's trunk, and supports the client's leg by placing her legs around his.*

tioned too far back, the client may slide forward off the board and if the board is too far forward, the client may fall backward off the back end of the board. The transfer sequence should be the same as the modified depression transfer. The client should be discouraged from sliding across the board. The board may provide extra support, but the goal is still to transfer the weight forward onto the lower extremities, unweighting the pelvis before the client attempts to move (Figures 55–57). The nurse may also need to adjust positions to assist the more physically dependent client.

Other suggestions may assist the rehabilitation team members in managing the physically dependent client. Often, the nurse may need to stand in front of the client and flex the client forward at the hips until the client is resting against the nurse's body. The nurse can then lean over the top of the client's trunk, reaching under the client's ischial tuberosities or around the trunk. The nurse then has more leverage to unweight the pelvis. Do not assist the client by grabbing onto clothing. If a nurse feels that he or she is unable to manage a client alone, a sheet can be wrapped around the client's body so that the nurse does not need to control each extremity separately. If the nurse still feels unsafe, then

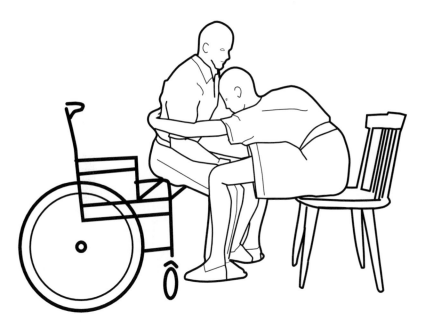

Fig 55. *The client should be discouraged from sliding across the board. The client should go through the same sequence as the modified depression transfer moving in smaller increments. The sliding board provides a bridge for the client to inch across to the bed.*

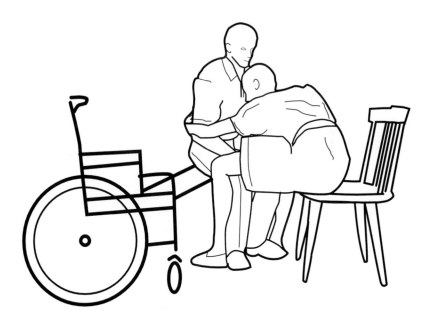

Fig 56. *The client's hand and foot position may need to be adjusted periodically as the client moves across the board. The nurse should also move her chair as needed to ensure that she remains directly in front of the client.*

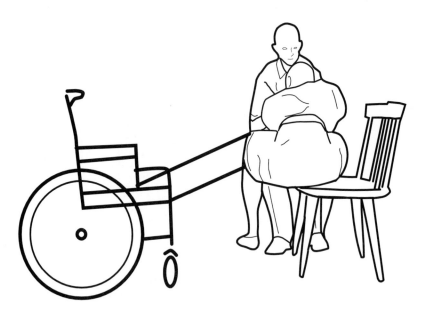

Fig 57. *Once the client is safely on the bed, the client should be positioned in a neutral sitting posture. The sliding board can be removed with the nurse always keeping one hand on the client for support. If the nurse lets go of the client to pull the board out, the client will fall off the bed.*

as additional team member should be called on to assist with the transfer. The second person should be positioned behind the client and assist by reaching under the client's ischial tuberosities. As the client leans forward, the second team member can lift the pelvis, shifting more of the client's weight forward onto the legs.

Sitting to Standing Transfers

In a **sitting to standing transfer,** the client should scoot forward to the edge of the surface and assume the proper upright sitting position. If the client is standing up without an ambulatory device the nurse can assist the client by sitting or standing in front of the client (Figure 58). If the client is using an ambulatory device such as a front-wheeled walker, the nurse should assist the client from the involved side. This will encourage awareness of the hemiplegic side and allow the nurse to assist the weaker extremities. The weight shift onto the legs is done the same as in the modified depression transfer. The client should maintain neutral trunk alignment and flex forward at the hips. Remember that the client must have the weight distributed symmetrically between both lower extremities. When

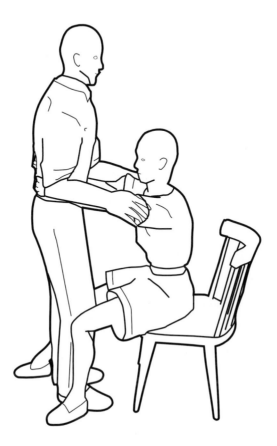

Fig 58. *Sit to stand transfers. If the client is not using an ambulatory device, the nurse should sit in front of the client. The nurse should support the involved lower extremity to keep it from buckling forward or hyperextending. Both hands should support the client's trunk and pelvis.*

the weight is transferred to the feet and the pelvis unweighted, the client can slowly lift up from the chair (Figure 59). The nurse should cue the hips to extend by applying pressure over the gluteus maximus and then at the trunk to bring the shoulders back until full trunk extension has been achieved. Last, the nurse may need to assist full extension of the involved knee. This motion of "unfolding" the trunk as the client comes to a stand must be done slowly to ensure that the client does not extend the legs first against the surface the are standing from (Figure 60). Watch that the client also does not allow the involved lower extremity to snap back into hyperextension (Figure 61). If the client requires con-

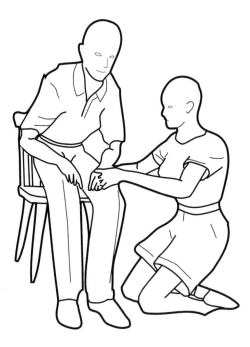

Fig 59. *Sit to stand transfers in preparation for ambulatory device. If the client is using an ambulatory device such as a walker, the nurse should assist the client on the hemiplegic side. (The walker is not pictured here to show the position of the client.) Note that the nurse assists the hemiplegic upper extremity by encouraging the client to weight bear through the hand. The client slowly flexes at the hips, transferring the weight from the pelvis onto the feet. The nurse can reach around behind the client to assist the client at the pelvis or trunk.*

siderable physical assistance, then one person may need to sit in front of the client to keep the lower extremities from buckling while a second team member maintains an upright trunk. The client should never be suspended from under the arms or forced to stand if the legs are not actively supporting the client's weight. Once the client is standing it is possible to perform a standing pivot transfer, or take a step forward to begin ambulation.

Standing Pivot Transfers

A **standing pivot transfer** is often performed with little attention to the symmetry of the transfer. Most clients will stand with all of their weight over the uninvolved leg and pivot around the stronger leg without transferring any weight onto the involved lower extremity. To initiate the standing pivot transfer cor-

rectly, the client should be guided throughout the sequence discussed in the preceding section (Sitting to Standing Transfers). Once the client is standing with
the weight equally distributed on both legs, the client is now ready to pivot toward the wheelchair (Figure 58). The nurse can stand in front of the client or to
the side if an ambulatory device is used. Support can be given at the pelvis or
trunk. The involved upper extremity should be placed in a weight-bearing position on the nurse's shoulder. If the client is transferring to the right, the transfer
is initiated by a weight shift to the left. Once the weight is centered over the left
lower extremity, the right leg is unweighted and free to move. The client should
then pivot the right heel out to the side, keeping the ball of the foot in the same
place. After the right foot has been repositioned, the nurse should then assist the
client in turning the trunk so that the client's back is starting to face the chair
and the client is shifting weight onto the right leg. Now the left leg is un-

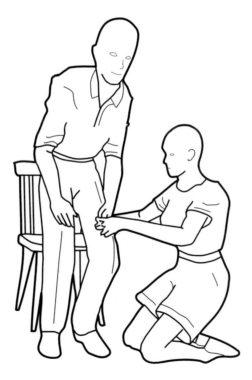

Fig 60. *Note that the nurse can half-kneel or stand next to the client to assist the transfer. As
the client lifts away from the chair, the nurse allows the hemiplegic hand to slide up the front
of the client's thigh while the client's trunk slowly unfolds. Do not allow the client to
hyperextend the involved knee back against the chair.*

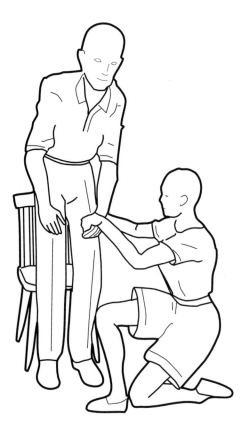

Fig 61. *As the client stands, the knees and hips slowly extend, as the client's trunk erects to a neutral position. Remember to always keep the client in a midline position, with equal weight bearing on the lower extremities. Do not allow the client to stand with the weight centered over the uninvolved lower extremity.*

weighted and free to move. The client should then slide the left foot backward toward the right foot until it is in the original starting position. The process is repeated as the client then shifts weight laterally onto the left foot again, while the right heel is pivoted out toward the surface the client is transferring to. It is critical that the client shifts weight completely onto the stance leg before attempting to move the unweighted limb. Do not allow the client to attempt to step before the weight shift is completed, or to pivot with his or her weight centered over the stronger leg. If the client cannot perform this transfer correctly, it may be more beneficial to use the modified depression technique to ensure that the appropriate movement patterns are reinforced.

Sitting from a Standing Position

If a standing transfer was performed, the nurse should guide the client back toward the wheelchair until the client is standing directly in front of the wheelchair. The nurse can cue the client to feel for the chair to contact the back of the legs, but the client should not reach back for the armrest before sitting down. This will only promote asymmetrical weight shifting onto the uninvolved extremity and reinforce abnormal movement patterns. Instead, the client should be cued to flex forward slowly at the hips, maintaining a neutral trunk and pelvis. As the trunk flexes, the knees should also flex. The shoulders should always stay forward of the hips to prevent the client from falling over backward. The client should slowly lower down onto the surface in a controlled manner. Once sitting, the shoulders can be realigned over the hips.

Scooting Back into the Chair

The client should assume the proper upright position, with the nurse sitting or standing in front of the client. The nurse cues the client to maintain a neutral trunk and pelvis as the client flexes forward at the hips until the weight is transferred over the feet. Once the pelvis is unweighted the client gently pushes backward with the legs, moving the pelvis back into the chair. The client should not be allowed to extend the trunk or forcefully push backward with the legs. This may need to be repeated several times before the client is all the way back in the chair. If the client requires considerable physical assistance, then the nurse may need to stand over the client to assist the weight shift forward. Once the pelvis is unweighted the nurse can apply a backward force at the client's knees to assist the client in moving the pelvis back into the chair. Once seated, the client should assume an upright position.

A Note on Wheelchair Positioning

Some specific comments on **wheelchair positioning** are warranted, as many of our clients spend a considerable amount of time sitting in wheelchairs. Therefore, the client's position in the wheelchair should reinforce the proper upright position and the appropriate movement patterns. The wheelchair itself should be lightweight to allow for easy propulsion. The seat and back of the chair should form a 90-degree angle. Reclining wheelchairs will only encourage a slouched position of the trunk and pelvis. The seat should be constructed of a firm material to increase the proprioceptive input through the ischial tuberosities, promoting symmetrical weight bearing of the pelvis and lower extremities. If the cushion is too soft, the client will sink into the cushion, encouraging a slouched posture and all proprioceptive input will be greatly reduced. A firm surface will also allow the client to scoot and transfer out of the chair with greater ease. If skin breakdown is a concern or already present, then a softer material must be used for appropriate **pressure release** and wound healing. A small towel roll or lumbar support can be added to encourage trunk extension. If the wheelchair back is worn out, a solid backing should be added to keep the client from slouching. The height of the seat must be adjusted so that the client can position both feet flat on the floor. If the seat height is too high, the client will slide the pelvis forward into a slouched position to bring the feet closer to the floor for wheelchair propulsion. A seat belt can be used to secure the client; however, it should be fastened over the client's thighs, not over the pelvis, as this will only encourage the client to slouch. A lapboard can be attached to most wheelchairs to support the upper extremity, especially if the arm is flaccid. This will keep the glenohumeral joint approximated and encourage early weight bearing through the arm.

Amyotrophic Lateral Sclerosis

Amyotrophic lateral sclerosis (ALS), more commonly known as Lou Gehrig's disease, is a disease of insidious onset that affects more men than women, usually after the age of 50 (Kandel and Schwartz, 1985). The disease is characterized by progressive degeneration of the anterior horn cells and cortical motor pathways. Both upper and lower motor neuron involvement is present. Asymmetrical weakness of the upper and lower limbs with atrophy of the small intrinsic muscles of the hands and feet are noted. Initially, the client will usually report difficulty manipulating small objects, tripping during ambulation, fatigue, muscle spasms, and weakness of the limbs. The disease eventually leads to bulbar and respiratory dysfunction (dysarthria and dysphagia). The prognosis is poor, with death usually occurring within 6 years from respiratory failure (Kandel and Schwartz, 1985).

Several precautions must be observed when managing a client diagnosed with ALS. Because of the progressive weakness of the muscles controlling swallowing and respiration, the head of the bed may need to be elevated to prevent aspiration and to make it easier for the client to breathe, especially in the later stages of the disease. The nurse must also be careful to listen to the client because the dysarthria may make it difficult for the nurse to understand what the client is saying. As the client becomes more physically disabled and immobile, special care must be taken to ensure that the client changes position frequently to avoid pressure sores. The bed positioning techniques used are similar to those reviewed in the section on stroke. Muscle spasms are common and may necessitate position changes more frequently. If the client is positioned in a bedside chair, it is important to remember that clients suffering from ALS fatigue quickly. Sitting upright even if supported requires muscular control of the head and trunk. The client should be transferred back into bed when tired and never forced to sit up when fatigued.

Guillain-Barré Syndrome

Guillain-Barré syndrome, or idiopathic polyneuritis syndrome, is a lower motor neuron disease characterized by demyelination and occasional axonal degeneration of the peripheral nerves. The exact cause of the disease is unknown although it is thought to be related to some viral infectious agent. The client will often report flulike symptoms before the onset of the disease. The onset can be rapid, occurring in one explosive episode, or a slow progression of symmetrical muscular weakness may occur, usually starting distally and progressing proximally. In addition to the weakness, paresthesias, numbness, pain, and fatigue are noted. The disease at its worst will leave the client a quadriplegic, often with respiratory dysfunction requiring the use of a ventilator. Steroid treatment, human immunoglobulin infusion, and plasmapheresis are three forms of treatment that can be used during the acute phases of the disease, although no treatment has been proven completely effective for all Guillain-Barré clients. Recovery from the disease is variable and begins anywhere from 2 to 4 weeks after the onset of the disease. Some clients can expect a full recovery; however, approximately half of the clients diagnosed with Guillain-Barré syndrome are left with some type of residual neurological deficits.

During the early stages of the disease, the head of the bed may need to be elevated secondary to respiratory and swallowing complications. The client may complain of pain, so the extremities should be moved slowly when the client is positioned either in the bed or wheelchair. A positioning program must be strictly followed to avoid joint contractures and pressure sores. Because the client has potential for a full recovery it is critical that mobility be maintained in all extremities, so that the client can resume all previous activities once motor function returns. The client should be encouraged to get out of bed as much as possible and to do as much as possible with each activity; however, caution should be taken not to overfatigue the client. The nurse may need to assist more during transfers and bed mobility at the end of the day if the client is tired or if the room temperature is elevated, because Guillain-Barré clients can be sensitive to heat. The nurse should allow the client to take extra rest breaks if needed.

Multiple Sclerosis

Multiple sclerosis is a chronic progressive demyelinating disease that affects the central nervous system. It is the most common demyelinating disease of young adults, affecting slightly more women than men (Hickey, 1992). The disease attacks the white matter, leaving an asymmetrical spotty distribution of plaques throughout the central nervous system. Because of the nature of the disease, there is great variability in clinical presentation. Some symptoms may include muscle weakness, spasticity, dysarthria, dysphagia, cognitive deficits, fatigue, motor and sensory deficits, impaired balance and co-ordination, and impaired bowel and bladder dysfunction. Clients may experience episodes of exacerbation or slow progressive degeneration leading to severe physical disability.

The approach used to manage the client diagnosed with multiple sclerosis will depend on the clinical presentation of the individual client. If the client presents with hemiparesis, then the techniques discussed previously for CVA clients will be appropriate. If all four extremities are involved, the techniques discussed subsequently in the sections on spinal cord injury may be more appropriate for meeting the client's needs. Whatever approach the nurse uses, the nurse must remember to change the client's position on a regular basis to prevent skin breakdown and to avoid joint contractures, especially in the presence of spasticity and severe immobility. Cognitive impairments may also be present, so the nurse should watch for deficits in safety judgement and reasoning.

Parkinson's Disease

Parkinson's disease results from a dopamine deficiency in the striatum and from loss of neurons in the substantia nigra and other pigmented nuclei. The disease affects older individuals, usually in their mid-fifties or above, and slightly more males than females. Clinically, the client will present with rigidity, bradykinesia, resting tremors, and postural deformities usually in flexion. The client may have a *festinating gait,* that is, short, stuttering steps are taken instead of normal-length strides. The client may also speak in a soft or monotone voice (see Chapter 18 on dysphagia).

The client with Parkinson's disease is at high risk for developing joint contracture because of the rigidity. This is especially true if the client is bed ridden or wheelchair dependent. The client should always be encouraged to move throughout full range of motion with all activities. Every opportunity should be taken to encourage trunk extension in all positions. A lumbar support can be added to the client's wheelchair and to the bed when the client is lying supine. Often, the client will have difficulty initiating movement. Rhythmic or reciprocal movements can be used to start a weight shift, making it easier for the client to begin to move. To initiate an activity, the client can be instructed to rock back and forth, count out loud with a weight shift, or swing the arms reciprocally before attempting the movement. Using reciprocal movements will also promote trunk rotation, which the majority of Parkinson's clients lack. The techniques used for Parkinson's clients are the same as those discussed previously; however, the nurse should emphasize trunk extension and as much motion as possible with all activities.

Traumatic Brain Injury

Traumatic brain injury is the leading cause of death and disability for children and young adults between the ages of 15 and 24. The incidence is higher for males than for females by 2 : 1 (Umphred, 1995). The leading cause of traumatic brain injury is motor vehicle accidents for adults and child abuse for children. Accidental falls, assault, and sporting accidents also account for adult traumatic head injury.

There are three types of head injuries: open head injury, closed head injury, and minor head injury. An open head injury occurs when the skull is fractured. This would include penetrating injuries; compound, linear, or depressed fractures; and lacerations. A closed head injury occurs when no skull fracture is present. The brain damage results from various forces of compression, tension, or shear acting on the brain. A concussion or minor head injury involves a transient loss of neurologic function that resolves without permanent damage.

The primary injury is the force that creates the direct trauma to the brain. In motor vehicle accidents acceleration and deceleration forces can add on the insult to the brain. An example would be a client who is driving and then suddenly hit by another car. The client is thrown forward, hitting the head on the steering wheel. This first point of impact is called the *coup*. As the car comes to a stop, the client's head is thrown back against the seat; this rapid change in direction can cause the brain to impact the inside of the skull, creating a *contrecoup* injury, that is, another injury directly contralateral to the zone of impact.

Secondary injuries are conditions that arise after the primary injury, adding further insult to the brain. They include

> *Intracranial hematomas (epidural, subdural, or intracranial):* A collection of blood is trapped between the tissues, creating compression on the structures around the hematoma
>
> *Brain swelling:* An increase in intravascular blood within the brain as a result of vasodilation
>
> *Brain edema:* An increase in extravascular brain fluid
>
> *Increased intracranial pressure:* Greater the 20 mm Hg
>
> *Hypoxia or ischemia:* Lack of oxygenated blood supply to the brain as a result of aspiration, obstructed airway, or chest wall injuries; can be local or diffuse

The clinical manifestation of a traumatic head injury is dependent on the severity and location of the head injury. An immediate alteration in the state of consciousness is noted with almost all head injuries. With minor concussions, the loss of consciousness may be brief with little or no posttraumatic amnesia. In moderate or severe head injuries, posttraumatic amnesia is present, and the loss of consciousness can last over a prolonged period of time. The Glasgow Coma Scale is a 15-point scale used to rate the level of consciousness on the basis of motor response, eye opening, and verbal response. A person is said to be in a coma if a score of 8 or less is given on the Glasgow Coma Scale, indicating unresponsiveness and paralysis of cerebral functions (Umphred, 1995). During this time it is critical that the nurse position the client in a variety of positions to prevent pressure sores and to increase arousal by giving sensory input to the nervous system. The nurse should also talk to the client and touch the client as much as possible. The nurse may note abnormal posturing such as decorticate or decerebrate posturing. Decorticate posturing is a combination of abnormal flexion of the upper extremities and abnormal extension of the lower extremities. In decerebrate posturing, abnormal extension of both upper and lower extremities is seen with weak flexor responses in the legs. The nurse should try to position the client out of these postures when the client is in bed. If left for a prolonged period of time in these postures, the client may develop contracture.

As arousal increases, the medical, behavioral (or *affective*), cognitive, and physical deficits will become more apparent. The physical disturbances may include hemiplegia, loss of motor control, impaired balance, impaired sensation, and alterations in muscle tone. Visual-perceptual problems, aphasia, dysarthria, and dysphagia may also be present. Cognitive impairment such as decreased memory, decreased safety judgment, poor problem-solving, decreased reasoning, impulsivity, and distractibility may occur. Behavioral problems may also be present, such as inappropriate social behavior, mood disorders, episodes of verbal or physical aggressiveness, restlessness, and irritability. The Rancho Los Amigos Levels of Cognitive Functioning Scale can be used as a descriptive tool to categorize the client's cognitive and behavioral status. It is important for the nurse to recognize that the cognitive and behavioral deficits that the client has will affect every aspect of the client's rehabilitation. Therefore even the rehabilitation of motor function will incorporate the necessary cognitive retraining needed to allow the client to be successful.

The strategies for assisting physical function are the same as those covered in the section on stroke. However, special attention must be given to the safety of the client if cognitive deficits are present. If a client demonstrates restlessness or agitation, a posey may be needed to secure the client in bed to prevent the client from falling or climbing over the bed rails. Wrist restraints may be needed if the client is pulling IV lines or nasogastric tubing out of place. If possible, the minimum amount of restraint should be used, as additional restraints will tend to increase the client's level of agitation. Use of a four-sided floor bed with padded walls will allow the client to roll around freely without endangering his or her safety. An extra team member should be available to assist with transfers if the client is likely to be physically aggressive or if the client is unable to follow commands. The client may physically be able to complete the transfer, but may not cognitively be able to perform the appropriate activity. Extra time should be given when instructing the client because cognitive processing deficits may delay motor responses. Consistency is critical for the brain-injured client if modification of a behavior is to occur. Therefore, all team members must follow the same sequence of verbal and physical commands when assisting the client with any physical activity. It is best to write the appropriate treatment program out on a piece of paper, step by step, and post it where it is easily accessible to all team members. This will give the client the best opportunity for carryover of new skills into his or her functional activities.

Spinal Cord Injury

A spinal cord injury can occur as a result of traumatic or nontraumatic conditions, although the majority of spinal cord injuries are traumatic. Approximately 47 percent occur from motor vehicle accidents, 20 percent from falls, and 15 percent from assault and sports activities. Of the 15 percent from sports-related injuries, 66 percent are diving accidents (Maddox, 1987). Nontraumatic injuries to the spinal cord include circulatory problems, compression, demyelinating diseases, congenital diseases, inflammatory processes, and psychological conditions such as hysterical paralysis. Approximately 80 percent of spinal cord-injured clients are young males, with the majority of the incidents occurring in the summer months.

A spinal cord injury is named by the level of the damage and can be classified as *quadriplegia,* which is a result of damage to the cervical spine affecting the trunk and all four extremities, or *paraplegia,* which is the result of damage to the thoracic and lumbar spine affecting the trunk and lower extremities. The lesion itself can also be classified as complete or incomplete. A *complete* lesion is characterized by complete loss of all reflexes, sensory and motor function below the level of injury. This occurs when there is complete transection of the spinal cord, extensive vascular compromise, or severe compression. In an *incomplete* spinal cord injury, there is some preservation of sensory and motor function below the level of injury. This is usually the result of contusions, swelling within the spinal canal, or partial transection of the cord. The clinical manifestations of incomplete injuries will be determined by the location and extent of the damage. Some can be identified as specific syndromes:

> *Brown-Séquard syndrome:* Hemisection of the spinal cord resulting in ipsilateral loss of motor function, with contralateral loss of sensation. Usually the result of a stabbing or gunshot wound
>
> *Anterior cord syndrome:* Flexion injury resulting in loss of pain and temperature sensation below the level of injury
>
> *Central cord syndrome:* Hyperextension injury characterized by greater impairment of the upper extremities than in the lower extremities
>
> *Cauda equina syndrome:* Damage to the cauda equina below level L1, resulting in a lower motor neuron injury with flaccid paralysis and no reflexive activity
>
> *Spinal cord concussion:* A condition that occurs as a result of fluid build-up, soft tissue or bony compression of the spinal cord presenting as either a complete or incomplete injury; usually resolves within a few hours after injury if the cause of injury is removed

The site of the fracture may be stabilized with either an internal or external device or both to allow healing of the fracture. Internal fixation of unstable fractures of the cervical spine includes surgical stabilization by anterior or posterior stabilization protocols. Externally, the client may be placed in a halo traction vest, which is a device that attaches directly to the skull and is held by four metal uprights bolted to a plastic vest. The halo limits any motion of the cervical spin. If less stabilization is required a Philadelphia collar made of polyethylene is used to limit motion of the neck. For the paraplegic client, a wide variety of jackets made from plastic or metal can be used to stabilize the trunk.

When caring for the spinal cord-injured client, the nurse should be aware that several secondary conditions may exist that can seriously affect the client's rehabilitation. Special attention should be given to the following:

Spinal shock: A period of generalized loss of motor and sensory function and areflexia immediately following the spinal cord injury; may last several hours to several weeks

Closed head injury: Approximately half or more of all traumatic spinal cord injury clients suffer some form of closed head injury; clients may need to be screened for cognitive deficits

Pressure sores: Immobility, decreased blood flow, muscle atrophy, and impaired sensation make the spinal cord injury client a prime candidate to develop sores; great care must be taken to ensure that sores do not develop

Autonomic dysreflexia: Uninhibited reflex response to noxious stimuli characterized by headache, flushing, extremely high blood pressure, increased pulse, profuse sweating above level of injury; occurs with injuries above level T6, a medical emergency if not resolved

Postural hypotension: Rapid onset of low blood pressure caused by peripheral venous pooling with position changes; the nurse should fit the client with TED hose and abdominal binder before getting the client out of bed

Heterotopic ossification: Abnormal bone growth in extra-articular tissues adjacent to large joints below the level of the injury; aggressive range of motion must be encouraged

Contracture: Progressive shortening of muscles most commonly in the flexor muscle groups; it is critical that the nurse position the client in a variety of positions, especially prone

Deep vein thrombosis: Development of a blood clot in the vessel as a result of decreased blood flow and loss of normal pumping action provided by active muscle contractions

Pain: Musculoskeletal pain, nerve root pain, dysesthesias

Osteoporosis: May be a result of lack of stress on skeletal system of nonambulatory clients

Edema: Result of loss of voluntary muscle contraction

Heat stroke: Impaired temperature-regulating systems, resulting in the inability to perspire below the level of injury; watch for dizziness, nausea, headache, thirst

Spasticity: Occurs with injuries at level T11 and above; characterized by hypertonicity, hyperreflexia, and clonus

Spinal deformity: A result of muscular imbalances that necessitate compensatory postural changes to maintain sitting balance

Bowel, bladder, and sexual dysfunction: Upper motor neuron, spastic, T11 and above; lower motor neuron, flaccid, T12 and below

Treatment   The approach used with the spinal cord injury client differs from the techniques used for the hemiplegic and brain-injured client, especially for the client with complete spinal cord injury. In the hemiplegic and brain-injured client, the goal is to promote use and eventual re-integration of the involved extremities. With the client suffering from complete spinal cord injury, there is no longer potential for recovery of the involved trunk and extremities. Therefore, the techniques used will emphasize using whatever motor control the client has left to compensate for the loss of motor control in the involved extremities. These techniques may not be appropriate for the client with an injury at level C4 or above. The goal of treatment for the C4 quadriplegic is to educate the client in all aspects of his or her care so that the client can direct other individuals in the appropriate procedure.

Bed Positioning

The client should be positioned in a variety of positions including supine, side-lying on both sides, and prone. The nurse should make sure that all joints are positioned neutrally and comfortably supported with pillows. The prone position should be emphasized as much as possible, with the eventual goal of having the client sleep in the prone position (Figure 62). This will stretch the hip flexors, relieve all pressure from the ischial tuberosities, encourage weight bearing through the upper extremities, and promote trunk extension. Maintaining mobility in the hips and trunk is critical if the client has potential to return to a partial or full ambulatory status. Tolerance to this position will have to be increased gradually. Alternate positions can be used for comfort until the client is able to maintain a prone position. External fixation devices such as body jackets and halo traction vests should not deter the nurse from encouraging the prone position.

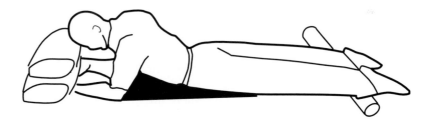

Fig 62. *Bed positioning, prone. The client should be positioned on a wedge with the upper body completely supported. The head should rest comfortably on pillows. The client can turn the head to the side if it is more comfortable. The upper extremities can be placed on the sides of the wedge or down at the client's side. A small towel roll can be added under the client's ankles to avoid overstretching into plantar flexion. Remember, tolerance to this position must be achieved gradually.*

To position the client prone, the nurse should have the client scoot or use a draw sheet to pull the client to one side of the bed. A pillow or wedge should be placed in the center of the bed to support the client's trunk once prone. The client's upper extremity can be placed overhead or at the client's side. Never force the client to roll over an extremity that is placed in the overhead position if the client does not have enough available range of motion. Instead, the client's arm can be placed at the side of the body when rolling. The client should then be rolled over the pillow or wedge into the prone position. The nurse can assist at the pelvis or reach under the client's arms around to the front of the chest to help lift the client over. The nurse should avoid lifting the client by the shoulders because this will restrict upper extremity movement. The pillow under the client should end up under the chest area. If it is too low under the pelvis, it will promote hip flexion. Once the client is prone, a pillow should also be placed under the dorsum of the ankles to avoid a plantar flexed position of the ankles. The upper extremities can be placed overhead, off the sides of the bed, or comfortably at the client's sides.

Bed Mobility

If a client is using an external fixation device, the nurse must make sure that the device is securely in place before the client is moved. If a collar is applied the nurse must keep the client in a neutral position and slide the collar around the back of the neck without moving the cervical spine. If a paraplegic is using a body jacket, the client must be log rolled onto his or her side, keeping the spine in a neutral position. A towel roll may need to be placed on the bed at the client's waist to prevent sagging into lateral flexion once the client is on his or her side. More than one team member may be needed to ensure that the trunk remains straight. Any uncontrolled or unwanted movement may disrupt the fracture site, necessitating further surgery or resulting in additional damage to the spinal cord.

The nurse should review the proper body mechanics before assisting the client with any functional activity. Remember, if the long sitting position is going to be used in any portion of bed mobility, the client must have 100 degrees of straight leg raise. If the client has tight hamstrings and attempts to long sit, the back extensors will be overstretched. The client will then lose further passive stability of the trunk provided by normal muscle and ligamentous tightness. The components of bed mobility for the spinal cord-injured client reviewed in this section include

1. Rolling
2. Supine to sit
3. Scooting
4. Lower extremity management

Rolling. The client should start slightly to one side of the bed or mat. Before starting, the client's outside lower extremity should be crossed over the other or flexed up. Eventually, the client should work toward rolling without any additional support or positioning. A pillow may also be used in back of the client to lift the client off the bed, making it easier to complete the roll. The client starts in a supine position with both hands clasped together. If the client does not have adequate hand function, the client can hook the backs of the wrists together (Figure 63). The quadriplegic or paraplegic client with a high level of injury will start by swinging both upper extremities in an arch across the body. Client's should be encouraged to look at their arms and follow the motion with their head (Figure 64). This motion is continued with increasing speed until the momentum of the motion carries the head, shoulders, and upper trunk over into side-lying and into a prone position (Figure 65). The lower trunk will follow the upper trunk (Figure 66). The nurse should stand on the side that the client is rolling to and assist the roll by guiding the client at the shoulder and pelvis. If the client does not use the head and shoulders along with the arms, the client will not create enough lift and will not be able to roll over. If the client's injury is low, or incomplete, the client may have enough trunk and upper extremity function to pull up off the bed and onto his or her side without needing to use momentum to complete the motion. A client wearing a halo traction vest may need additional assistance, because the halo can restrict upper extremity movement.

Supine to Sitting. There are three methods that the spinal cord injury client can use to move from the supine to a sitting position. For the quadriplegic or paraplegic with a high level of injury, the wrist extension method and the rolling to semiprone method will be used, depending on what works best for the client. The paraplegic will use the triceps/abdominal method. To use the wrist extension

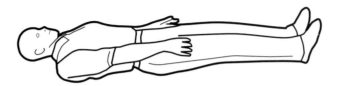

Fig 63. *Bed mobility for the spinal cord injured client. The client starts supine. If the client is first learning this technique, the lower extremities should be crossed, placing the outside leg over the other. Initially, the client is instructed to clasp the hands together. During the later stages of the client's rehabilitation, the hands can remain apart.*

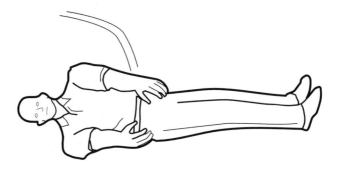

Fig 64. *The client starts the roll by swinging both upper extremities in an arch across the body. The client should be strongly encouraged to follow the motion of the arms with the head.*

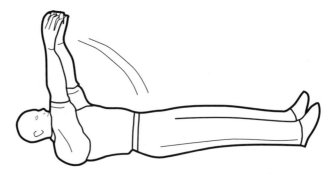

Fig 65. *The client swings the arms back and forth, pulling as much as possible with the head, neck, and shoulders. This motion is continued with increasing speed.*

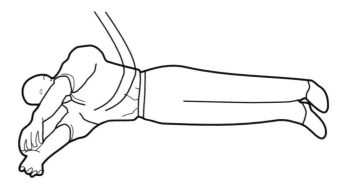

Fig 66. *As the speed and size of the arc of motion increases, the momentum carries the head, shoulders, and upper trunk over to a side lying position. Even though the width of the bed may be narrow, the client should be encouraged to perform safely as much of the motion as possible. The nurse can assist by guiding the shoulders and trunk. The nurse should stand on the side the client is falling to.*

method for quadriplegics, clients should start supine and wedge their hands under their hips, or hook their thumbs into their pants pockets, or belt loops (Figure 67). The C5 quadriplegic will not have wrist extension and will need to wedge his or her hands under the hips or use pants with deep pockets. The C6 quadriplegic will be able to extend the wrists to assist with the motion. The client then forcefully contracts the biceps and wrist extensors to initiate the lift and pull up into a reclined position on both elbows (Figure 68). The client immediately begins a weight shift from side to side, gradually repositioning the elbows back until they are under the shoulders (Figure 69). The client then increases the magnitude of the weight shift until one arm is unweighted (Figure 70). The opposite arm is immediately thrown back and locked into elbow extension, shoulder extension, and external rotation (Figure 71). The client repeats the weight shift onto the straightened arm and throws the other upper extremity back into a locked position until the client is resting back on both extremities (Figure 72). Remember that the entire sequence is completed in one smooth motion (Figure 73). Maintaining the momentum of the movement is critical to allow the client to weight shift enough to move the upper extremities. The nurse should assist from behind the client by helping to lift the upper body off the bed as the client props up on the elbows. The nurse can now reach under the trunk and scapula to give additional support as the client throws the arms back into a locked position. The nurse may also needs to help the client position the hands and arms. If the client is a C7 quadriplegic, triceps will also be available to assist with the motion and may be used to push up into elbow extension instead of throwing the arms back.

The second method for quadriplegics is the rolling to semiprone method. The client uses the method described previously to roll to a semiprone position. The nurse must now be positioned behind the client, assisting at the trunk as the client's weight is supported on the elbows (Figure 74). The progression to sitting

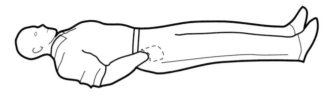

Fig 67. *Supine to sit for the spinal cord injured client-wrist extension method. The client starts in a supine position, placing the hands in the pockets of the pants, belt loops, or under the thighs.*

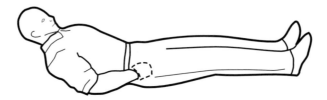

Fig 68. *The client then forcefully contracts the biceps and wrist extensors to initiate the head lift. The client should simultaneously tuck in the chin and pull up with the neck and shoulders. This action may need to be repeated several times. The nurse can assist by standing at the side of the bed facing the client. The nurse should reach behind both scapulae, assisting the upper trunk off the bed. Never pull the client up by the shoulders.*

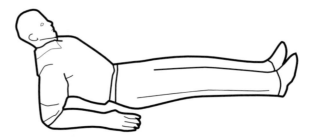

Fig 69. *As the client pulls up into a reclined position, a weight shift from side to side begins immediately, and the elbows are gradually repositioned until they are under the shoulders.*

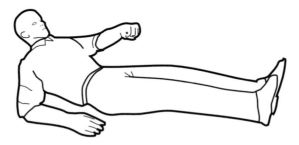

Fig 70. *The client then increases the magnitude of the weight shift until one arm is unweighted. The nurse can assist the lift off the pillow from the front, but should move to the back of the client once the client begins to swing the arms to avoid getting in the client's way. The best position is to kneel behind the client on the bed. The nurse should support the client's upper trunk up off the bed until the client is able to support the body independently.*

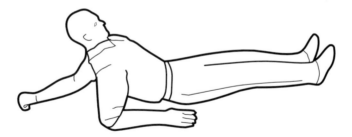

Fig 71. *The client immediately throws the unweighted arm back, positioning the upper extremity in elbow extension, shoulder extension, and external rotation. The nurse may need to assist the client with hand placement and correct positioning of the upper extremity.*

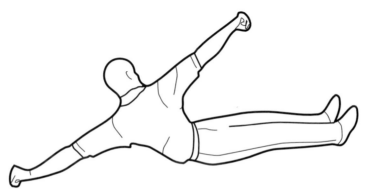

Fig 72. *The client immediately repeats the weight shift and throws the other extremity back. The nurse may need to support the client's trunk and assist the hand and arm position of the moving extremity.*

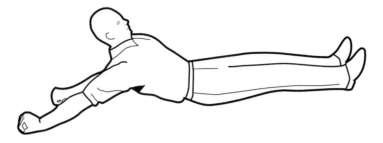

Fig 73. *The client should end with both extremities extended back, supporting the trunk in a reclined position. (Remember that this entire sequence is completed in one smooth motion.) The client can then shift back and forth, drawing the hands closer to the body, raising the trunk to a more erect position.*

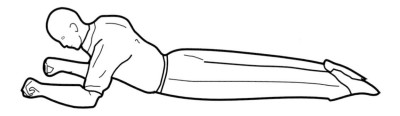

Fig 74. *Prone to sit for the spinal cord injured client. The client starts in a prone position, with the client's upper trunk supported on the elbows.*

starts as the client "walks" the elbows around to position the trunk in flexion in the long sitting position (Figures 75–77). The client throws back the opposite upper extremity and locks it in external rotation and extension. The same is repeated for the other arm (Figures 78–81). The nurse will need to assist the client to the upright position and help place the hands and arms to allow the client to prop back on the arms (Figure 82). If the client has triceps strength, then once the semiprone position is reached the client can fully extend the arms and walk the hands around until a long sitting position is reached.

Using the triceps/abdominal method for paraplegics, the client can pull straight up and prop on elbows. The client will extend the arms, pushing up into an upright position. The nurse can stand in front of the client and help pull the client forward by reaching over the shoulder to the scapula. The nurse should never pull forward on the client's neck or arms. Pulling the neck can cause seri-

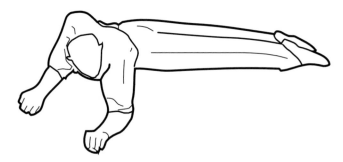

Fig 75. *The client begins by walking the elbows around to position the trunk to one side. The nurse can assist by kneeling behind the client's trunk and reaching under the sides of the client's trunk or over the scapula to the front of the shoulders. The nurse should never pull on the client's head, neck, or arms.*

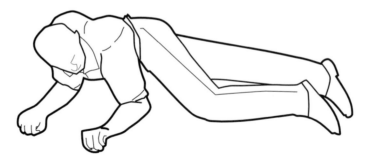

Fig 76. *The client continues to walk the trunk around as the trunk and pelvis begin to rotate backwards and the front lower extremity flexes at the hip and knee.*

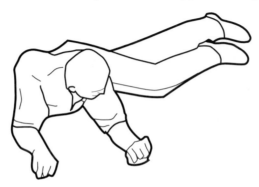

Fig 77. *The client walks the arms all the way around until the lower trunk and pelvis are in a sidelying position. The client in this picture then supports the upper trunk on the right upper extremity, unweighting the left.*

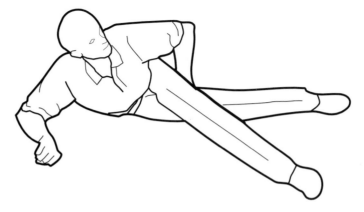

Fig 78. *The client then grabs the top leg, hooking the thigh with the wrist or hand.*

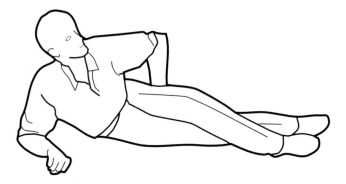

Fig 79. *The client then contracts the biceps of the left arm, pulling the upper trunk towards the leg. At the same time, the client is pushing away from the bed with the right upper extremity moving the trunk toward an erect position.*

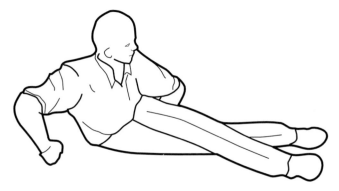

Fig 80. *As the client moves away from the bed, the right arm can be repositioned to allow the client to push the upper trunk up to a sitting position. The nurse can kneel behind the client supporting the upper trunk guiding the client to a sitting position. The nurse should not hold onto the client's shoulders or arms, as this restricts the client's ability.*

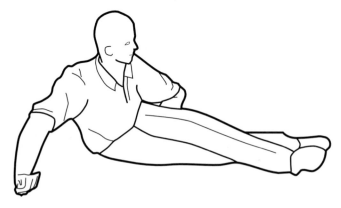

Fig 81. *As the trunk moves to an upright position, the client can position the arms in back of the trunk to allow the client to recline back on the arms.*

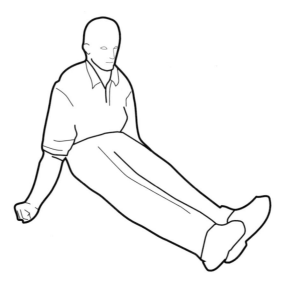

Fig 82. *Once the client has reached a long sitting position, the nurse can assist in uncrossing the legs. The nurse can also assist scooting in this position. The nurse should always assist the client from behind. If the client's arms collapse, the nurse will be in position to support the upper trunk. The nurse reaches under the ischial tuberosities as the client performs a depression and the nurse helps to unweight the pelvis and slide the pelvis forward. If the client is scooting backward, the legs should be flexed slightly to reduce the drag on the bed.*

ous injury to the client and pulling on the arms will restrict upper extremity mobility.

Scooting. The bed should be flat with the client long sitting in the bed. The nurse can assist with scooting from behind the client. To scoot forward in the bed, the quadriplegic client balances in a tripod position, propped back on the arms. The client performs a depression and pushes the buttocks away from the hands. The nurse assists by reaching under the ischial tuberosities and helps the client to unweight and move the buttocks forward. The client repositions the hands and repeats this motion until the client has moved forward in the bed. To scoot backward, the client assumes the same long sitting position with the nurse assisting from behind. There will be less drag of the lower extremities if the legs are bent up slightly and allowed to fall out to the side (Figure 82). The client performs a depression and pulls the buttocks back toward the hands. The nurse assists the unweighting and backward movement of the buttocks. The client repositions the hands and repeats the same motion until the client has moved back in bed.

Lower Extremity Management. To move the lower extremities on and off of the bed, the quadriplegic client must balance on one elbow and use the opposite upper extremity to pull or walk the legs toward the direction that the client wants to go. To pull the legs up onto the bed, the client will prop on one elbow. The other arm hooks onto the leg that is closest to the bed by using wrist extensors, or a thigh strap (Figure 83). As the client leans away from the leg, the opposite arm is used to pull the leg along until it is on the bed (Figure 84). The nurse will assist with pulling the leg up onto the bed. The client then hooks onto the other leg and pulls it onto the bed as well (Figures 85 and 86). To move the legs off the bed, the client will perform the same sequence of movements in the opposite direction. Because hospital beds are small, most clients will choose, if possible, to push their legs off of the bed instead of pulling them off to avoid leaning over the edge of the bed.

Transfers

To transfer off the bed onto a wheelchair, the wheelchair must first be positioned next to the bed at a 20- to 30-degree angle from the side of the bed. Make sure that the brakes are locked and all armrests and footrests are out of the way. If the

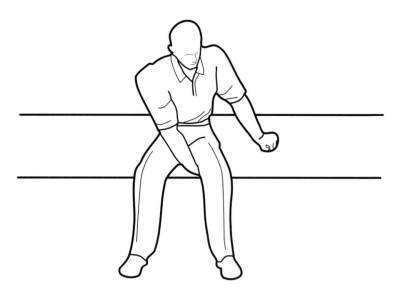

Fig 83. *Lower extremity management. To move the legs up onto the bed, the client first balances supporting the trunk on one extremity. The other arm hooks onto the leg that is closest to the bed.*

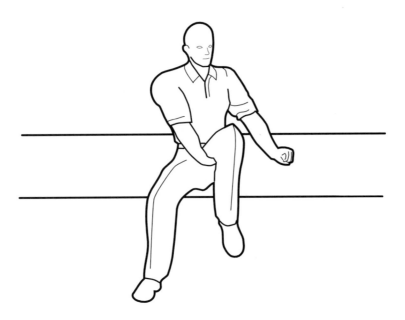

Fig 84. *As the client leans onto the supporting upper extremity, the opposite hand is used to lift the leg onto the bed.*

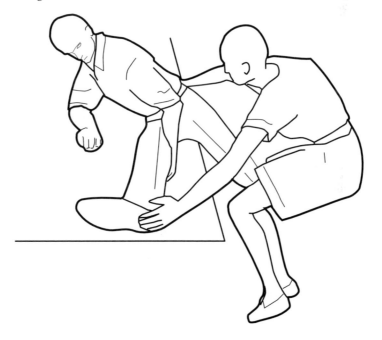

Fig 85. *If the client is quadriplegic and cannot lift the leg, the client can hook the leg and lean onto the supporting elbow dragging the leg up onto the bed. The nurse should assist the leg up onto the bed sitting close to the edge of the bed to prevent the client from falling if the client should lose balance.*

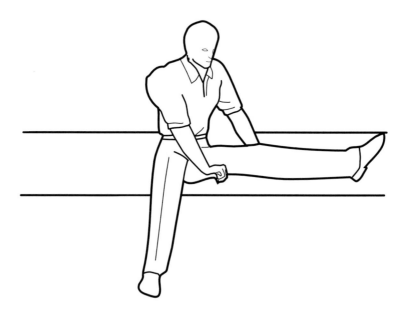

Fig 86. *Once the leg is positioned securely on the bed, the same sequence is repeated for the opposite lower extremity. Straps may be placed around the client's thighs to give the client something to hook onto if unable to grab the thigh.*

client is transferring from the wheelchair to the bed, he or she should be enycouraged to remove the wheelchair features and set up the transfer. This can be done by hooking the wrist of one arm under the thigh of the opposite leg and lifting the foot off of the wheelchair. The client can then lean forward to remove the footrests. There are two types of transfers that the complete spinal cord injury client will use: the depression transfer and the sliding board transfer.

The sliding board transfer will be used by clients with C6 quadriplegia or above. To make the transfer easier, the height of the bed can be raised slightly above the chair. The client will start by placing the sliding board under the thigh bridging the gap between the bed and the wheelchair. The board should not be placed too far back under the buttocks or the client will slide forward off the edge of the board. If the board is too far forward the client will slide off the back of the board during the transfer. Both feet should contact the floor (Figure 87). The nurse should assist the client from the front by reaching around to the back of the client's trunk or under the ischial tuberosities. The nurse can also lean the client forward and reach over the top of the client's trunk to the ischial tuberosities. The nurse should make sure that the client's head is facing the trailing leg. The nurse can also sandwich the client's lower extremities between their legs, but should never "block" the knees. The client should place both hands down, one on each surface, placing the trailing hand close to the trailing leg. The client will proceed across the board by twisting the upper trunk toward the trailing shoulder and pushing with the trailing arm as the forward arm pulls (Figure 88). To assist the client, the nurse should hold onto the client and rock backward to unweight the pelvis and assist the lateral movement across the board. The nurse should never attempt to lift the client up. The client's upper extremities are repositioned and the process is repeated until the client is safely onto the new surface (Figure 89). If a second team member is needed to assist, he or she will be positioned behind the client. To assist the client in scooting back, the nurse should lean the client forward to unweight the pelvis. At the same time, pressure should be applied through the lower extremities to move the client back into the seat. This may be repeated as many times as needed.

The depression transfer will be used for clients with C7 quadriplegia and below. If the client is severely physically dependent or if the transfer is between two surfaces positioned far apart, the sliding board may still be used for these clients as well. The set-up for the depression transfer is similar to that of the depression transfer without the board. The nurse can assist the client from the front. The cli-

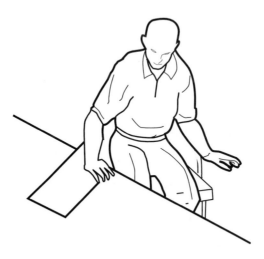

Fig 87. *Sliding board transfer. The client should be encouraged to remove the armrest and footrest and position the chair next to the bed with as little help as possible. The nurse must assist the client from the front. The nurse should assist the client in scooting to the edge of the chair and place the sliding board under the client. Once the nurse assists the placement of the sliding board, the nurse should stand in front of the client, supporting the lower extremities by placing their legs around the outside of the client's legs.*

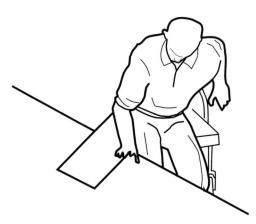

Fig 88. *The nurse should then reach around to the back of the client under the ischial tuberosities or the trunk. The client's head should be facing the trailing leg. The client above then pushes with the left upper extremity and pulling with the right. At the same time, the client twists the head and upper trunk to the left, pushing the lower trunk and pelvis across the sliding board. The nurse helps to unweight the pelvis and move the client laterally across the board.*

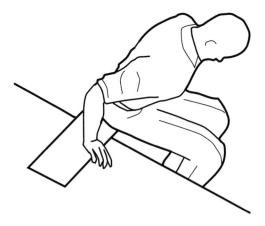

Fig 89. *Each time the client moves, the hands and arms are repositioned to give the client more leverage. This process is repeated until the client is safely onto the bed. Remember that the nurse should always hold onto the client, supporting the trunk once the client is seated on the bed to avoid falling.*

ent will position both hands down with the trailing hand close to the trailing thigh. The client will then lean forward slightly to unweight the pelvis (Figure 90). As the client performs a depression, the trailing arm pushes as the forward arm pulls the body over to the new surface. The client's upper body should always twist toward the trailing shoulder. The nurse should assist the lift off the chair and onto the new surface (Figure 91). The client should not be allowed to drag the buttocks from one surface to the other. Special care must be taken to ensure that the client does not land on top of the wheel of the wheelchair. The client should then be scooted to the back of the chair.

Pressure Release

Once the client is safely in the chair, the client must be encouraged to perform a pressure release to prevent skin breakdown. The quadriplegic client should lean all the way forward, resting their trunk in their lap. The nurse will have to assist the client from the front by gently lowering the client forward until he or she is in the correct position. The client can also lean to the side, unweighting one ischial tuberosity. The same must be done to unweight the other side. The client

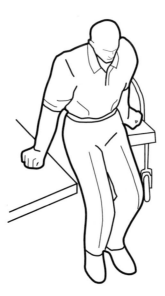

Fig 90. *Depression transfers. The client scoots to the edge of the chair by performing a depression and moving the pelvis forward. The client must be positioned with both feet flat on the floor with the feet positioned back under the knees. The client flexes forward at the hips and performs a depression. The nurse assists from the front.*

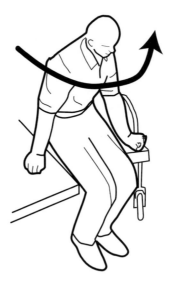

Fig 91. *To move laterally onto the new surface, the client pushes with the trailing arm and pulls with the opposite arm, twisting the upper body to the left. The nurse should assist the unweighting of the pelvis and the lateral movement onto the new surface.*

needs to maintain the pressure relief position for 1 minute. The nurse should assist the client back up to an upright position. The procedure should be repeated every 30 minutes to 1 hour during the time that the client is in the chair.

Summary

The nurse plays a crucial role in the rehabilitation of the neurologically involved client. Because of the amount of time that members of the nursing staff spend with each client on a day-to-day basis, they become a valuable source of continuity during the time that the client is in the hospital. In this chapter a variety of bed mobility and transfer techniques have been presented to assist the nurse in managing the neurologically involved client. These techniques will allow the nurse and client to maximize safety and efficiency while reinforcing skills that the client will need to successfully transition back into a home setting. As hospital stays become shorter, it becomes increasingly important for all team members to work together to create a quality treatment delivery system that will allow client's to reach their full potential during their hospitalization.

References

Hickey, J. V. (1992). *The clinical practice of neurological and neurosurgical nursing* (3rd ed., p. 630). Philadelphia: Lippincott.

Kandel, E. R., & Schwartz, J. H. (1985). *Principles of neuroscience* (2nd ed., pp. 202–204). New York: Elsevier.

Maddox, S. (1987). *Spinal network.* Boulder, CO: Sam Maddox.

Umphred, D. A. (1995). *Neurological rehabilitation* (3rd ed.). St. Louis, MO: Mosby–Year Book.

Suggested Readings

Charness, A. (1986). *Stroke/head injury: A guide to functional outcomes in physical therapy management.* Rockville, MD: Aspen.

Fisher, B. (1987). *Journal of Head Trauma Rehabilitation, 2*(2), 72–79.

Fisher, B., & Woll, S. (1992). *NDT (Bobath) approach to adult hemiplegia.* Downey, CA: Rancho Los Amigos Medical Center.

Fisher, B., & Yakura, J. (1993). *Orthopaedic Physical Therapy Clinics of North America,* 1059–1516.

Nixon, V. (1985). Spinal cord injury: *A guide to functional outcomes in physical therapy management.* Rockville, MD: Aspen.

O'Sullivan, S. B., & Schmitz, T. J. (1988). *Physical rehabilitation: Assessment and treatment* (2nd ed.). Philadelphia, PA: F.A. Davis.

CHAPTER 27

Communication Processes: Disorders and Strategies

Wendy E. B. Perez

Key Words *Alternative/Augmentative Communication (AAC)*
Alzheimer's Disease
Amyotrophic Lateral Sclerosis (ALS)
Aphasias
Apraxia
Articulation
Attention
Auditory Comprehension
Cerebrovascular Accidents (CVAs)
Cognition
Communication Process
Cueing
Dysarthria
Executive Functions
Impulsivity
Initiation
Judgment
Language
Larynx
Learning
Memory
Multiple Sclerosis (MS)
Neurogenic
Parkinson's Disease
Pragmatics
Problem Solving
Reasoning
Speech
Speech/Language Pathologist
Traumatically Brain Injured (TBI)
Verbal Expression

Objectives 1. Describe important cognitive, language, and speech production processes involved in normal communication.

2. Explain how various common neurologic disorders disrupt these processes and cause communication problems.

3. Provide principles for facilitating the clearest possible level of communication in people who have communication disorders.

Introduction

People communicate in varied ways and for many purposes: Two friends meet for a conversation over coffee, a mother rocks her baby and sings a lullaby, an executive writes e-mail correspondence to a co-worker, a student reads a textbook . . . the list could go on indefinitely. Communication, in its many forms, is a part of daily life that is usually done naturally and nearly effortlessly. However, many **neurogenic** disorders, including stroke, traumatic brain injury, Parkinson's disease, and Alzheimer's disease, cause problems that disrupt communication and bring frustration and isolation in their wake. The purpose of this chapter is to suggest ways to approach persons with communication disorders that will facilitate the best possible level of communication. Unfortunately, there are no easy answers, no simple explanations of disorders and their treatments. In fact, although our knowledge base continues to grow, our understanding of how the brain and nervous system actually perform the complex processes that result in communication behaviors is still very limited. However, there are some basic principles that can provide guidance when working with people who need help to communicate. To provide an understanding of these principles, this chapter presents an overview of some of the important cognitive, language, and speech production processes involved in communication, describes common communication deficits arising from various neurogenic disorders, and discusses techniques for facilitating communication.

Although some techniques for improving communication are universally applicable, others are unique to particular clients. To provide the best care for a communicatively impaired client, a **speech/language pathologist** should be consulted. The speech/language pathologist performs a complete evaluation, determines whether a communication therapy program is indicated, and provides specific recommendations to the medical staff on how best to facilitate communication with the client. Because nurses need to communicate with patients frequently throughout the day and in a wide variety of situations, they have the opportunity to observe how the client attempts to communicate and how often he or she is successful. When the nurse is able to share these observations with the speech/language pathologist and in return receive suggestions on how to better facilitate communication, the two disciplines work together as a team. Both the nurse and the speech pathologist can gain important insight into the patient's abilities when they share their observations and concerns. The client will benefit from this by receiving more efficient and effective nursing care, as well as opportunities to practice communication skills in functional settings. The nurse who has a basic understanding of normal communication processes, common communication disorders, and principles of communication facilitation will be both a more effective nurse and a stronger contributor to the medical care team.

Processes Involved in Normal Communication Thought and Language

The normal **communication process** involves three major and complex processes: thought (cognition), language, and speech production. Although the relationship between thought and language has been an issue of extended investigation and debate, both common sense and clinical experience indicate that at least some ideas (such as mathematical or spatial reasoning, emotions, etc.) are nonverbal and, when they are expressed in words, must somehow be mentally "translated" into verbal form. Most people have, at one time or another, experienced difficulties putting some "nonverbal" ideas into words. Also, as is discussed in more detail later, certain communication disorders demonstrate that thought can be disordered without affecting language ability (e.g., some traumatic brain injuries), and that at least some forms of thought (e.g., visual memory) can remain unimpaired in the presence of severe language disorder. However, in order to have normal, clear communication, both cognitive processes (thinking) and language processes must be intact.

Language and Speech

In addition to recognizing the distinction between thought and language, it is important to understand the difference between language and speech. **Language** is a symbolic communication system. For example, American Sign Language and ancient Latin are both languages, even though they are not spoken. **Speech,** on the other hand, refers only to the physical process of producing verbal sounds. While language is a thought process, speech is an anatomical and mechanical process. To use a musical analogy, language could be compared to the musical ideas that a composer creates in his or her head, whereas speech would be analogous to the sounds made by the musicians playing the symphony the composer writes. Given this distinction, it becomes apparent that although cognition and language are necessary to communication, speech is a typical but not necessary feature. That is, one can communicate through written language that is never spoken aloud (just as the composer can write music that is never performed), because the ideas, whether encoded mentally as linguistic or musical symbols, exist separately from their physical production (which is speech production or production of sound from a musical instrument). A person who for some reason is unable to speak, but continues to have normal cognitive and language skills, can communicate complex ideas through other methods (such as writing, sign language, or charades). However, problems with any of the processes involved in cognition, language, or speech production will affect the quality of communication. In addition, problems in each of the areas may occur together, in a variety of combinations. However, to simplify this discussion, the areas of cognition, language, and speech production are considered in turn, with some examples provided of clinical situations in which these problems often overlap.

Role of Cognitive Skills in Communication

Because cognitive skills are necessary to develop intent and meaning in communication, they are considered first. In general, **cognition** refers to the thinking skills through which individuals acquire knowledge of the world and continue to process this knowledge. It is an inclusive term referring to a wide range of skills including attention, memory, learning, conceptualization, abstract reasoning, problem solving, judgment, visual processing, initiation, goal formulation, self-regulation, planning, and others. Although language is an aspect of cognitive functioning, it is considered separately and in more detail, because of its special role in communication. Cognitive skills, then, allow us to process information and formulate appropriate behavioral responses. Any cognitive deficit may affect the appropriateness and effectiveness of communication behavior; but because of the limitations of this chapter, just a few of the most common cognitive disorders are discussed.

Attention

Of all the cognitive skills, **attention** is perhaps the most basic and essential, not only to communication, but to the ability to be alert and aware of one's surroundings. Being able to pay attention to what the conversational partner is saying is obviously necessary for effective communication. In fact, "paying attention" is not a single process, but rather a combination of complex processes critical to information processing. In the world around us, sights, sounds, smells, tastes, and textures bombard our senses. Because of the limitations of human sensory processing, certain stimuli, from among the myriad of information available at any one time, must be selected for processing. This most basic alerting and selection process, in which certain stimuli are attended to at the expense of others, occurs unconsciously, at the level of the reticular activating system (RAS) in the midbrain.

Beyond this basic level of alertness, attention involves a cluster of higher level capacities. *Focused* or *selective attention* refers to the ability to pay conscious attention to a particular stimulus at a given time without being distracted by competing stimuli. This is clearly important when engaged in a conversation, because the information may be lost if the listener becomes distracted by irrelevant stimuli in the environment. *Sustained attention* refers to the ability to continue to maintain selective attention over a period of time. Sophisticated attention skills include *alternating attention* (the ability to shift attention back and forth between activities, such as when watching a television program and doing homework during the commercials) and *divided attention* (the ability to engage in more than one activity at a time, such as driving a car and listening to the news on the radio). These higher level attention skills are mediated primarily in the prefrontal cortex.

Because the characteristic pattern of damage caused by closed head injury typically involves frontal lobe damage, attention deficits are a very common symptom in traumatically brain-injured people. Depending on the severity and nature of the attention deficits, and on what additional deficits the person has, a variety of communication problems may result. Severely injured people may be too lethargic to respond to simple questions, whereas mildly injured people may seem normal in conversation, but be unable to perform previously familiar tasks that require higher level attention skills (such as driving or cooking a meal). No matter what the severity of deficit, the best strategy for improving communication is to provide a simpler environment free of distractions and, when appropriate, use physical or visual cues to help focus attention on the topic under discussion. Unfortunately, medical care professionals often adapt to distracting environments and fail to notice how noisy or visually overwhelming a room or area can be.

One typical scenario involves a nurse who arrives to give a client his medications after breakfast. The television is on, the client's roommate has a visitor, the breakfast tray has not yet been cleared away, the client needs to use the toilet, and the nurse, in a hurry to pass medications and oblivious to the distractions, asks the client to list the medications and their functions. In this situation, the client's response will probably not be reflective of his actual knowledge. It would be most effective for the nurse to begin the interaction by minimizing the internal and external distractions, in order to enable the client to perform at his best. This simplification would include taking the client to the bathroom (to eliminate discomfort which causes internal distraction), turning the television off (to reduce external visual and sound distractions), and clearing the breakfast tray out of the way (visual distractor). In addition to simplifying the environment, the nurse might consider simplifying the task she is presenting to the client. That is, instead of asking him to name all his medications and their purposes, she could make it simpler by giving the name of the medication and then asking its purpose. Clients with attention deficits will frequently be unaware of their deficits or how best to compensate for them, so nurses need to be particularly aware of how best to assist them. Intervention to assist clients with attention deficits would include simplifying and organizing the environment, simplifying the activities presented, breaking activities into shorter sessions (with quiet times provided in between), and providing physical and verbal cues to direct attention to important information. Certain interventions will be more effective with different clients, depending on their needs.

Memory

Memory and the ability to learn new information are also cognitive functions that are fundamental to normal communication. Like attention, memory actually involves multiple functions, and the theoretical analysis of these functions is controversial. For the purposes of this discussion, memory is divided in the following hierarchy of functions:

1. Short-term or immediate memory
2. Long-term memory
   a. Procedural (implicit) memory
   b. Declarative (explicit) memory
      (1) Semantic memory (general knowledge)
      (2) Episodic memory (personal timeline)
   c. Prospective memory

Short-term memory has many names including immediate, working, or primary memory. This is a limited memory, both in terms of time (approximately 2 minutes) and capacity (approximately seven items). It is perfect for remembering a new telephone number just long enough to dial it, but if the number is to be used more than once, it must be either written down or memorized, that is, transferred to long-term memory.

Long-term memory, which is used generally to describe what is remembered for longer than that brief interval of short-term memory, has several other subdivisions. One way of describing different types of long-term memory is to make a distinction between those memories that involve information that can be verbally described (called declarative memory) and those memories which involve a process that is nonverbal (called procedural memory). Declarative memory is the familiar type of memory in which one can verbally describe what is remembered. A test taken in school is an examination of the declarative memory for the information studied. In contrast, procedural memory involves the ability to gain knowledge about a procedure and improve skill in performance without necessarily being able to verbalize the skill. For example, a person may learn the route to a friend's house and be able to find his way there repeatedly, without being able to give clear verbal directions about how to do it. This example demonstrates that the same kind of information can be remembered in more than one way. That is, the person may initially learn how to get to the house by following written directions. Later, the person may memorize the street names and turns and recall them as he drives, perhaps looking for familiar landmarks. Later still, the person becomes so familiar with the route that the drive becomes nearly automatic and the street names are forgotten. At the point in the process when the street names are necessary, this route is held in declarative memory, and requires conscious effort to perform. At the point when the drive is made almost without thinking about it, it is held in procedural memory, and it requires very little conscious effort to perform. Another typical example of procedural memory is the process of learning to drive a car with a manual transmission. This distinction between remembering how to do something (procedural memory) and remembering how to explain how something is done (declarative memory) becomes significant for many people who experience memory problems, because procedural memory for simple tasks (such as how to dress, groom, and bathe) tends to be better preserved than declarative memory. In addition, the ability to learn simple new tasks (e.g., putting a puzzle together) tends to be better preserved than the ability to learn simple verbal information (e.g., reciting a shopping list). Studies have shown that, given repetition, patients with severe memory problems can show improved performance on simple tasks, even when they cannot recall ever having previously performed the task (Bondi & Kaszniak, 1991). Therefore, in rehabilitation, where the focus is on learning and relearning skills, it is important to assess a client's ability to actually do an activity, rather than his or her ability to describe it. A patient who is unable to learn and repeat verbal information may still demonstrate ability to benefit from rehabilitation training in activities that are simple, repetitive, and routine (such as self-care).

Just as long-term memory is subdivided into procedural and declarative types, declarative memory is further divided into semantic and episodic memories. Semantic memory is the ability to recall general facts. That George Washington was the first president of the United States and Abraham Lincoln was president during the Civil War are generally well-known facts of American history. These questions are often used to assess integrity of semantic memory. Semantic memory also includes personal general information, such as a home address, a spouse's name, and the city of birth. Episodic memory, on the other hand, is memory for specific events that have been personally experienced. (Although city of birth is related to a personal event, it is not a piece of information that is remembered because of the experience. Rather, it is remembered because it was learned at a later date!) Episodic memory appears to involve a mental time line on which events are related to each other. Your ability to describe what you did over the weekend is an example of recent episodic memory, whereas the story you can tell about a favorite childhood birthday party is an example of a past episodic memory. In patients who experience memory problems, both semantic and episodic memory appear to function on a temporal gradient. That is, the earlier the memory was stored, the more likely it is to be preserved. Facts learned in elementary school tend to be easier to remember than who the current president is, and memories of vivid childhood experiences may be more easily recalled than the events of the previous day (or hour). When communicating with persons who have memory problems, then, it is often helpful to build rapport by first introducing familiar topics from the past, before attempting to assess their ability to recall new information. Similarly, family members who are impressed that the client can remember the address of the house where he lived 50 years ago should be cautioned that this is not indicative of functional memory for new information.

Although memory is most often tested by requesting that information learned in the past be recalled and recited (declarative memory), this is probably not the most frequently used or most important type of memory. On a daily and even moment-to-moment basis, we are recalling what we are in the process of doing and what we need to be doing next. This kind of memory, the memory for what is to be done at a particular time or in a particular sequence, is referred to as *prospective memory.* Instead of remembering what happened in the past, it is the remembering of what is to be done now or in the future. In familiar terms, this includes remembering to turn in a completed assignment on the due date, remembering to send a birthday card to a friend, and remembering to pick up groceries on the way home from work. Of all the memory skills, prospective memory or "remembering to remember" is probably the most complex, because it requires attention, short-term memory, long-term declarative memory, episodic memory, as well as other cognitive skills, in order to function. It is also probably the most critical skill for organizing and completing daily activities.

All of these memory functions can be damaged by a variety of neurogenic disorders including traumatic brain injury, anoxia, chronic long-term alcohol abuse resulting in Korsakoff's syndrome, and other forms of dementia, such as *Alzheimer's* disease. Although each of these etiologies tends to differentially affect aspects of the neuroanatomical systems involved in memory and thus produce somewhat different functional deficits, this chapter again focuses on several guiding principles to improve communication with memory-impaired clients.

First, to facilitate communication, and particularly if it is necessary to teach new information, it is important to have a general understanding of a client's memory skills, including both strengths and weaknesses. Although formal assessment by a neuropsychologist is very helpful, it is not necessary in order to gain a working knowledge of the client's needs. A combination of structured questioning and behavioral observations can suggest how best to assist the client. Natural conversation that includes questions regarding the client's recent medical history and activities (so long as there is a way to check the answers for accuracy) will provide a general picture of the client's ability to recall and describe recent personal experiences (declarative, episodic memory). Questions regarding past personal information (such as date and place of birth, family members, etc.) tap into areas of memory that should be relatively well preserved even in clients with relatively severe memory deficits. Depending on the length of time the nurse is able to spend with the client, more sophisticated but subtle assessment of prospective memory skills can be carried out by asking the client to remind the nurse to do something at the end of the interaction. For example, at a bedside intake interview, the nurse might say, "Before I leave, I need to take your blood pressure one more time. Remind me, if I forget, okay?" Later, the nurse is ready to leave and signals this with "Okay, I guess that's about it. I'll see you later," and pauses, to see if the client will remind her to take the blood pressure again. If not, another cue can be given to the client, such as "Let's see, I think there was something else I was going to do . . . what was it?" If the client still doesn't remember to remind the nurse, then the nurse should "remember" on her own and go ahead and take the blood pressure. Of course, in an informal assessment such as this, one failure should not be taken as conclusive evidence of a memory deficit, but it is one indicator that a particular client may need assistance to perform prospective memory tasks (such as taking medications, doing exercises, or reviewing educational materials). If it is possible to make behavioral observations over the course of more than 1 day, these will be very revealing.

Because procedural and declarative memories are qualitatively different, it is particularly important to observe whether the client is able to perform certain tasks, verbally explain how to do them, or both. Some clients (such as those who have experienced right hemisphere strokes) may have intact verbal skills and be able to give a general explanation (e.g., "I have to take medication in the morning and at night") without being able to follow through and perform the task (e.g., if told to call the nurse in order to request medications at a certain time, the client would be unable to remember to do it). Others (such as those who have experienced left hemisphere strokes) may have impaired verbal skills and be unable to state what should be done, but will seek out the nurse passing medications and nonverbally identify the correct medications. Through this kind of observation and conversation with the client, the nurse can gain a better understanding of the kind of assistance the client needs.

Clearly, whenever an informal memory screening suggests that deficits are present, the client should be referred for evaluation by a neuropsychologist and/or speech/language pathologist. Therapists with experience in assessment and treatment of clients with memory deficits can determine whether a client may benefit from training to use external memory aids such as calendars (for orientation and/or prospective memory tasks), lists, or signs with explanations (e.g., "turn right to go to the dining room"). The therapist will work with the treating team to determine the client's needs and to demonstrate how to assist the client to use the memory aids.

Whether or not the client receives formal treatment, the nurse must modify his or her approach in order to provide the most appropriate care and teaching. When memory deficits are severe, the client is often disoriented. Environmental cues, including calendars, photographs, and simple signs (such as "John's room"), can help the client be more comfortable in, and aware of, the current environment. Most clients who have memory deficits, of whatever type or severity, can benefit from repetition of predictable routines and a well-organized environment. The old adage "a place for everything and everything in its place" describes an organized and simplified environment, which can assist a memory-impaired client in locating needed items in a familiar place. Similarly, if certain activities, and the daily schedule, are always carried out in the same way, the repetition of the sequence of steps may eventually allow the client to use relatively intact procedural memory to perform the activities, even if he or she can't describe how to do them. However, the nurse should be careful not to assume that a client recalls and understands the purpose for a particular procedure just because it has been performed numerous times. Until it is clear that the client recognizes the procedure and understands what it is for, the nurse should always provide a simple statement explaining what is happening. On the other hand, it is important that this information be presented in a matter-of-fact way, not in a condescending or patronizing manner. Clearly, in order to carry out assigned responsibilities for the client's basic care and teaching, the nurse needs to have a good general understanding of the client's memory and learning skills.

Overestimation of a client's memory skills can have dangerous consequences. For example, a nurse tells a **traumatically brain-injured (TBI)** client who is sitting on the toilet to call her when he is finished and ready to transfer back to his wheelchair. He states that he will call her when he needs her. She then leaves him in order to assist another client. The TBI client finishes, attempts to stand up, and falls. There are several possible causes of this communication problem. First, the TBI client may have forgotten the instruction he was given, or he may have forgotten how to use the call system. The nurse could have asked the client to actually demonstrate how he would use the call system when he needed her. However, even if the client were able to use the call system, he might not have initiated using it, because he failed to recognize that he needed assistance in this situation, owing to a deficit in judgment. Or, he may have realized that he needed assistance, initiated using the call system, but, instead of waiting for the nurse to arrive, impulsively attempted the transfer without assistance. In this scenario, memory, self-monitoring, initiation, impulsivity, and judgment are all possible causes of the communication problem. Clearly, clients with any of these cognitive problems are at increased risk for falls and other accidents. To provide the extra assistance needed by clients who have memory deficits, the nurse needs to present information in a simplified, repetitive manner, check understanding and recall by having the client both perform the activity and verbalize the information, provide visual cues in the environment, and use external memory aids, such as calendars and lists, as appropriate.

Executive Functions

In the scenario described above, the traumatically brain-injured client may have had a variety of cognitive deficits in addition to his memory problem. Initiation, planning, self-monitoring, self-regulation, goal formation, and judgment are frequently impaired following traumatic brain injury. These cognitive processes, which all involve self-regulation, are called **executive functions.** Just as a business executive is responsible for planning, monitoring and organizing the corporation's behavior, so executive functions are the processes involved with organizing the individual's behavior. The cognitive skills described as executive functions are typically discussed as a cluster of processes dealing with aspects of purposeful behavior that involve intention, planning, acting, monitoring effectiveness of action, and modifying action accordingly. Deficits in executive function are common in clients with neurogenic disorders such as TBI, right cerebral vascular accident, Parkinson's disease, and anoxia. Frequently, clients whose deficits appear to be moderate in severity will demonstrate discrepancies between their verbal skills and their performance skills. Although they may be able to describe verbally how to solve a hypothetical problem situation (such as, "What would you do if you locked your keys in your car?"), they may have difficulty solving problems in real life, such as figuring out what to do if they get lost on the way from their own room to the dining room. To have an accurate understanding of a client's actual skills, and need for supervision, it is very important to observe both verbal skills and behavioral patterns, in a variety of settings and at different times.

As with other cognitive deficits, the presentation of executive function problems is highly variable. Ironically, a single client may have a seemingly contradictory combination of deficits. For example, it is fairly common for clients who have sustained right hemisphere **cerebrovascular accidents (CVAs)** to display both initiation and impulsivity problems. For example, when provided with a breakfast tray, they may sit and do nothing for a long period of time. Then, when handed the spoon, they may start feeding themselves large spoonfuls of cereal, one after another, without stopping to chew and swallow. When cued to slow down, they may put down the spoon and stop eating for a long period of time, until they are again given the spoon. Their behavior in conversation may reveal similar difficulties. They may not initiate any simple social interaction with other patients, but when asked a question, they may launch into a long, complex, tangential story and continue talking indefinitely until interrupted.

Although executive function deficits may at times seem complex and frustrating, a common sense approach will often be effective. As with cases of attention and memory deficits, clients with executive function deficits will perform better in a calm, organized environment. In a sense, these clients need external direction to do what they are unable to direct themselves to do, because of their difficulties with self-regulation. However, the goal should always be to set up the task so that the client can do as much of it him- or herself as possible. In the case of the breakfast example, it might be helpful to put only one dish of food, rather than a whole tray, in front of the client. If the initiation/impulsivity problem persists, a verbal cue, along with a simple explanation, can be provided. For example, "In order to eat without choking, you need to take a small bite, chew and swallow before you take another bite. . . . Put down your spoon between bites." After this instruction, if necessary, the nurse can verbally cue the client at each step, intervening physically only as needed. The nurse should attempt to fade out the cueing, while checking to make sure the client maintains the appropriate behavior. This approach is based on the therapeutic principle of providing the least amount of **cueing** (or assistance) needed to elicit the desired behavior. As the client practices producing the target behavior given one level of cueing, the cueing is gradually diminished while the client attempts to sustain the same level of performance. The level of assistance required is easier to visualize in the case of activities of daily living than in the case of conversational skills, but the principles are the same. For example, maximum assistance for eating may involve hand-over-hand guidance as the client puts food in his or her mouth. Maximum assistance for communicating basic needs may mean observing nonverbal behaviors indicating that the client is hungry (e.g., client reaches for a snack on the bedside table) and then asking, "Are you hungry?" as you provide the snack, and encouraging the client to verbalize or use a head nod to indicate yes. In comparison, minimal assistance for eating might mean setting up the meal tray. In the case of verbal interaction, a minimal level of cueing might include guessing the word a client is searching for and then providing the initial sound in order to help them retrieve it (e.g., "Are you trying to tell me about your vacation to Fr____" and the client fills in "France, yes, I went to Paris for a week last year.").

When intervening to increase initiation or reduce impulsivity in conversation, the target behaviors may seem more abstract, but the intervention approach is basically the same. No matter what the communication deficit, it is important to give clear supportive feedback with a model or suggestion of alternative, more effective behavior. It is often helpful to emphasize the two-way nature of conversation. For example, if the client has **initiation** problems and does not make requests to fulfill basic needs, it can be helpful to try to elicit verbal requests by giving multiple choices such as "Do you need to go to the bathroom or would you like something to eat?" If the patient can respond with a single word answer, such as "eat," the nurse can then encourage the client to say a little more by giving a sentence completion cue, "Tell me what you'd like. Try starting with, 'I would like to eat ____.' " If the client has **impulsivity** problems and tends to interrupt when the nurse is trying to provide education, the nurse can respond with, "I know you have a lot of important things to say, and I want to give you time to say them, but right now I need you to listen carefully . . . you need to know ____. Now, I need to make sure you understood that, can you show me how ____." The emphasis on communication as a mutual process of give and take must be sincere. It is important that the listener (or nurse) provide clear feedback regarding what he or she does and doesn't understand when the client is trying to communicate. It is equally important that when the client is able to get his point across, he receive a response to the content of the message rather than a response to the quality of his speech. Effective communication takes time, but ineffective communication is a waste of time.

Of course, there are limits on the amount of time a nurse can spend with any particular client. It is important to be clear about this. It is fine to say, "I wish I could take the time to listen to the whole story you want to tell me, but I can only spend five more minutes with you. In order to better understand what you need, I need to know _____. " Even if clients cannot understand everything you say to them, they will generally appreciate a respectful tone and manner, and recognize that you have other responsibilities. It is also helpful to involve others in providing feedback to the client about the effectiveness of their communication attempts. Clients who are impulsive and tangential can often benefit from participating in group conversations in which equal turn-taking is encouraged. Clients may be more open to feedback from their peers than from medical professionals. Although the nurse is probably not involved in group treatment sessions (although educational classes may fall in this category), he or she is in a good position to observe which clients may benefit from introductions and informal opportunities to socialize. Whether the client's cognitive deficits are in the areas of attention, memory, executive functions, or some other domain, opportunities to practice daily activities and communication skills in a supportive atmosphere will be therapeutic.

Language

Whereas cognitive deficits impair communication skills by disrupting abilities to organize ideas and actions, aphasia impairs communication by disrupting language skills. The primary processes involved in language use are auditory comprehension, verbal expression, and gesture, while the secondary processes are reading and writing. **Auditory comprehension** is the ability to understand spoken language. **Verbal expression** involves the ability to retrieve words mentally and use them to formulate meaningful sentences. *Gesture* is the production of head, hand, or body movements that are associated with specific meaning (e.g., a head nod for yes, a "thumbs up" for OK). At a holistic level of analysis, involving the interaction of linguistic and other cognitive skills, is the function of pragmatics. **Pragmatics** involves the ability to use language within real situations to accomplish a variety of different purposes (e.g., requesting information, giving directions, describing events, expressing emotions). Knowledge of pragmatics is also involved in determining the socially appropriate way to interact in conversation, such as when to maintain eye contact, how to take turns, and even how close to position yourself in relationship to your conversational partner. *Reading* and *writing* are secondary language processes because they are learned skills that involve ability to interrelate internal language symbols and their graphic representation.

Aphasia

In most humans, language skills appear to be localized in the left hemisphere. (Apparently, a very small percentage of the population, typically left-handed persons, have right hemisphere or bilateral language representation.) Any trauma or disease process that causes damage to these areas will result in language impairments. These language impairments are termed **aphasias.** Benson (1996) provides five helpful aphorisms regarding brain damage and aphasia:

1. Aphasia is a product of brain damage.
2. It is the neuroanatomical location of brain damage, not the etiology, that determines aphasic symptomatology.
3. When aphasia is prominent, focal structural pathology involving language area structures must be suspected.
4. Different pathological states can produce identical aphasic syndromes.
5. Damage to nonlanguage areas of brain produces little or no aphasic symptomatology.

Although several aphasia classification systems have been developed, it is primarily important to understand the difference between fluent and nonfluent aphasias. *Fluent aphasia,* also called receptive or posterior aphasia, results from damage in the postrolandic language areas (including the parietal-insular area, temporal isthmus, superior and middle temporal gyri, temporal-occipital area, parieto-occipital area, and angular gyrus). Although symptoms vary depending on the particular areas involved, the typical language deficits seen in these clients include relatively severe auditory comprehension deficits and fluent, relatively grammatical verbal output marked by nonsense words. Depending on the severity of the disorder, clients with fluent aphasia have difficulty following simple verbal directions, answering yes/no questions, and identifying, from a group of common objects, the one named by the examiner. In addition, the client has difficulty monitoring his or her own verbal output. Thus, although the disorder is sometimes called receptive aphasia, it also disrupts the client's expressive skills. The fluent aphasic person's speech is often characterized by excessive talking that includes a variety of complex sound combinations, but is lacking in specific meaningful content. For example, the speaker may begin an utterance, "The whisbies and lootbies hustled but only shortly . . . "; the speaker might then continue indefinitely, without being able to respond relevantly to a simple question, because he or she does not understand the question, nor is the speaker able to monitor his or her verbal output. These "made up" words, which sound as though they should make sense but are not real words, are termed *jargon.* Wernicke's aphasia, named after the neurologist Carl Wernicke who first described this verbal behavior in a person who had damage to the left temperoparietal region, is the classic example of a fluent aphasia.

In contrast, the client with *nonfluent aphasia* presents a very different clinical picture. The classic example of a nonfluent, anterior or expressive type of aphasia is called Broca's aphasia, named after Paul Broca, a French neurologist. He not only described this pattern of language disorder, resulting from damage to the left supplementary motor area, he also broke theoretical ground by arguing that this and other deficit patterns could be used to localize functions to different parts of the brain. A client with nonfluent aphasia has relatively intact receptive skills and thus is able to follow simple directions and identify items named by the examiner. However, he has limited ability to produce speech. If severely affected, the client may struggle to produce even familiar single words such as his own name, or the names of common objects such as "pen" and "watch." At a moderate level of severity, the client may be able to get simple ideas across in effortful, so-called agrammatic or telegraphic speech (because of its superficial resemblance to the economic speech of old-time telegrams). However, telegraphic speech typically involves breakdown of grammatical relationships and, therefore, the client's utterance involves not just the omission of small function words (such as *a, and, the,* etc.), but may also involve failure to use word order to signal meanings. Thus an aphasic's utterance of "daughter . . . husband . . . clothes . . . wash" may mean "My daughter and her husband will take my clothes home to wash." or it may mean, "My daughter has to wash her husband's clothes and so she doesn't have time to wash mine." These two different interpretations obviously convey different circumstances and different needs. At a milder level of severity, the client may be able to produce sentences, but these may be interrupted by long pauses as the client searches to retrieve the intended word. For example, the client might say, "Yesterday I took my . . . uh sis . . . no uh, daughter, no, uh, granddaughter, to uh, uh, Disneyland to ride the, uh, roller-coaster." Difficulty retrieving words, called *anomia,* is a frequent feature of aphasia. Semantic substitutions (e.g., sister for granddaughter) are common in both expressive and receptive aphasia.

The question of whether language errors result from loss of linguistic knowledge or just from difficulty accessing that knowledge remains controversial. From a neurological perspective, either one is possible. Clinical experience would suggest that in milder cases there is a discrepancy between knowledge and performance, but depending on the specific location and extent of the brain damage, certain types of linguistic knowledge may be partially or completely lost. Those clients who can inconsistently comprehend or produce more intact or complex language are more likely to have intact linguistic knowledge that they are having difficulty accessing. It is also probable that these clients are more likely to benefit from therapy.

Although many aphasic clients demonstrate a predominant pattern of either nonfluent aphasia with relatively intact comprehension or fluent aphasia with impaired comprehension, severely aphasic clients, who have experienced left hemisphere damage in both anterior and posterior portions of the brain, will demonstrate both comprehension deficits and difficulty producing simple utterances. These clients may be able to follow simple commands only inconsistently or when provided with visual cues, and they may be unable to say their own names, verbalize yes/no responses, or name common objects. When aphasia involves both receptive and expressive components, it may be termed "global" aphasia, although this term is not particularly helpful in describing its specific features or severity. These clients present great communication challenges, but once the basic principles for approaching these clients are understood, they can be modified to assist less severely involved clients, as well.

Facilitating Communication with Aphasic Clients. First, it is important to determine the client's general level of comprehension. This will determine how conversational partners need to modify the way information is presented. It will also provide a general indication of severity of communication impairment. Comprehension is typically assessed by asking the client to follow directions of increasing length and complexity. However, if the client has difficulty carrying out simple motor movements volitionally, this method may underestimate his comprehension because he is physically unable to follow some commands which he actually comprehends. **Apraxia,** a breakdown in ability to perform patterned motor functions, is a common deficit in aphasic patients. Apraxia may involve the whole body, the arms, or just speech movements. Although it is a speech disorder rather than a language disorder, it so frequently accompanies aphasia, and makes it more difficult to assess the client's ability to comprehend directions, that it is mentioned here. Obviously, the difficulty of both comprehension and performance increases as the length and complexity of the directions increase. For example, two-item commands (touch the pillow and your shoulder) are simpler than two-action commands (point to the door and tap your knee twice), which are in turn simpler than commands that require processing temporal or spatial relationships (before you touch your nose, point to the ceiling).

Because the client's ability to respond to commands depends on motor and attention skills in addition to auditory comprehension, it is important to assess comprehension in a variety of ways. In addition to following commands, clients are often asked questions that involve yes or no responses. Responses to yes/no questions can be given verbally, or through head nod/shake. Both of these modalities should be tested. Often, the aphasic person will find the head gestures easier and these responses will be more consistent. In this case, it is helpful to encourage the client to use only the best modality, as his listeners will be confused by responses that involve conflict (e.g., the client verbalizes no as he nods his head, and he actually means yes). Because responses to yes/no questions can yield a 50 percent accuracy rate even when the client responds at no better than a chance level, the assessment of yes/no reliability requires careful presentation of a variety of questions. As with commands, yes/no questions may be formulated according to a hierarchy of complexity, ranging from basic personal questions ("Is your name Jack? Are you married?") to basic factual questions ("Are we outside now? Are we in a hospital?") to complex factual questions ("Do apples grow on trees? Should children disobey their parents?") and abstract or comparative questions ("Is a horse bigger than a dog? Do you eat a banana before you peel it?"). Many clients are able to answer basic personal questions reliably but have difficulty with abstract questions. Understanding a client's basic level of comprehension allows the nurse to provide the client with information at the appropriate level of complexity. Reducing the level of linguistic complexity, along with slowing the rate of presentation of information and using nonverbal cues to augment verbal input, are the three most important strategies nurses and other professionals can use to enhance the comprehension of clients who have receptive language problems.

Once the client's general level of auditory comprehension has been established it becomes easier, not only to provide the client with the information needed, but also to facilitate the client's ability to express him- or herself as effectively as possible. Often, the efficiency with which the client can communicate needs depends on how well the nurse can organize the questioning process and can respond to nonverbal as well as verbal forms of expression. If the client is able to comprehend simple questions and has some reliable mode of response (yes/no gestures, pointing to written choices, or saying some simple words), it is possible, using an organized pattern of questioning, to carry on a surprisingly complex conversation. An organized pattern of questioning involves starting with general categories, eliminating irrelevant topics, and eventually confirming specific details. This is the sort of questioning involved in the old parlor game, Twenty Questions, in which one competitor must guess what the other person is thinking of in fewer than twenty questions. In the case of aphasic clients, it is important to begin the general questioning with simple, immediate needs such as, "Do you need to use the bathroom?," "Are you hungry?" and "Are you in pain?" Although using the context (e.g., whether the client is in the hospital, is currently an outpatient, has family visiting, etc.) can provide invaluable clues as to possible topics to pursue, it is important to look beyond the immediate context to general concerns (e.g., is the patient religious, concerned about family members, worried about money, etc.). When the client's ability to respond in a consistent manner is unclear, it is important to ask questions in more than one form, and when possible, to use actual objects during the questioning process. Consider the following hypothetical dialog:

Nurse: "Are you cold?"–Client: "Yes."
Nurse: "Do you want your sweater?"–Client: "No."

Nurse: "Do you want a blanket?"–Client: "No."
Nurse: "Are you hot?"–Client: "No."
Nurse: "Do you want your slippers?"–Client: "Yes."

It is also important to remember that as stress and frustration increase, response accuracy tends to decrease. When the patient feels pressured to respond, the responses tend to become less accurate. In addition, although yes/no responses can often be helpful when the client is unable to verbalize words, comprehension of yes/no questions may require a level of abstraction that the client has difficulty making on a reliable basis. These clients may require more visual input. For these clients, a choice between two or three actual items (e.g., orange juice to drink or a cracker to eat) is most effective. When it is not feasible to present actual items, it is sometimes helpful to write down simple words or short phrases as possible responses. For example, the nurse can say to the client, "Do you want to sleep, go the bathroom, or go outside?" while simultaneously writing the possible choices "sleep," "bathroom," and "outside" on a piece of paper and pointing to the corresponding word as he or she says the option. The patient can then be encouraged to point to the preferred item. Even clients who cannot read simple information can sometimes benefit from this pairing of verbal and written information and indicate simple preferences. Clients who have emerging verbal expressive skills can also be encouraged to verbalize as well as point to the chosen response. Just as clients with comprehension deficits benefit when verbal input is augmented by visual aids, clients with expressive deficits may benefit from having visual cues to assist them with verbal output. Finally, it is important to remember that although a client's aphasia may be described as receptive or expressive, almost all aphasias involve some difficulties with comprehension and with expressive skills.

Speech Production

In contrast to language, which is an abstract symbolic function, the production of speech involves motor functions and interaction of several anatomical systems including the lungs and respiratory system, larynx, pharynx, mouth, nasal cavities, and associated structures. Obviously, each of these structures serves important physiological functions such as breathing and eating, in addition to speaking. However, the demands of speech production are different, and, in some ways, significantly more complex than the capacities required for basic life support functions. For example, the simple resting breathing pattern typically involves muscular exertion for inhalation and relaxation for exhalation and is physiologically regulated according to blood gas levels. However, during speech production, muscles of inspiration must regulate the rate of exhalation to maintain an appropriate air pressure to drive the larynx. Thus the typical ratio of inhalation to exhalation used for resting breathing is changed in order to provide extended time of exhalation during which voice can be produced. Because exhalation is the driving force necessary to produce voice at the level of the larynx, strength and coordination of muscles of the *respiratory system* are the first prerequisites for normal speech.

The **larynx,** located at the top of the trachea, contains the vocal folds. These two tiny shelves of muscle fiber form a valve. Physiologically, the valving function of the larynx (which also involves the epiglottis and ventricular or false vocal folds) is important for airway protection during swallowing and as a pressure valve mechanism during forceful lifting, urination, defecation, vomiting, and childbirth. To serve the valving function, the vocal folds are adducted to close off the airway. During normal respiration, the vocal folds are abducted to allow for uninterrupted inspiration and expiration. During speech, the vocal folds are fully (or almost fully), adducted and exhalation produces a pressure below them that momentarily forces them apart. Vibration of the vocal folds is set in motion and sustained by the build-up of air pressure below the level of the vocal folds, rather than by muscular movement of the vocal folds themselves. This happens in much the same manner as the noise made by a blown-up balloon when the air is allowed to escape through the neck of the balloon. If the opening is stretched, the releasing noise is higher in pitch. The vocal folds are analogous to the opening (neck) of the balloon, and the lungs are analogous to the balloon. From this analogy, it can be seen that, unless muscular force is exerted to control and slow the rate of exhalation, air will escape so rapidly that phonation (noise production) can be sustained for only a few seconds at a time. As with the balloon, changes at the level of the vocal folds (in the larynx) determine the pitch and, at least partially, the quality of phonation. The physical characteristics of the vocal folds, such as size and texture, also affect the vocal pitch and quality. Because, on average, men have longer and thicker vocal folds, their voices tend to be lower pitched than women's voices. Physical changes caused by pathology (e.g., inflammation, presence of polyps) also cause audible changes (usually in the form of hoarseness or breathiness). In addition, muscular changes such as increasing the tension of the folds, or shortening the length of fold allowed to vibrate, can also be used to control the pitch and vocal quality.

Above the level of the vocal folds, the quality of the voice is further modified through *resonance* in the vocal tract. As the voice ascends through the pharynx, mouth, and nose, certain aspects of the vocal quality may be enhanced or dampened. The velum, also called the soft palate, functioning in coordination with the pharynx, is one of the most important anatomical structures affecting resonance. Velopharyngeal closure, in which the velum elevates and pharynx constricts, provides a valve between nasal and oral cavities. During swallowing, its closure allows a pressure gradient to build, which assists in the swallowing process and prevents food from entering the nasal passages. In normal speakers, the velum is relaxed to allow air flow through the nasal cavity in order to produce nasal resonance required for sounds such as *m, n,* and *ng.* When the velum is elevated (for all other sounds), air flows through the mouth and nasal resonance is reduced. When looking inside a client's mouth, elevation of the velum can be observed as a client says "ah ah ah." Although vocal resonance is affected by a variety of factors, including size and shape of the pharynx, the difference between nasal and nonnasal resonance is of primary importance in speech production.

The most obvious aspect of speech production is articulation. **Articulation** involves the interactive movements of the lips, jaw, teeth, palate, tongue, and velum that produce the discrete sounds of speech. The distinctions between the numerous sounds involved in speech, including vowels and consonants, involve a multitude of tiny, rapidly coordinated muscular movements. Although articulation is probably the most familiar and easily observable aspect of speech production, its complexity is often underestimated.

Dysarthria

When neurological damage results in paralysis, paresis, abnormal tone, or incoordination of the muscles involved in speech, the resulting disorder is called **dysarthria.** Of course, because neurological damage varies greatly in its nature and extent, dysarthria is a varied disorder that may involve a variety of different problems. The traditional classification of dysarthrias, developed by Darley, Aaronson, and Brown (1975) at the Mayo Clinic, includes flaccid, spastic, ataxic, hyperkinetic, hypokinetic, and mixed dysarthrias. Although these classifications have theoretical importance, current speech language pathology tends to emphasize assessment of a dysarthria according to its effects on respiration, phonation, resonance, and articulation rather than on its classification. Therefore, this discussion briefly describes each classification, but focuses on hypokinetic and mixed dysarthrias, because clients with severe dysarthria resulting from a neurogenic disorder often fall into these two categories.

Flaccid dysarthria results from disease of the lower motor neurons and is characterized by weakness. Myasthenia gravis, a myoneural junction disease, is the classic example of a flaccid dysarthria. Spastic dysarthria results from disease of the upper motor neuron system and is characterized by spasticity, weakness, limitation of range, and slowness of movement. Although spastic hemiplegia is a common syndrome following unilateral upper motor neuron disease, such as CVA, the dysarthria that may accompany it is typically mild, with imprecise articulation being the primary problem. Ataxic dysarthria results from disorders of the cerebellar system, which may be caused by a variety of problems including tumors, multiple sclerosis, CVA, or trauma. It is characterized by inaccurate, slow, and arrhythmic movements resulting in speech that has been compared to the slow, careful but thick-tongued speech of a drunk person. The hyperkinetic dysarthrias result from some disorders of the extrapyramidal system such as chorea, Tourette's syndrome, athetosis, dyskinesia, and dystonia and have varied presentations.

Hypokinetic dysarthria results from certain disorders of the extrapyramidal system. The extrapyramidal system involves the basal ganglia, the substantia nigra and subthalamic nuclei of the upper brainstem, and their interconnections. Although this area can be affected by CVA, tumor, trauma, and other neuralgic problems, **Parkinson's disease** is the classic example of an extrapyramidal disorder. Parkinson's disease is a progressive condition of unknown cause that usually results from degeneration of cells in the substantia nigra, which are important in the synthesis of the neurotransmitter dopamine. Although the progression and relative severity and onset of various symptoms are variable, the classic descriptions of parkinsonism include resting tremor, difficulty in initiating movement, general slowing of movement, masklike face, and slow shuffling gait. Dementia may be evident as the disease progresses. The hypokinetic dysarthria that is characteristic of Parkinson's disease is obviously related to the motor symptoms described. The voice is monotonous and soft while articulation is limited in range, with a tendency toward fast rushes of speech, hesitations, and false starts. Parkinson-like symptoms may be present whenever damage to the basal ganglia occurs, such as in carbon monoxide or manganese poisoning, encephalitis, and repeated head trauma in boxers.

Because clinical cases of neurogenic disorders often involve damage to more than one motor system, many dysarthrias fall into the category of mixed dysarthria. For example, CVAs may be bilateral or may affect both corticospinal and basal ganglia motor control, whereas disease processes such as **multiple sclerosis (MS)** and **amyotrophic lateral sclerosis (ALS)** cause widespread neural degeneration. Thus the term *mixed dysarthria* is a broad category that cannot be associated with a particular cluster of speech characteristics, owing to the variable nature of nervous system involvement implied by the name. The speech characteristics apparent in any particular case of mixed dysarthria are dependent on the extent, severity, and etiology of the damage to the nervous system. For example, ALS is a progressive fatal disease involving degeneration of the upper motor neurons from the precentral gyri of the brain and the lower motor neurons of the pons, medulla, and spinal cord. While cognition, sensation, and autonomic functions remain intact, progressive weakness gradually overtakes the client. The progression of weakness may begin with either upper or lower motor neurons, but as the illness progresses both are involved and affect speech production. Articulation is imprecise and vowel quality is hypernasal owing to weakness of the velum and pharynx and resulting in difficulty achieving adequate velopharyngeal valving. The voice may be harsh and breathy owing to poor adduction of the vocal cords. The intensity of the voice and ability to sustain phonation for more than a short phrase are limited by the weakness of respiratory support. Because all of the components of speech production systems may be affected, speech intelligibility is eventually severely affected. As the disease progresses, the client may become totally unintelligible, in spite of the fact that all cognitive skills are intact. ALS provides a tragic, but classic, example of a disease in which dysarthria (i.e., disruption to the motor systems necessary for speech) is the only factor interfering with communication. Because it is a progressive disease, there is no suggested treatment for improving clarity of speech production. However, there are many compensatory strategies and devices (called augmentative and alternative communication, or AAC) that can be used, depending on the severity of the dysarthria, with ALS or other dysarthric clients.

For the dysarthric client whose speech is mildly to moderately affected, but who is still able to use speech as the primary method of communication, it is often helpful to encourage the client to slow down, take a breath just before speaking, and try to say only one or a few words at a time. It usually saves time for the listener to repeat the understandable portions of the message and have the client repeat only the unclear words or phrases. Some listeners are hesitant to interrupt and ask for clarification, but it is very important not to feign understanding. It is usually easier to repair misunderstandings as they occur, rather than wait for the context to make it clearer.

It is also important to be aware of how the setting influences the communication process. As much as possible, communicate in a quiet, distraction-free environment. In everyday life, people adapt to a variety of communication settings. Some settings are naturally more stressful than others. Typically, people find it more difficult to talk about technical issues (such as medical problems) than to talk about familiar topics (such as daily activities or favorite hobbies). Similarly, it is usually more stressful to talk with people who are perceived as experts (such as nurses and doctors) than it is to talk with friends and family. People with communication impairments often have even more difficulty adapting to stressful communication situations. They tend to be able to perform communication functions best in a quiet, calm, unhurried environment, with one or only a few familiar people at a time.

Providing a quiet communication environment is obviously important when speech intelligibility is reduced because the client cannot produce a loud voice. In this situation, listeners sometimes put their ears close to the speaker's mouth in order to hear better. This is usually not effective. It is usually better to watch the client's mouth carefully for articulatory clues. Although the average listener may not realize it, most native speakers of a language can "lip read" to a limited extent, and it is important to take advantage of these clues. As the listener gains familiarity with a particular dysarthric speaker, he or she will likely begin to recognize certain ways of saying words that were at first unintelligible but later become recognizable. If the client's articulation skills are relatively unimpaired, and the intelligibility problem is primarily due to weakness at the level of the vocal folds, speech amplification may be an option the speech/language pathologist will explore.

Finally, and perhaps most importantly, the listener should pay attention to the context of the utterance or conversation. In any communication situation, the listener is constantly (usually unconsciously) using experience to predict what the speaker is about to say. This is possible because of the knowledge shared by listener and speaker and the built-in redundancy of language (due to the multiple layers of meaning provided by phonemic, morphologic, semantic, syntactic, and pragmatic aspects of language). For example, yxx mxxxt bx xblx tx xndxrstxnd thxs sxntxncx even though the vowels are replaced by x's. Most people, and particularly nurses, could probably predict what the words missing from these sentences would be: "_____ head hurts. _____ need _____." In addition to the linguistic context, the physical, psychological, and social context of the situation can provide important clues to the probable content of the message. Again, the more familiar the listener is with the speaker, the more personal context will be available. Of course, the danger involved in this process of prediction is that a misunderstanding occurs because of a wrong prediction. (This happens in "normal" communication settings when someone "jumps to a conclusion.") To avoid this, it is important to check the accuracy of the prediction with the speaker. It is also important to check with the dysarthric speaker regarding his or her comfort level with prediction. Most people resent having their sentences finished for them. Unless the speaker is struggling, and would prefer to be interrupted as soon as the message can be predicted, it is better to make the prediction internally, but allow the speaker to finish, and then confirm the accuracy of the interpretation.

When verbal output is impaired, whether because of aphasia or dysarthria, the listener must pay particular attention to nonverbal aspects of communication. There are a variety of ways of communicating any message. For example, a greeting can be transmitted verbally ("hello"), gesturally (a wave), or through facial expression (smile, nod), in writing, or even in a drawing. Although it may occur at an unconscious level, people engaged in conversation pay as much, or more, attention to nonverbal messages as they do to what is actually said. Facial expressions, body language (a raised eyebrow, a wink, a touch on the shoulder), gestures, tone of voice, and silence often communicate much more than words. When speech is very difficult to understand, these nonverbal aspects of communication can provide important clues in facilitating conversation. For example, a client who sounds as though he is saying "deebee" may be unintelligible, but if the listener recognizes that the client is looking in the direction of the television, the request to turn on the TV may suddenly become clearer. Instead of focusing only on speech as a means of communication, it is important to recognize all of the possible modalities a client may be able to use.

Alternative/ Augmentative Communication

When dysarthria is so severe that speech becomes nearly or completely unintelligible, the speech/language pathologist may introduce the client to the use of **alternative/augmentative communication** devices such as picture, word, or alphabet boards; or computer communication devices. The selection of a particular communication device depends on a professional evaluation of the client's cognition, language, and speech production and motor strengths and weaknesses, as well as the client's communication environment and needs. For example, a client with advanced ALS would have intact cognitive and language skills, but would have severely impaired speech production and motor skills. A communication assessment would involve identifying the best yes/no motor response. Although it is most practical to begin with a motor response that is most automatic and familiar to both the client and family, such as head nod/shake, as motor control declines other possible responses may be explored. These might include hand squeezes (e.g., one for yes, two for no), finger movements, eye blinks, or whatever movement can be reliably produced and observed without fatiguing the client. If the client is so motorically impaired that eye gaze is the only reliable response, he or she is not necessarily limited to yes/no responses. For example, the therapist might develop a gaze system in which the listener holds up a communication board shaped like a picture frame, with often-used phrases written in each corner. The client would then indicate the message by looking toward the corner where the phrase is written, while the listener watches the client's eye movement through the picture frame. Clients and listeners who are adept at this system can use it to identify letters of the alphabet in order to spell out novel and complex messages. In contrast, a client with MS who still has some intelligible speech and ability to move his or her fingers and hands for pointing, may be able to use a basic alphabet board, pointing to the first letter of each word, to clue the listener as the client speaks. If the listener still can't understand the word when given the first letter clue, the client can then spell out the word. These are just two types of communication boards that can be fabricated by the speech/language pathologist. Of course, there are many new computer technologies available and in development that are able to produce stored words, phrases, and sentences and even synthesize speech. However, these sophisticated devices are appropriate for a relatively small population of clients. A client's ability to benefit from an AAC approach can best be determined by the speech/language pathologist in consultation with the client and family. This determination is based on both the communication skills and current and future communication needs, depending on the living situation of the client.

Introduction of an AAC device is a sensitive process because of the social, psychological, and emotional implications of using an artificial communication process. Because speech is a natural, efficient, effective way to communicate, and an important part of each individual's identity, losing the ability to produce speech is a devastating loss. For some clients, acceptance of an artificial means of communication is an admission of that loss. For example, to a client with ALS, beginning to use a communication device may feel like an admission of defeat to the ongoing and irreversible progression of the disease. Similarly, the family of a client who has sustained massive head trauma resulting in severe dysarthria may feel that the use of a communication device somehow reduces the client's incentive to practice speech and thus reduces the possibility of improvement in speech production. It should be clearly explained to the family that use of a communication device, because it increases the number of attempts to communicate, actually enhances attempts at speaking, rather than reducing them. Typically, a client who has experienced severe frustration in the struggle to communicate simple messages through speech, and then experiences significant success with a communication device, readily accepts the device and expands his or her communication activities. Although professional caregivers may immediately see the advantages of AAC approaches, they need to be sensitive to the perceptions of the client and family. To facilitate acceptance of AAC approaches, it is often helpful to present the approach as a tool that can be used in addition to speech, only as much as it is necessary or useful.

Unfortunately, AAC is not a panacea. Devices tend to be helpful only for those clients who are primarily dysarthric or have, at most, mild cognitive or language deficits. There are many nonspeaking clients who, because of cognitive and/or language deficits, are unable to use even simple communication devices such as picture boards. These clients are often very frustrated communicators and they are frustrating to work with because they want to communicate, and yet they can't produce any functional speech. Well-meaning nurses often request communication boards for these clients. However, they are rarely able to use them effectively, usually because they have difficulty with symbolic functions. Thus it is not just that their ability to use language symbols is impaired (aphasia); their ability to link a picture to an object or an action is also impaired. Although many of these clients may have intact attention, and visual memory and the ability to solve simple functional problems that arise during their daily activities, they are unable to consistently link abstract symbols with real items or events (e.g., a drawing of a glass of water to their need for a drink). Determination of appropriate candidates for AAC approaches relies heavily on the important distinctions between dysarthria (disorder of speech production), aphasia (disorder of language and symbolic function), and cognitive deficits (disorders that may involve problems with attention, memory, **problem solving, reasoning,** and executive functions, among others). Although dysarthria may not be amenable to treatment (i.e., therapy may not enable the client to produce speech that sounds normal, or even intelligible) there are many more options for compensating for this disorder, when the client has intact cognitive and language skills to support alternative approaches to communication.

Conclusion
Although communication disorders are frustrating, isolating, and confusing for clients, their families, and caregivers, there are many techniques available to facilitate communication. The nurse who has a basic understanding of normal communication processes and how these can be disrupted by deficits in cognitive, language, and/or speech production processes will be able to apply principles of communication facilitation to particular patients in a more effective manner. Successful communication will result in more empathetic care and more positive patient outcomes.

Summary
The normal communication process involves cognitive, language, and speech production processes. Neurologic deficits may cause deficits in any of these domains, which will, in turn, cause communication deficits. Communication problems arising from cognitive deficits have a variable presentation and may include difficulties in understanding information, organizing ideas or responding appropriately in conversation owing to attention, memory, reasoning, executive function, or other related problems. Language deficits resulting from neurologic damage are called aphasias and involve auditory comprehension, verbal expression, gesture, reading, and writing problems. Dysarthrias arise from neurologic damage causing muscular weakness, abnormal muscle tone, or incoordination. Severely dysarthric clients may benefit from the use of augmentative/alternative communication devices. Although some techniques are most helpful with particular communication deficits, generally applicable principles include the following:

1. Communicate in a quiet, nondistracting environment.
2. Present information in a simple, direct manner and check for understanding and recall by having the client answer questions about the information presented.
3. Provide the least amount of cueing (physical, verbal or visual) needed, while assisting the client to do as much as possible independently.
4. Provide simple, honest feedback regarding the clarity or successfulness of the client's communication attempts. Never pretend to understand when you do not.
5. When possible, use visual input to supplement verbal information.
6. Observe for possible discrepancies between verbal skills and performance abilities; do not over- or underestimate actual skill level based on language skills.
7. Use the context or situation to help predict what a client may need to communicate.
8. Learn to ask yes/no questions in an organized manner to arrive at information through process of elimination.
9. Pay attention to nonverbal forms of communication including eye gaze, facial expression, and gesture.
10. Allow the client extra time for processing input or formulating output.

Each client with a communication disorder is a unique individual who deserves respect and sincere effort on the part of health care professionals to facilitate communication.

Review Questions

1. List five cognitive skills involved in communication.
2. Describe how language is different from speech.
3. Describe how you might assess whether a nonfluent aphasic client can recall his or her medications.
4. Describe several ways to reduce distractions in a medical setting.
5. Describe a communication problem that might be addressed through the use of an alternative/augmentative communication approach.
6. Describe how dysarthria is different from aphasia.

For Further Discussion: A Case Study

Mr. Brown is a 62-year-old man with a history of hypertension who was living at home with his wife. He awoke early one morning and when he attempted to get out of bed to go to the bathroom, he was alarmed to find that he was having difficulty moving his right leg. When he woke his wife, to tell her about his problem, his speech didn't make sense to her. She immediately called the paramedics. On arrival at the ER, Mr. Brown was diagnosed with a left middle cerebral artery thrombotic CVA. After transfer to acute care, Mr. Brown has a nasogastric tube, a Foley catheter, and requires total assistance for all daily activities. The nursing needs of this patient are great, and he has severely limited ability to communicate.

Are Mr. Brown's communication problems the result of cognitive deficits, aphasia, or dysarthria? What kinds of problems would you predict Mr. Brown would have, and how could communication be facilitated?

References

Bondi, M. W., & Kaszniak, A. W. (1991). Implicit and explicit memory in Alzheimer's disease and Parkinson's disease. *Journal of Clinical and Experimental Neuropsychology, 13,* 339–358.

Suggested Readings

Benson, D. F., & Ardila, A. (1996). *Aphasia: A clinical perspective.* New York: Oxford University Press.

Darley, F. L., Aronson, A. E., & Brown, J. R. (1975). *Motor speech disorders.* Philadelphia: W.B. Saunders.

Dickson, D. R., & Maue-Dickson, W. (1982). *Anatomical and physiological bases of speech.* Boston: Little, Brown.

Dworkin, J. P. (1991). *Motor speech disorders: A treatment guide.* St. Louis, MO: Mosby–Year Book.

Fromkin, V., & Rodman, R. (1978). *An introduction to language.* New York: Holt, Rinehart and Winston.

Holland, A. L. (1984). *Language disorders in adults: Recent advances.* San Diego, CA: College Hill Press.

Johns, D. F. (1985). *Clinical management of neurogenic communicative disorders.* Boston: Little, Brown.

Lezak, M. D. (1995). *Neuropsychological assessment* (3rd ed.). New York: Oxford University Press.

Pinker, S. (1995). *The language instinct.* New York: Harper-Perennial.

Solberg, M. M., & Mateer, C. A. (1989). *Introduction to cognitive rehabilitation: Theory and practice.* New York: The Guilford Press.

Wilkinson, I. M. S. (1993). *Essential neurology.* Oxford: Blackwell Scientific.

CHAPTER 28

Altered Sexual Functioning

Darlene N. Finocchiaro and *Michael V. Finocchiaro*

Key Terms *Artificial Devices*
Autonomic Dysreflexia
Coitus
Ejaculation
Electroejaculation
Erection
Excitement Phase
Exhibitionism
Fertility
Hypersexuality
Impotence
Incontinence
Infertility
Intensive Therapy
Intracavernosal Injection
Libido
Limited Information
Lower Motor Neuron (LMN) Lesion
Masturbation
Orgasm
Penile Implant
Permission Giving
Pharmacologically Induced Ejaculation
Plateau Phase
PLISSIT Model
Positioning
Priapism
Reflex Arc
Resolution Phase
Sexuality
Spasticity
Specific Suggestions
Stuffing
Upper Motor Neuron (UMN) Lesions

Vacuum Pumps or Systems
Vaginal Lubrication
Vibratory Ejaculation

Objectives

1. Describe "sexuality" and how it relates to one's health state.

2. Describe the male and female sexual response cycles.

3. Discuss the male and female sexual functioning capacity when neurological damage is not present.

4. Identify the five factors that affect the sexual response of individuals.

5. Identify 10 factors that can alter the sexual response of individuals.

6. Compare and contrast alterations in sexual functioning in the following population groups: clients with spinal cord injury, multiple sclerosis, cerebrovascular accident, acquired brain injury, and arthritis.

7. Identify appropriate questions to ask the client during an interview for assessment of sexual functioning.

8. List four possible nursing diagnoses for the client experiencing sexual concerns and changes resulting from disability or disease.

9. List at least seven nursing interventions for the client with sexual dysfunction.

10. Identify the four levels of the PLISSIT model and describe the nursing role in each.

Introduction

Sexuality is one of those words that has many different meanings, depending on how one perceives oneself or others. "Human sexuality is a broad concept that includes how one thinks, feels, and acts as a sexual being" (Santora, 1989, p. 407). These actions and feelings contribute to an individual's identity as either male or female. Society also contributes to this identity by its standards and expectations regarding how a female or male should act, think, and feel. At times, with some individuals, this can bring personal conflict, characterized by quesitons such as "Who am I?" and "Am I normal?" Often adolescents have these questions, but individuals with chronic illnesses and long-term disabilities also question their human sexuality.

Besides having sexual feelings and desires, disabled individuals are concerned about their sexual capacity. There are concerns about how their disability limits their functional ability to perform sexual acts and how society and loved ones see them as "sexual beings." It is a myth to think that "sexuality" and "sexual capacity" are no longer concerns for disabled clients, or that they are "asexual." In fact, on interview, more often than not, being able to perform sexually and having reproductive capabilities rank higher than being able to walk again.

The effects of disability will be different for each individual, depending on gender, and age of onset. An early onset could alter one's sexual orientation, sexual identity, and biological capacity for reproduction. Disabilities occurring later in life can result in a distorted body image, along with sensory, cognitive, and motor changes (Cole & Cole, 1993).

Sexuality is also an important component of optimum health. Having a positive view of one's own sexuality leads to feeling good about oneself. The World Health Organization (1975) defined sexual health as an integration of somatic, emotional, intellectual, and social aspects of sexual being, in ways that are positive, enriching, and that enhance personality, communication, and love. The person should have the ability to enjoy sexual and reproductive behavior according to personal and social ethics; freedom from fear, guilt, shame, and false information that impairs a sexual relationship and inhibits sexual response; and freedom from organic diseases and disabilities that present barriers to sexual and reproductive functions (World Health Organization, 1975).

Part of rehabilitation following a disability includes planning for the future and promoting a good quality of life. The physical needs are always addressed, but the emotional needs of the client must also be addressed: the need to be loved and to belong. Maslow (1954) identified the sexual drive as a basic human need that must be satisfied before higher needs can emerge. As such, the human sexuality of the disabled client must be part of the rehabilitation program. Nurses must not be afraid to ask the client about sexual concerns postinjury. Sexual capacity concerns should be part of the client's history and physical data on admission, during hospitalization, and at discharge.

This chapter looks at the sexual response cycle and functioning of the nondisabled client and compares it with that of the disabled client. Special attention is given to those clients with spinal cord injury, multiple sclerosis, brain injury, cerebrovascular accident (CVA), and arthritis conditions. Appropriate client outcomes and nursing interventions are identified and discussed.

Sexual Response Cycles

The sexual response is the physiological ability to experience genital sensations, erection, ejaculation, vaginal lubrication, pelvic thrusting, and other responses to stimulation (Zejdlik, 1983). It consists of four phases: excitement, plateau, orgasm (male), and orgasm (female), and resolution (Masters & Johnson, 1966).

The **excitement phase** in the male consists of **erection** (vascular engorgement of the corpora cavernosa in the penis), testicular elevation, and flattening of the scrotal skin (Boone, 1995). There is also an increase in muscular tension, the beginning of scrotal elevation, and the beginning of a cardiovascular response when the pulse and blood pressure increase. The **plateau phase** includes secretions from the urethral Cowper's glands and further accelerated cardiovascular responses. During male orgasm, the perineal musculature contracts rhythmically, the bladder neck closes, and seminal fluid is deposited into the posterior urethra from the prostate vas deferens, and seminal vesicles (Boone, 1995). There is a total body response consisting of involuntary muscular contractions, tightening of the rectal sphincter, and the heightening of cardiovascular activity. The total body response results in an **ejaculation** (pelvic event) and **orgasm** (cerebral event). During the **resolution phase,** there is a final contraction followed by a refractory period before erection and ejaculation can occur again.

The excitement phase in the female includes vaginal lubrication, clitoral enlargement, upper vaginal dilation with constriction of the lower third of the vagina, and uterine elevation (Boone, 1995). There is also breast enlargement with nipple erection, and the beginning of a cardiovascular response. During the plateau phase, the clitoral shaft and glans retract against the pubic symphysis, and an increase occurs in muscle tone, heart rate, respiratory rate, and blood pressure (Boone, 1995). The vagina, clitoris, and labia are fully engorged; the vagina is fully expanded. The orgasm phase consists of simultaneous contractions involving the uterus, fallopian tube, the outer portion of the vagina, and rectal sphincter. There is a total body response. Females may experience one or multiple orgasms, or they may experience none, progressing from the excitement to the plateau phase until resolution. During the resolution phase, the female experiences an involuntary reduction of sexual tension.

For an individual to progress through the sexual response cycle and perform sexual acts, there must be stimuli present that initiate a reaction, nerve tracts to carry stimuli to centers in the nervous system, nerve tracts to return messages to appropriate body parts, and sexual organs that react to the messages carried. A psychological desire must also be present (Santora, 1989). Looking at sensual pictures, movies, or at someone who is attractive and desirable can elicit a sexual response psychologically. Physiologically, a sexual response can occur when touch stimuli are applied to erotic zones of the body, such as the breasts, penis, and inner thighs. Massaging or rubbing the genitalia in a constant manner for a period of time usually leads to a successful sexual response. Direct touch stimulation is carried to sacral segments 2 through 4 (S2–S4) of the spinal cord by the pudendal nerve. The messages are conducted to the brain through the lateral spinothalamic tracts (Zejdlik, 1983). Messages are conducted down through the pyramidal tracts to thoracic segments 11 and 12 (T11–12) and sacral segments 2 through 4, resulting in erection in the male and vaginal lubrication in the female (Santora, 1989).

Male Sexual Functioning

When neurogenic damage is not present, a male client usually experiences an erection, ejaculation, and orgasm. Erection may be mediated by either the sympathetic or parasympathetic nervous system. Erection can be activated reflexively by physical stimuli such as touch sensations to the genitals travel through the pudendal nerve to sacral segments 2 through 4 of the spinal cord. Motor impulses leave these segments, causing vasodilation and congestion and resulting in an erection.

A psychogenic erection is controlled at thoracic segments 11 and 12 and at lumbar segments 1 and 2 (L1–2) of the spine. Psychogenic erections occur when stimuli travel from the brain to the sacral area. The brain sends messages in response to the stimuli received (sight, sound, smell) that either excite or inhibit sexual activity.

Ejaculation is a complex, co-ordinated series of reflexes. The first set of reflexes occurs at the T12 through L2 segments of the spine. Preganglionic neurons at these segments are activated to cause smooth muscle contraction in the vas deferens and epididymis (Boone, 1995), also known as seminal emission. The second set of reflexes occurs at sacral segments 2 through 4. True ejaculation results as there is an expulsion of fluid from the posterior urethra. Contractions of the bulbocavernous and ischiocavernous muscles via pudendal nerve activity compress the urethra to propel the ejaculate. Sympathetically mediated closure of the bladder neck occurs with ejaculation to prevent back flow of semen into the bladder (Boone, 1995). "Orgasm is a sensation coinciding with seminal emission and ejaculation" (Santora, 1989, p. 409).

During the resolution phase, the male begins a refractory period in which erection may continue but further ejaculation is not possible. A rapid loss of pelvic vasocongestion occurs (Santora, 1989).

Female Sexual Functioning

Sensory pathways from the clitoris and vagina are present in the pudendal nerves. The sensory level for the uterus occurs at the T6 spinal segment. Stimulation at the T11–12 level results in tumescence of the labia and clitoris, along with vaginal lubrication via the pelvic hypogastric nerves. Psychogenic lubrication occurs with stimulation of the thoracolumbar sympathetic nervous system and sacral parasympathetic nervous system. Reflex vaginal lubrication involves the sacral parasympathetic nerves. In addition, T11–12 and L1–2 segments regulate uterine smooth muscle contraction. Activation of the somatic pudendal nerves causes contraction of the vaginal wall and pelvic floor musculature (Boone, 1995).

Psychosocial Factors

There are several psychosocial factors that can affect the sexual response of individuals. These factors include love, communication, surroundings/mood, timing, and sensory stimulation/fantasy.

> Love is patient, love is kind. It does not envy, it does not boast, it is not proud. It is not rude, it is not self-seeking, it is not easily angered, it keeps no record of wrongs.

Love does not delight in evil, but rejoices with the truth. It always protects, always trusts, always hopes, always perseveres. Love never fails. (1 Cor. 13:4–8a)

Love is based on sharing, affection, trust, involvement, and togetherness (Masters, Johnson, & Kolodny, 1986). It entails commitment to one another. Sexual desire without love can be meaningless and have selfish intentions. It cannot withstand times of illness, fatigue, and distress. Love, however, responds to change and adapts. It is constant and can endure the hard times. "Love is a more complex and constant emotion with respect for the loved one as a primary concern" (Greco, 1996). Sexual activity with love is more fulfilling and satisfying to the individual.

Communication is often the secret key to satisfying sexual activity between partners: telling the loved one what is pleasing, what elicits sexual satisfaction, and what perhaps causes displeasure. A useful technique to determine what areas of the body feel good to the individual through touch is called "sensate focus," developed by Masters and Johnson (1970). Partners, before having sexual intercourse, explore different parts of each other's body (not resulting in intercourse or orgasm), letting the partner know what feels good and what does not. Communicating one's needs and concerns is an absolute must for a healthy positive sexual relationship. Setting aside special time to know each other's feelings and interests, during which just touching and holding each other take place, can greatly improve the sexual relationship.

Surroundings/mood: The environment that is pleasing can add to a successful sexual experience. The use of candles, soft music, a clean environment, flowers, and/or a fireplace can arouse sexually stimulating feelings. The use of mirrors when the partner has limited sensation can enhance visual enjoyment. Waterbeds can stimulate mobility when the partner has immobility (Greco, 1996). Creating a romantic setting, using one's imagination, can make all the difference. Privacy must also be assured.

Timing: The time for sexual activity is best when partners are rested, not ill, and not rushed. Some partners prefer the morning hours, whereas other couples prefer the later hours. Also to be considered is whether or not other activities or physical needs will interfere during the experience. The ideal time is when there are no interruptions expected.

Sensory stimulation/fantasy: The use of scented oils, creams, or lotions while massaging the body can enhance sexual arousal through touch and smell. Having visual awareness of where the partner is touching can increase sexual desires for the client who has limited or absent sensation.

Foreplay can stimulate a psychological desire for sex. This can start with holding hands and then slowly progressing to lightly touching and kissing the erogenous zones of the genitalia, breasts, neck, ears, lips, thighs, back, buttocks, anus, palms, and feet. Clients with disabilities require more time of foreplay.

Fantasy is what the client imagines to be sexually appealing. This can include viewing sexually explicit books, magazines, and movies. "Daydreaming," i.e., looking back at a previous positive sexual experience, can also elicit sexual desire.

Alteration in Sexual Functioning

Clients who have a chronic illness or long term–permanent disability are at high risk for sexual dysfunction. Examples of such conditions include spinal cord injury, multiple sclerosis, CVA, acquired brain injury, and arthritis. Problems of increased or decreased sensation, immobility, and incontinence are just a few reasons why disabled clients have difficulty with sexual functioning, despite having healthy sexual organs. Other possible problems include pain, fatigue, changes in libido, genital dysfunction, fertility (male spinal cord injury [SCI]), endocrine dysfunction (acquired brain injury), effects of medication, social isolation, and poor self-concept.

Pain has been identified as a greater barrier to sexual intimacy than disabling characteristics (Conine & Evans, 1982). Pain can be such a focus that having a pleasurable sexual experience becomes impossible. With pain, movement becomes unbearable and positioning limited. Constant chronic pain can also lead to depression.

Incontinence occurring during the sexual act can be a major concern. It is best to plan for sexual activity after the client completes his or her bowel program. Other preparation includes emptying the bladder, padding the bed, and adding pleasant scents in the environment and on the person (Greco, 1996). Limiting fluids and foods that stimulate bowel activity ahead of planned sexual activity should also be considered.

Acquired brain injury, spinal cord injury, CVA, rheumatic disease, and multiple sclerosis have *fatigue* as a major side effect. These conditions also require a great expenditure of energy to manage activities of daily living, such as performing bladder and bowel programs (Greco, 1996). After a long day of managing self, there is often little time, energy, or desire for sexual activity. The client might prefer to just rest comfortably in his or her partner's arms.

With *impaired physical mobility* the client will have difficulty transferring, dressing and undressing, inserting or applying birth control methods, performing personal hygiene, and performing the thrusting motion inherent during intercourse.

A client with *increased or decreased sensation* may no longer derive stimulation from some of the erogenous zones of the body. In the female, a decrease in sensation around the genital area may alter the orgasm experience. In some cases hypersensitivity occurs, resulting in pain (Greco, 1996).

Changes in **libido** can occur when there are lesions in the thalamus or limbic system; bitemporal injury can result in **hypersexuality.** A decreased desire for sexual activity tends to be associated with involvement of the paralimbic and neocortical frontotemporal areas (Greco, 1996). It is believed that hypersexuality qualities include (1) insatiable sexual activity that may interfere with other everyday functioning, (2) impersonal sexuality having no emotional intimacy, and (3) unsatisfying sex despite frequent orgasms (Masters, Johnson, & Kolodny, 1986). A decreased sex drive can be caused by organic affective disorders, reactive depression, cognitive dysfunction, stress, and anxiety (Greco, 1996). Factors that affect libido include medications, depression, aging, and specific diseases. The use of tranquilizers, antihypertensives, diuretics, hormones (increased estrogen in the male), barbiturates, and anticholinergics needs to be evaluated because they tend to decrease libido.

Medications can have adverse effects on sexual functioning. Analgesics can have the same result on the client as alcohol. Alcohol can inhibit arousal, reduce erectile capacity, and decrease ejaculation. It weakens male masturbatory effectiveness and decreases the intensity of male orgasm. Psychologically the person might be sexually aroused due to lack of inhibition (Masters, Johnson, & Kolodny, 1986). Ejaculation problems can occur from diazepam (Valium), methyldopa (Aldomet), ranitidine (Zantac), phenytoin, and baclofen (Lioresal). Baclofen also causes problems with erection (Greco, 1996). "**Priapism** is an uncontrolled, persistent erection of the penis" (Smeltzer & Bare, 1996, p. 1357). This can occur with the use of hydralazine (Apresoline), prazosin (Minipress), and labetalol (Trandate) (Greco, 1996).

Genital sexual dysfunction includes problems of **impotence** (erectile dysfunction) and premature ejaculation for the male. Female genital dysfunction may involve libido, vaginal lubrication, and orgasm (Greco, 1996).

Social isolation is likely to be experienced by disabled clients for many reasons. Often the client might feel "unnormal" and choose not to socialize with others. The client must find a partner who can accept him or her "sexually" with a disability. This might take several relationships before a sexually satisfying relationship is obtained. Society favors someone who is slim, youthful, and mobile. This perception and expectation can make the disabled feel hopeless about achieving positive sexual relationships. The client needs to be assured that the possibility of a mutually fulfilling sexual relationship with a significant other is strongly present. The client needs only to go out and find that special someone.

Other times social isolation is due to lack of transportation or accessibility to where the client might want to go. When family members work and the client is left at home alone all day (not by their choice), this can lead to social isolation. Disabled individuals may find it difficult to meet partners of the opposite sex when opportunities are limited. Sometimes family members don't encourage socialization outside "protective" activities or family functions. Often they feel sex is out of the question for their loved one and believe they are only protecting him or her.

Self-concept includes all the beliefs people hold with regard to themselves; beliefs concerning the ideal self, the value of self or self-esteem, and internal feelings about body parts and body image (Greco, 1996). During one's lifetime, a self-concept is developed through relationships with others. How another person responds to you and interacts with you determines a lot about how you see yourself. Clients with chronic illnesses or disabilities start to question their self-concept and whether or not it has changed. The ability to adjust to these changes varies between clients, but almost always there is some loss in body image and self-concept (Hirsch, Seager, Seldor, King, & Staas, 1990). Usually clients who had a positive body image and self-concept before illness or injury adjust to the changes experienced over time and maintain or re-establish a positive self-concept and body image. Encouraging the client to be independent in their care and praising the client for success, whenever possible, help enhance a positive self-concept. Encouraging the client to "take care of themselves" through dress, make-up, and hygiene, and commenting on "how good they look" promote a positive body image.

Fertility and *endocrine dysfunction* are discussed below, in relationship to specific diseases or disabilities.

Spinal Cord Injury

Clients who suffer a spinal cord injury with a complete lesion experience paralysis below the level of injury. In the beginning, the paralysis is flaccid; at a later stage, postspinal shock, it becomes spastic if the reflex pathways below the level of the lesion remain intact. The paralysis will stay flaccid if the reflex pathways have been severed, and also in spinal injuries affecting the medullary cone and/or the cauda equina. Loss of all feelings below the level of injury occurs. The senses of touch and pain, as well as the deep sensations, are reduced or disappear. (See Chapter 17 on spinal cord injury.)

Erections can be classified as reflexogenic and psychogenic. Psychogenic stimuli can be both facilitatory and inhibitory, and the degree of tactile stimulation necessary to produce a reflex erection can be diminished by psychic stimulation (Yarkony & Chen, 1995). The spinal centers related to erection are in the sympathetic preganglionic fibers from T11 to L2 and the parasympathetic fibers from S2 through S4 (Krane & Siroky, 1981; Weiss, 1972). Studies done by Comarr (1977) on 150 clients showed that 93 percent of reflexogenic erections occurred in complete **upper-motor neuron (UMN) lesions.** These are lesions above L1. With this diagnosis, there is also an absence of genital sensation, psychogenic erection/lubrication, and orgasm. Vaginal lubrication does occur in the female. Studies by Higgins (1979) showed the ability to ejaculate was lower than 10 percent for these clients. The reproductive potential is less than 6 percent (Comarr, 1977). However, fatherhood is possible. Improving ejaculation is the key and using the sperm for artificial insemination is an option.

In general, ejaculates from spinal cord-injured men have decreased volume, decreased sperm counts, decreased overall and progressive sperm motility, impaired sperm membrane integrity, and poor oocyte-penetrating capabilities of the sperm (Hirsch, Sedor, Callahan, & Staas, 1992). The emission of sperm is reflexic. A contraction of the smooth muscles of the seminal vesicles, the testicular duct and the prostate gland occurs, resulting in the sperm being transported to the posterior urethra. The center that regulates this lies in the lateral horn of the thoracolumbar spinal cord. This is followed by the ejaculation reflex. The sperm are ejaculated from the seminal vesicles, ampulla, and prostate.

Possible causes of poor semen quality in spinal cord-injured men include elevated scrotal temperatures; intrinsic damage to the testicles related to atrophy of the seminiferous tubules; subtle changes in serum follicle-stimulating hormone (FSH), lutetinizing hormone (LH), and in serum testosterone levels; the presence of sperm antibodies; chronic use of specific injury-related medications; and urine contact with sperm due to retrograde ejaculations (Yarkony & Chen, 1995).

The spinal cord-injured male with an *incomplete UMN lesion* (injury above L1) has reflexogenic erections, psychogenic erections, ejaculation, and successful intercourse 98, 45, 36, and 83 percent of the time, respectively (Comarr, 1977). Ejaculation is more common with lower motor neuron lesions and with most caudal lesions (Yarkony & Chen, 1995). Because of the high incidence of reflexogenic erections and a better chance of ejaculation, the occurrence of successful intercourse greatly increases.

With spinal cord-injured men who have a *complete lesion below L1,* i.e., a **lower motor neuron (LMN) lesion,** where the **reflex arc** is not intact, there will be no erection possible, because there is no reflex activity present. Lower motor neuron lesions result from cauda equina lesions. In SCI, absence of rectal tone and the bulbocavernosus reflex indicate this type of lesion (Gatens, 1984). The possibility of a psychogenic erection in clients with complete LMN injury is 26 percent (Comarr, 1977). Ejaculation can occur 18 percent of the time (Bors & Comarr, 1960). Ejaculation generally is more common with lower motor neuron lesions and more so with caudal lesions (Yarkony & Chen, 1995). Orgasms are possible, but are poorly defined in studies (Higgins, 1979). Successful coitus occurs 24 to 50 percent of the time (Comarr, 1977).

Even though reflexogenic erections are generally not possible with LMN lesions, clients with an *incomplete LMN lesion* have psychogenic erections 83 percent of the time (Comarr, 1977). Comarr and Vigue (1978) reported that the ability to achieve psychogenic lubrication is possible in the woman with incomplete SCI; that it may be related to the preservation of the ability to perceive pin-prick sensation in T11 through L2 dermatomes. The ability to ejaculate for clients with incomplete lesions can be as high as 32 percent (Higgins, 1979). Comarr (1977) reported ejaculation with orgasm to be as high as 56 percent, and coitus to be successful 75 percent of the time.

Women with spinal cord injury have concerns about their sexuality and whether or not they can still have enjoyable sexual encounters. Unfortunately, there has been limited information and literature available. There are several reasons this has occurred. Approximately 82 percent of the SCI population are males and only 18 percent are females. Also, the sexual functioning of the female is generally not impaired, in contrast with the male client. There is also the belief that women are often passive regarding sexual concerns and that sexual functioning is not as high a priority, in comparison with the male (Cole, 1975).

Even though there is less information on changes occurring in females with SCI, the pathways are thought to be the same as for the male (Poorman, Smith, & Robertson, 1988; Weinberg, 1982). Lubrication parallels erection and can occur reflexogenically or psychogenically, depending on the type of lesion. Lubrication occurs reflexogenically above T10 and is psychogenic with lesions at S2–4. Even though vaginal lubrication occurs, it often is limited. This can result in painful intercourse. As with the male, orgasm with a complete lesion is not due to genital stimulation, but may occur as a cerebral event (Goddard, 1988). A study by Sipski, Alexander, and Rosen (1995) showed that a large percentage of SCI women achieved orgasm regardless of pattern or degree of neurological injury. Subjects who achieved orgasms had a higher sex drive and greater sexual knowledge. Charlifue, Gerhart, Menter, Whiteneck, and Manley (1992) noted genital or genital and breast stimulation are most frequently used.

For many spinal cord injury clients, the questions of **fertility** and **infertility** arise. Generally, *male fertility* is poor owing to low sperm count and decreased motility resulting from hyperthermia. There is also considerable debris (dismembered sperm). Another problem present is that the internal sphincter fails to close as the sperm travels to the bladder (retrograde ejaculation). Weinberg (1982) identified four barriers that may interfere with fertility in this population: inability to ejaculate or retrograde ejaculation, inability to obtain or sustain an erection, reduced sperm count, and urethral scarring associated with frequent urinary tract infections. Owing to these problems, pregnancies caused by clients with SCIs are rare (Amelar & Dubin, 1982). Fortunately, there are several procedures and options available within the areas of semen retrieval, improvement of semen quality, and fertilization (discussed below).

Female fertility is good and eventually the client returns to pre-injury status. Menstruation may be interrupted for 6 to 12 months and irregular cycles may continue after injury. Ovulation may occur before the menstrual cycle returns. Therefore, the concern of an unwanted pregnancy is present and discussion of birth control methods may be necessary. Because of increased incidence of phlebitis with SCI and oral contraceptives, oral contraceptives are not recommended for birth control. Owing to the spinal cord injury, the client will not have the symptom of pain associated with a clot and may not notice symptoms of redness and swelling (Goddard, 1988). Another option for birth control consists of intrauterine devices. Because of absent or decreased sensation, insertion is painless. However, it becomes a problem when pelvic inflammation is not recognized owing to lack of pain sensation. The client must be taught to observe for irregular periods or spotting, an elevated temperature, or increased spasticity (Goddard, 1988).

Diaphragms with jelly can be used, but if the client has limited use of hands, her partner will need to assist with the insertion. Potential problems include adductor spasms (interfering with insertion) and dislodgment due to weak pelvic floor muscles or use of the Credé method for emptying the bladder (Goddard, 1988).

The ability of the female SCI client to conceive has not changed. This should not be discouraged if this is truly the client's desire. Preferably this is mutually decided on between the client and the partner. Potential complications of pregnancy include urinary tract infections, anemia, and autonomic dysreflexia (Carroll, Tempkin, & Worth, 1986). Close monitoring by an obstetrician who is knowledgeable about spinal cord injury is necessary. Because contractions may not be felt, delivery could come quickly and unexpectedly (Mendius, 1989). The nurse needs to instruct the client on how to palpate for abdominal contractions and to be aware of other signs of labor such as increased spasticity or a bloody discharge (Mendius, 1989). In most cases vaginal delivery is possible.

The major problem to be concerned about with spinal cord injury clients with an injury at the T6 level or above is **autonomic dysreflexia.** This can occur during sexual activity (male and female), labor, delivery, and lactation. During labor, uterine contractions elicit profound reflex responses of the autonomic mechanism, resulting in intermittent hypertension and bradycardia (Guttman, Frankel, & Paeslack, 1965). Other symptoms include a sudden pounding headache due to a rapid increase in blood pressure, chills, and sweating above the level of injury. (See Chapter 17 on spinal cord injury.) Sometimes this life-threatening situation can be confused with pregnancy-induced hypertension. McCunniff and Dewan (1984) stated that all women with spinal cord injury who are prone to autonomic dysreflexia should receive an epidural block during labor. A "nonpush" attitude with women who have chosen epidural anesthesia should be practiced (Craig, 1994).

Common sexual functioning problems for the client with a UMN spinal cord injury include ejaculation and poor semen, resulting in infertility. Other concerns include spasticity and incontinence.

Ejaculation with semen production can be achieved through masturbation, pharmacologically induced ejaculation, vibratory ejaculation, electroejaculation, and, as a last option, surgical management.

Masturbation can, for some men with SCI, be sufficient for retrieval of semen and may even be better than electroejaculation (Rawicki & Lording, 1988).

Pharmacologically induced ejaculation has been used since 1946. Since that time, intrathecal neostigmine and subcutaneous physostigmine have been used. Owing to serious complications, the use of intrathecal neostigmine is no longer recommended. A more recent technique that may prove to be useful and safer for clients with SCI is the intrapenile injection of vasoactive drugs (Walbroehl, 1987).

Vibratory ejaculation can produce semen specimens if a vibrator is fitted with a collection cup. Vibratory stimulation of the penis may induce reflex ejaculation, and pregnancies have been reported from this technique (Yarkony & Chen, 1995). Comarr (1970) described a client using a "Swedish massager" to obtain sperm and then inseminating his wife with the condom-collected ejaculation. There are several types of vibrators available, such as the Ling vibrator and the Pifco vibrator for home use. Autonomic dysreflexia is a complication for clients with a T6 level or higher SCI.

With **electroejaculation,** a probe is inserted into the man's rectum and the nerves controlling ejaculation are electrically stimulated (McCarren, 1991). Brindley (1981) described the goal of electroejaculation to be stimulation of the proper nerve fibers and as few as possible of the wrong ones, with the least possible risk of thermal and electrolytic damage to the rectal mucosa occurring. Electroejaculation may be more appropriate when vibratory stimulation fails because there is a greater success rate. However, it has been shown to be more successful in conus, caudal lesions (Yarkony & Chen, 1995).

Another method to obtain spermatozoa is by direct aspiration from the vas deferens (Sonksen & Biering-Sorensen, 1992). Brindley, Sauerwein, and Hendry (1989) reported that an additional method to induce an ejaculate was by providing direct stimulation of the hypogastric nerve using an implanted nerve stimulator. These surgical methods are considered only if the other options discussed have failed.

Spasticity can be a positive by helping the client transfer and position as necessary. However, when spasticity is so severe that transferring and positioning are painful and/or impossible to perform, intervention must be taken. Possible solutions are a low dose of Valium or Lioresal. Range-of-motion exercises before sexual activity can also be helpful by stretching the muscles. Positioning for sexual intercourse requires experimentation. The client's trunk and arm muscles are used for balance and positioning is limited only by the amount of energy each partner is willing to use. With spasticity, **positioning** with hip and knee flexion will help counteract the hypertonicity (Mendius, 1989). Positioning options and techniques are addressed further in connection with the client with CVA.

Bowel and bladder incontinence is also a major problem. Teach the client to empty the bladder before and after intercourse, empty the bowel before intercourse, decrease fluid intake 2 to 3 hours before intercourse, and prevent dislodgment of catheter (if in place). "An indwelling catheter need not stand in the way of physical intimacy. It should be positioned out of the way so that no action accidentally pulls the catheter out of the bladder" (Mendius, 1989, p. 72). The catheter should be taped to the inner thigh of the female. One's partner may feel the catheter through the wall of the vagina during intercourse. Some men have reported that this sensation is pleasurable (Becker, 1976). For the male client with a catheter in place, it is advised to fold back the catheter along the penis and cover it with a condom. Ideally, it is better not to have a catheter in place during intercourse, if this can be tolerated by the client. Bowel programs should be scheduled, to assure successful bowel emptying. If a bowel or bladder accident occurs during sexual interaction, it is not an emergency. It is best to prepare the partner of this possibility and perhaps have a sense of humor about it (Mendius, 1989).

Spinal injury clients with an LMN lesion have problems with ejaculation, poor semen, and incontinence, but the most prevalent problem is in establishing an erection. There are several suggestions to increase the possibility of erection, such as "stuffing," artificial devices, vacuum devices, pharmacological management, and penile implants.

With **stuffing,** the female positions the soft penis into the vagina, contracts the vaginal (pubococcygeal) muscles, and holds the penis in the vagina (Griffith & Trieschmann, 1983). In a dominant position, the woman may perform a rotary or circular motion, which is helpful when the client is impotent (Greco, 1996).

Artificial devices include using either a vibrator or a phallus-like device (plastic penis) that is held in place with a belt.

Vacuum pumps or systems are external devices that produce or maintain an erection. There are different types from which to choose. Erection can be maintained for up to 30 minutes (Greco, 1996). The penis is placed in a rigid tube, a pump creates the needed vacuum and fills the corpora with blood, and a constricting band maintains the erection (Yarkony & Chen, 1995). Complications include damage to the penile shaft, internal penile tissue damage, and infection or irritation to the urinary tract (Greco, 1996). Pain and pain with orgasm have also occurred (Cookson & Nadig, 1993). The use of the vacuum pump should always be under the supervision of a physician. This method is contraindicated with clients who are on anticoagulant therapy or have blood dyscrasias (Witherington, 1988).

Pharmacological management includes the use of dopamine agonists (L-dopa and yohimbine) to increase erections, testosterone injections to increase libido and erectile function, and intracavernosal injections. The **intracavernosal injection** consists of papaverine, phentolamine, and prostaglandin E, which are injected into the corpus cavernosum of the penis to stimulate erection through vasodilation (Greco, 1996). Those with neurological damage, such as the client with an SCI, are more prone to sustained erections lasting more than 6 hours (priapism) (Smith & Bodner, 1993). Besides possibly adversely altering erectile activity, intracavernosal injections can result in transient pain and paresthesias, ecchymosis, and fibrotic changes at the site of injection (Yarkony & Chen, 1995). More than 30,000 men are successfully using some type of penile injection therapy to treat impotence (Leslie, 1990).

Penile implants are effective for counteracting impotence due to spinal cord injury, diabetes, or long-term use of antihypertensives. There are several types of penile prostheses available. Semirigid prostheses can be hinged, malleable, or articulating. The inflatable penile implants can be multicomponent or self-contained (Yarkony & Chen, 1995). Green and Sloan (1986) suggest combining psychosexual counseling with surgical treatment. Green recommends the implantation when the client has a stable bladder program, a recent urological x-ray examination, sterile urine, and no skin breakdown. From 1981 through 1994 a retrospective study was done to assess the incidence of complications with a penile implant. Green, Killorin, Foote, Bennett, and Sloan (1995) reported that 49 of 117 implants (41 percent) were associated with complications. These included penile erosion of the prosthesis, infection, mechanical malfunction, and insufficient rigidity. The most common complication observed (15 percent) was erosion through the glans or the urethra. Infection occurred in 12 percent of the implants studied, and 21 percent resulted in mechanical failure. The majority of complications occurred in the group using inflatable implants. Penile prostheses should be reserved for clients who are not satisfied or have failed with less invasive treatments. They are also recommended for those clients who require prostheses to keep condom catheters on the penis (Smith & Bodner, 1993).

Beside concerns with positioning, spasticity, incontinence, and possible autonomic dysreflexia depending on the level of injury, female clients with SCI, have poor **vaginal lubrication.** A client with a UMN lesion usually has vaginal lubrication. The client with an LMN lesion usually does not. Because the penis does not emit enough fluid to maintain necessary moisture for comfortable intercourse, a water-soluble lubricant (not petroleum jelly) may be needed (Mendius, 1989).

Another option for men and women would be to engage in oral-genital activity, which may be considered a viable alternative to penile-vaginal stimulation (Mendius, 1989).

With all the methods described, there is more hope today for the SCI male to father a child. A touching, successful story is that of Stacy and Jimmy Green (Hudson & Green, 1995); as of this writing Stacey is expecting twins. An entire decade of ups and downs preceded this outcome, and the couple have commented that "electroejaculation combined with in vitro fertilization made something possible for us that 10 years ago was unthinkable."

Multiple Sclerosis

Multiple sclerosis is an autoimmune disease in which the myelin sheath insulating the nerve fibers of the central nervous system (CNS) is damaged. As the myelin sheath is disrupted, firm, dense tissue called plaque, or sclerosis, forms at the damaged site (Whitaker, 1983). Because these plaques can form at any place throughout the nervous system, sexual functioning becomes impaired.

Normal sexual function requires intact nervous and circulatory systems. These systems become impaired as the parasympathetic and sympathetic fibers are affected with MS. The ability to be sexually stimulated requires intact pathways from the cortex to the appropriate cord level and from there to the effector muscle involved (Fogel & Laiver, 1990). Sexual function also involves emotional and psychogenic components necessary for sexual arousal and desire. This is also affected in the MS client (Weiss, 1992).

Multiple sclerosis tends to affect young adults, especially at the time in their life when sexuality and sexual relationships become significant. Problems encountered by female clients with MS include fatigue; decreased sensation; decreased vaginal lubrication; and decreased libido, arousal, and ability to reach orgasm. Male clients experience impotence, decreased sensation, fatigue, decreased libido, and difficulty in reaching orgasm. Other sexuality problems common to the client with MS include incontinence, spasticity, pain, and stiffness. Problems with sexual functioning occur owing to the effects of MS, which progressively increase. The use of multiple medications also adds to the dysfunction.

Fatigue can be controlled by planning for sexual activity ahead of time. Planning for rest periods before the event is advisable, so as to conserve energy. The morning hours might be best for sexual activity, when the client is well rested.

Many of the problems encountered by the client with MS also occur for the client with an SCI, as previously discussed. Interventions are the same relative to the problem(s) identified. Fatigue, pain and depression tend to be of higher concern for the client with MS, sometimes hindering sexual desire altogether.

Cerebrovascular Accident

Most clients who suffer from a CVA are elderly. Understanding the physiological changes of aging and sexuality in the elderly is the prerequisite to any discussion regarding sexuality in stroke clients. Even though it is often believed that sex is of little interest to the elderly, it has been well documented that sex continues to play an important role in the lives of many elderly people (Monga & Ostermann, 1995).

Clients who suffer a CVA have difficulties in sexual functioning. Problems that may occur include a decline in libido, decline or cessation of coital activity, lack of or poor erection, absence of ejaculation, poor vaginal lubrication, orgasmic difficulties, poor satisfaction with sexual activity, lack of enjoyment with sexual activity, and hypersexuality (Monga & Ostermann, 1995).

Sexual impairment in CVA clients can be due to dysfunction, disfigurement, or both. The severity of the disease correlates with the degree of sexual impairment. However, it has been shown that clients who had a higher frequency of sexual activity before the stroke were more likely to resume sexual intercourse after the stroke (Hawton, 1984).

In clients with a CVA, in whom a decline in sexual functioning is apparent, there are several factors to consider: poor coping skills; psychosocial adjustment to the impairment and disability; fear of having another stroke; and sensory, motor, and cognitive deficits.

In having to deal with the stress of a stroke, the client usually experiences role change, dependency on others for care, and social isolation. According to Sjogren, Damber, and Liliequist (1983), a stroke client may become distressed and less willing to initiate a sexual encounter while the spouse assists him or her with toileting and other self-care activities. There is also the concern of a different role in the family; perhaps no longer being the head of the household. This results in the questioning of one's self-concept. Once self-concept turns from positive to negative, the client will also question his or her desirability as a sex partner. When there is hemiplegia and one side of the body is flaccid, the client worries about self-image; how do others look at me?

Psychosocial factors also include problems of communication, cognitive dysfunction, and use of alcohol and necessary medications. Aphasia makes it difficult to express what feels good and what does not. With cognitive dysfunction, there is lack of understanding of what is occurring (sexual activity) and why. Alcohol, as a central nervous system depressant, can cause erectile problems. Hawton (1984) reported that up to 80 percent of chronic alcoholics experienced a decreased sex drive and ejaculation dysfunction. All of these psychosocial factors can result in depression. Depression is common among clients with a CVA, especially those with a left hemisphere lesion and right-sided paralysis. Antidepressants can increase libido if depression is reduced but they also cause central nervous system depression, impotence, inhibited ejaculation, and orgasmic difficulty (Ebersole & Hess, 1994).

Stroke clients are usually on multiple medications. Antihypertensives, antidepressants, and hypnotics can contribute to erectile difficulties and ejaculatory dysfunction. Sexual dysfunction, particularly impotence, has been reported with the use of antihypertensives (Monga & Ostermann, 1995). The use of thiazide diuretics can lead to decreased libido, difficulty in gaining and maintaining an erection, and difficulty with ejaculation (Chang, Fine, Siegel, et al., 1991).

As soon as the client with a CVA is considered medically stable and has clearance by a physician, sexual activity can resume. Having another stroke during sexual activity, especially during orgasm, is a common fear. There is an elevation of blood pressure that occurs with sexual activity, but several studies have indicated that the elevation of blood pressure that occurs is no greater than the elevations that accompany normal daily activities of living (National Stroke Association, 1993).

Clients with a CVA usually exhibit some sensory and motor deficits. Paralysis and spasticity can make positioning difficult. The muscles can become very stiff and rigid, increasing difficulty in movement (National Stroke Association, 1993). If the loss of sensation extends to the genitalia, this can result in impotence or poor vaginal lubrication. *Apraxia* (inability to perform purposeful acts or to manipulate objects) and *ataxia* (inability to coordinate movement) can limit the initiation of movement or the co-ordination of movement (Greco, 1996).

Interventions include assessing for causes of sexual impairment, removing communication barriers, reassuring clients with a CVA that they are "acceptable," that they can "perform" sexually and that it is "safe," adjusting medication, managing depression, teaching the client coping skills, and suggesting alternate positions (Monga & Ostermann, 1995).

Besides assessment of sexual functioning and allowing the client to express concerns (permission giving), the nurse can instruct the client on how to cope with the CVA more effectively. The nurse can also inform the client of alternative positioning techniques.

Teaching needs to be given regarding side effects of medications taken and how to intervene with spasticity. If spasticity is present, the partner should avoid quick, jerky movements. If lack of muscle tone is present, the partner should avoid overstretching the joints.

There are several positions the CVA client and his or her partner can consider for sexual activity. Conine and Evans (1982) and Fugl-Meyer and Jansko (1980) suggest that the client should lie on the affected side so that the unaffected arm is free to caress the partner. In this position, with a pillow wedged behind the male's back, a rear entry is easiest. Another option is for the man to lie supine during intercourse and the woman can adopt a top superior position (Monga & Ostermann, 1995). If the client with a CVA has shoulder pain, it would be best to avoid the side-lying position in favor of the female top superior position.

The client with a CVA can also consider nontraditional coital positioning, such as the sitting position (see Figure 1).

Figure 1A shows **coitus** in the male-superior position. This position requires much upper body strength and body balance. Figures 1B and C display two different female-astride coital positions. This is best if a male client has the CVA. Figures 1D and E portray coital possibilities while the client with a CVA is sitting in a wheelchair. Figures 1F and G show positions to be considered when the male has good balance and lower body strength. Figure 1H portrays how the female can lie on her back with the male perpendicular to her body trunk, minimizing the sensory and motor limitations imposed by a male CVA client's hemiplegia or hemiparesis (McCormick, Riffer, & Thompson, 1986). The partner may need to assist or direct movements. The partner also may need to be reminded that the client may neglect stimuli from the affected side because of perceptual and sensory deficits (Monga & Ostermann, 1995).

Acquired Brain Injury   Acquired brain injury can result in sexual problems due to several factors including genital and nongenital dysfunction. Genital dysfunction can result in erectile dysfunction, ejaculatory problems, orgasmic dysfunction, problems with vaginal lubrication and vaginismus. Nongenital dysfunctions include sensory and motor deficits, perceptual deficits, limited range of motion, neurogenic bowel and bladder functioning, motor dyspraxias, posttraumatic behavioral deficits, and alterations in self-image and self-esteem (Zasler & Horn, 1990).

Disturbance of libido is a frequent finding after brain injury. Most clients with this type of disturbance will have decreased or even absent sex drive and interest (Griffith & Lemberg, 1993). Hormonal abnormalities and brain chemical neurotransmitter deficiencies or imbalances can alter libido. When there is brain damage, the endocrine system is affected, resulting in hormonal imbalance. Testosterone levels lower and fertility becomes poor. As testosterone levels decrease, libido decreases and impotence occurs (Greco, 1996). Infertility is a rare occurrence, however. Other reasons why the brain-injured client has reduced libido include fatigue, pain, depression, and anxiety; all characteristics the client may experience (Griffith & Lemberg, 1993).

Impotence and unsustained or partial erections may occur as well. This can be caused by neurotransmitter and/or hormonal deficits but usually impotence is due to the side effects of medications taken or psychosocial factors, such as depression, anxiety, "performance" anxiety, reduced self-esteem, and a perceived decline in personal sex appeal (Griffith & Lemberg, 1993; Kreutzer & Zasler, 1989).

Medications that can result in impotence and a decreased sex drive include tranquilizers, antidepressants, sedatives, hypnotics, antihypertensives, anticholinergics, anticonvulsants, illicit drugs, alcohol, and hormones, especially progesterones (Griffith & Lemberg, 1993).

In most instances decreased sexual activity is due to psychological and cognitive factors. Studies have shown disinterest on the part of brain-injured clients (Lezak, 1978), but often it is due to partner disinterest. The client displays memory dysfunction, impaired learning, communication difficulty, and personality changes (Levin, Benton, & Grossman, 1982). Personality changes such as childishness, emotional lability, irritability, and restlessness are common 10 to 15 years postinjury (Thomsen, 1984). Cognitively, the client can have a decreased attention span, memory deficits, and lack of initiative.

Some clients with brain injury will experience an increase in sex drive, exhibiting loss of impulse control and **exhibitionism.** This occurs in a low percentage of clients, usually those with frontal lobe damage (Ducharme, 1987). This impulsivity results in sexually inappropriate behavior. Crewe (1984) defines sexually inappropriate behavior as behavior that is explicitly sexual in nature or the product of an underlying sexual conflict, that is harmful physically, mentally, or emotionally to the individual or to persons in one's environment. Hypersexuality can also

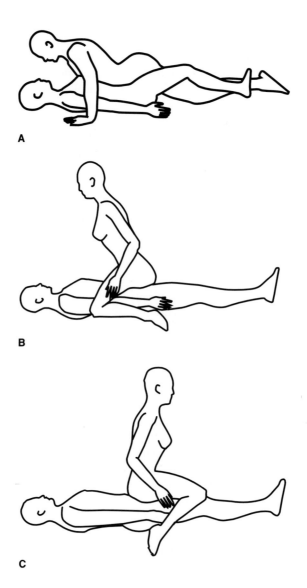

Fig 1. *Nontraditional coital positioning. (A) Male-superior position; (B and C) female-astride positions; (D and E) client-in-wheelchair position; (F and G) positions for client with lower body strength; (H) position minimizing limitations of hemiplegia and hemiparesis.*

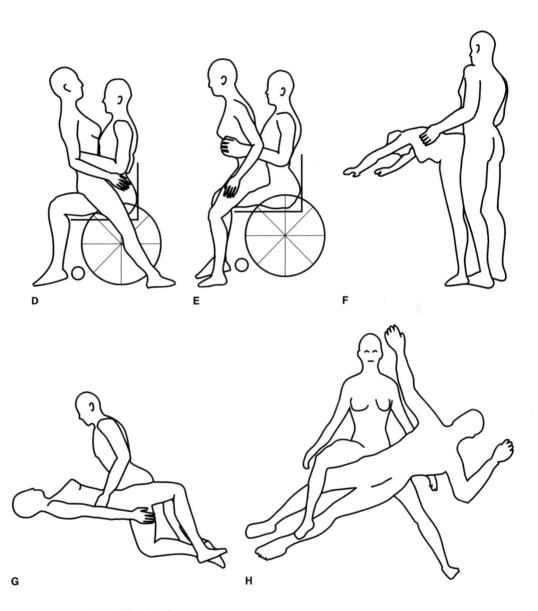

Fig 1. (*Continued*)

occur with either temporal lobe seizures or surgical removal of the temporal lobe limbic structures (Lusk & Kott, 1982).

Very little has been documented on the effects of brain injury to the female client. Cognition and psychosocial factors need to be considered as possible causes of sexual dysfunction, as presented with the male client. Vaginal lubrication has been noted to be a problem. The woman's ovarian endocrine function is also affected. Menstrual irregularities and more androgen production occurs, resulting in symptoms of hirsutism, ache, obesity, and polycystic ovaries (Greco, 1996). Amenorrhea occurs immediately after brain injury, but menstrual periods resume in 4 to 6 months. If amenorrhea continues after 6 months, hypothalamic-pituitary injury or dysfunction is possibly present (Griffith & Lemberg, 1993).

Other disorders that can result from brain injury and lead to sexual dysfunction include deficit in mobility, self-care, sensation, oral communication, disfiguration, and mental disorders (behavioral, emotional, and personality changes) (Griffith & Lemberg, 1993).

Spasticity, fear of a seizure, apraxia, ataxia, and/or poor equilibrium can make movement and positioning difficult. These conditions also limit a client's ability to dress, bathe, and perform other self-care functions. Slow movement, rigidity, tremors, and other involuntary movements often impede motion, balance, and positioning. Lack of interest in initiating activity or behavior, or apraxia, may make a person totally passive during sexual activity (Griffith & Lemberg, 1993). Deficits of mobility and self-care can be reversed by a caring, understanding partner.

The brain-injured client can experience decreased or increased sensation. Half of the body, as with the CVA client, might become insensitive to touch, therefore not feeling pleasurable acts in sexual activity. The opposite may also occur: The affected side may be hypersensitive to touch, resulting in severe pain. If the external genitalia become insensitive, local touch stimulation may be ineffective in producing erection or vaginal lubrication. Painful genital sensations may also interfere with sexual responses (Griffith & Lemberg, 1993).

Communication deficits make it difficult for the client to express his or her needs and desires. Also, problems in understanding what his or her partner needs or wants sexually can occur. Nonverbal communication can also be misleading to the partner, leading to frustration and hurt feelings.

Intervention with the brain-injured client is similar to that with the CVA client; however, the focus is more on cognition deficits. Teaching the client and partner various positioning techniques and how to control or adjust to spasticity is necessary. Strategies for the problems of incontinence, poor vaginal lubrication, impotence, poor ejaculation, and sensation alterations are discussed in earlier sections in this chapter.

Medroxyprogesterone acetate has been used successfully to suppress aggressive behavior and excessive sexual arousal. Serotonergic agents such as trazodone hydrochloride have also been effective in increasing libido. Selective serotonergic reuptake inhibitors (SSRIs) such as peroxetine and sertraline have also been effective (Zasler, 1995). Noradrenergic agonists and/or hormonal supplementation have been used for hyposexuality, especially in males (Zasler, 1995).

Interventions for the client with hypersexuality include immediate feedback to decrease inappropriate touching. Another strategy is to schedule massage to shift stimulus control to an appropriate setting. In the situation of exhibitionism, a combination of self-monitoring, private self-stimulation, and dating skills training has been successful in suppressing inappropriate sexual behavior (Zencius, Wesolowski, Burke, & Hough, 1990). A client can use a self-monitoring notebook to record all sexual urges and feelings. Whenever clients have the urge to expose themselves, they should record the urge in the notebook and then masturbate to fantasies of situations presented in a dating skills training class. Dating skills training includes role-playing. Scenarios of asking someone for a date, initiating conversation, and telephoning someone are examples (Zencius, Wesolowski, Burke, & Hough, 1990).

Scheduled massage has been helpful in decreasing episodes of inappropriate touching. In a case study done by Zencius, Wesolowski, Burke, and Hough (1990), treatment consisted of giving the client the opportunity to give back rubs under certain stimulus conditions. The client was allowed to give back rubs during a scheduled relaxation class. All clients and staff enrolled in the class could receive back rubs during the daily half-hour session. Whenever the client attempted to touch peers or staff outside the relaxation class, he was reminded that back rubs were to be given during the relaxation class only.

Arthritis Conditions

When a client has a rheumatic disease, such as rheumatoid arthritis (RA), it is imperative that the nurse be familiar with the signs and symptoms that can threaten fulfillment of a satisfying and intimate relationship, such as pain, stiffness, and deformities (see Chapter 23 on degenerative joint disease).

With RA, articular inflammation often progresses to joint destruction, deformity, and varying degrees of functional impairment. The synovium becomes edematous and protrudes into the joint space, with the periphery of the cartilage sustaining the greatest articular destruction. Ultimately, the pannus erodes the underlying cartilage, ligaments, tendons, and bone (Harris, 1983; Schumacher, 1993).

As RA progresses, pain and stiffness become worse, resulting in less range of motion and decreased ability to perform activities of daily living independently. Pain can interfere with genital intercourse when the hips and pelvic joints are affected, or with kissing and caressing when the temporomandibular or hand and arm joints are painful (Conine & Evans, 1982). Arthroplasties can decrease pain and improve the client's range of motion, and thus reduce physical limitations and make sex more gratifying (Swinburn, 1976).

Problems encountered by arthritis clients with sexual functioning include pain (major problem), limited range of motion and movement, fatigue, use of antirheumatic and steroid drugs, and genital lesions. Psychosocial problems include depression, anxiety, and loss of self-esteem (Lim, 1995).

Dealing with pain must be the highest priority. The client with RA is aware of when the pain is likely to occur and, therefore, planning ahead of time for intimacy versus spontaneous sex might be better. Taking an analgesic before sexual activity might be helpful. Joint discomfort may decrease after a brief resting interval, but prolonged rest periods can result in joint stiffness. Sharing a warm shower or bath can relieve the client's pain while also enhancing the sexual experience (Barbach, 1982). Clients with inflammatory arthritis experience Sjögren's syndrome, which may lead to a dry atrophic vaginitis, causing painful intercourse and dryness of the mouth, inhibiting oral-genital activity (Erlich, 1978).

Sexual activity can be a pain reliever in itself. After sexual intercourse there can be relief of pain and depression for up to 6 to 8 hours (Erlich, 1978). This may be due to endorphins or to the psychological benefits of caring and being cared for (Cole & Cole, 1995).

Another intervention for pain and range-of-motion limitations is to consider nontraditional coital positioning during sexual activities (Figure 1). In choosing a position, weight bearing on affected joints must be avoided. The use of pillows with positioning to increase comfort can also be helpful.

Arthritic hip involvement can limit abduction and external rotation. This limitation is especially significant when flexion contractures in adduction have occurred or when there is fusion of the hip by disease or surgery (Erlich, 1978). Following surgery, such as an open reduction and internal fixation of the hip, teaching the client how to prevent dislocation of the prosthesis is a must. Maintaining abduction with pillows will be necessary. The client can be positioned on the unaffected side, facing toward or away from the partner, while the affected leg can be partially flexed at the hip and/or knee and supported on a pillow (Fuchs & Salvati, 1989). Avoid hip flexion of more than 60 degrees. Avoid hip abduction of more than 30 degrees and external rotation of more than 45 to 60 degrees in unilateral hip disease. It should be advised that the client avoid vigorous thrusting during sexual intercourse until 6 to 8 weeks after surgery (Emick-Herring, 1993). Usually, the physician will clear the client of these restrictions 3 to 6 months postsurgery (Fuchs & Salvati, 1989).

The side effects of drugs to treat arthritis, including corticosteroids, have been implicated in causing fatigue and decreased libido (Erlich, 1978). The use of corticosteroids can cause physical changes, such as moon face, truncal obesity with buffalo hump and thin extremities, ecchymoses, acne, hirsutism, and osteoporosis (Erlich, 1978). Besides the loss of physical attractiveness, corticosteroids can result in impotence for the male client on prolonged use. Immunosuppressants can lead to hair loss. Gold compounds and immunosuppressants can produce both mouth and genital ulcers (Erlich, 1978).

These physical changes make the client feel unattractive, resulting in poor body image and negative self-esteem. In a world where beauty and physical perfection are emphasized, the client with arthritis should be reminded of his or her positive traits. These clients should be taught to focus on their strengths, rather than on their physical limitations. Nurses should also encourage the client to express the need for love and intimacy. A heightened self-image may actually increase libido (Dale, 1996).

If a female client with RA desires pregnancy, it will be necessary to discontinue antirheumatic drugs, because most of these medications cross the placental barrier. Salicylates should also be discontinued just before delivery to help control bleeding. RA goes into remission during pregnancy, but the client should be informed of the likelihood of an anticipated flare-up postpartum (Dale, 1996).

The Nursing Process: Assessment

Besides assessing the client's medical history and condition, the nurse will also want to address the client's sexual-reproductive pattern by taking a history. The history must be taken in private and with good time allotment. It is recommended that the client and the partner be interviewed separately, and then together.

The interview will consist of questions examining the client's and partner's moral and religious values and whether parenting or birth control is desired. Included are questions that will evaluate the psychological and emotional status of the client. Examples of "open ended" questions are the following: "How do you feel about the way your disability or disease has affected your sexual functions?"; "Do you feel as sexually attractive since your stroke?"; "What ways do you feel less attractive?"; "What are your concerns about sexual functioning once you go home?" The key is to use open-ended questions (Emick-Herring, 1993).

The nurse should also assess the client's psychosexual development. What knowledge does the client have about sexual functioning, reproduction, contraception, and the effects from his or her disability/disease? How are the client's social skills in dating, relationships, and communication with partners postdisability/disease? How do the client's current sexual patterns differ from premorbid patterns?

Many medications, as previously discussed, affect sexual functioning; therefore a review of what drugs the client is currently taking, including alcohol, is necessary.

Although the nurse does not order laboratory or diagnostic testing, it is helpful to be aware of possible tests that might be done or referred. The testosterone test (for males) can rule out organic reasons for a decreased libido or erectile dysfunction. The glucose test can rule out diabetes-induced erectile dysfunction (Emick-Herring, 1993). Other tests can include sensorimotor testing, a genitourinary (GU) examination/studies, pharmacologic erection testing, a penile cavernosogram and/or cavernosometry, and nocturnal penile tumescence monitoring (Emick-Herring, 1993).

Nursing Diagnoses, Goals/Outcomes, and Interventions

Nursing diagnoses listed are accepted by the North American Nursing Diagnosis Association (NANDA).

Nursing Diagnosis

- Sexual dysfunction, altered sexuality patterns related to altered body structure or function; motor/sensory deficits; knowledge deficit regarding sexual functioning and effects of disability or disease; values/cultural conflict; lack of privacy; role changes; body image disturbance; pain or discomfort; medication side effects or reduced activity intolerance (Mumma, 1987)

Goals/Outcomes

See Carpenito (1993).

- The client will identify factual limitations on sexual activity caused by disability or disease.
- The client will identify and perform appropriate modifications in sexual practices in response to these limitations.
- The client and partner will report satisfying sexual activity.

Nursing Interventions

The following are general nursing interventions for all clients (see interventions previously discussed for specific diseases or disabilities).

- Provide an uninterrupted intimate time for the client and partner.
- Provide information on alternative methods to achieve sexual intercourse, such as touching, caressing, massage, use of a vibrator, masturbation, penile implants, use of lubricants, music, waterbed, or erotic movies.
- Be aware of and comfortable with your own sexuality.
- Develop a trusting relationship with the client.
- Introduce the topic of sexuality in a nonthreatening, caring manner.
- Encourage open communication between the client and partner regarding sexual concerns and practices.
- Give permission for the client to verbalize feelings and concerns without being judgmental.
- Teach the client in the areas of sexuality and sexual function, offering educational materials when available.
- Teach the client regarding the side effects of medications affecting sexual function.
- Teach the client regarding bladder control and bowel program regulation.

- Inform the client about opportunities for social contact, such as clubs, church, and school functions.
- Advise the (severely disabled) client to obtain household/attendant help because it is difficult to combine lover and caregiver roles.
- Refer the client to experts as necessary if sexuality concerns cannot be answered or resolved successfully, or if considering ways to conceive such as artificial insemination or *in vitro* fertilization.
- Use the PLISSIT model, consisting of conceptual levels of interventions (Table 1).

The **PLISSIT model,** developed by Annon (1976), is useful in guiding the nurse in the role of sexual counseling. Conceptual levels include permission giving, limited information, specific suggestions, and intensive therapy.

Permission giving must be practiced by nursing. This first level is expected from all nurses. The nurse gives the client permission to be a sexual being. The nurse encourages the client to ask questions and assures the client that being concerned about his or her sexuality is normal and that his or her current sexual hab-

Table 1
The PLISSIT Model

Level	Intervention
P: Permission giving	The nurse lets the client express feelings/concerns. The nurse encourages open discussions, is a good listener, is nonjudgmental, and sanctions the subject of sexuality
LI: Limited information	The nurse provides verbal and/or nonverbal teaching on human sexuality and how sexual functioning is affected by disability or disease. The nurse should impart only information that he or she is knowledgeable about and comfortable with. Providing pamphlets, diagrams, and articles can be helpful
SS: Specific suggestions	The nurse proposes a planned course of action to reach specific goals determined by client and partner. The nurse helps the client find solutions and alternatives: possibilities include joining a support group, doing certain exercises, or trying different positioning techniques
IT: Intensive therapy	The nurse refers the client to an appropriate expert in sexual functioning or a specialized clinic for assistance and counseling. A highly individualized program, provided by specially trained professionals, is necessary when levels of P, LI, and SS do not solve the client's concerns

its are appropriate and healthy (Greco, 1996). This may not be true with the brain-injured client. This level also gives permission to the nurse to refer the individual to another professional when there is lack of knowledge or conflict in comfort or values (Hodge, 1995). Permission includes allowing the client to grieve for the loss acquired from disability in order to accept possible alternatives (Goddard, 1988).

Limited information should answer basic questions regarding the client's sexual functioning following disability or disease; only specific questions by the client are addressed at this level. Group sessions are an option for sharing this information with clients who have the same type of medical diagnosis.

An area of limited information relates to assertiveness by the client. Clients with disabilities need to be assertive in dealing with personal questions, stares, negative comments, indifference or apathy, and inappropriate assistance. They also need to be assertive with their partner, being certain that the partner has his or her questions answered as well (Goddard, 1988).

Specific suggestions may be offered by the nurse to address specific concerns such as alternative positioning methods for the client with a CVA or total hip replacement. Specific suggestions involve direct problem-oriented strategies or referral for specific medical interventions (Greco, 1996). Suggestions specific to each problem are offered to help the individual alter behavior to achieve stated goals. Inclusion of a urologist or physiatrist might be appropriate at this level (Hodge, 1995).

Intensive therapy is a referral mechanism used to meet the needs of a client whose problems cannot be solved using the previous levels of intervention. Intensive therapy may be necessary to deal with sexual problems existing before injury or disease or arising afterward (Goddard, 1988). A full sex history is required at this level.

Nurses who are uncomfortable with any of the levels should refer the client to other team members who are skilled and knowledgeable in specific areas of counseling and education. Team members who may be skilled in sexual counseling include the clinical nurse specialist, psychologist, social worker, therapy staff, gynecologist, physiatrist, urologist, and sex therapist (Greco, 1996).

Other *nursing diagnoses* that should be considered include

- Body image disturbance, personal identity disturbance, self-esteem disturbance related to loss of a significant other; unrealistic self-expectations; repeated negative interpersonal experiences with significant others; separation from support systems while hospitalized; or inability to adjust to and integrate body changes (Mumma, 1987)
- Social isolation related to physical disability; cognitive impairment; fear of embarrassment; rejection by partner; incontinence; body image disturbance, or disfigurement (Mumma, 1987)

- Knowledge deficit regarding alternative means to sexual functioning; positioning techniques; birth control methods or side effects from medications. The knowledge deficit could be related to new onset of disability; low readiness to receive information; lack of interest or motivation; psychomotor limitations or cognitive impairment (Mumma, 1987)

Conclusions

The ability to function as a sexual being is a basic need for all individuals. This need occurs also in clients with chronic illness or disability, for whom sexual concerns sometimes become a major focus. Disability has demonstrable impact on sexuality and must be taken into account by nurses working with rehabilitation clients. The nurse's role as it relates to sexuality in people with disabilities is to assist clients to find, implement, and integrate their beliefs and behaviors into a healthy and satisfying lifestyle (Rieve, 1989). We all have the desire to be loved and close to another human being. Sexuality is one way that individuals express that need. Nurses can help clients to be open about their sexual concerns and needs. A positive sexual relationship is possible when love is present and when the client and partner are open to trying different alternatives. This requires a change from the traditional way, but through open communication, patience, and encouragement by nurses and the whole rehabilitation team, change can be good and sexually rewarding.

References

Amelar, R. D., & Dubin, L. (1982). Sexual function and fertility in paraplegic males. *Urology, 20,* 62–65.

Annon, J. S. (1976). The PLISSIT model: A proposed conceptual scheme for behavioral treatment of sexual problems. *Journal of Sex Education Therapy, 2,* 1–15.

Barbach, B. (1982). *For each other: Sharing sexual intimacy.* New York: Anchor Press/Doubleday.

Boone, T. B. (1995). The physiology of sexual function in normal individuals. *Physical Medicine and Rehabilitation, 9*(2), 313–323.

Bors, E., & Comarr, A. E. (1960). Neurological disturbances of sexual function with special reference to 529 patients with spinal cord injury. *Urology Surgery, 10,* 191–222.

Brindley, G. S. (1981). Electroejaculation: Its technique, neurological implications and uses. *Journal of Neurological Neurosurgery Psychiatry, 44,* 9–18.

Brindley, G. S., Sauerwein, D., & Hendry, W. F. (1989). Hypogastric plexus stimulators for obtaining semen from paraplegic men. *British Journal of Urology, 64,* 72–77.

Carpenito, L. J. (1993). *Nursing diagnosis: Application to clinical practice* (5th ed.). Philadelphia: J. B. Lippincott.

Carroll, M., Tempkin, T., & Worth, W. (1986). In N. Woll (Ed.), *Nursing spinal cord injuries.* Totowa, NJ: Rowman & Allanheld (pp. 89–105).

Chang, S. W., Fine, R., Siegel, D., et al. (1991). The impact of diuretic therapy on reported sexual function. *Archives of Internal Medicine, 151,* 2402–2408.

Charlifue, S. W., Gerhart, K. A., Menter, R. R., Whiteneck, G. G., & Manley, M. S. (1992). Sexual issues of women with spinal cord injuries. *Paraplegia, 30,* 192–199.

Cole, S., & Cole, S. C. (1993). Sexuality, disability, and reproductive issues through the life span. In F. P. Haseltine, S. S. Cole, & D. B. Gray (Eds.), *Reproductive Issues for persons with physical disabilities.* Baltimore: Paul H. Brooks (pp. 3–21).

Cole, T. M. (1975). Sexuality and physical disabilities. *Archives of Sexual Behavior, 4,* 389–403.

Comarr, A. E. (1970). Sexual function among patients with spinal cord injury. *Urology International,* *25,* 134–168.

Comarr, A. E. (1977). Sexual function in patients with spinal cord injury. In P. S. Pierce & V. H. Nickel (Eds.), *The total care of spinal cord injury.* Boston: Little, Brown.

Comarr, A. E., & Vigue, M. (1978). Sexual counseling among male and female patients with spinal cord and/or cauda equina injury. *American Journal of Physical Medicine, 57*(5), 215–229.

Conine, T. A., & Evans, J. H. (1982). Sexual reactivation of chronically ill and disabled adults. *Journal of Allied Health, 11,* 261–270.

Cookson, M. S., & Nadig, P. W. (1993). Long-term results with vacuum constriction device. *Journal of Urology, 149,* 290–294.

Craig, D. I. (1994). Spinal cord injury and pregnancy: The stories of two women. *SCI Nursing, 11*(4), 100–104.

Crewe, N. M. (1984). Sexually inappropriate behavior. In D. S. Bishop (Ed.), *Behavioral problems and the disabled: Assessment and management.* Malabar, FL: Robert E. Krieger.

Dale, K. G. (1996). Intimacy and rheumatic diseases. *Rehabilitation Nursing, 21*(1), 38–40.

Ducharme, S. (1987). Sexuality and physical disability. In B. Caplan (Ed.), *Rehabilitation psychology desk reference.* Rockville, MD: Aspen.

Ebersole, P., & Hess, P. (1994). *Toward healthy aging: Human needs and nursing response* (4th ed.). St. Louis: Mosby–Year Book.

Emick-Herring, B. (1993). Sexuality—Reproductive pattern. In A. E. McCourt (Ed.), *The specialty practice of rehabilitation nursing: A core curriculum* (3rd ed.). Skokie, IL: Rehabilitation Nursing Foundation.

Erlich, G. E. (1978). Sexual problems of the arthritic patient. In A. Comfort (Ed.), *Sexual consequences of disability.* Philadelphia: George F. Stickley.

Fuchs, M. D., & Salvati, E. A. (1989). Sexual counseling following a total hip replacement. *Medical Aspects of Human Sexuality, 23*(4), 55–57.

Gatens, C. (1984). Sexuality and disability. In N. F. Woods (Ed.), *In health and illness.* St. Louis: Mosby.

Goddard, L. R. (1988). Sexuality and spinal cord injury. *Journal of Neuroscience nursing, 20*(4), 240–244.

Greco, S. B. (1996). Sexuality education and counseling. In S. Hoeman (Ed.), *Rehabilitation nursing: Process and application* (2nd ed.). St. Louis: Mosby–Year Book.

Green, B. G., & Sloan, S. L. (1986). Penile prostheses in spinal cord injured patients: combined psychosexual counseling and surgical regimen. *Paraplegia, 24,* 167–172.

Green, G. G., Killorin, E. W., Jr., Foote, J., Bennett, J. K., & Sloan, S. (1995). Complications of penile implants in spinal cord injured patients. *Topics in Spinal Cord Injury Rehabilitation, 1,*(2), 44–52.

Griffith, E. R., & Lemberg, S. (1993). *Sexuality and the person with traumatic brain injury: A guide for families.* Philadelphia: F. A. Davis.

Griffith, E. R., & Trieschmann, R. B. (1983). Sexual dysfunctions in the physically ill and disabled. In C. C. Nadelson & D. B. Marcotte (Eds.), *Treatment interventions in human sexuality.* New York: Plenum Press.

Guttman, L., Frankel, H. L., & Paeslack, V. (1965). Cardiac irregularities during labor in paraplegic women. *Paraplegia, 3,* 144–151.

Harris, E. D. (1983). Evaluation of pathophysiology and drug effects on rheumatoid arthritis. *The American Journal of Medicine, 75*(4B), 56–61.

Hawton, K. (1984). Sexual adjustment of men who had strokes. *Journal of Psychosomatics Research, 28,* 243–249.

Higgins, G. E. (1979). Sexual response in spinal cord injured adults: A review of the literature. *Archives of Sexual Behavior, 8,* 173–196.

Hirsch, I. H., Seager, S. W., Seldor, J., King, L., & Staas, W. E., Jr. (1990). Electroejaculatory stimulation of a quadriplegic man resulting in pregnancy. *Archives of Physical Medicine and Rehabilitation, 71,* 54–57.

Hirsch, I. H., Sedor, J., Callahan, H. J., & Staas, W. E. (1992). Antisperm antibodies in seminal plasma of spinal cord-injured men. *Urology, 39,* 243–247.

Hodge, A. L. (1995). Addressing issues of sexuality with spinal cord injured persons. *Orthopaedic Nursing, 14*(3), 21–24.

Hudson, L. M., & Green, S. (1995). Parenthood after spinal cord injury: The personal side. *Topics in Spinal Cord Injury Rehabilitation, 1,*(2), 62–67.

Krane, R. J., & Siroky, M. B. (1981). Neurophysiology of erection. *Urology Clinics of North America, 8,* 91–102.

Leslie, S. W. (1990). *Impotence: Current diagnosis and treatment.* Lorain, OH: Geddings Osbon, Sr. Foundation.

Levin, H. S., Benton, A. L., & Grossman, R. G. (1982). *Neurobehavioral consequences of closed head injury.* New York: Oxford University Press.

Lezak, M. L. (1978). Living with the characterologically altered brain injured client. *Journal of Clinical Psychiatry, 39,* 592–598.

Lim, P. (1995). Sexuality in patients in musculoskeletal diseases. *Physical Medicine and Rehabilitation, 9*(2), 401–415.

Lusk, M. D., & Kott, J. A. (1982). Effects of head injury on libido. *Medical Aspects of Human Sexuality, 16,* 22–30.

Maslow, A. (1954). *Motivation and personality.* New York: Harper & Row.

Masters, W., & Johnson, V. E. (1966). *Human sexual response.* Boston: Little, Brown.

Masters, W., & Johnson, V. E. (1970). *Human sexual inadequacy.* Boston: Little, Brown.

Masters, W. H., Johnson, V. E., & Kolodny, R. C. (1986). *Masters and Johnson on sex and human loving.* Boston: Little, Brown.

McCarren, M. (1991). Where are all the babies? *Spinal Network Extra,* Fall, *41,* 22–27.

McCormick, G. P., Riffer, D. J., & Thompson, M. M. (1986). Coital positioning for stroke afflicted couples. *Rehabilitation Nursing, 11*(2), 17–19.

McCunniff, D. E., & Dewan, D. (1984). Pregnancy after spinal cord injury (letter to the editor). *Obstetrics and Gynecology, 63*(5), 757.

Mendius, R. A. (1989). Female sexuality and spinal cord injury. *SCI Nursing, 6*(4), 68–74.

Monga, T. N., & Ostermann, H. J. (1995). Sexuality and sexual adjustment in stroke patients. *Physical Medicine and Rehabilitation, 9*(2), 345–359.

Mumma, C. (Ed.). (1987). *Rehabilitation nursing: Concepts and practice—A core curriculum* (2nd ed.). Evanston, IL: Rehabilitation Nursing Foundation.

National Stroke Association. (1993). There is sex after stroke. Be stroke smart (client education handout). Englewood, CO: Author.

Poorman, S. G., Smith, J. G., & Robertson, L. L. (1988). Changes in sexuality related to physical and emotional illness and disability. In S. G. Poorman (Ed.), *Human sexuality and the nursing process.* Norwalk, CT: Appleton & Lange.

Rawicki, H., & Lording, D. W. (1988). Assisted fertility in complete paraplegia: Case report. *Paraplegia, 26,* 401–404.

Rieve, J. E. (1989). Sexuality and the adult with acquired physical disability. *Nursing Clinics of North America, 24*(1), 265–277.

Santora, J. (1989). Sexuality and sexual function. In S. Dittmar (Ed.), *Rehabilitation nursing: Process and application.* St. Louis: Mosby.

Schumacher, H. R. (1993). *Primer on the rheumatic diseases.* Atlanta: Arthritis Foundation.

Sipski, M. L., Alexander, C. J., & Rosen, R. C. (1995). Orgasm in women with spinal cord injuries: A laboratory-based assessment. *Archives of Physical Medicine Rehabilitation, 76,* 1097–1102.

Sjogren, K., Damber, J. E., & Liliequist, B. (1983). Sexuality after stroke with hemiplegia. *Scandinavian Journal of Rehabilitation Medicine, 15,* 55–61.

Smeltzer, S. C., & Bare, B. G. (1996). *Brunner and Suddarth's textbook of medical-surgical nursing* (8th ed.). Philadelphia: Lippincott-Raven.

Smith, E. M., & Bodner, D. R. (1993). Sexual dysfunction after spinal cord injury. *Urologic Clinics of North America, 20*(3), 535–542.

Sonksen, J., & Biering-Sorensen, F. (1992). Penile erection in men with spinal cord or cauda equina lesions. *Seminars in Neurology, 10*(2), 98–105.

Swinburn, W. R. (1976). Sexual counseling for the arthritic. *Clinics in Rheumatic Diseases, 2,*(3), 639–651.

Thomsen, I. V. (1984). Late outcome of severe blunt head trauma: A 10–15 year second follow-up. *Journal of Neurology and Psychiatry, 47,* 260–268.

Walbroehl, G. S. (1987). Sexuality in the handicapped. *American Family Physician, 36*(1), 129–133.

Weinberg, J. S. (1982). Human sexuality and spinal cord injury. *Nursing Clinics of North America, 17*(3), 407–419.

Weiss, J. (1992). Multiple sclerosis: Will it come between us? Sexual concerns of clients and their partners. *Journal of Neuroscience Nursing, 24*(4), 190–193.

Witherington, R. (1988). Suction device therapy in the management of erectile impotence. *Urology Clinics of North America, 15,* 123.

World Health Organization. (1975). *Education and treatment in human sexuality: The training of health professionals.* WHO Technical Report Series No. 572. Geneva: Author.

Yarkony, G. M., & Chen, D. (1995). Sexuality in patients with spinal cord injury. *Physical Medicine and Rehabilitation, 9,*(2), 325–344.

Zasler, N. D., & Horn, L. J. (1990). Rehabilitative management of sexual dysfunction. *Journal of Head Trauma Rehabilitation, 5,* 14–24.

Zejdlik, C. M. (1983). *Management of spinal cord injury.* Monterey, CA: Wadsworth Wealth Sciences Division.

Zencius, A., Wesolowski, M. D., Burke, W. H., & Hough, S. (1990). Managing hypersexual disorders in brain-injured clients. *Brain Injury, 4*(2), 175–181.

CHAPTER 29
Medical-Surgical Complications in the Rehabilitation Client

Lorise Rodriguez

Key Terms
Cardiovascular Assessment
Cardiovascular Complications
Functional Limitations
Gastrointestinal Complications
Hypotension
Immobility
Physical Assessment
Pulmonary Assessment
Pulmonary Complications
Renal Complications

Objectives

1. Identify the medical-surgical complications in the rehabilitation client.

2. Assess for major medical-surgical complications of the rehabilitation client.

3. Discuss medical interventions used for managing medical-surgical complications.

4. Discuss nursing interventions used for managing medical-surgical complications.

5. Determine outcomes for evaluation of management of medical-surgical complications.

It is impossible in a book to teach a person in charge of sick how to manage, as it is to teach her how to nurse. (Nightingale, 1969, p. 35)

Introduction
The nurses' role for the rehabilitation client is most significant in identification, prevention, and management of complications arising from an altered health status and altered bodily functions. This compromised health status may be related to a multitude of causes, including trauma, stroke, head injury, or burns, and may affect multiple organ systems including the cardiorespiratory, urinary, musculoskeletal, and gastrointestinal systems. In addition to assessing and managing the physical and/or medical condition of the client, consideration must be given to

the client's **functional limitations** and age. The young and the old adapt differently to the rehabilitative process: physically, psychologically, and developmentally (Matteson & McConnell, 1988).

Many complications encountered by the rehabilitation client arise from immobility. The nurses' management of medical-surgical complications will determine the success of the rehabilitation program and patient efficiency for self-care. Assessment by a multidisciplinary team is crucial in the patient's ongoing care. Inclusive in the **physical assessment** is a review of body systems. Information is needed on the integumentary system, for example, skin integrity, and the presence of casts, incisions, and wounds. A baseline assessment of the patient's musculoskeletal and neurologic systems, including functional ability, cognitive capacities, orientation, the presence of weakness or dizziness, muscle strength, and range of motion, should be obtained. The **cardiovascular assessment** should include the stability of blood pressure and other vital signs and the assessment for deep vein thrombosis (DVT). **Pulmonary assessment** is necessary to determine the patient's ability to cough, clear secretions, and safely maintain the airway. Information on the patient's nutritional status and bowel function should be ascertained. The functioning of the urinary system should include the patient's ability to void and potential risks of developing urinary tract infections and renal calculi. Diagnostic procedures and laboratory tests are additional tools to aid the nurse's assessment.

Important in a holistic assessment is the client's psychosocial status. Is the patient able to communicate to make his or her needs known? Confusion, pain, sedatives, and tranquilizers may alter the client's perceptions (Holloway, 1984). With altered perceptions, patients may not be able to communicate their needs or express their fears, concerns, or questions.

Cardiovascular Complications

Cardiovascular complications can arise from restricted activity and altered mobility experienced by rehabilitation clients, resulting in detrimental effects on the cardiovascular system, namely in altered cardiac output and/or altered tissue perfusion. These are manifested by cardiovascular deconditioning, orthostatic **hypotension,** and increased thrombus formation (Holloway, 1984; Underhill, Woods, Sivarajan Froelicher, & Halpenny, 1989).

The effects of immobility are most acutely exhibited by the deconditioning of the cardiovascular system to the extent that it is unable to support physical activity. Cardiovascular deconditioning becomes evident as the myocardial workload is increased through altered stroke volume, tachycardia, and Valsalva's maneuver.

Supine positions add strain to the myocardium by promoting the pooling of central blood volume. When clients are in a supine position, approximately 8 percent of the blood volume may move from the lower extremities to the heart and lungs (Holloway, 1984). This pooling of blood subsequently increases preload. With an increase in preload, stroke volume also increases due to the Starling's law, which causes an increase in the volume of blood being pumped.

Studies have demonstrated that clients on bedrest will have an increase of their resting heart rate by 0.5 beats per minute per day (Underhill, Woods, Sivarajan Froelicher, & Halpenny, 1989). Cardiac output is determined by heart rate times stroke volume. When cardiac output is increased due to increases in the resting heart rate and increases in stroke volume, myocardial workload is definitely compromised.

Simple client movements, such as turning in bed or straining for a bowel movement, can compromise the myocardium. Valsalva's maneuver places additional strain on the myocardium by increasing the intrathoracic pressure and by decreasing the venous blood return to the heart. When intrathoracic pressure decreases, a "rebound effect" is created. What follows is an increase in venous return to the heart (Holloway, 1984; Underhill, Woods, Sivarajan Froelicher, & Halpenny, 1989).

Orthostatic hypotension is another common cardiovascular complication secondary to prolonged immobility. Clients experience orthostatic hypotension when there are abrupt position changes that cause a drop in blood pressure and syncope. This hypotension is related to venous pooling and loss of muscle tone. A fall in blood pressure is manifested by an increase in heart rate, a decrease in venous return, and a decrease in stroke volume. Essentially, even though the heart rate increases, it is not sufficient to maintain cardiac output. Similarly, there is an increase in the systemic vascular resistance, but that too is not enough to maintain the blood pressure (Underhill, Woods, Sivarajan Froelicher, & Halpenny, 1989).

Another cardiovascular complication faced by the rehabilitation team is the prevention and detection of thrombus formation. Thirty-five percent of all hospitalized clients develop deep vein thrombosis. Clients at risk for the development of thrombi may have decreased venous flow to the lower extremities, an altered fluid status as in dehydration, pressure on veins (especially those in the lower extremities), and immobility, which leads to the pooling of blood in the lower extremities. Pulmonary emboli are also associated with thrombus formation, particularly as the clot breaks and travels to the pulmonary artery.

Deep vein thrombosis is usually characterized by a positive Homans' sign, swelling, tenderness, and pain in the lower extremity, particularly the calf. Some clients experience redness and warmth in the lower extremity. Clients at risk for developing thrombosis have a history of cardiac disease and may have had recent orthopedic and neurosurgical surgery.

Nursing Interventions for Cardiovascular Complications

One of the most significant interventions that will minimize cardiovascular deconditioning and thrombus formation is early mobilization (Underhill, Woods, Sivarajan Froelicher, & Halpenny, 1989). Mobilization is effective if done gradually through progressive activity. Active and passive range-of-motion exercises, especially for the lower extremities, serve to decrease the risk of thrombus formation and to stimulate venous return (Underhill, Woods, Sivarajan Froelicher, & Halpenny, 1989). Gradual elevation of the head of the bed and dangling the legs over the side of bed will minimize orthostatic hypotension and syncope. Early activity is integral in preventing cardiovascular deconditioning and thrombus formation. Teaching patients to avoid Valsalva's maneuver by exhaling when turning, exercising, or having a bowel movement will decrease intrathoracic pressures, which strain the myocardium.

Medical management of thrombus formation is accomplished by anticoagulation through the administration of intravenous heparin and oral agents. Antiembolitic stockings, pressure cuffs, early mobilization, and range-of-motion exercises are other nursing interventions that may be used to prevent and treat DVTs.

Pulmonary Complications

One challenge for the rehabilitation staff is the management of respiratory complications, specifically hypostatic pneumonia. Factors that heighten a client's risk for the development of pneumonia include the inability to mobilize secretions, hypoventilation, and atelectasis (Underhill, Woods, Sivarajan Froelicher, & Halpenny, 1989). When the respiratory muscles are weak and clients fatigue easily, hypoventilation and atelectasis may ensue. Respiratory acidosis may develop as the patient takes in less O_2 and retains more CO_2. Consideration should be given to the client's medication regimen, such as narcotics, which depress the respiratory effort. Likewise, assessment and management of the client's pain, if not done adequately, may inhibit the client from turning, coughing, and breathing deeply.

The client's ability to be mobile may contribute to the development of **pulmonary complications.** In healthy individuals, secretions are mobilized naturally through coughing and activity. For the immobile client, recumbency contributes to the development of hypostatic pneumonia. The pooling of secretions to the dependent side of the bronchiole leads to the shunting of blood past unventilated alveoli. Bacteria in the mucous pools proliferate, as they are no longer in contact with the phagocytes, resulting in the development of hypostatic pneumonia and/or atelectasis. Medications that depress the ability of the client to cough and participate in pulmonary toilet, as well as the client's pain level, should be assessed.

Nursing Interventions for Pulmonary Complications

Preventive nursing measures, such as turning, coughing, and deep breathing and teaching clients the importance of these functions, are essential in maintaining good pulmonary toilet. Early mobilization and ambulation also contribute to the prevention of complications. Assessing the client's fluid status and hydration is necessary to maintain moist mucous membranes and to liquefy secretions. Determining the client's respiratory status before administering a sedative or analgesic is necessary to avoid hypoventilation. Chest physiotherapy, postural drainage, and the use of breathing treatments are adjuncts to care in the management of respiratory complications.

Renal Complications

Among the renal complications that the rehabilitation client faces are kidney stone formation, urinary tract infections, and urinary retention. The effects of **immobility** and recumbency take their toll on the urinary system with a rise in the concentration of urinary calcium, magnesium, and phosphates (Underhill, Woods, Sivarajan Froelicher, & Halpenny, 1989). The rise in calcium, magnesium, and phosphate is primarily related to demineralization and protein breakdown secondary to immobility. With demineralization and protein breakdown, urine changes from an acidic concentration to a more alkalotic environment, lending itself to the development of infection and stone formation. In addition, recumbency promotes the pooling of urine in the renal pelvis and, therefore, the formation of renal calculi.

Urinary retention associated with bladder distention contributes to the development of urinary tract infections. Stasis of urine, weakened urethral sphincters, incomplete bladder emptying, and the presence of an indwelling catheter are also cited as risk factors for infection (Holloway, 1984).

Nursing Interventions for Renal Complications

There are three main nursing interventions to prevent complications of the urinary system. Assessment of the client's hydration status is paramount through accurate monitoring of intake and output. Urine that is dilute and acidic will minimize the formation of renal calculi. If not contraindicated, patients should be encouraged to drink at least eight glasses of fluid per day.

Activity plays a role in preventing protein breakdown and demineralization of bone. Range-of-motion exercises, turning, weight-bearing exercises, and ambulation encourage proper bladder emptying and the development of urinary tract infections.

Complete bladder emptying prevents urinary stasis and the development of infection. Assessing the bladder for distention and monitoring urinary output will aid the nurse in an accurate assessment. Although urinary catheters have the benefit of complete bladder emptying, they do carry with them the increased risk of infection. Maintaining a sterile, closed urinary drainage system is a basic nursing function.

Gastrointestinal Complications

Gastrointestinal complications can occur subsequent to illness, injury, and hospitalization, which increase the nutritional demands for the rehabilitation client. Factors that can create altered nutrition include nausea, decreased appetite, the inability for self-feeding, an altered swallowing reflex, medications, and inactivity. Stress increases the body's caloric requirements. If caloric needs are not met, catabolism will lead to protein breakdown and, ultimately, a negative nitrogen balance. Early intervention and an accurate assessment of the client's nutritional status are integral for the rehabilitation client. Nutrition drives the client's energy level and ability to participate in the rehabilitation program.

In addition to nutrition, the gastrointestinal assessment should include assessment of bowel function. Inactivity contributes to the development of constipation. Often, bedbound clients lose the defecation reflex or are too weak to use the abdominal muscles for defecation. Prevention is the key to minimizing constipation.

Nursing Interventions for Gastrointestinal Complications

Assess the client's usual bowel pattern and nutritional status. Encourage the client to eat foods high in fiber. To promote normal bowel activity, patients should maintain an adequate fluid intake. Although the use of suppositories, enemas, and laxatives may be necessary, regular use of these methods should be avoided as they disrupt a regular bowel pattern.

Clients should avoid straining with a bowel movement. Valsalva's maneuver is contraindicated in clients with cardiac disease and stroke. Teaching clients to exhale while tightening the abdominal muscles will prevent straining. Other nursing interventions, such as providing privacy and/or a bedside commode, will assist patients in promoting or maintaining normal bowel function.

Outcome Evaluation

Although all complications cannot always be avoided, taking measures to minimize the occurrence of untoward effects is within the realm of nursing. Evaluating patient outcomes measures nursing effectiveness. Outcomes such as clear breath sounds, bowel movements that are of normal consistency and frequency, absence of a urinary tract infection, and a resting heart rate that has been constant represent nursing effectiveness. Implementing medical and nursing interventions in a timely manner will hopefully hasten the patient's recovery.

References

Holloway, N. M. (1984). *Nursing the critically ill adult* (2nd ed.). Menlo Park, CA: Addison-Wesley.
Matteson, M. A., & McConnell, E. S. (1988). *Gerontological nursing.* Philadelphia: W.B. Saunders.
Nightingale, F. (1969). *Notes on nursing.* New York: Dover.
Underhill, S. L., Woods, S. L., Sivarajan Froelicher, E. S., & Halpenny, C. J. (1989). *Cardiac nursing* (2nd ed.). Philadelphia: J.B. Lippincott.

Suggested Readings

Bullock, B. L., & Rosenthal, P. P. (1984). *Pathophysiology: Adaptations and alterations in function.* Boston: Little, Brown.

Grindel, C. G., & Costello, M. C. (1996). Nutrition screening: An essential assessment parameter. *MedSurg Nursing, 5*(3), 145–156.

Lubkin, I. M. (1986). *Chronic illness: Impact and interventions.* Boston: Jones & Bartlett.

Martin, N., Holt, N., & Hicks, D. (1981). *Comprehensive rehabilitation nursing.* New York: McGraw-Hill.

Recker, D. (1992). Overcoming the obstacles to caring for the long-term critical care patient. *Critical Care Nurse, 12*(5), 40–48.

Thornlow, D. K. (1995). Is chest physiotherapy necessary after cardiac surgery? *Critical Care Nurse, 15*(3), 39–48.

Wirtz, K. M., La Favor, K. M., & Ang, R. (1996). Managing chronic spinal cord injury: Issues in critical care. *Critical Care Nurse, 16*(4), 24–35.

GENERATIONAL ISSUES

CHAPTER 30
Pediatric Rehabilitation

Carol Lea Melvin, Mary Lee Lacy, and *Linda E. Swofford-Ten Eyck*

Key Terms   *Agnosia*
Aphasia
Attention Deficit Disorder
Blunt Trauma
Cerebral Palsy (CP)
Children's Coma Scale (CCS)
Cognitive Remediation
Designated Health Nursing Services
Diplegia
Hemineglect
Hypertonicity
Hypotonicity
Individual Education Plan (IEP)
Individual Family Service Plans (IFSPs)
Individual Transition Plan (ITP)
Nonaccidental Trauma
Posttraumatic Amnesia (PTA)
Spastic Quadriparesis
Special Education

Objectives   1. Describe the difference between habilitation and rehabilitation.

2. Define pediatric rehabilitation, the role of the pediatric rehabilitation nurse, and the components of practice.

3. Describe the developmental model and apply it to common pediatric disabilities.

4. Describe common pediatric disabilities, i.e., spina bifida, cerebral palsy, muscular dystrophy, head injury, and juvenile rheumatoid arthritis. Apply common nursing diagnoses against the background of developmental theory to these common disabilities.

5. Describe the four main types of cerebral palsy.

6. Define cerebral palsy and discuss its incidence and etiology.

7. Discuss nursing care approaches to specific developmental stages.

8. Discuss common family concerns associated with cerebral palsy.

9. Identify and describe the incidence of traumatic injury in the pediatric population of the United States.

10. Describe the different types and causes of injury as differentiated by sex and age.

11. Describe the Children's Coma Scale and its use in assessing pediatric brain injury.

12. Compare the use of the Children's Coma Scale with posttraumatic amnesia as a prognostic indicator in pediatric brain injury.

13. Describe how the clinical picture of a child with a brain injury differs from the clinical picture of an adult with a brain injury.

14. Identify two common long-term problems of a child with a brain injury.

15. Identify the community agency primarily responsible for the postdischarge rehabilitation of the child with a brain injury.

16. Describe the evolution in the past 75 years of educational services for children with disabilities.

17. Describe how this evolution has affected the delivery of health services to children with disabilities.

18. List and describe Designated Health Nursing Services provided by school nurses.

19. List five disabling conditions that might be found among students at a school site and describe a nursing intervention for each condition.

Definitions

Habilitation: A comprehensive, interactive process, the goal of which is to enable an individual with a disability of dysfunction (usually congenital or acquired shortly after birth) to develop new abilities and to achieve his or her maximum potential (Bramadat and Melvin, 1987)

Concept of dependence, independence, and interdependence: Concept in which one knows when to rely on others, ask for help, and delegate responsibility (Peterson, Rauen, Brown, & Cole, 1994, p. 229)

Spina bifida: Common term used by parents and professionals to identify the disability that falls in the broad category of myelodysplasia.

Myelodysplasia: Condition that results from the failure of the neural tube to close during embryonic development, resulting in a dysplastic spinal cord with impaired neurological function

> *Hydrocephalus:* An abnormal accumulation of cerebrospinal fluid in the ventricles within the brain. The abnormal accumulation results in increased intracranial pressure that squeezes the brain and can result in tissue atrophy and cell death
>
> *Ventriculoperitoneal (VP) shunt:* Tiny tube that is placed in the ventricle of the brain to drain excess cerebrospinal fluid from the ventricle into the peritoneal cavity, where it is reabsorbed

Introduction

Pediatric rehabilitation nursing is the specialty practice committed to improving the quality of life for children, adolescents, and their families. The mission of this subspecialty is to provide a continuum of nursing care from injury and diagnosis to productive adulthood in collaboration with the interdisciplinary team. It is both specialized and diverse. Pediatric rehabilitation nurses care for a variety of disabling conditions in a variety of settings, including the home and the school. In fact, most nurses who deal with children with disabilities are not based in the hospital or a rehabilitation center. They are school nurses, community health nurses, home health nurses, public health nurses, and case managers for programs that serve disabled children. Many of these nurses did not intentionally become pediatric rehabilitation specialists but their chosen practice area demanded that they learn the content. For many years, these individuals have functioned well without the benefit of knowing their peers in rehabilitation nursing. Many of them do not understand that rehabilitation concepts serve them well and help them to understand where to turn next when facing a difficult problem. Developmental theory is the cornerstone of their practice. These nurses are experts in theory and well-child care. Their clients are children first and disabled incidentally. These nurses actively advocate for the child and not the disability.

Pediatric rehabilitation draws from both the conceptual basis of habilitation and rehabilitation. *Habilitation* is defined as a comprehensive, interactive process, the goal of which is to enable an individual with a disability of dysfunction (usually congenital or acquired shortly after birth) to develop new abilities and to achieve his or her maximum potential (Bramadat & Melvin, 1987). Infants who have never walked cannot be rehabilitated to relearn walking because they did not know how to walk before becoming disabled. Obviously, the younger the child, the more the process is one of habilitation rather than rehabilitation. The older the child, the more the process is composed of the concepts of both processes. *Rehabilitation,* on the other hand, is defined as a dynamic process in which a disabled person is aided in achieving optimum physical, emotional, psychological, social, or vocational potential in order to maintain dignity and self-respect in a life that is as independent and self-fulfilling as possible (Hickey, 1986, p. 179). All of the components of the rehabilitative process are contained within the process of habilitation. Pediatric rehabilitation nurses use both concepts within their practice unconsciously as they work with disabled children.

Family involvement is imperative. The child and the family are the core of the rehabilitation team, more than in any other practice area (Association of Rehabilitation Nurses, 1993, p. 19). The family is the environment that provides the child with the framework in which to try out newly learned skills and to witness its effect on others. Adjustment to the disability is colored by the family's adjustment to raising a child with a disability.

Developmental Model
Infancy

Many children with chronic illness or developmental disabilities are treated by an interdisciplinary team. These teams are composed of physicians and other health care professionals as well as child development specialists, educators, and behavior management specialists. The components of the team are tailored to the unique problems caused by the disability. The goal is to address all aspects of the child's development as well as the physical aspects of the disability. The role of the rehabilitation nurse is to demonstrate proper care techniques while supplying the family with the information they need to understand and comply with the treatment plan. The focus of the interdisciplinary team is to address the multisystem aspects of the disorder. The nurse must assure that the family understands the overall effects of the disability and its effects on their child as well as the child's achievement of developmental milestones.

Frequently, the diagnosis of the disability is not apparent at birth but evolves over time as the parents realize that their infant is not developing normally. This phenomenon occurs most frequently in children with cerebral palsy, neuromotor disorders, encephalopathies, and other disabilities. As the infant develops, neurological maturation does not follow the normal sequence. Primitive reflexes do not fade but become fixed and interfere with normal movement. These reflexes are the involuntary actions that are the newborn's earliest movements. Reflex testing is the neurologic examination for the neonate. Reflex patterns are quintessentially developmental: Early primitive brainstem and spinal reflexes, such as asymmetrical tonic neck reflex (ATNR) and palmar grasp, disappear after a few months and midbrain reflexes, such as neck righting, appear after a few months and peak around 10 to 12 months of age. Three factors determine whether a reflex can be elicited: (1) maturational level of the nervous system, (2) structural integrity of the nervous system, and (3) the infant's physiologic condition at the time of testing, i.e., sedation from medications and other conditions that contribute to decreased arousal. As the child matures neurologic dysfunction is suspected when the reflex continues too long, the next sequential reflex fails to appear at the anticipated time, or a certain reflex does not appear at all. Thus reflex development forms the theoretical framework for the physiological mode of normal development. Other developmental issues are those of cognitive development (Piaget, 1970, Table 1) and social development (Erickson, 1963, Table 2). Maslow's (1970) hierarchy of needs (Table 3) provides another useful way of conceptualizing development. The

Table 1
Piaget's Stages of Intellectual Development

Stage	Age	Characteristics
Sensorimotor	Birth to 2 years	Reflex action to environment; gains object permanence
Preoperational: Preconceptional thought	Two to 4 years	Develops conceptual system through exploration of environment
Preoperational: Intuitive thought	Four to 7 years	Advances toward concrete operations but cannot hold two points of view when problem-solving
Concrete operational	Seven to 11 years	Can problem-solve, but reasoning tied to concrete experience
Formal operational	Eleven to 15 years	Thinks abstractly, uses theories and logic

framework of dependence-independence-interdependence (Table 4) provides a useful way of evaluating the child's adaptation to the disability.

Developmental issues for infancy are object permanence (Piaget, 1970) and nurturing (Erikson, 1963). According to Piaget (1970), play is necessary for the developing child to explore his environment and act on it in a way that sets the stage for the direction and course of mental development. Progression through the stages is cumulative and provides indicators for educational programs. Object permanence provides the basis for symbolic representation and thus the concept of space, time, causality, and intentionality. According to Erikson (1963), the focus for nurturing is the maternal figure. Through a secure and dependable relationship with the maternal figure, the infant learns to trust the world and others. Without this basic trust, the infant learns to mistrust and becomes frustrated, angry, and suspicious. This can lead to depression and paranoia as adults. Thus it is of paramount importance that the nurse foster a nurturing relationship with the family, helping them to feel adequate and secure in the care of their child. Questions must be answered honestly and realistic expectations for the child's future fostered. Individual conferences should be held when necessary and written materials given so the parents can review the information at their own pace. Parents often benefit from meeting other parents who have "walked in the same moccasins," and from participation in the local parent support group. Parents must be allowed to grieve the loss of the ideal infant. The need for a lifetime of

Table 2
Erickson: Eight Stages of Social Development

Stage	Age	Characteristics	Focus
Trust vs. Mistrust	Birth to 1–2 years	Learning to trust the world and others leads to security and dependence. Mistrust leads to frustration, anger, and suspicion; can lead to depression and paranoia as adults	Maternal person
Autonomy vs. Shame and Doubt	$1\frac{1}{2}$–2 years to $3\frac{1}{2}$–4 years	Physical abilities lead to feelings of autonomy and independence—tantrums. Shame and doubt from thwarted attempts lead to timidity, feelings of loss of control or no control, fear of choices	Parental persons
Initiative vs. Shame and Guilt	4–5 years	Imagination, active play, curiosity, social training. Too much training and control destroys spontaneity and curiosity; child becomes immobilized by guilt, fearful, afraid to try new things, people, foods, ideas	Nuclear family
Industry vs. Inferiority	6–11 years	Formal skills of life, rules, schoolwork, homework, need for self-discipline. Too many failures leads to inferiority; do not force into situations where they can't be successful	Peers
Identity vs. Role Confusion	12–18 years	Integrating self into one identity; talents, skills, social and sexual identity point them toward college or career	"Shoulds" defined by family; fear that decisions are irrevocable
Intimacy vs. Isolation	Young adulthood	Intimacy and lasting partnership: Sharing everything from sex to work to play—child rearing. Isolation leads to shallow relationships, lack of meaning in life	Putting down roots; discontent is normal
Generativity vs. Stagnation	Middle age	Reproduce, generate, or be productive, generate works or ideas, care for self, family, society. Stagnation occurs when people sit back and do not continue to grow and develop socially, leading to self-centeredness, complacency	Fear that this is the last chance
Integrity vs. Despair	Maturity	Ego integrity, sense of achievement. Despair occurs when they feel their life has no meaning or was useless or wasted	Equilibrium regained

Table 3
Maslow's Hierarchy of Needs

Assumption	Habilitation Implication
Human behavior is driven by the need of the individual	Developmental stage of child determines level of self-initiating activity
Need is hierarchical: Physiologic needs take precedence over safety, then love and belonging, then esteem and recognition, then self-actualization	Drives prioritization in developing habilitation plan
Meeting need reduces tension until next level emerges	Motivation to obtain objectives is tension driven

support should be acknowledged. The family needs to be linked to appropriate emotional and financial assistance.

Parents need guidance in bonding with the "less than perfect" child. Handling a hypertonic infant is challenging, as the expectations of cuddling and visual interaction are often not met. Sucking and feeding difficulties require special positioning and handling. These concerns frequently interfere with the natural bonding that usually occurs at feeding times. In the case of dysphagia, the family will need to cope with dysphagia testing and the possibility of nasogastric or gastrostomy tube feedings. The mother frequently becomes the expert caregiver and

Table 4
Concept of Dependence, Independence, and Interdependence

Concept	Description
Dependence	Relying on others for support (meets need for nurturing, normally this occurs in infancy)
Independence	Not requiring or relying on others for support
Interdependence	Recognizing and distinguishing situations in which one needs to rely on others and situations in which one needs to rely on oneself Knows when to rely on others, ask for help, and delegate responsibility

Source: Peterson, Rauen, Brown, and Cole (1994, p. 229).

has no one to relieve her from the chore of feeding her struggling infant. The understanding of a supportive nurse or another parent with a disabled child can help the mother vent her frustration. It is important that she try to find another person who can handle the child and his special needs.

Recognizing the grief that the parents and family members are feeling is of paramount importance. Hope and support from a variety of sources will help the family develop coping skills and adjust to life with their disabled child. It is important for the entire team to recognize the high potential for child abuse that occurs from the frustration of dealing with an irritable or unresponsive child. Frustration also results from the high number of visits to health care providers, feeling of loss of control of one's life, and the grief of losing the expected "perfect" child.

Toddler/Preschool

For toddlers and preschoolers with chronic illness and/or developmental disabilities, the focus shifts to mobility issues. The team's energies are directed toward getting the child moving independently whether that is accomplished with braces, braces and crutches, mobile stander, or wheelchair. The child must be able to explore the environment and interact with it in order to meet developmental milestones. Parents are often fearful as the child attempts to explore his environment despite his limitations. The child's developmental need often outstrips the limitations of the prognosis. Parents often need reassurance as they begin to embrace the concept of the child's achieving the beginnings of independence. The stage is set for the beginnings of behavior management and the parent's conviction that their child will experience as much of a normal life as is possible within the limits of the disability. When a child has a developmental disability, the usual childhood experiences are many times parent-driven rather than child-driven as the physical constraints may limit the child's world. Parents need encouragement in setting up experiences for their child so that his natural abilities are stimulated. Discipline is important and behavior should be age appropriate as well as socially appropriate. Issues of safety become important, as the child is encouraged to acquire independence. Nursing interventions focus on helping the parents to trust their own instincts as they identify developmental goals and expect their child to reach those goals. The nurse provides information and encouragement in the areas of safety, nutrition, self-care, mobility, and socialization with peers. At these early ages, the parents can begin to identify the child's unique style and learning abilities. Play with peers is vital as the child learns the give and take of friendships. Friends provide fertile soil for first-hand experiences in problem solving and decision making. It is within these early relationships that the foundation is laid for important social and cultural values.

During the toddler/preschool years, the nurses' primary focus is on the achievement of bowel continence. Toilet training does not differ radically from that of a nondisabled child. Constipation should have been ameliorated in infancy. If not, the program is begun with a clean bowel. Water consumption is stressed to improve stool consistency. Fiber supplements may be needed. They are best taken 15 to 20 minutes before meals with water. Any one from the large selection at the grocery market or pharmacy may be used as long as the child will take it. A fruit purée may also be made and spread on toast or served with cereal. Anything that increases the dietary fiber is helpful. Peanut butter usually works fine but is not stressed as the only one because of it high caloric content. With the stools of the correct consistency, "long and cigar shaped," a program of toilet sitting after meals is begun. Most children with disabilities involving their neuromotor system must be taught to push. Feet should be flat on the floor or a stool with the knees slightly higher than the hips. The parents should be encouraged to notice the child's inherent pattern and toilet sit the child at their unique time. The child should be given special activities reserved for toilet sitting time to encourage them to sit and push for 15 or 20 minutes or less if they produce a stool in a shorter interval. Some children need to sit on the toilet twice a day after meals. Parents need to know that success is measured in tiny achievements and that it may take months before they are consistently "catching" most of the stools. Nurses spend many hours helping the parents adjust the child's bowel program to achieve the desired results.

If the child has a neurogenic bladder and develops a mild form of vesicoureteral reflux, a catheterization program may be necessary to relieve the pressure on the kidneys. Toddlers are usually resistant to clean intermittent catheterization (CIC) just as they are resistant to diaper changes. They do not want to be still for the 20 to 30 minutes it takes to empty their bladders with the tiny catheters (#6 or #8). Bladder capacity should be 60 to 180 milliliters. As the child gets older and more aware of what is happening, he needs to know that only certain people can catheterize him. Privacy needs to be assured and modesty needs to be encouraged. Interest in the procedure should be encouraged and sets the stage for the acquisition of self-catheterization. Some children as young as 3 years have learned self-catheterization although most of the children are 5 or 6 years old or older. If there is no medical indication for the introduction of CIC, the program is not introduced until the child is ready to achieve bladder continence. The child should be aware that others void in the toilet and wear underwear. The caregivers also must be interested in achieving continence. They are responsible for the program for many years until the child is able to assume the responsibility himself.

Acquisition of the usual activities of daily living is important. Toddlers should learn to feed and begin to dress themselves. Preschoolers should be close to dressing themselves independently. They should learn when and how to ask for help if they are unable to dress their lower extremities or put on their braces. Children with trunk instability may wear a body jacket and be able to assist with its donning and doffing. Training and techniques are very similar to those used in teaching an adult with a spinal cord injury, except that the expectations are tailored to the child's developmental level. If the disability involves cognition and attention, the techniques used resemble those for adults with brain injuries. Preschoolers should actively participate in their bathing and grooming. As children with altered sensation learn to dry themselves, they should be taught skin checks simultaneously. Skin checks taught in this manner become a habit, as it is part of the drying routine. These children must also be taught about safety precautions for their insensate skin. Now is the time to instill those lifelong habits that lay the foundation for prevention of secondary disability.

School Age   As the child enters school, the focus of the team turns to psychosocial concerns and prevention of secondary disability. It is imperative that the child attend school or an appropriate educational program. Sometimes incontinence is the issue that prevents the child from attending regular classes with his peers. Occasionally, it is the concern cited by the educators as the reason the parents' or child's desires are not acted on in the educational setting. Continence should never be the reason for a special education classroom but the issue is very important. When the child enters school the team focuses on achieving both bowel and bladder continence if not previously achieved. Continence has a great effect on the child's self-image. Lack of it frequently limits the choices and experiences of the child. It decreases opportunities for socialization with peers. It is often cited as the reason for not spending the night with his peers or not getting invited to pajama parties.

Skin problems often become the primary reason why the child with altered sensation is brought to the doctor. Problems with fitting malformed, spastic, or flaccid feet with braces and mechanical problems with the degree of physical activity cause shearing and friction. The activity should not be abandoned. The activity may need to be modulated if frequent skin checks, change of socks, and scrupulous skin care do not ameliorate the problem. The child should take increasing responsibility for the appearance of his skin. He should also learn that his skin will ultimately cause him the most time and concern if it is not properly cared for throughout his life.

Mobility issues facing children with disabilities are varied. Children with mid- to high lumbar spinal cord lesions frequently become focused on function versus preference. This area is particularly volatile for parents as their desire for their child to walk clouds their ability to see the functional advantages of wheelchair mobility. Their children, on the other hand, adapt quite quickly and some are able to tell their parents that walking with braces above their hips and crutches requires too much energy and is too slow. For children with neuromotor disorders, wheelchairs become a part of their lives. Electric chairs often provide an appropriate degree of independence. For children with increasing developmental delay, the chair may provide the parents with relief from carrying the growing child. Mobility issues are pervasive and parents may have a difficult time dealing with them. Knowing other parents helps but not all family members will experience the reality of limited mobility to the same degree. Frequently, counseling is needed to help the family through this stage.

As the child enters school, his style of learning becomes apparent. According to Piaget, this is the age of concrete operational thought. Reasoning is tied to concrete experience. Thought is action oriented. Intuitive thought is less rigid, but he is still unable to use secondary concepts. Children of this age are able to think about what will happen without having to experiment with the object. Erickson labels the stage "Industry versus Inferiority." Formal skills of life, rules, schoolwork, homework, and the need for self-discipline are the important issues of this stage. Too many failures lead to feelings of inferiority. Parents must be aware of this as they monitor their child's experiences. Difficulties with perceptual motor skills and attention or hyperactivity need to be identified and remedied quickly. School-age children are usually excited about learning. Learning problems must not dim that excitement. Children of this age engage in many activities at school, church, and in the community. Parents must direct their child's participation in these activities so that the experiences will be positive. The developmental focus is on decision-making and problem-solving. The child needs to experience the repercussions of his behavior and assume responsibility for it. He can make simple decisions and be accountable for household chores. Some children with disabilities have difficulty initiating and maintaining goal-directed behavior and need structure and routine. Lack of initiation and motivation responds to the same management plan as programs for the brain injured. Learning disabilities within the backdrop of a specific disability respond to the same educational programs as those learning disabilities occurring alone. Adaptations may be needed to accommodate the pervasiveness of the physical problems.

School-age children are submersed in the socialization process. The child with a disability often needs assistance from parents or other adults. Self-care is frequently time consuming and takes the child away from his peers. Efforts should be directed toward helping the child to perform those tasks that can be done independently at times that least interfere with peer interactions. The child needs assistance to recognize when he needs help and how to ask for it. Learning this important concept helps the child achieve good self-esteem. Peer interaction more than anything else paves the way for socially appropriate behavior and for learning how their behavior influences others. Children who have experienced many interactions with their friends and peers learn socially appropriate behavior easily. Friends should be encouraged to make allowances for the physical aspects of the disability only. The child must not be protected from the consequences of unruly or obnoxious behavior. Self-esteem grows within the child through his successes and failures. The parents need only assure that the failures do not exceed the successes. Once again it is important that expectations be appropriate to the limits of the disability.

The school-age child is aware of his own health. He should be given explanations at his level about his disability. He should be able to discuss it with both peers and adults. He should understand his treatment regimen and have a voice in the determination of his short-term and long-term goals. He should know the signs and symptoms of problems associated with his condition. He must be taught to report the symptoms to an appropriate adult.

Age-appropriate information regarding sexuality and physical sexual development needs to be given within the context of the disability. The prevention of sexual abuse is of paramount importance, as many of the treatment regimens (especially catheterization and bowel programs) place the child at risk for inappropriate behavior by caregivers. The phenomenon of precocious puberty accompanies several of the developmental disabilities that affect the brain and hormonal system. This phenomenon adds to the risk for these affected children. Parents must be made aware of the problem and be alert for signs of abuse. Weight control can become an important issue for children with paralysis and eating disorders. Physical exercise may not be feasible for controlling weight gain. Hopefully, food was not used as a reward or punishment as it now becomes a health issue.

Adolescence

For all children, adolescence means the transition to independence. According to Piaget, it is the age of formal operational thought. The adolescent is able to solve problems, think abstractly, develop and use theories, and use logic and math in problem solving. He can be responsible for total self-care. In Erickson's model, adolescence is the age of "Identity versus Isolation." This is the stage when the child's concept of himself is molded into one identity. His talents and skills, and social and sexual identity, point him toward college or an appropriate career. Adolescents fear that their decisions are irrevocable and need the support of their family and friends when circumstances do not work out as anticipated. For children with chronic illnesses and disabilities, the road to independence often means knowing what they can do independently and what they need to ask for help with and how to tell the difference. Self-care may mean learning to direct someone else in helping them with, for example, applying their braces and shoes. A sense of humor becomes a valuable asset when asking for help with intimate aspects of self-care. They need to be aware of and protected from problems of physical, sexual, and social abuse. Self-care also includes self-medication. Adolescents need to learn everything that is generally taught to patients even though they may have been taking the medication for years. They should also learn how to refill their prescriptions. Many interdisciplinary teams are based in children's hospitals and, therefore, stop caring for the adolescent at 21 years of age. The team must teach him what each specialist does, the reason he sees that specialist, and when he need to consult with another physician in that specialty. Continued surveillance of health is necessary throughout their life span.

During adolescence, the focus of the team changes to prevention of secondary disabilities such as skin breakdown, compromised kidney function, and nutritional concerns. Sex education includes fertility, sexually transmitted diseases, and pregnancy. Fertility issues must be addressed. Boys with spinal cord dysfunction need the same sex education, including erectile aids, as clients with spinal cord injuries. Young men should be taught testicular self-examination. Young women need information regarding menstruation, gynecological examinations, breast self-examinations, and other preventive health practices. Both sexes should experience their first examinations by the professionals who will care for these aspects of their health throughout their lives.

If school placement has not included vocational training, it must begin immediately. Questions, concerns, and plans must be addressed. Plans must be consistent with abilities. Opportunities must be available for trying out career choices. If learning problems are present, they must continue to be addressed so that the adolescent can become as independent as possible. School placement can be a combination of mainstreaming and special education known as *combined placement*. The most important factor is that the adolescent has the chance to interact with his peers and learn from them as all adolescents do. Peers are vital to the development of healthy self-esteem. The potential for isolation and loneliness is great.

Issues of physical mobility now broaden to include driving. The potential for each adolescent must be assessed. If driving is not feasible, then independence in alternative transportation methods must be fostered. The adolescence must be given the opportunity to try to manage all forms of public transportation. He must be given the experience of coping with environments not necessarily friendly to the disabled so that he can problem-solve his dilemma while still in the protection of others.

Opportunities for interaction with peers must be assured. All teens need to form friendships and relationships with others. Many teens with disabilities need assistance with socialization. They need to experience the give and take of friendships and begin dating. These early experiences provide the foundation for future long-term relationships. The development of realistic expectations for the future is easier against the backdrop of peer experiences.

Some teens experience social isolation. The impact of this must be minimized. Relying on others for providing care and limited opportunities impact the adolescent's ability to launch out on his own in his peer group. A lifetime of restricted choices, physical barriers, and avoidance by others contributes to social isolation and must be addressed as the child matures. If necessary, he must be helped to develop the courage and skills to find opportunities for his social development. This will help build the foundation for healthy self-esteem. When teens with disabilities experience repeated obstacles in these areas, parents and professionals need to assist them in identifying positive achievement in the dependence-interdependence-independence cycle. Managing this cycle becomes the job of the adolescent as he moves toward self-reliance. A balance in this cycle allows achievable goals to be set that foster growth of the individual. This provides the foundation for mastering independence in identifying and meeting physical, social, and emotional needs and allows the emergence of a young adult ready to accept responsibility for himself and his health care needs.

Neuromotor Diseases

The most common neuromotor diseases in children are the muscular dystrophies, with Duchenne's muscular dystrophy being the most common form. Werdnig-Hoffmann's dystrophy (SMA-1) and Kugelberg-Welander's dystrophy (SMA-2) are together classified as progressive spinal muscular atrophy and make up the bulk of the remaining forms. A discussion of these will allow the reader to generalize the information to other neuromotor diseases such as myotonic dystrophy and limb girdle dystrophy (Eng, 1992).

Duchenne's muscular dystrophy is a sex-linked genetic disorder occurring in 0.2 per thousand live births in the United States. There are several forms ranging from mild to severe. Males are affected, with females being the carriers. Infants appear to be normal at birth. Developmental gains outstrip the disease until about the third year of life, when symptoms begin to appear. Pain in the legs, especially the calves, is usually the presenting symptom. The progression of symptoms usually includes difficulty in running, a waddling gait, prominence of the calves, and exaggerated lumbar lordosis. Gowers' sign is diagnostic. The prone child uses his arms, extended in front of him on the floor, to "climb up his legs" by pushing on his thighs with his hands. Weakness of the upper extremities appears late in the progression. Laboratory values show elevated creatine phosphokinase (CPK), which results from dying muscle cells (Eng, 1992).

About half the children with Duchenne's are mentally retarded. Schooling usually begins with a combined placement and progresses to a self-contained special education classroom as the physical limitations as well as the mental retardation progress. Socialization is encouraged as long as it is possible.

Management of the disability includes exercise and stretching to prevent contractures. Deconditioning is frequent, particularly after orthopedic surgery. Surgery is usually only done in young children with the prospect of continued ambulation. Diaphragmatic action is usually well preserved. Cardiomyopathy and restrictive pulmonary disease are common. Scoliosis further compromises the respiratory function. Spinal fusion is often done in adolescence before the onset of severe respiratory compromise. End-stage respiratory failure is currently being managed with intermittent positive pressure devices in combination with other means of ventilatory support.

Progressive spinal muscular atrophy (Werdnig-Hoffmann or SMA-1, Kugel-berg-Welander or SMA-2) is an autosomal recessive disorder occurring in 1 in 15,000 to 25,000 live births in the United States (Molnar, 1992). The disorder selectively involves the large anterior horn cells at all levels of the cord, eventually including the diaphragm. There is muscle wasting because of lower motor neuron dysfunction.

Werdnig-Hoffmann's form frequently has its onset *in utero* with rapid progression after birth. Most victims die within the first 2 years of life. When clinical manifestations do not occur until after the first 2 months, the disease has a slower progression. The children can live for quite a number of years. This form is called Kugelberg-Welander's dystrophy. The victims are often unable to sit unsupported and rarely can walk. In both forms of spinal muscular atrophy, there is an absence of reflexes, progressive proximal weakness, recurrent respiratory infections, osteoporosis, scoliosis, and fixed contractures. Unlike Duchenne's muscular dystrophy, intellectual capabilities are rarely affected. Keeping the child stimulated and in school becomes a challenge as the deterioration progresses.

Management is with judicious physical therapy and occupational therapy. Therapy can prolong some activities of daily living, minimize deformities, and retard development of osteoporosis. Respiratory support is a case by case decision. Some of these children become ventilator dependent at night during the late school-age years. Respiratory failure may progress to complete ventilatory support in some cases. Interestingly, there are a number of cases in which the respiratory failure arrests and the person lives many years without progression of the dependence on ventilatory support.

The diagnosis of any neuromotor disorder is devastating for the entire family. The family often feels a profound sense of guilt, as is often the case in genetic disorders. The family will have many questions and concerns. Genetic counseling must be provided. The incidence rate must be addressed. Grieving must be expected, as the family must deal not only with the disability, but with the shortened life span of the child, and the potential for future children to be affected. The affected child must be allowed to develop what new skills he can while he is still able. Parental guilt interferes with the child's ability to explore his environment. The parents fear for the child's safety, and they mistakenly think that helping him preserves the "strength" of his wasting muscles. The child's life span is shortened because involuntary muscle, including the cardiac muscle and the diaphragm, is affected. Death usually occurs in adolescence. Support groups often provide the child and his family with a forum for grieving, and provide examples of the coping mechanisms of others dealing with similar issues.

Spina Bifida

Spina bifida is the term used by parents and children for the broad category of spinal dysraphism or myelodysplasia. Technically speaking, spina bifida applies only to the bony defect of the spinal column in which the vertebrae is bifid or missing the spinous process. Myelodysplasia refers to the dysplastic spinal cord that impairs neurological function. In normal embryonic development, the neural tube closes on about the twenty-first day after conception. Failure of the neural tube to close can present in several forms. In the most common form, the malformed spinal cord is contained in a sac on the infant's back (myelomeningocele). The sac may leak cerebral spinal fluid or be covered with a thin layer of skin. Another common variation occurs when the dysplastic spinal cord contains fatty deposits and is skin covered (lipomeningocele). Associated abnormalities of the brain include hydrocephalus, microcephaly, and/or a learning disability. Some children with spina bifida have no apparent problem with brain function. During the early 1960s, delicate surgical procedures and shunting increased the life span beyond infancy. Today, with the introduction of a small plastic catheter to drain their bladder, these children grow into adulthood and can approximate normal life span (McLone, 1990).

Nursing interventions are designed to demonstrate proper care techniques while supplying the family with the information they need to understand and comply with the treatment plan. The interdisciplinary team addresses problems associated with the multisystem disorder. These children are not just little spinal cord injury clients. The defect is often asymmetrical and assails the kidneys, the urinary tract, the brain, and the spinal cord. Tests are done to determine the normalcy of the urinary tract. If anomalies, such as ureterovesical reflux or ureteropelvic junction obstruction, exist measures are taken to protect the upper tracts from further damage. Clean intermittent catheterization may relieve the pressure of a full bladder, ameliorate the cause of the reflux, and allow the kidney to heal. If the reflux is massive, a vesicostomy may be done to preserve the kidneys. Rarely is the damage so massive that ureterostomies must be done to save what function there is. Kidney failure significantly shortens the life span of these youngsters.

Child/family teaching includes a brief synopsis of genetic counseling information and the role of folic acid in the development and recurrence rate of the anomaly. The parents must know that their infant must always receive well-child check-ups and immunizations. They must be told about hydrocephalus and/or Chiari II malformation and shunt malfunction. Manifestations of Chiari II include pressure on the brainstem. Symptoms may include stridor, respiratory distress, dysphagia, and feeding problems. Another common associated abnormality is strabismus. Without correction, the child will not develop depth perception, which causes increased difficulty with mobility. The prevention of secondary disability is another nursing concern. The nurse teaches the family about insensate skin and its care; nutritional guidance to prevent constipation and obesity; signs and symptoms of urinary tract infection, retention, and reflux; and the prevention or correction of orthopedic deformities (Peterson, Rauen, Brown, & Cole, 1994).

The nurse should counsel the parents and caregivers regarding the high risk of the child developing latex allergy. All children with spina bifida need to be treated in a latex-free environment. They are the most common group of people to develop the most severe form of the allergy (Leger & Meeropol, 1992; Getchufsky, 1997).

The most important determinant of outcome is the achievement of their developmental milestones. Socialization is important. Success in the parameters of educational opportunities and appropriate professional/vocational placement helps secure a productive and fulfilling adulthood.

The care of these children is most appropriately achieved by an interdisciplinary clinic in which the child makes one visit to see the team of specialists, who then consult with each other and co-ordinate their care. This approach, although expensive, can be very cost effective in facilitating communication among the individual practitioners, the family, and the child. The co-ordination of surgeries, diagnostic tests, and consultations with specialists outside that of the regular team assures that the child remains in school for the maximum number of days and does not fall behind his classmates.

The stage for this scenario is set in infancy with the reaction of the staff members who first care for the newborn. It can take the treatment team years to replace an offhand negative comment about the child's future intelligence or ability to achieve continence with the true realistic expectations that most children with spina bifida can achieve continence and can function appropriately in the classroom. The Spina Bifida Association of America through their information and referral service can help the family locate others in their geographical area if there is not a group associated with the clinic.

Prevention of secondary disability is the focus during the school-age and adolescent years. Assessment is done to look for symptomatic tethered cord and scoliosis as well as kidney and bladder function. Skin breakdown and compromised kidney function are the primary causes that prevent the adult with spina bifida from living a full life. Both can shorten the life span and increase the cost and suffering of the individual and his family.

Cerebral Palsy

Cerebral palsy (CP) is a diagnostic category with varied presentations; however, the thread between these various clinical pictures lies in its definition. CP may be defined as a disorder of movement and posture caused by a nonprogressive lesion or injury that affects the immature brain (Molnar, 1992). It is either a pre- or perinatal event. The key term in the definition is "nonprogressive." The damage is done. The patient must live with a lifetime of consequences that define the individual disability. The injury itself is static and fixed in time. As the injured nervous system grows and develops the process of growth and development is continually impaired, and frequently results in increasing and nonstatic functional impairment (Molnar, 1992).

Incidence

An examination of trends of incidence in western industrial nations produced an interesting conclusion. Incidence fluctuates depending on the nation, study, and time. For the past 20 years the incidence has held grossly steady at 2 to 3 cases per 1000 live births. Of course the obvious question is why no overall progress toward improvement in decreasing this number has been made, given the medical scientific technological advances of the last 20 years. Clearly, socioeconomic political factors such as failure to provide preventive health care or proper education for women of the childbearing age come into play. When consideration is given to the fact that the rise of neonatal intensive care units (NICUs) promoted the survival of premature infants one would actually expect an overall increase in the incidence of CP. An increase did initially occur. With improved NICU care and proper management of the immature nervous system, the incidence of CP decreased. Only time will determine whether further advances can contribute to an overall decline in the incidence of CP (Groholt & Nordhagen, 1995; Jorch, 1995; MacGillivray & Campbell, 1995; Meberg & Broche, 1995; Molnar, 1992; Suzuki, Ito, & Tomiwa, 1996).

Etiology

The known antecedents to CP are many, including maternal illness, socioeconomic factors, genetic disposition, and congenital factors; but prematurity is the most common. Prevalence is inversely related to birth weight and gestational age. Although the actual cause of CP is unknown, it is theorized that as prematurity is accompanied by an immature cardiopulmonary system, brain hypoxia/anoxia occurs, resulting in brain injury. Clinicopathological correlations with CP include the following (Molnar, 1992):

- Ischemic hypoxic encephalopathy
- Periventricular leukomalacia
- Intraventricular hemorrhage grades II and IV
- Bilirubin encephalopathy

The two major subtypes of CP are spasticity and dyskinesia. Spasticity is the most common presentation, resulting from motor strip lesions, and accounts for 75 to 85 percent of the cases. Potential involvement is from one to four extremities, but **diplegia** is the most common type. Dyskinesia is less common and ensues from extrapyramidal lesions. Dyskinesia is thought to be associated with episodes of complete anoxia.

Diagnosis

Diagnosing CP is difficult because of the requirement of waiting for it to "emerge." Early signs include "floppy baby," poor suck, weak cry, asymmetric tone, tremor, clonus, overly brisk deep tendon reflexes, and excessive sleep. These clinical signs are commonly associated with other conditions. In the early stages it is important that other conditions such as anterior horn cell disease, myopathies, and spinocerebellar disease be ruled out (Molnar, 1992).

Diagnostic tools include the computed tomography (CT) scan, magnetic resonance imaging (MRI), cranial ultrasound, the positron emission tomography (PET) scan, the single-photon emission computed tomography (SPECT) scan, evoked potentials, and the clinical examination. The failure of primitive reflexes to disappear and midbrain reflexes to appear is an essential marker in the diagnostic process. Clinically CP is characterized by tone abnormalities, reflex abnormalities, postural abnormalities, and delayed motor development/atypical motor performance. The degree to which one or more of these abnormalities present is a product of the type of brain injury sustained. Thus, the clinical picture varies extensively (Molnar, 1992; Steele, 1985; Nelson, 1995).

Standards of Care   CP is essentially a process of brain injury. Accordingly, the deficits that can accrue are those of brain injury or its complications. The following standards of care both articulate and address those deficits:

- Address visual deficits.
- Address hearing deficits.
- Address communication deficits.
- Address cognitive concerns.
- Enhance mobility.
- Address feeding/nutrition issues.
- Promote skin integrity.
- Prevent/alleviate deformity.
- Address tone, postural, reflex and motor abnormalities.
- Promote bowel/bladder continence.

The basis of treatment for cerebral palsy is the concept of habilitation. CP, although not always strictly a congenital problem in nature, is nonetheless for functional purposes a perinatal event. If the cornerstone of the approach to treatment is habilitation, the "cement" so to speak, is the interdisciplinary to transdisciplinary team approach. Efficacious treatment must be eclectic but co-ordinated.

The organization and setting of CP treatment depends on state and local modalities. Clinic-based settings that can provide integrated pediatric services are the most efficient treatment settings, as both efficiency in cost and quality of care can be achieved. The United Cerebral Palsy Association is instrumental in setting national standards of care and providing services at the local level. Similarly, Shriners' Hospital for Children and California Childrens' Services provide services for CP patients.

The actual "product" of treatment can include the following:

- Functional training
- Adaptive devices/orthoses
- Therapeutic exercises/aggressive stretching
- Home exercise and positioning programs
- Pharmacological intervention
- Orthopedic surgery
- Neurosurgery
- Neuromuscular electrical stimulation

A Developmental Approach to Nursing Care

The nursing care of the CP patient follows the developmental model. The goal of care is to transition into adulthood on the basis of successful completion of developmental stages of infancy into young adulthood. The nurses' role in addressing developmental and emotional issues is much the same as those noted in the section on spina bifida. Instructions for issues of physical care and the prevention of secondary disability are dependent on the clinical presentation of CP.

As CP emerges, physical care issues begin to present. Tone abnormalities include both **hypotonicity** and **hypertonicity.** Reflex abnormalities become evident by age 4 to 6 months with hyperreflexia (asymmetrical tonic neck reflex, symmetrical tonic neck reflex, Moro reflex, tonic labyrinthine reflex, positive supporting reflex, palmar reflex, and plantar grasp). Postural abnormalities include extensor posturing with scissoring, plantar flexion, fisted hands, strap hangar design, asymmetrical arm position, pithed frog position, and athetosis of the hands (spooning). Delayed motor development such as failure to roll, sit, crawl, stand, cruise, and eventually ambulate starts to unfold in this period. Finally, symptoms such as atypical motor performance (combat crawling), abnormal stance of gait, asymmetrical upper extremity use in the first year (often confused with precocious handedness by parents), facial grimacing, writhing of the tongue, fingers, and toes (athetosis), and sucking and feeding difficulties (lack of jaw and lip closure, and tongue thrust) emerge.

Given the nature of these emerging clinical movement characteristics, positioning, handling, feeding, and nutrition issues become key concerns during infancy. The initiation of a treatment plan that includes family training for proper exercise, positioning, handling, and feeding needs to begin to prevent joint and head deformity, and malnutrition.

Parents need guidance in bonding with the "less than perfect" child. Handling a hypertonic infant is challenging, as the expectations of cuddling and visual interaction are often not met. Managing increased extensor tone and posturing is best achieved by handling and positioning that facilitates flexion through a process of internal rotation of the extremities, proning, and avoidance of upright postures with foot placement on hard surfaces.

It is important for the nurse to recognize the grief that parents are possibly feeling and to provide the hope and support that can help them through this period. It is equally important to recognize the high potential for child abuse that is also present in this period that can ensue from the frustration of handling an excessively irritable or unresponsive child.

Prevention of Secondary Disability

Prevention of secondary disability is addressed with development of a treatment plan that provides handling (range of motion) and positioning techniques to decrease joint deformity and a feeding regimen that prevents malnutrition. Special nipples, formula, and handling during feeding may be indicated. In cases of dysphagia, families will need preparation for dysphagia studies and may need to learn nasogastric feeding techniques.

Another component of prevention is the assessment of the need to control/prevent seizure activity. Approximately 50 percent of patients with CP have seizure disorders. The initiation and adjustment of pharmacologic regimens that control seizures can be a time-consuming but imperative process. Seizure medications must be administered carefully as side effects of misadministration can be either lethal or result in uncontrolled seizure. The importance of family training is self-evident.

As the child moves into the toddler/preschool developmental stages, CP completes its emergence. By age 3 years the particular picture of disability for the child has become clearer. The implication of this fact for the habilitation plan is profound. The all-encompassing planning for the life of the child must be taking shape; otherwise secondary disability will start to "run rampant."

Continuing the efforts that hopefully started in infancy, feeding, mobility, and seizure precautions are addressed and "fine-tuned." Acquisition of a gastrostomy tube, dietary changes such as adding solid foods, use special feeding devices (nipples, utensils), and possibly the initiation of self-feeding can occur during this period.

Mobility, fine motor activity, and prevention of joint deformity are addressed or further addressed through splinting and bracing programs. Common orthotic devices are the ankle foot orthosis (AFO) and the knee foot orthosis (KAFO). The latter decreases extensor tone and the former provides stability for ambulation when children present with hypotonia.

Extraocular movements and visual deficits are assessed and treated. Failure to do so impairs learning of motor activities, leading to an inability to focus properly, or to insufficient depth perception for motor planning. Strabismus presents more frequently than other abnormalities and is more common in spastic diplegia and **spastic quadriparesis** (Molnar, 1992).

Impaired skin integrity often accompanies impaired mobility. Children in this age group are not at as great a risk for impaired skin integrity as older children who weigh more and exert more pressure on their skin. The process of monitoring and teaching families to monitor skin integrity should begin. In the spirit of habilitation, early patterning of behavior to address lifelong problems is desirable and effective. Skin integrity will be a lifelong problem. Any individual wearing an orthotic device is at risk for impaired skin integrity.

As the client approaches the age for toilet training, the presence of bowel/bladder dysfunction may emerge. Dysphagia may lead to decreased fluid intake that in turn may lead to constipation. Tone alterations may impair bowel elimination. Impaired mobility, fine motor coordination, and mental retardation can impair bowel/bladder continence. The source of dysfunction must be determined so that the appropriate approach to toilet training can be implemented.

Communication disorders may result from a variety of sources such as hearing loss, visual deficits, and mental retardation. Most children with athetosis and half of the children with diplegic spasticity have some dysarthria (articulation impairment) (Molnar, 1992). The nurse collaborates with the multidisciplinary team for family training for use of communication and augmentive devices (hearing aids, glasses).

Scoliosis related to postural abnormalities interferes with seating and movement. In its more severe presentations it becomes a cause of restrictive pulmonary disease. On the other hand, obstructive pulmonary disease occurs secondary to ineffective control of pulmonary muscles. It is incumbent on the nurse to teach families pathophysiology and management of pulmonary hygiene.

Surgical intervention for the correction of joint deformity (tendon releases) may be initiated in this period. New splinting and bracing regimens and exercise programs may follow surgery. The nurse collaborates with the team to ensure proper family education regarding positioning, splint/brace-wearing schedules, and skin checks.

Developmental Issues

The individual with hearing, speech, visual, perceptual, and intellectual disability will need special educational services. The rate of mental retardation among the CP population is significantly higher than in the population at large. Approximately 50 percent of patients with CP have some degree of mental/intellectual impairment. One of the most valuable services that the nurse can provide for the family/client with CP is mentoring regarding their rights and privileges with respect to the educational system.

During school age the natural developmental tendency to blossom toward independence, "industry," mastery of the environment, and competence in efforts can be complicated by the impairments of the disease process. The assumption that needs to underlie the relationship between the nurse and the client/family is that of a team effort to promote the highest level of independence possible for the child in all areas. Self-feeding, mobility, skin checks, bowel program, and medication administration are areas that can be mastered with the right attitude and equipment. Children want to engage in learning, and want to make decisions for and take responsibility for themselves during this period. This window of opportunity, if missed, can close to the development of lifelong patterns of dependency, low self-concept, and failure.

This period also presents another window of opportunity for medical intervention to prevent deformity and immobility. Orthopedic surgeries performed during this stage include spinal fusion, tendon release, and muscle transfer. Until recently the neurosurgical procedure sometimes elected was the dorsal rhizotomy, a complex procedure that involves the severing of the dorsal nerve roots to relieve hypertonicity and spasticity. Owing to the complexity of the nervous system the ability to obtain the desired outcome was often less than desired. A more promising procedure has been the use of a baclofen pump that is implanted intra-abdominally and releases the antispasmodic medication intrathecally. The recent approval of this intervention by the Food and Drug Administration (FDA) is promising in terms of improving mobility outcomes and decreasing spasticity for the CP population.

In adolescence the team continues to focus on preventing secondary disability and encouraging the independence of the client. Spinal fusion is most frequently done in this period, because bone maturity has been achieved. Seating systems will usually need adjustment because of the growth spurt. Maintenance of skin integrity becomes a greater challenge owing to increased growth and weight.

Joint Disease

There are several types of joint disease with childhood presentations, including dermatomyositis, scleroderma, ankylosing spondylitis, systemic lupus erythematosus, Kawasaki disease, infectious arthritis, and hemophiliac arthropathy. The most common is juvenile rheumatoid arthritis (JRA) (Koch, 1992).

JRA is defined as an objective synovitis lasting six or more consecutive weeks. Its prevalence in the United States is 60,000 to 200,000 children. The etiology is unknown (Koch, 1992).

There are four subtypes of JRA: systemic onset with fever, rash, and organ involvement; polyarticular disease (involvement of five or more joints); pauciarticular disease (involvement of four or more joints); and monoarticular disease (involvement of one joint).

The diagnosis of JRA is based on clinical examination; history; and laboratory results on rheumatoid factor (RF), anti-nuclear antibody (ANA), human leukocyte antigen-B27 (HLA-B27), white blood cell count (WBC), and erythrocyte sedimentation rate (ESR). x-Rays are initially negative (Koch, 1992).

The life of the child with JRA is characterized by periods of remission and exacerbation. Early onset can occur in toddlerhood. Early implementation of the habilitation model is recommended because coping with pain, fatigue, and joint deformity may be a lifelong process. Children with severe cases of disease often have impaired growth patterns related to steroid use and poor nutrition. Many of these children are "picky eaters." Others have weight control problems related to steroid use and/or inactivity. Excess weight exacerbates joint deterioration. Finding an appropriate activity level without placing undue stress on the joints is challenging. Many children become sedentary. Another challenge is to ensure the correct school setting for the child. Because the disease carries no cognitive impairment, success in school is achievable under conditions in which the functional impairments of the child are addressed. The nurse plays an instrumental role in family education and training as the habilitation or rehabilitation plan is developed for the child.

The goal of treatment is to limit joint deformity and induce remission to prevent crippling disability. The standards of care that contribute to that goal attainment include the following:

- Address functional limitations.
- Address preservation of range of motion.
- Address maintenance of muscle strength and endurance.
- Control joint inflammation.
- Control and manage pain.
- Address nutrition.
- Address activity intolerance and rest needs.

The treatment "product" includes medications (nonsteroidal anti-inflammatory drugs, steroids, and methotrexate); rest; heat; massage; exercise; posture; functional training; and orthotics, splints, and adaptive devices (self-dressing and eating aids, as well as assistive devices useful in the classroom). Guiding the child successfully through periods of remission and exacerbation requires a team approach. Adjustments to the treatment plan are based on the presentation of impairments related to the disease process.

Pediatric Traumatic and Injury
Traumatic Injury

In the United States and in most industrialized nations, traumatic injury is the leading cause of death for children and adolescents. Whereas 8000 to 10,000 children in the United States under the age of 15 years die from injury each year, according to National Center for Health Statistics, for each death another 34 are admitted to a hospital for treatment of injury, and for every child admitted to hospital another 30 are treated in emergency departments. These numbers equate to approximately one child out of five in this country sustaining an injury that necessitates seeking medical assistance (Gallagher, Finison, Guyer, & Goodenough, 1984).

The types and causes of these injuries vary widely. Under the age of 1 year, **nonaccidental trauma** (child abuse) is the leading cause and injuries are fairly evenly distributed by sex. After infancy males are at a higher risk for injury than females (Rivara, Bergman, LoGerfo, & Weiss, 1982).

Blunt trauma is the most common cause of injury in children from 1 to 15 years of age, with motor vehicle accidents being the leader and falls second (Centers for Disease Control, 1990). Penetrating trauma becomes increasingly frequent in the 15- to 19-year-age range, and nearly five times as many males as females become victims of firearms (Rouse & Eichelberger, 1992). Burns and suffocation, including drowning, range from 5 to 50 percent in each category according to age group (National Center for Health Statistics, 1988).

Children who sustain significant trauma rarely have only one type of injury. Because of the comparatively large head in young children and the "javelin affect" secondary to this anatomical construct, head injuries with concurrent brain injuries cause the majority of traumatic deaths among children. Even though medical advances are providing increasing rates of survivorship, the incidence of head injury, in children younger than 15 years, sufficiently severe as to require hospitalization is 2 per 1000 (Grzankowski, 1997). Other associated traumatic injuries such as amputations or long bone fractures, injuries to the spine or pelvis, or thoracic or abdominal injuries are often associated with severe trauma and are concurrent with a brain injury (Rouse & Eichelberger, 1992).

Traumatic Brain Injury

There are few experiences more devastating to a family than the sudden traumatic brain injury of a child. It is one of those events that can result in the sensation of entering a parallel universe, similar in appearance, yet inexorably, irrevocably changed. People will never be the same, and hopes, dreams, aspirations, and plans are put on hold or vanish. It is at this time that the injured child and his family most need the expertise of a comprehensive care team, from emergency department to rehabilitation unit, that is skilled in the care of the unique physical, social, developmental, and emotional needs of children.

While the resuscitation and medical management of the injured child is similar to that of the adult (as discussed extensively in Chapter 15 on acquired brain injury), it should be directed and delivered by health care providers who know the anatomical and physiological differences of children. Although the mechanisms of injury in children are similar to those seen in adults—shearing, axonal injury, bruising, bleeding, and swelling—the responses are different.

The common instrument for initial evaluation of brain injury, the Glasgow Coma Scale (GCS), has been revised into the **Children's Coma Scale (CCS)** (Table 5) for assessing pediatric brain injury. The pediatric version of the GCS has not proven to be as accurate a predictor of outcome as the regular GCS has been for the adult brain injury population. A better indicator for the pediatric brain injury population is the duration of **posttraumatic amnesia (PTA).** PTA is used to classify an injury as mild, moderate, severe, or very severe. A mild injury

Table 5
Children's Coma Scale

Parameter	Score
Eye opening	
Spontaneous	4
Reaction to speech	3
Reaction to pain	2
No response	1
Best motor response	
Spontaneous (obeys verbal command)	6
Localizes pain	5
Withdraws from pain	4
Abnormal flexion response to pain (decorticate)	3
Abnormal extension to pain (decerebrate)	2
No response	1
Best verbal response	
Smiles, oriented to sound, follows objects, interacts	5
Crying—interacts	5
Consolable—inappropriate	4
Inconsistently consolable—moaning	3
Inconsolable—restless	2
No response	1

is one with a PTA of 1 hour or less, a moderate injury has a PTA of 1 to 24 hours, and a severe injury has a PTA of 24 hours to 1 week. A PTA of more than 1 week indicates a very severe injury. Neither the GCS, the length of time of impaired consciousness, or the site of the lesion has been an accurate predictor of memory loss (Levin, Goldstein, High, & Eisenberg, 1988).

Complicating the prognostic assessment of a child's brain injury is the inability of children to recognize their own deficits and the parents' often unrealistic belief, especially in the case of a mild to moderate brain injury, that the event is over and that everything is fine. This situation is further complicated by the picture presented by the child with a brain injury, which can be very different from that presented by an adult with a brain injury. Disorders such as **aphasia,** unilateral **hemineglect,** or **agnosia,** which are frequently permanent in adults with brain injuries, are often less severe or are of shorter duration in children. More common as long-term problems are **attention deficit disorder** and neurobehavioral problems. A middle-aged child (6 to 9 years old) with a mild to moderate brain injury may appear to recover adequately until he or she advances to a point where more abstract reasoning or executive functioning is required, and then begin to manifest academic and social difficulties. For youngsters with brain injuries sufficiently severe to require rehabilitation hospitalization (moderate to severe), 50 percent require **special education** or **cognitive remediation** (Edwards, 1987).

Because most children with traumatic brain injuries return home to receive ongoing care and support services in the community, they present a challenge to multiple levels of nursing service. Children with brain injuries are often discharged from hospital when they have reached Rancho Los Amigos Scale level 4+/5, necessitating the advent of discharge planning on admission. The integration of public health nursing, state children's services, and the educational system into the plan of care well before discharge is essential. At the time of discharge the responsibility for on-going rehabilitation services is transferred to community agencies, primarily the educational system. Under current education statutes, even the most impaired youngsters receive services. Rehabilitation nurses play a key role by providing transition care, orientation, and education about traumatic brain injury to community agencies.

Nursing in the Exceptional Education Services Definitions

PL 94-142—The Education for the Handicapped Act: This law established as a national policy that education is a fundamental right that must be extended to all children with disabilities.

PL 101-476—The Individuals with Disabilities Education Act (IDEA): This law made significant changes in PL 94-142, including terminology, addition of new classifications pertaining to students with disabilities, listing of additional services required to be provided, and establishment of transition services.

One area of distinction in pediatric re/habilitation is that much of it takes place in partnership with the educational system. Although a small percentage of youngsters with special needs will have a brief period of hospitalization in a rehabilitation facility, the majority of care and follow-up is community based and usually associated with a school system in some way.

Earlier in this century, most children with disabilities who received any education did so in state schools, large residential institutions where they were separated from their families and society, or in self-contained classrooms on occasional school sites, classrooms that often had schedules different from those of the rest of the school and were de facto segregated.

Beginning in the late 1930s and increasing with the surge of interest in rehabilitation after World War II, center-based education became the model. Many children with special needs, especially those with orthopedic and/or severe disabilities, could stay at home with their families, but were transported to special schools or "centers" that often had physical and occupational therapy treatment units on site. They provide for comprehensive, albeit incomplete, education and therapy from age 3 until age 21 or high school graduation.

In 1973 Section 504 of the Federal Rehabilitation Act provided that no program, including educational programs, that received federal money could exclude any person with a disability from the program on the sole basis of the person's disability.

On November 29, 1975, the Education for the Handicapped Act (PL 94-142) was passed. This law established as a national policy that education was a fundamental right that must be extended to all children with disabilities. This law mandated that all children with disabilities shall be

1. Provided with a free and appropriate public education
2. Educated in the least restrictive environment based on individual needs

PL 94-142 required provision of services with these conditions:

1. Each individual with exceptional needs is guaranteed a culturally unbiased, valid assessment.
2. Each individual with exceptional needs is to have an **Individual Education Plan (IEP).**
3. Due process procedures will be established to ensure parent and child rights.

Subsequently, PL 98-456 extended these services to the 0–3 years age group and established **Individual Family Service Plans (IFSPs).**

In 1990 several amendments were made to Part B of PL 94-142. These amendments, contained in PL 101-476, made significant changes, including the following:

1. PL94-142 was revised and was now titled the Individuals with Disabilities Education Act.
2. The term "handicapped" in the act was changed to the preferred term "disabled" and, in accordance with the trend to "people first" language, terminology under the act has been changed. For example, "handicapped children" are now referred to as "children with disabilities."
3. The amendments recognized some new classifications pertaining to students with disabilities, including autism and traumatic brain injury.
4. The amendments listed additional services required to be provided under the act, such as social work services and rehabilitation counseling.
5. The amendments also added as related services: assistive technology devices—any item, piece of equipment or product system, whether acquired commercially off the shelf, modified or customized that is used to increase, maintain, or improve functional capabilities of persons with disabilities; and assistive technology services—any service that directly assists an individual with a disability in the selection, acquisition, or use of assistive technology.

6. Potentially of the greatest impact is the amendment that requires that, where appropriate, transition services must be addressed in the IEP once the child reaches 14 years of age. Transition services, as delineated in the **Individual Transition Plan (ITP),** are defined as

A coordinated set of activities for a student designed within an outcome-oriented plan which promotes movement from school to post-school activities, including post-secondary education, vocational training, integrated employment (including supported employment), continuing and adult education, adult services, independent living, or community participation.

Many states have laws such as California Assembly Bill 3632, which develop interagency agreements in order to maximize and coordinate services to children with disabilities. Examples of services that are added to the child's educational program by the IEP team are as follows:

1. State children's services or equivalent state agency shall be responsible for providing occupational and physical therapy assessments and services.
2. The public mental health agencies shall be responsible for psychotherapy and other mental health assessments.

These changes in the educational system have had sweeping rebound effects on the health care system, including nursing. Children with disabilities remain in, and receive services in, their communities rather than in sequestered state schools, and are now integrated into their neighborhood school sites, fully included in regular classrooms with their age-appropriate peers. These changes, as well as the changes in goals and expectations for youngsters with disabilities, have impacted all levels of nursing, especially community-based nurses and school nurses.

Keeping children with disabilities in their homes and maintaining close family involvement has led to higher levels of health care for these clients, longer life expectancies, and increased numbers of hospitalizations for corrective surgical procedures to maximize their level of function. Knowledge of rehabilitation concepts and techniques such as positioning, feeding, skin care, mobility, and elimination is required of general staff nurses at levels that far exceed those of a generation ago. Hospital-based nursing practice as well as community-based nursing practice have been affected by these educational system changes.

Of those nurses in community-based practices, the school nurses have been most affected. It is the school nurse who is the medical case manager for all students with disabilities within his or her jurisdiction. She or he must provide **Designated Health Nursing Services** to these students or ensure that they are done. Designated Health Nursing Services are the services required to assist an individual with special needs to benefit from special education as defined by each state's education code. These services include managing the student's health problems on the school site, consulting with school staff members regarding management of the student's health problems, doing group and individual counseling with students and parents regarding health problems, and making appropriate referrals to and communicating with health agencies providing care to students with disabilities. The school nurse is the health officer on each school site and sits on the IEP team. She or he is responsible for identification and certification of students with disabilities and for the determination and implementation of the necessary supplemental health services for each of these students. These duties require that the school nurse counsel and confer with students and parents, school staff, physicians, other health care providers, and community agencies. The school nurse also must provide individual teaching or inservices to any or all of these groups to ensure that the child's individual health care and safety goals are met.

It is not uncommon to find a student who is ventilator dependent, gastrostomy fed, and quadriplegic in a public school setting. An example of a typical school nurse's day might include catheterizing a child with spina bifida, suctioning the tracheostomy of a child with myotonic dystrophy, giving an inservice on tube feedings to a group of health aides, calling a physician's office as a reminder to renew a medication order, contacting a physical therapist about a wheelchair seating problem of a child with spinal muscular atrophy, attending an annual IEP for a child with cerebral palsy, conferring with parents on a behavior modification plan to address inappropriate behavior of a child with precocious puberty, and calling a nurse coordinator of a specialty clinic to schedule an assessment of a skin lesion on a child with a spinal cord injury, and continue to maintain the highest level of professional documentation and communication while following all legal requirements of confidentiality.

As the educational system strives to provide a full continuum of services to students with disabilities from self-contained classrooms to full inclusion, it is evident that the school nurse will continue to play a vital role in the process.

References

Association of Rehabilitation Nurses. (1993). *The specialty practice of rehabilitation nursing: A core curriculum.* Glenview, IL: Rehabilitation Nursing Foundation.

Bramadat, I., & Melvin, C. L. (1987). Habilitation: Application of a concept. *Clinical Nurse Specialist,*

Centers for Disease Control. (1990). Childhood injuries in the United States. *American Journal of the Diseases of Children, 144,* 627–646.

Edwards, P. A. (1987). Rehabilitation outcomes in children with brain injury. *Rehabilitation Nursing, 12*(3), 125–127.

Eng, G. D. (1992). Rehabilitation of children with neuromuscular diseases. In G. E. Molnar (Ed.), *Pediatric rehabilitation* (pp. 363–399). Oakland, CA: Williams & Wilkins.

Erikson, E. (1963). *Childhood and society.* New York: Norton.

Gallagher, S. S., Finison, K., Guyer, B., & Goodenough, S. (1984). The incidence of injuries among 87,000 Massachusetts children and adolescents: Result of the 1980–81 Statewide Childhood Injury Prevention Program Surveillance System. *American Journal of Public Health, 74*(12), 1340–1347.

Getchufsky, M. (1997). Issues and answers in latex sensitivity. *Ostomy/Wound Management, 43*(3), 42–53.

Groholt, E. K., & Nordhagen, R. (1995). Cerebral palsy in light of old and new research results—In what direction does the pendulum swing? *Tidsskrift for Den Norski Laegeforening, 17,* 2095–2099.

Grzankowski, J. A. (1997). Altered though processes related to traumatic brain injury and their nursing implication. *Rehabilitation Nursing, 22*(1), 24–31.

Jorch, G. (1995). Causes of perinatal brain damage. *Zentralblatt fur Gynakologie, 4,* 175–180.

Koch, B. M. (1992). Rehabilitation of the child with joint disease. In G. E. Molnar (Ed.), *Pediatric rehabilitation.* Oakland, CA: Williams & Wilkins.

Leger, R. R., & Meeropol, E. (1992). Children at risk: Latex allergy and spina bifida. *Journal of Pediatric Nursing, 7,* 371–376.

Levin, H. S., Goldstein, F. C., High, W. M., Jr., & Eisenberg, H. M. (1988). Disproportionately severe memory deficit in relation to normal intellectual functioning after closed head injury. *Journal of Neurological and Neurosurgical Psychiatry, 51*(10), 1294–1301.

MacGillivray, I., & Campbell, D. M. (1995). The changing pattern of cerebral palsy in Avon. *Paediatric and Perinatal Epidemiology, 2,* 146–155.

Maslow, A. (1970). *Motivation and personality.* (2nd ed.). New York: Harper and Row.

McLone, D. (1990). *Information about children with spina bifida.* Washington, DC: Spina Bifida Association of America.

Meberg, A., & Broche, H. (1995). A changing pattern of cerebral palsy: Declining trend for incidence of cerebral palsy in the 20-year period. *Journal of Perinatal Medicine, 5,* 395–402.

Molnar, G. E. (1992). *Pediatric rehabilitation.* Oakland, CA: Williams & Wilkins.

National Center for Health Statistics. (1988). *Vital Statistics of the United States, 1986* (Vol. 2, Mortality, Pt. A). Washington, DC: U.S. Government Printing Office.

Nelson, C. A. (1995). Cerebral palsy. In D. A. Umphred (Ed.), *Neurological rehabilitation* (pp. 263–286). St. Louis: Mosby.

Peterson, P., Rauen, K., Brown, J., & Cole, J. (1994). Spina bifida: Transition into adulthood begins in infancy. *Rehabilitation Nursing, 19*(4), 229–238.

Piaget, J. (1970). *Structuralism.* New York: Basic Books.

Rivara, F. P., Bergman, A. B., LoGerfo, J. P., & Weiss, N. S. (1982). Epidemiology of childhood injuries. II. Sex differences in injury rates. *American Journal of the Disabled Child, 136*(6), 502–506.

Rouse, T. M., & Eichelberger, M. R. (1992). Trends in pediatric trauma management. *Surgical Clinics of North America, 72*(6), 1347–1364.

Steele, S. (1985). Young children with cerebral palsy: Practical guidelines for care. *Pediatric Nursing,* July/August, 259–267.

Suzuki, J., Ito, M., & Tomiwa, K. (1996). Incidence patterns of cerebral palsy in Shiga, Japan, 1977–1986: An epidemiological study. *No to Hattatsu, 1,* 60–65.

Suggested Readings

Barker, E. (1994). *Neuroscience nursing.* St. Louis, MO: Mosby.

Block, K., Brandt, P., & Magyary, D. (1995). A nursing assessment standard for early intervention: Family coping. *Journal of Pediatric Nursing, 1,* 28–39.

Clubb, R. L. (1991). Chronic sorrow: Adaptation patterns of parents with chronically ill children. *Pediatric Nursing, 17,* 461–465.

DeLisa, J. A., & Gans, B. M. (1993). *Rehabilitation medicine: Principals and practice.* Philadelphia, PA: J.B. Lippincott.

Edwards-Beckett, J., & King, H. (1996). The impact of spinal pathology on bowel control in children. *Rehabilitation Nursing, 21*(6), 292–297.

Hickey, J. V. (1986). *The clinical practice of neurological and neurosurgical nursing* (2nd ed.). Philadelphia, PA: J.B. Lippincott.

Hoeman, S. P. (1996). *Rehabilitation nursing* (2nd ed.). Long Valley, NJ: Mosby.

Kurtz, M., Van Zandt, D. K., & Sapp, L. (1996). A new technique in independent catheterization: The Mitrofanoff catheterizable channel. *Rehabilitation Nursing, 21*(6), 311–314.

Morota, N., Abbott, R., Kofler, M., Epstein, F. J., & Cohen, H. (1995). Residual spasticity after selective posterior rhizotomy. *Child's Nervous System, 3,* 161–165.

Rawlins, P. (1995). Intrathecal baclofen for spasticity of cerebral palsy: Project coordination and nursing care. *Journal of Neuroscience Nursing, 3,* 157–163.

Rehabilitation Nursing Foundation Nursing Diagnosis Publications Taskforce. (1995). *21 rehabilitation nursing diagnoses: A guide to interventions and outcomes.* Glenview, IL: Rehabilitation Nursing Foundation.

Spoltore, T., & O'Brien, A. M. (1995). Rehabilitation of the spinal cord injured patient. *Orthopedic Nursing, 14*(3), 7–14.

Zickler, C. F., & Dodge, N. N. (1994). Office management of the young child with cerebral palsy and difficulty in growing. *Journal of Pediatric Health Care, 3,* 111–120.

TRANSITION TO THE COMMUNITY

SECTION
TRANSITIONS TO THE COMMUNITY

CHAPTER 31
Rehabilitation Case Management

Lynda Jones

Key Terms *Case Management*
Continuum
Discharge Planning
External Case Manager
Internal Case Manager
Life Care Planning

Objectives 1. Identify components of the case management process
2. Discuss the direct care nurses' role in case management

Introduction This chapter covers aspects of case management as it relates to the direct care rehabilitation nurse. Rehabilitation nursing is practiced in many settings including acute care, home health, and long-term care facilities. In all of these health care continuum points it is the direct care nurse who is able to provide the client and significant others with the information, education, and support to assist them in planning their future. This is the essence of case management. Mullahy (1995) states the focal point of case management in all of its roles is to empower patients and give them and their families access to a greater understanding of their disability or disease, a larger voice in the delivery of their care, and more personalized attention to their particular needs.

Rehabilitation focuses on client self-determination, achievability of goals, and the team process. This is in concert with the definition of **case management** from the Certification of Insurance Rehabilitation Specialist Commission: "Case management is a collaborative process which assesses, plans, implements, coordinates, monitors, and evaluates the options and services to meet an individual's health needs, using communication and available resources to promote quality, cost effective outcomes" (Mullahy, 1995, p. 5). Rehabilitation nurses have in their scope of practice all components of case management. Hanlon and Sharkey (1989) outline some of the roles of the rehabilitation nurse as caregiver, coordinator, educator, advocate, collaborator, facilitator, and discharge planner. The Association of Rehabilitation Nursing (1994) lists the Standards of Care and Standards of Professional Practice to include assessment, diagnosis, outcome identification, planning, implementation, evaluation, ethics, collaboration, and resource utilization.

The direct care rehabilitation nurse is able to assess, diagnose, set the client specific outcomes, co-ordinate the plan of care in collaboration with the client and other team members, implement the plan of care including education and resource utilization, and evaluate the plan. Although the direct care rehabilitation nurses are able to carry out the case management process as listed here, they will lack expertise in one or more of the components. It is for this reason that most agencies have dedicated case managers to assist with this process.

Overview of Case Management

It is important to remember that all institutions have their own titles and job descriptions. The term "case manager" has been used to describe hospital discharge planners, insurance review nurses, and social workers. This has led to confusion over the role of case manager and case management.

What was formally known as **discharge planning** is now referred to as case management in many institutions. Social work, workers compensation, insurance companies, vocational rehabilitation, utilization review, and hospital discharge planners have all contributed to the management of the rehabilitation client. Two terms are used to describe case managers: internal and external.

An **internal case manager** is one who is hired by an agency to manage the care of the clients served by the agency. Usually the relationship ends when the client is discharged from service. The **external case manager** can be an employee of the insurance company or be contracted to provide the service. The external case manager follows the client at all points along the **continuum** of service. The external case manager is also familiar with the client's health care benefits. The external case manager involvement ranges from telephone reviews to active participation in the rehabilitation process, including planning and arranging for continued services and equipment.

Life Care Planning

One other area of case management is that of **life care planning.** This is necessary and useful for clients with chronic conditions that will require continuous resource utilization. Many of these clients are receiving monetary settlements for their disability claims. To assure the moneys are appropriate, they may enlist the assistance of a life care planner to assess accurately the financial impact their disability will have now and in the future. To predict accurately the cost of care over a lifetime the life care planner makes a detailed list of expected lifetime expenditures. The life care planner can then assist the client, family, or insurance company in setting aside funds to be used as the needs arise.

Components of Case Management
Assessment

Assessment includes the medical status, functional status, psychosocial status, family issues, coping skills, home environment, and financial state. This assessment is ongoing as new information becomes available and as the client status changes over time.

Diagnosis

From the assessment the nursing diagnosis can be formed. Although each client is unique and can have multiple nursing diagnoses related to their medical condition and health status, many rehabilitation clients have one or more of the following:

- Knowledge deficit related to the medical condition, the functional status, the use of equipment, and the rehabilitation process
- Self-care deficit related to mobility and/or cognition
- Body image disturbance related to changes in physical abilities and/or appearance
- Role modification related to physical condition

Outcomes

As a client advocate, the nurse assists the client/family in setting realistic short-term goals. From these goals, the rehabilitation plan is developed.

Coordination and Implementation

The direct care rehabilitation nurse must use the goals set by the client and work with the team to initiate the client's rehabilitation program or plan of care.

If independence is most important, then working on independent dressing—no matter the energy expended or length of time necessary to perform the task—is important. For a client who will be returning to work or school, it may be more important to work on mobility issues and allow family/caregivers to be trained in bathing and dressing techniques.

Education and Resource Utilization

The first issue with all clients is that of education. If case management is to succeed, the client and family must be empowered not only to advocate for their needs, but to make appropriate choices related to care. If they are unaware of what their choices consist of, how can we as health professionals expect them to make adequate, appropriate, and informed choices? Rehabilitation nurses need to educate themselves as to resources that are available in their community as well as the myriad of options available to the client for durable medical equipment and other health care supplies. Initiating and maintaining a resource book for their practice setting is one way to accomplish this.

The second area of education is that of long-term consequences and care needs associated with the client's diagnosis. Appropriate plans for the client must take into account the length of time the client will need a specific service or treatment, cost associated with it, and who the payer source will be as well as alternatives. Many of these clients have needs that will extend beyond their payer source's abilities. Planning from the beginning for the treatment option that is both financially and clinically reasonable avoids the unnecessary and difficult transition to another option when money is no longer available. Although technology allows us to make environmental controls for even the most disabled client, not everyone will have the resources necessary to access these options.

Once the family knows what is needed, assisting them with choosing how that treatment, service, or item will be provided is another way the direct rehabilitation nurse can assist families and clients in their case management. A simple example is that of bowel programs. Using suppositories and medication, although effective, can become financially burdensome.

Initiating a bowel care routine that includes consistent time of day, high-fiber foods, and digital stimulation before adding medications is one way the direct care rehabilitation nurse can assist with the delivery of cost-effective care.

Ensuring that the client is able to train others in their care is the major way the direct care rehabilitation nurse provides for the successful transition of the client from one continuum point to another.

Evaluation

The final step in the case management process leads us in a circle back to the beginning. Evaluation or reassessment of the client's health status and response to the rehabilitation program allow modification as needed for the goals, interventions, and plans. The evaluation should be ongoing, making changes as needed in their program to move them along the continuum from a dependent state to their maximal independent state.

Levels of Client Need

Many institutions use a system of risk identification or prioritization of their clients. One health care network uses five categories to decide the degree of case management involvement. The categories are based on the client's health status and anticipated resource utilization (Brown, Mayer, & Jackson, 1992).

The following is another example of using categories to identify clients on the bases of potential resource utilization:

Category 1: The short-term client with limited need for continued equipment, supplies, and education. Two examples of this type of client are those who have joint replacement surgery and surgical repair of a fractured hip and who have no other medical conditions.

Category 2: The intermittent client with the potential for ongoing needs for equipment, supplies, and education. Examples include amputees, clients with a mild cerebrovascular accident (CVA) with limited deficits, and incomplete paraplegics.

Category 3: The continuous need client who is being maintained at home with family and caregivers. These patients can include anyone who requires assistance with activities of daily living (ADLs). Examples include quadriplegics and clients with a CVA, multiple sclerosis (MS), brain injury, and severe arthritis.

Category 4: The continuous need client who has been institutionalized to receive care.

Successful rehabilitation requires input from the direct care nurse, assigned case managers, and a variety of other team members. The bedside nurse who does not take into account the client's situation in total and leaves the "case management" to others is not providing complete rehabilitation to her client.

Case Study

Category 2: A 50-year-old female client who is an insulin-dependent diabetic has entered rehabilitation following a below-the-knee amputation (BKA).

Assessment

Focus of the assessment is on the client and family's ability to assist with home care, home safety, knowledge of disease process, surgery, rehabilitation, and economic resources. Particular attention should be focused on the client's perception of how the BKA will impact her lifestyle. Another area of concern is the client's prior and future ability to manage independently all aspects of her chronic illness and disability.

Outcomes

On the basis of the assessment, the long-term goal is to have the client return to the home setting, able to care for herself independently and to require health care resources on a planned intermittent basis.

Diagnosis

- Body image disturbance related to limb amputation
- Knowledge deficit related to diabetes, insulin, and/or equipment use
- Self-care and mobility deficits related to amputation

Coordination and Implementation

The client and nurse will collaborate with other team members to facilitate the rehabilitation program. This may include blood sugars, insulin administration, meal planning, and mobility training with equipment and prosthesis. Having the program approximate the client's home situation is a good way to utilize resources appropriately and provide cost-effective care.

Education and Resource Utilization

Education is best provided on the basis of the individual client's ability. Frequent, short sessions provide the client with the opportunity to integrate the information into her daily routine. For example, education on blood glucose monitoring and insulin dosage, including return demonstrations, should be done at the same time the client will be doing it at home.

Specific needs for this client include

- Medical follow-up including prescriptions for medication, syringes, blood glucose monitoring equipment
- Prosthesis and ambulation aids
- Short-term home health follow-up
- Referral to community support groups

Evaluation/Reassessment

During the rehabilitation process the continual monitoring of both her medical status and ability to be independent in self-care activities are equally important. This will be a predictive indication of her ability to manage independently at home. The program is modified on the basis of her meeting progress toward her specific goals.

Summary

In summary, the rehabilitation direct care nurse, regardless of practice setting, has many responsibilities and opportunities to participate in the case management process.

As rehabilitation nurses, with the knowledge and skills related to team process, client advocacy, education, and the nursing process, they are able to provide cost-effective and quality care.

Acknowledgments

Jacque Vance, RN, CRRN, MSN is gratefully acknowledged for her comments and contributions regarding this chapter.

References

Association of Rehabilitation Nurses. (1994). *Standards and scope of rehabilitation nursing practice* (3d ed.). Skokie, IL: Author.

Brown, N. P., Mayer, G. G., & Jackson, K. L. (1992). Case management. In A. E. Barnett & G. G. Mayer (Eds.), *Ambulatory care management and practice* (pp. 363–370). Rockville, MD: Aspen.

Hanlon, D., & Sharkey, E. L. (1989). Professional practice of rehabilitation nursing. In S. Dittmar (Ed.), *Rehabilitation nursing: Process and application.* St. Louis, MO: Mosby.

Mullahy, Catherine M. (1995). *The case manager's handbook.* Rockville, MD: Aspen.

Suggested Readings

Certification of Insurance Rehabilitation Specialists Commission. (1993) *CCM certification guide.* Rolling Meadows, IL: Author.

McCollom, P. L., & Sager, D. (1996). Case management. In S. P. Hoeman (Ed.), *Rehabilitation nursing: Process and application* (2nd ed., pp. 101–113). St. Louis, MO: Mosby.

CHAPTER 32
The Stress of Relocation

Patricia A. Chin

Key Terms   *Relocation Stress*
Relocation Stress Syndrome

Objectives
1. Discuss relocation stress and relocation stress syndrome.

2. Identify the types of relocation confronting the rehabilitation client and family members.

3. Identify factors associated with relocation stress in the rehabilitation setting.

4. Identify characteristics and indicators that might indicate that a rehabilitation client is experiencing actual or potential relocation stress or relocation stress syndrome.

5. Identify specific nursing interventions for the client experiencing actual or potential relocation stress or relocation stress syndrome in the rehabilitation setting.

6. Identify the expected outcomes of nursing interventions for the client experiencing actual or potential relocation stress or relocation stress syndrome in the rehabilitation setting.

Relocation

Stress is associated with any life event requiring an adaptive response (Selye, 1956). The rehabilitation process constantly exposes the client to numerous demands for adjustment and adaptation. There is stress and anxiety associated with initial hospital stabilization and treatment, possible surgical interventions and invasive procedures, and the transitions of entering and leaving the rehabilitation settings. McDaniel and Sexton (1970) found that all indicators of stress increased dramatically just before discharge from the rehabilitation center. When the rehabilitation center provides complete care and assumes responsibility for all aspects of the person's treatment and life it is understandable that entry and termination become stressful episodes in the client's and family's life.

The clients in the rehabilitation setting are in a constant state of physiological and psychological adaptation and adjustment. They must cope with the onset of an illness, disease, an injury, or disability that was sudden and neither expected nor anticipated; and the resulting complex change to self and life. Unpredictable, sudden, and life-threatening stressors resulting in serious or multiple consequences may become catastrophic for the individual. Events that do not occur when or as they are expected may be perceived as stressful. Although transitions are often anticipated changes experienced by individuals and families as they adjust, adapt, and cope with normalcy they are still stress producing. Andreasen and Wasek (1980) observed that continuous exposure to stressors over a period of time was identified more often as the precipitant of maladaptive functioning than sudden-shock stressors. Relocation will be stressful even when it is perceived to be a sign of client progress.

Relocation forces the client into a transitional period. Transitional periods can be considered a personal crisis: The past must be integrated into the new. During relocation the client must adapt past life structure into the new and must consider a series of new choices. Much of what occurred before must be reworked in a new way. Learning must be evaluated for its use in the new environment. Each transition involves a leave-taking from the past ideas and view of life (Carson & Arnold, 1996).

Relocation Stress and Relocation Stress Syndrome

Relocation stress is a time-limited emotional response resulting from a situational stressor—specifically, the need to transfer from one health care environment to another environment. Relocation is stressful for both the client and the family. Relocation can be very disruptive and damage family patterns. The manifestations of relocation stress are extremely varied. The response will be dependent on the client's personality, adaptation and adjustment strategies, past life experiences, the availability of support for the client, the client's perceptions of physical and physiological strength and needs, and the degree of disruption relocation will present for the client and family. Relocation is especially stressful for clients experiencing cognitive disturbances, sensory deficits, altered levels of consciousness, and general limitation in adaptation and coping. Common behavioral responses may include sleeplessness, loss of appetite, restlessness, tension, irritability, and depression.

Relocation stress syndrome is the consequence of catastrophic injury or debilitating disease, often augmented by a required transfer from one health care unit or living arrangement to another. Relocation stress syndrome is classified as a maladaptive reaction to an identifiable psychological stressor (APA, 1994; Townsend, 1997). Clients with relocation stress syndrome can respond with physical complaints, tearfulness, social withdrawal, work or learning inhibition, depression, hopelessness, anxiety, anger, and conduct disturbance. The impairment is corrected when the client adapts to the stressor or when the stressor disappears (Townsend, 1997).

Types of Relocation Associated with the Rehabilitation Experience

The precipitant stressor for relocation stress or relocation stress syndrome is the need to uproot oneself and move on to a new environment. The types of relocation that would be an important consideration for the rehabilitation client and family members might be

1. Transfer from an acute care environment to the rehabilitation environment
2. Transfers to and within long-term care facilities (Rantz & Egan, 1987)
3. Transfers from critical care to step-down or subacute care (Harkulich & Brugler, 1991)
4. Transfer from the rehabilitation unit to a community setting

Factors Related to Relocation Stress in the Rehabilitation Setting

Reasons that rehabilitation clients may experience stress associated with relocation include the following:

- Transfer is stressful when the client and family members have developed a sense of security, trust, and confidence in the therapeutic triad of client-family-nurse and this is disrupted by relocation.
- When confronted with relocation the client and family members are faced with another unpredictable unknown. This is stressing even if the relocation is a signal of physical improvement for the client.
- If the transfer is related to a worsening of the client's condition, stress and anxiety are magnified for the client and family members.
- Clients and families will experience stress if there has been inadequate or no preparation for the impending move.
- Relocation will be more stressful when there is a moderate to high degree of environmental change. This can be a geographical change, such as a transfer from a hospital in one community to a hospital in a neighboring community. Stress will also be heightened if the new environment is perceived by the client to significantly differ in its level of technology. An example would be transferring a client from the intensive care unit directly to the rehabilitation unit within the same facility.
- Relocation is stressful when there are losses involved in the decision to move.
- Prior feelings of powerlessness or loss of control will increase the stress associated with relocation.
- Clients who have experienced past, recent, and current losses will experience greater levels of stress.
- Clients and family who lack an adequate support system to assist in relocation and deal with any losses will experience additional stress of relocation.
- The client's and family's history with previous transfers and the types of previous transfers will influence the nature of stress associated with relocations.
- Impaired psychosocial health status will be an additional stressor for the client coping with relocation.
- Decreased physical health status will be an additional stressor for the client coping with relocation.
- Patients who have a limited capacity to comprehend the move will be confused and see the move as a major threat to them and their security.

Nursing Process

Nursing diagnosis: Relocation stress syndrome—A state in which the client experiences physiological or psychological disturbances as a result of transfer from one environment to another (Townsend, 1997, p. 304).

Assessment

Areas to be included when assessing to determine if the client has an actual or potential reaction of relocation stress or relocation stress syndrome are the following:

- Behavioral responses: sleeplessness, loss of appetite, restlessness, anxiety, tension, irritability, apprehension, social isolation, and depression
- The client's or family members' symptoms of apprehension, stress, or anxiety
- The client's or family members' expressions of negative feelings about the future relocation
- The client's or family members' willingness or refusal to discuss the future relocation
- The client's or family members' feelings of powerlessness or loss of control regarding the relocation
- Increased desire for independence or dependency
- Regression in self-care skill mastery and self-management
- Nonadherent and rebellious behaviors
- A sense of loneliness
- Insecurity about the new surroundings and personnel
- Feelings regarding the future

Interventions

Planning for relocation should include attempting to minimize physiological and/or psychological disturbances triggered by the move. Interventions focus on the client's progress toward independence and the prevention of rehabilitation setbacks. Nursing interventions are determined by the source of the client's stress associated with the relocation. General interventions could include

- Informing the client and family members about goals, programs, and resources of the new environment
- Exploring the relocation with the client and family, emphasizing that the relocation is uncomfortable but necessary for progress through the rehabilitation process
- Encouraging visitation by the family members, and the client if possible, to explore the new environment and meet the personnel prior to client's transfer
- Communicating the client's physical, psychological, social, and spiritual needs to new health care professionals who will be caring for the client
- Encouraging the verbalization of feelings and perceptions about the meaning of and any problems or concerns associated with the relocation
- Encouraging the client and family to discuss how the relocation will affect their lives
- Communicating with family members regarding the client's adjustment to the relocation

- When possible and appropriate, encouraging the participation of the client and family members in the choice and decision-making regarding relocation issues
- Assisting the client and family to identify people within the new environment who can provide them with assistance and services

Outcomes The long-term outcome of nursing interventions for a client experiencing relocation stress or relocation stress syndrome is that the client exhibits positive adaptation to the new environment.

Expected Outcomes
- The client no longer exhibits signs of anxiety, somatic symptoms, or depression.
- The client verbalizes satisfaction and makes positive statements concerning both acceptance of new environment and reasons for the relocation.
- The client and family members are motivated by goals of rehabilitation and reentry into the community.
- The client and family members willingly participate in social and rehabilitation activities within the new environment.
- The client expresses feelings of control and self-confidence when confronted with relocation.
- If relocation stress does occur the client successfully demonstrates stress management techniques.
- Client and family members will express trust in new care providers and confidence in the program of the new facility.

Conclusion Stress is associated with any life event requiring an adaptive response. Relocation stress is an acute maladaptive emotional response, the result of specific, intense environmental stress. The precipitant stressor for relocation stress or relocation stress syndrome is the need to uproot oneself and move on to a new environment. The response is considered maladaptive when there is impairment in social or occupational functioning or the client's behaviors are exaggerated beyond the usual response associated with such a stressor. Planning for relocation should include attempting to minimize physiological and/or psychological disturbances triggered by the move. Intervention should focus on the client's progress toward independence and the prevention of rehabilitation setbacks.

References American Psychiatric Association (APA). (1994). *American Psychiatric Association: Diagnostic and statistical manual of mental disorders* (4th ed.). Washington, DC: Author.

Andreasen, N. C., & Wasek, P. (1980). Adjustment disorders in adolescents and adults. *Archives of General Psychiatry, 37,* 1166–1170.

Carson, V. B., & Arnold, E. N. (1996). *Mental health nursing: The nurse–patient journey.* Philadelphia: W. B. Saunders Company.

Harkulich, J., & Brugler, C. (1991). Nursing diagnosis: Relocation stress. In K. Gettrust (Ed.), *Interventions for nursing diagnosis: Guides for comprehensive care planning* (pp. 461–468). Albany, NY: Delmar Publishing.

McDaniel, J. W., & Sexton, A. (1970). Psychoendocrine studies of patients with spinal cord lesions. *Journal of Abnormal Psychology, 76,* 117–122.

Rantz, M., & Egan, K. (1987). Reducing death from translocation syndrome. *American Journal of Nursing, 87,* 1351–1352.

Selye, H. (1956). *The stress of life.* New York: McGraw-Hill.

Townsend, M. C. (1997). *Nursing diagnoses in psychiatric nursing: A pocket guide for care plan construction* (4th ed.). Philadelphia: F.A. Davis.

CHAPTER 33
Community Re-entry

Patricia A. Chin

Key Terms   *Community Integration*
Community Re-entry
Community Resources
Discharge Planning
Educational Programs
Housing
Vocational Rehabilitation
Workplace Disability Management

Objectives   1. Discuss the principles underlying community re-entry and integration for persons with disabilities.

2. Discuss the importance of early discharge planning for community re-entry.

3. Discuss issues that can affect the quality of life for those re-entering the community with disabilities: housing, transportation, education programs, vocational rehabilitation, assistive devices.

Community Re-entry

The primary purpose of rehabilitation is to assist clients with disabilities to adapt to living with the disability and to promote **community re-entry**: independent living. When the clients are physically ready to re-enter the community they continue to encounter numerous factors that influence their functional adaptation, including family support, geographical location, community resources, financial resources, public policy, and attitudes of society toward those with disabilities. Clients must develop a number of skills to complete successfully the transition from life in an institutional setting to re-entry to the community.

Discharge Planning

Successful re-entry into the community does not happen without preparation and efforts by those involved: the client, family members, interdisciplinary treatment team, and the community. The goal of community re-entry is for the client to achieve the highest level of independence possible. Re-entry into the community should be a central component of **discharge planning** and that plan should be designed as soon as the client's functional abilities are determined. Issues that arise related to that successful transition include safe living, working, and recreational environments. Clients with disabilities will have to be able to access housing, transportation, and educational opportunities. They may require vocational rehabilitation, disability management in the workplace, or adaptive equipment to facilitate community living. Once in the community the client will need working knowledge and skills for networking support services, advocacy groups, and community resource availability.

Once community re-entry becomes a reality the treatment team may be expanded to include additional resources from the Department of Human Services staff, neighbors, or community network persons, and extended family members (Buchanan, 1996). Families may feel unprepared or uncertain about their abilities to provide care at home. Their concern may include medication administration, following instructions, inability to provide direct physical care, and inadequate awareness of community services and resources that might be required by the client (Rhoads, Dean, Carson, & Blaylock, 1992). Many of these issues can be successfully addressed through preparatory instruction and practice. This is best accomplished by allowing the client to go home on pass before discharge. The client and caregivers will be able to practice skills in the home setting. This can boost client and caregiver confidence and morale. These excursions into the community can help in the identification of actual or potential difficulties that were not anticipated in the institutional environment. Home passes will also give the treatment team an opportunity to assess the client's ability to function in the home environment, and the client's mood and motivation during community re-entry (Henderson & Pentland, 1991).

Reflections of Community Integration

Taylor, Racino, Knoll, and Lutfiyya (1987), in a seminal work on **community integration** for those with developmental disabilities, have articulated a set of basic principles that can also be applied to those with physical limitations or disabilities. The principles they described are as follow:

- All people, regardless of any differences, belong in a community.
- People with differences can be integrated into typical neighborhoods, work situations, and community social situations.
- Support is necessary for all people and their families. This support should be offered in regular places in the community, not in specialized settings designed for peoples who are "different."
- The development of relationships between people with and without labels is crucial.
- Service users and families should be involved in the design, operation, and monitoring of all services. They should also hold those services accountable (Taylor, Racino, Knoll, & Lutfiyya, 1987).

It is essential for rehabilitation clients and those with disabilities to have access to the workplace, medical services, shopping, support services, recreational facilities, churches, public buildings, banks, post offices, and grocery and clothing stores. Taylor, Racino, Knoll, and Lutfiyya (1987) concluded that preparatory programs are not effective; instead, people need to learn in the community setting, in homes, and at jobs. They also proposed that community acceptance of those who are different follows community integration; it is not a prerequisite for integration. The most effective way to meet the complicated needs of the disabled is a highly individualized approach attending to home, jobs, friends, and human connectedness.

The movement to regard community integration as a right stems from experience with those with disabilities and from the civil rights movement. The basic belief of community integration is that all people, including those with disabilities, have a right to community participation and membership. The goal of community integration will be achieved through peer support and self-help, as well as through physical access, vocational training, jobs, and relationships with nondisabled peers. The goal will be achieved when those with disabilities exercise full control over the services and supports they need (Carling, 1995).

Carling (1995, pp. 23–24) identified the following assumptions when reflecting on community integration of the mentally ill.

- Success in housing, work, or social relationships is primarily a function of whether the person possesses the skills and support relevant to the environment or relationship.
- Relationships with service providers change over time and should depend on the clients' needs, not on how they get along with the care providers.
- Peoples' needs change over time, so support and services should be available at the appropriate level of support as long as the services are needed.
- Family members require and deserve substantial support while supporting the disabled person.
- Family members should not be blamed for their relative's disability.
- The legitimate target of family advocacy is for family needs.

Carling was writing about community integration of the mentally disabled but it seems logical that these assumptions also apply to the rehabilitation client and to those with physical disabilities as well.

Clients terminating rehabilitation services and clients with a disability who are re-entering the community need to be aware of the community resources available to them. The comprehensive assessment of the continuing and changing needs of persons with disabilities across their life span will result in directing adequate funding and support services to ensure the most efficient use of resources. Furukawa and Shomaker (1982) defined **community resources** as new, or existing, support services that fulfill the health and social needs of the community's residents. Communities will differ in the ability to provide services for their residents. Factors that will affect resource delivery in a community include the commitment of the community to ensuring the rights of the disabled, financial resources available to provide services, the community's geographical location, and the availability of caregivers able and willing to learn the care required.

The rehabilitation nurse plays a vital role in identifying client needs and developing the knowledge base necessary for successful transition to the community. The nurse can assist clients with community re-entry by encouraging the client and family members to be active participants in discharge planning. The nurse should monitor the progress of discharge planning to ensure that all elements for success will be available and ready for implementation when the client is ready to take advantage of them. The nurse should also provide the client and family members with opportunities to discuss feelings and concerns they may have as preparations for community re-entry become a reality.

There are numerous issues related to successful re-entry into the community. The purpose of the following discussion is to look at several significant issues (housing, transportation, workplace management, educational programs, adaptive equipment, and vocational rehabilitation) that have a direct influence on the quality of life for the disabled client after re-entry into the community.

Accessible Housing

Clients should be made aware of the options for **housing** available to them on discharge from the rehabilitation setting. There are a number of laws governing housing availability and accessibility for the disabled:

1. The Housing Act (1959) provides funding for the development of housing for the elderly and the disabled.
2. The Architectural Barriers Act (1968) mandates physical accessibility to any federally funded building.
3. The Rehabilitation Act (1973) prohibits discrimination against the disabled when renting or purchasing federally subsidized property.
4. The Rehabilitation, Comprehensive Services, and Developmental Disabilities Amendment of 1978 provides for housing grants.
5. The Americans with Disabilities Act (1990) established new laws governing physical access to the community.

There are housing alternatives available for persons with disabilities. The choice of residence will depend on the client's functional ability, support system, needs, and goals. Some client will return to their prior residence following termination of rehabilitation services or during the final stage of rehabilitation. Other clients may have to consider alternative housing situations if they are unable to remain in their previous residence. Their options will include independent living programs, residential living arrangements, congregate housing, or extended care facilities.

Clients who cannot return to their prior residence without assistance might be encouraged to connect with an independent living program. These programs allow individuals with disabilities to remain in their own residences while offering, but not managing, support services. A variety of support services related to activities of daily living, personal health management, and counseling assistance are provided through independent living programs (see Table 1).

An alternative housing option for those clients who are unable to remain in their previous residence is residential living. *Residential living* refers to housing arrangements that group people with disabilities in the same building or geographic area. Clients can share support services and assist each other in meeting needs. Residential living arrangements present several challenges: finding accessible housing, securing attendant services, and obtaining rent subsidies.

Several option for clients with major care needs or who require the services of licensed medical personal are also available. Those options include 24-hour care institutions, subacute rehabilitation programs, neurobehavioral programs, skilled care facilities, and board and care homes.

Residential units, whether the client's prior home or a new residence, may require necessary adaptations, including access ramps, wider doors, or modifications of the kitchen and bathroom so that all facilities and appliances are easily accessible. Alterations may also be necessary in parking arrangements.

Whatever the housing option chosen, several factors need to be considered when assessing housing. Home assessment is usually the role and responsibility of the occupational therapist, but nurses need to address these issues in client teaching and discharge planning. The nurse also needs to coordinate the team's efforts in preparing the client for community re-entry.

Housing assessment should include a review of

- The appropriate type of living quarters given the client's functional abilities

Table 1
Types of Independent Living Support Services

Activities of Daily Living	Personal Health Management	Counseling Support
Communal meals	Sexuality and family relationships counseling	Advocacy services
Emergency procedures		Consumer and legal information
Housing options	Management of attendants	
Recreational opportunities	Training in communication techniques	Peer counseling
Training in communication techniques		Personal business management
Training in homemaking skills		
Supervision of and guidance in transportation skills		

- The design of the building and accessibility in multistory buildings
- Lighting in the living quarters and at the entrance
- Heating, running water, electrical outlets, and toilet facilities
- Access to the residence and whether there is a need for wider doors or assistance with door openings; automatic door openings
- The need for bathroom and kitchen modifications
- Assistive devices needed to facilitate mobility and safe participation in the environment
- The client's level of independence in transfers, homemaking skills, personal care, food preparation, and household maintenance
- The adequacy of communication devices, and the client's ability to hear doorbells, fire alarms, and door bells
- Safety issues—e.g., handrails, clutter, cords, rugs, carpets, toys, and animals that could pose safety risks
- The arrangement of furniture, its functionality, and any need for adaptive equipment (e.g., chair lifts)

Accessible Transportation

It is important that persons with disabilities have access to the workplace, medical services, support services, shopping, recreational facilities, churches, and public buildings in order to increase independence in self-care and community participation. The person must be mobile to accomplish this. The person can get around the community using private or public transportation. If public transportation is used, contact should be made with the system before use to ensure that assistive services and accommodations are available for the client.

Legislation mandates that public transportation systems and buildings be designed to ensure equal access to public transportation for all people. It also mandates the modification of airplanes, transportation terminals, buses, subways, and railroad systems to facilitate use by the disabled and elderly. Other issues that have been addressed through legislative action include space accommodation for wheelchairs, wider doorways and aisles for ease of movement of those with wheelchairs or other assistive devices, and the incorporation of ramps, lifts, and elevators into the design of new buildings.

Many persons with disabilities or limitations can provide their own transportation if their vehicles are appropriately modified with hand controls, lifts, customized seats, and transfer mechanisms in and out of the vehicle. Educational programs and evaluation are available to facilitate client vehicular operation with modifications. Federal and state funding for vehicle modifications is available. The Chamber of Commerce in most cities provides information booklets regarding community accessibility for the disabled. The Department of Transportation provides information to the disabled regarding highways and airport use.

Issues that will have to be determined before community re-entry include the following:

- What are the client's transportation needs?
- What type of transportation is available to the client?
- What is the distance from the client's residence to public transportation?
- How accessible are medical or therapy services to major public transportation lines?
- What will be the cost to the client for both private, modified vehicles and public transportation?
- How much assistance is needed by the client to access transportation, and is that assistance available for the client?
- Does the client require adapted driver education and evaluation?

Disability Management Program in the Workplace

The focus of most **workplace disability management** programs is on prevention. These programs emphasize early identification of disabled workers and focus on the prevention of work-related injuries. They attempt to identify conditions in the environment that could result in worker disability, and provide evaluations to identify the medical, social, and physiological assistance that would enable the worker to return to work. They also provide case management services in the form of job analysis, job modifications, and job placement monitoring to address problems that arise after job placement occurs.

Businesses are motivated to develop disability management programs to lower workers' compensations costs, reduce employee absenteeism, and increase employee retention. By focusing on the prevention of work-related injuries or illness the health care system is able to reduce costs of rehabilitative services and reduce medical costs.

Educational Program Consideration

Educational programs are available to ensure the attainment of educational goals. Special services are offered for the disabled to facilitate access to educational services. Educational materials can be adapted to meet special needs: talking books, Braille books, textbook recordings, cognitive software, and so on. Special equipment can be obtained for home or classroom use: reading machines, audiology services, communication augmentation devices, and voice-activated computers. Some colleges and universities have resources for evaluating the needs of disabled students and providing assistive services to enhance their learning experience: taking notes, typing papers, providing assistance with movement around campus, and so on.

To take advantage of these special programs and services the client needs to be able to have access to classrooms, cafeteria, dormitories, chapel, library, book store, and parking. School and educational facilities may need modifications so that the client has access to adapted bathrooms and shower facilities. To be a full participant in the educational community the client will need to have access to social activities and to entertainment, recreational, and sporting events.

Issues that will have to be determined before re-entry into education programs include the following:

- What are the client's special education needs?
- What support services are available for a particular program?
- Is there financial assistance available for the client?
- What types of attendant services are available for students residing on campus? (*Campus* refers to school grounds: K-12 as well as postsecondary education facilities.)
- What health care services are available on campus?
- What career planning and placement services are available to counsel those with disabilities?
- How accessible are the programs on campus for persons with disabilities?
- Are vocational or counseling services available on campus for those with disabilities?

Vocational Rehabilitation

Independent living is different from **vocational rehabilitation.** The independent living paradigm refers to those medical and social services that enable a disabled person to live in the community short of being gainfully employed. Vocational rehabilitation is for those clients who are perceived as able to attain vocational goals. Vocational rehabilitation focuses on issues of employment without regard for disability or medical rehabilitation. Some consider vocational rehabilitation objectives as an integral part of independent living (De Jong, 1984). The purpose of vocational rehabilitation is to provide support and training services that enable clients with disabilities to return to work. These services may include modification of home or vehicles, work-hardening programs, transportation resources, and job training and evaluation.

Traditional vocational rehabilitation programs have served clients with disabilities primarily in sheltered workshops and other sheltered environments. The Rehabilitation Act Amendments of 1986 defines the contents of supported employment programs. The perspective since 1989 is that providing services to the severely disabled is a priority, that disabled workers be paid for their services, and that work settings be integrated with both able-bodied workers and disabled workers.

Federal law mandates each state to have a public agency that provides vocational rehabilitation. This is the Office of Vocational Rehabilitation (OVR). Funding is available from the OVR for various aspects of vocational rehabilitation to facilitate the client's return to work or supported employment. Those funds can be used to make vehicle and home modifications, assess the client's work capacities and capabilities, determine the client's vocational limitations, and identify vocational interests and previous work experience. The OVR also funds the assessment of training facilities, employer education and development, and assessment of the current job market. The OVR provides services to match the disabled client's functional, cognitive, and emotional abilities with job training, modification, and placement.

Adaptive Equipment to Facilitate Community Reintegration

The client with a disability who is re-entering the community will need devices to facilitate activities of daily living and for mobility. The nurse should co-ordinate the assessment and obtaining of the client's specific requirements well in advance of discharge so that the equipment or devices are available for client education and practice in advance of their use in the community. Clients should also be familiar and comfortable with the equipment or devices before they become dependent on their use in the community.

- What specific type of devices will the client need for mobility: walker, stretcher, commode, braces, scooter, sliding board?
- What specific equipment or devices will the client need for independent living? Areas to consider include hygiene, dressing, and cooking.
- What specific equipment or devices will the client need for functional communication? Examples include amplification systems, assistive listening devices, telecommunication devices, vibrators for alarm clocks, visual alert systems, telephone amplifiers, around-the-clock relay services by telephone companies, communication boards, speech synthesizers, hearing-ear dogs for the hearing impaired, guide dogs for the visually impaired, and independence dogs.
- What devices will the client require to prevent medical sequelae after disability? Examples include wheelchair cushions, self-catheterization equipment, and so on.

The nurse will need to reinforce client and family member education regarding the use, repair, and replacement for equipment necessary for community re-entry and integration.

Conclusion

Those in need of rehabilitation services did not ask to be sick or injured. They dislike being defined by illness or by a set of limitations. They seek advocates who appreciate their humanness, and value them for their usefulness. They want others to appreciate the degree of strength required to pull themselves up alone, day after day in the face of something beyond their control. They perceive the primary objectives of the interdisciplinary treatment team as

- Helping the client continue with life
- Helping the client seek moments of joy
- Helping the client become active to make life better and maintain hope
- Helping the client create a life with meaning and fulfillment
- Helping the client simplify life in order to remain as functional as possible (Benet, 1996)

Community re-entry, community integration, and empowerment of people with disabilities are ideas whose time has come. Putting the ideas and strategies into practice will require more than providing information to the public. It will require clients, family members, professionals, client advocates, and policy makers to confront the challenges of making community integration the norm rather than the exception. The successful rehabilitation nurse will develop a knowledge base that includes (1) a philosophy of rehabilitation nursing; (2) anatomy and physiology; (3) family and group dynamics; (4) community services, resources, and funding for the rehabilitation client; (5) intervention, teaching, and case management skills; and (6) public policies and legislation that protect the legal rights of rehabilitation client (Buchanan, 1996).

References

Benet, A. (1996). A portrait of chronic illness: Inspecting the canvas, reframing the issues. *American Behavioral Scientist, 39*(6), 767–776.

Buchanan, L. C. (1996). Community-based rehabilitation nursing. In S. P. Hoeman (Ed.), *Rehabilitation nursing: Process and application* (2nd ed., pp. 114–129). St. Louis: Mosby.

Carling, P. J. (1995). *Return to community: Building support systems for people with psychiatric disabilities.* New York: The Guilford Press.

De Jong, G. (1984). Independent living: From social movement to analytic paradigm. In R. P. Marinelli & A. E. Dell Orto (Eds.), *The psychological & social impact of physical disability* (2nd ed.). New York: Springer.

Henderson, E. J., & Pentland, B. (1991). Home pass assessment in neurorehabilitation practice. *Journal of Advanced Nursing, 16,* 1439–1443.

Furukawa, C., & Shomaker, D. (1982). *Community health services for the aged.* Rockville, MD: Aspen.

Rhoads, C., Dean, J., Carson, C., & Blaylock, A. (1992). Comprehensive discharge planning. *Home Healthcare Nurse, 10,* 13–18.

Taylor, S. J., Racino, J., Knoll, J., & Lutfiyya, Z. (1987). *The nonrestrictive environment: A resources manual on community integration for people with the most severe disabilities.* New York: Human Policy Press.

Suggested Readings

De Jong, G. (1993). Health care reform and disability. *Archives of Physical Medicine and Rehabilitation, 74,* 1017–1024.

Eisenberg, M. G., Sutkin, L. C., & Jansen, M. A. (Eds.). (1984). *Chronic illness and disability through the life span: Effects on self and family.* New York: Springer.

Marinelli, R. P., & Dell Orto, A. E. (Eds.). (1984). *The psychological & social impact of physical disability* (2nd ed.). New York: Springer.

Resources for Rehabilitation, Inc. (1991). *Resources for people with disabilities and chronic conditions.* Lexington, MA: Author.

Roessler, R. T., & Schriner, K. F. (1991). Partnerships: The bridge from disability to ability management. *Journal of Rehabilitation, 57*(1), 53–58.

CHAPTER 34
Funding Resources

Patricia A. Chin

Key Terms *Accessing Health Care*
Alpha
Automobile Liability Policies
Diversification
Health Maintenance Organizations (HMOs)
Horizontal Integration
Medicare
Medicare Supplemental Benefits Plan (Medigap)
Medicaid
Preferred Provider Organizations (PPOs)
Public Health Department
Social Security Insurance
State Disability Programs
Vendor Services
Vertical Integration
Visiting Nurse Association
Within Market Consolidation
Workers' Compensation

Objectives 1. Discuss current issues regarding the health care delivery system.

2. Discuss costs associated with rehabilitative care.

3. Discuss issues of access to health care services and resources associated with rehabilitation and disabilities.

4. Identify public and private sector resources and funding sources of health care and rehabilitation services.

5. Identify nursing interventions to increase accessibility to health care services and resources for rehabilitation clients and families.

Health Care Delivery

Americans have come to expect a great deal from the health care delivery system. America's acute care system, the system on which Western health care delivery was built, can offer the premium in care and technology. Yet criticism of the current system has grown. The current health delivery system has been criticized as being a nonsystem; as highly fragmented, lacking coordination, and too focused on acute care. This criticism arises from growing dissatisfaction over the use of more complex and disjointed services, limited access, and rising costs that limit access (American Hospital Association, 1992).

The current delivery system, which is based on the "ability to pay," has created a two-tier system of delivery and resulted in the unaffordability of health care for many. Those most severely affected include the employed uninsured, uninsured children, the poor and near-poor, and the elderly poor. Historically, and politically, the public has communicated to national leaders that health care is considered a right, not a privilege. Wealth and health insurance have provided access and financial protection for many. However, many Americans continue to have inadequate or no health insurance to deal with the burden of illness, injury, or disease.

The cost of health care in America has risen almost twice as rapidly as the costs of general good and services (Congressional Budget Office, 1993), and four times greater than the "growth rate" of the country's general economy (Letsch, 1993). The per capita expenditures for health care, adjusted for inflation, have increased fivefold (Congressional Budget Office, 1993). The majority of these costs are associated with hospitalization, physicians and personnel, drugs, and nondurable medical goods and services.

Rehabilitation and Costs

Nurses must expand their knowledge beyond the clinical and psychological components of client care to include health care financing, economics, and insurance (Wieseke & Bantz, 1992). Rehabilitation clients confronted with serious financial problems and decisions about their health care look to the nurse for assistance and guidance. The rehabilitation nurse has an important role in supporting and educating clients about financial issues. The goal for both client and rehabilitation team should be cost-effective, quality care.

Medical rehabilitation is currently a $15 billion to $20 billion a year industry. This figure is expected to exceed $45 billion by the year 2000 (Meili, 1993). Historically, rehabilitative services were hospital-based programs; today, medical rehabilitation is provided in a variety of inpatient and outpatient settings, in skilled nursing facilities (SNFs), comprehensive outpatient rehabilitation facilities (CORFs), and the home. As medical rehabilitation has shifted its emphasis from the care of clients with major physical or cognitive impairments resulting from catastrophic injuries and chronic health conditions to providing services to clients requiring a wide array of restorative services that enhance residual functional capacities it has grown to be an essential component of care in Western society.

Four trends are emerging in the organization of medical rehabilitation service providers:

- **Diversification**—The trend among established rehabilitation providers to offer a greater variety of services in multiple settings. This trend is driven by Medicare and managed care polices forcing providers to develop cost-effective alternatives outside the walls of the hospital.
- **Vertical integration**—The trend among providers to become vertically integrated within a larger network of health care. This trend is driven by the desire of rehabilitation providers to have a steady stream of clients. This seems to be the best established tend.
- **Horizontal integration**—The trend of rehabilitation providers to be horizontally integrated into a national multihospital or multiprovider chain. This trend is driven by the desire of the providers of service to achieve economic scale and reduce costs in a more price-competitive economy.
- **Within market consolidation**—The trend of rehabilitation providers to consolidate, merge, or forge ad hoc partnerships with competitors. This trend is driven by the excess capacity of too many existing or similar providers in a given market.

Services to the individual following illness, injury, or disease resulting in major changes in health state or disability are provided in a variety of settings over a long period of time; perhaps over the person's life time. These services can include custodial care as well as medical health care services. The goal of medical rehabilitation is to enable clients to live in the least restrictive, least costly environment at their highest level of functioning (Melvin & Zollar, 1993). Approximately 64% of discharged clients requiring rehabilitation services are people with strokes and orthopedically related conditions. Other groups of clients requiring services are clients with spinal cord injuries, brain injuries, amputations, major multiple trauma, arthritis, congenital conditions, neurological conditions, and burns. Medical rehabilitation services are also used by clients with less severe impairments who have functional limitations (Granger & Hamilton, 1992). As the number of people living with functional limitations increases and the population ages the demand for medical rehabilitation services will continue to increase (De-Jong & Sutton, 1995; Farley, 1992; Lubkin, 1995).

The rehabilitative nurse needs to be familiar with the various programs available for possible health care resources, rehabilitation programs, and income support for persons with long-term care needs. These resources can affect the nature of the rehabilitation program and care the client receives as well as the client's treatment outcomes. The availability of personal wealth, private insurance, or access to health care can be a predictor of the need for services more than the ailment itself (Colter, 1996).

Currently the focus of health services in Western medicine is directed toward immediate or urgent symptom relief and the prevention of physical complications. The need for rehabilitative and long-term care is seen as less legitimate than the need for acute episodic care because of the subjectivity, variation, and unpredictability of the relationship between treatment and outcomes. However, through advances in medical knowledge and ever-widening areas of technology we have increased the life span and extended life for those born with birth defects and surviving serious injuries. We now possess the knowledge for the eradication of several communicable diseases, learned how to perform major repair of damaged body parts, and learned to successfully remove potentially lethal tumors from the body. As a result people are now having to live with the chronic health problems and physical and psychological sequelae of those medical interventions, increasing the demand for rehabilitative services and long-term care.

For the individual the injury, illness, or disability becomes a part of life. Clients requiring rehabilitative care will cycle through a series of services. These multiple services may be more or less linked together. An integrated delivery system would include prevention services, acute care services, intermediate care services, and home care services. The range of care should be culturally and linguistically appropriate and convenient and accessible to clients. A good strategy for developing a continuum of care encompassing all levels of care may be a partnership between health care providers and social service organizations. Generally, care outside the formal system is not insured. The less acute or the farther from the hospital setting care is provided the less the likelihood of insurance reimbursement for services. Clients prefer to remain in their own home and resist institutional settings. Eighty to 85 percent of the care provided to the elderly or relatives in need of long-term care is provided in the home. The care is provided primarily by family members without reimbursement.

Costs for rehabilitation services include initial stabilization, community care agencies, counseling services, educational facilities, respite care for caretakers, and day care and homemaker services. Indirect costs include medication prescriptions, over-the-counter drugs, and other nondurable medical costs, such as bandages. In *Healthy People 2000* (1991), it is reported that the first-year cost of caring for a client with coronary bypass surgery is $30,000.00; the cost for stroke hemiplegia treatment and rehabilitation is $28,000.00; and the treatment and rehabilitation cost for severe head trauma is $310,000.00. These figures do not include nonmedical costs, such as loss of productivity to society.

The current health care delivery system does provide for increased continuity for the patient and for record keeping. However, there needs to be the opportunity for long-term clients to develop a trusting relationship with care providers. Decisions about providing rehabilitative care or reimbursement for services need to be based on individual client evaluation rather than statistics. And an appreciation of important attributes such as the need for a few additional days of rehabilitation to regain strength or palliative care needs to be factored into clinical judgment.

The complex nature of rehabilitation care makes decisions regarding the determination of benefits difficult. Those who provide reimbursement for health care services generally have a short-term time frame orientation. Their perspective focuses on the meeting of health care expenses over a period of a year or two. Unfortunately, the benefits of health promotion, illness, complication, and disability prevention; social services; and education to clients are often achieved only over a longer period of time. In rehabilitation there appears to be a greater need to provide social services and other services, such as personal care for clients and respite care for family members, which has not been established in current reimbursement and compensation systems. Evaluation of the impact of medical rehabilitation is difficult to determine. The contribution of each professional team member is difficult to assess. The provider-driven method of financing, in which rehabilitation services are partitioned into and billed by discipline service units, undermines the foundation of the interdisciplinary rehabilitation model.

Effective management of care holds the key to providing the wide range of integrated services required by clients undergoing rehabilitation and long-term care, and people with disabilities and/or chronic illnesses. To better serve these populations America's health care system needs to

- Integrate primary, preventive, and specialty care
- Coordinate medical care with home care and community-based services
- Include the client and the family in decision-making processes
- Respond to the episodic nature of chronic care
- Adjust the indicators of legitimate need for care
- Remain flexible with regard to referral for care and the mix between medical and nonmedical services
- Shift the focus from prevalence of illness to a measurement of health care used

Several themes emerge:

- The importance of integration of the illness or disability in daily life
- The importance of listening to and hearing the pain, the need, and the suffering of clients
- The importance of making choices that provide a measure of hope and control for clients
- The importance of nontechnical services
- The inadequacy of the high-technology model to focus on the whole client and nontechnical needs

Access to Health Care Resources and Services

Accessing health care resources and services has always been a challenge for those who require rehabilitation services and for those with disabilities. It is important for the rehabilitation nurse to possess knowledge and strategies to assist clients in obtaining access to care. The rehabilitation nurse must be knowledgeable regarding strategies for obtaining health care services, able to identify financial resources available to clients, and have current knowledge regarding laws governing access to health care services. The rehabilitation nurse will play an important role in assisting clients to secure health care services.

Efforts to obtain access to health care services can be strenuous and result in frustrating experiences for clients, especially those with disabilities. Two of the most significant factors influencing this experience are obstacles to obtaining services and the limited availability of health care services, especially in rural areas. Obstacles to obtaining health care services include geographic location, the high cost of transportation, limited funding for vehicular modifications, architectural barriers to physical accessibility, attitudes of discrimination by health care providers toward the elderly and the disabled, the lack of understanding about the needs of the disabled, and economic constraints.

Economic constraints can be a major obstacle to accessing health care services. Disabled individual are encouraged to be dependent on the system. Clients may have lost their medical benefits, Supplemental Security Income (SSI) or Social Security Disability Insurance (SSDI) if they are employed and earn more than the specified allowable amount. If the disabled client marries, a reduction in Social Security benefits and medical benefits is assessed. Medicare medical benefits for clients with disabilities are not available until 2 years after the onset of the disability. This discourages clients from seeking health care services and raises the possibility that clients with disabilities are without medical benefits if they do not qualify for state assistance or Medicaid. The consequence of this is that often these clients will seek health care services only when the health problems are significant and require hospitalization.

Economic constraints may also limit the client's ability to obtain needed equipment, supplies, and medications. Rehabilitation clients and those with disabilities are very dependent on insurance coverage to pay for these expensive items. Frequently there are limits on what additional equipment insurance providers will allow and it is possible that the client may be unable to obtain necessary equipment that is not available through the insurance provider. Even if the insurance provided will cover the cost of a piece of equipment, when purchasing the equipment a cash down payment may be required that would have to come from the client's personal resources.

The availability of health care services also limits access to care for clients. There are limited counseling services, especially for community-based care. Medical social worker services are usually available only through hospitals and home care agencies. Reimbursement for counseling for psychological issues related to rehabilitation or disabilities is limited. Clients with disabilities have special care needs of which health care providers may be unaware, such as special examination tables for gynecological examinations or chairs for dental examinations.

Obtaining Access to Health Care Resources and Services

Access to resources and services can be obtained by contacting state and local governmental disability offices and agencies. These agencies and departments can assist clients to obtain a variety of services to address issues of housing, transportation, employment, supportive services, and education.

1. *Housing:* Referral systems for accessible housing and public housing offer technical assistance, development, and design and building assistance, and may provide funds for the modification of private residences. They also can assist in obtaining home mortgage loans.
2. *Transportation:* Designated parking is mandated in all public parking areas for individuals with disabilities, and parking passes are available for those who transport individuals with a disability. Private transportation services may be available in some areas, and there are reduced rates on public transportation for those with disabilities.
3. *Employment:* Training and placement assistance and services and funding for workplace modification are available. Affirmative action policies exist, mandating employment opportunities for the disabled.
4. *Supportive services:* Supportive services available through public agencies and departments include information and referral, counseling, personal care assistance programs, telecommunication devices, homemaker services, augmentative communication aids, adaptive toys, assistive technology, health screening services, and funding for rehabilitation technology services and adaptive equipment.
5. *Education:* The public provides services to facilitate accessibility to educational opportunities. This is accomplished through public funding, building accessibility, therapy available in school systems, programs for disabled children, acquisition of equipment to supplement special education and training, playground accessibility, school environment modifications, and special transportation services.

Various agencies receive state funding through appropriation of monies or grants or direct reimbursement. Those agencies include *visiting nurse associations,* proprietary agencies, the *Public Health Department,* elder and adult services, and *Alpha. Vendor services,* and selective professional services and programs are also available through state funding appropriations. The types of services these agencies can provide are listed in Table 1.

Some agencies receive federal funding through appropriations of monies, grants, or direct reimbursement for services. Many of these are agencies that also receive monies appropriated on the state level (see Table 2).

Funding Resources for Health Care and Rehabilitation Services

Because of the extremely dynamic state of the current health care delivery system it is possible to provide only a general overview of the available resources providing funding for health care and rehabilitation services. This section identifies existing federal and state public sources and private sector resources.

Federal Programs

Federal programs providing funding for rehabilitation programs include (1) Medicare and (2) Medicaid.

Table 1
State Funding Sources and Community Resources

Type of Agency	Services Provided through the Agency
Visiting nurse association (VNA)	Skilled nursing
	Physical, occupational, and speech therapy
	Medical social worker
	Hospice care
	Home health aid services
	Homemaker services
	Contracted services
Proprietary agency services (for profit)	Nursing, RN, LVN (LPN) aid
	Homemaker services
	Private duty nursing
Public Health Department	Nursing
	Food stamps
	Program for Women, Infants, and Children (WIC)
	Clinics
	Vocational rehabilitation services
	Adult and child protective services
	Mental health services
Elder and adult services	Information and referral
	Homemaker funding
	Transportation funding
	Nutrition program and funding for meals
	Sensor companion services
	Psychiatric services
	Nursing home assessments
Alpha: Member of National Council on Independent Living; funded through state and federal monies	Attendant programs
	Adaptive equipment loan program
	Independent living programs
	Access design consultation
	Environmental access loans and grants
	Client advocacy, peer support
	Adapted vehicle driving evaluation and education
	Monitoring of access issues
	Filing of complaints or litigation for violation in providing access for the disabled

Table 1
State Funding Sources and Community Resources (Continued)

Type of Agency	Services Provided through the Agency
Vendor services	Durable medical equipment
	Intravenous therapy
	Chemotherapy
	Medical supplies
	Oxygen and/or ventilator services
	Nutrition-related services
	Enteral feedings
Selective professional services	Physican office and home visits
	Inpatient and outpatient hospital services
	Mobile medical services
	Outpatient phlebotomy services
	Eye care cards
	Adult drug cards
	Counseling services
Special programs	Adult day care and day treatment programs
	Hospice care
	Prosthetic and orthotic devices
	Supervised environmental living

Medicare is a federal funding program created under Title XVIII of the Social Security Act of 1965. Medicare is the single largest payer of medical rehabilitation services and has been a driving force in shaping the delivery of medical rehabilitation services (DeJong & Sutton, 1995). Retired workers (and spouses) over 65 years of age and workers who have been disabled for two or more years are eligible for Medicare coverage. Since its creation in the mid-1960s the federal government has become the largest payer of health care in the United States (Letsch, 1993). The program operates under the authority of the U.S. Department of Health and Human Services (DHHS). There are three types of health insurance included in this federal program: a compulsory program of hospital insurance (Part A), a voluntary program of supplementary medical insurance (Part B), and special programs (e.g., for end-stage renal disease) (Part C). Each of the insurance plans included in Medicare is managed by the Health Care Financing Administration (HCFA). The HCFA designates regional intermediaries to process insurance claims.

Medicaid is a federal funding program created under Title XIX of the Social Security Act of 1965. Medicaid is the single largest payer of nursing home care

Table 2
Federal Funding Sources and Resources

Type of Agency	Services Provided through the Agency
Veterans Affairs services	Inpatient and outpatient hospital services
	Pharmacy services
	Nursing home services
	Home health services
	Orthotic and prosthetic devices
	Durable medical and adaptive equipment
	Services for the visually impaired
	Vocational rehabilitation services
	Home modifications
	Mortgage loans
Elder and adult services: Recipients must be more than 62 years of age	Respite care
	Light housekeeping
	Companion program
Assistance based on age, income, and disability	Health services at public clinic
	Adult drug cards
	Eye cards
	Subsidized housing
	Utility and telephone rebates
	"Meals on Wheels" program
	Talking books

in the United States (DeJong & Sutton, 1995). The purpose of the Medicaid program is to provide grants to state for medical assistance programs.

State Programs   State programs include Medicaid and Workers' Compensation systems.

Medicaid programs, unlike Medicare programs, are designed and operated by individual states. The programs are developed and administered by individual states under broad federal guidelines. Eligibility for Medicaid programs is established by each of the fifty states. Funds are distributed to those each individual state designates as those who are "medically needy." Certain groups are federally mandated for support (e.g., children from age 1 to 6 years of age are enrolled in Aid to Families with Dependent Children [AFDC] programs). These programs generally cover costs associated with hospitalization and visits to physicians. They also provide for care in skilled nursing facilities.

Financing for Medicaid programs is shared by both state and federal governments. States are reimbursed at a rate of 50–75 percent of actual cost of health care. Medicaid represents only one-third of federal health spending but Medicaid expenditures have been increasing. Because each state dictates income eligibility for Medicaid insurance only about one-half of the nation's poor receive Medicaid funding (Congressional Budget Office, 1992).

Workers' Compensation systems are administered by states. Workers' Compensation is available to workers disabled by work-related injury. It is also available to families of workers whose death was the result of, or occurred in the course of, their employment. The systems are administered within individual states. A state's Worker's Compensation law will be administered by that state's Department of Labor, an independent workers' compensation agency, or the court. The program provides both medical care related to the compensable injury and income benefits. Income sources can be provided through private commercial insurance companies, self-insurance from companies who can carry their own risk, or state injury funds.

Medical care compensation provided through Workers' Compensation includes treatment and rehabilitating programs for work-related injury and full (or, in certain states, partial) reimbursement according to a fee guide. Vocational rehabilitation benefits are also available through some Workers' Compensation systems. The majority of states do have provisions for education, job retraining, and job placement.

Private Health Care Insurance

Private health care insurance provides health care and rehabilitation services to those who are policyholders. A policyholder can be an individual who pays premiums or an employer who pays full or partial premiums to an insurance carrier. Various types of insurance plans are available: contractual plans with variable deductibles (Blue Cross), **health maintenance organizations (HMOs), preferred provider organizations (PPOs),** the **Medicare Supplemental Benefits Plan (Medigap),** and **automobile liability policies,** which cover medical care needs resulting from an automobile accident. Each of these insurance plans will have different eligibility requirements and benefits coverage. Clients who receive health care insurance through the private sector will have to investigate benefit options available to them through individual insurers.

Programs for Special Groups

Programs for special groups are also available. These include

1. Veterans of the armed forces (Veterans Affairs, VA): This program, administered by the Veterans Benefits Administration, provides coverage either for treatment of an armed service-related disability or for needy veterans who have non-service-related disabilities.
2. Federal government civilian employee workers' compensation programs.
3. Railroad Retirement Act Program

4. The Black Lung Act of 1972
5. The Longshoreman and Harbor Workers' Compensation Act

Income Support Programs and Supplemental Funding Resources

Many clients will require long-term or short-term funding resources and/or income support. These income and funding resources are also available from the federal and state public sector or the private sector.

Social Security Programs

Social Security is the primary federal income funding resource. *Social Security income insurance* consists of two programs. One program is the Old Age and Survivors Insurance (OASI) and Disability Insurance program. Retired workers who are 65 years of age are eligible for program benefits. The minimum age for benefit eligibility will increase to 66 years of age in the year 2009. Reduced benefits are available to workers who retire at 62 years of age and to a widow(er) or a surviving divorced spouse of a retired worker.

Retired workers are eligible for "fully insured status" if they have worked under the OASI program and have paid into the program for a minimum of 10 years. Under the OASI program 1 year of employment equals 4 credits with a total of 40 credits necessary for full benefits. Currently, benefits are paid as an earned right. There is no minimum income during active employment years to receive income benefits. Social Security income benefits are not influenced by the receipt of other income resources. There is also no limit placed on other income sources, including saving, pensions, or retirement plans.

The second income funding program is the Social Security Disability Insurance program. The regulations for administration of this program are established by the U.S. Secretary of Health and Human Services. The disabled worker must be under 65 years of age. To be eligible for income funding from this program the individual must be determined to be so severely impaired physically or mentally that there is the inability to perform substantial gainful work (Jehle, 1992). Individuals seeking Social Security Disability benefits must have attained "fully insured status." Applicants requesting benefits are referred to the state's health department and/or to agencies for vocational rehabilitation services. Specific benefits vary in individual states.

State Disability Programs

States also provide various forms of income and resource funding. Workers' Compensation insurance is available for individuals with conditions, disability, or death that are work related. The individual's benefits are usually calculated as a percentage of worker's weekly earnings at the time of injury or death. Some states make a stipulation of a maximum number of weeks for receiving benefits. There may also be a waiting period before the individual can begin receiving benefits.

The types of income benefits available under Workers' Compensation plans are numerous and vary by state. Specific levels of funding and benefits are established for each of the compensation catagories:

1. Temporary total disability—The worker is disabled for a temporary period but is expected to recover
2. Permanent total disability—The worker is disabled permanently and unable to perform any type of work
3. Temporary partial disability—The worker is able to work but has diminished capacity for productivity
4. Permanent partial disability—The worker is able to work but has a defined or estimated partial impairment
5. Survivor—Payments are made to a spouse until remarriage and to children until they are 18 years of age.

Federal and State Supplemental Programs

Several federal and state income programs are also available. These additional programs include Aid to Families with Dependent Children; food stamps; supplemental food for women, infants, and children (WIC); public housing and subsidized housing; and state general assistance and welfare programs.

Private Sector Income and Resource Funding Programs

Individuals can also invest in a variety of private retirement and/or disability income insurance plans. These plans are voluntary investments and the plans may be purchased by the individual, the individual's employer, or by a labor or professional union or association.

Certain types of automobile insurance benefits exist for injury, disability, or death resulting from incidents involving automobiles. These plans can provide no-fault automobile insurance, automobile liability insurance, and hospital indemnity insurance benefits. They can provide general liability benefits for personal injury, accidental death and dismemberment, or wrongful death. Some companies offer benefit plans that provide mortgage and credit disability insurance benefits in the event of injury, disability, or death related to an automobile accident.

Nursing Interventions

1. Identify agencies that provide free care or charge based on the client's ability to pay and duration of service needed.
2. Co-ordinate home care agency referrals between private and not for profit agencies.
3. Contact the state department of human services, and the state disability office, commission, or department to identify services available.
4. Educate the client and family members on issues of health care accessibility.
5. Promote interagency communication regarding rehabilitation needs.
6. Act as a community and political advocate.

Conclusion

The rehabilitation nurse must take an active role in assisting clients to maximize their access to health care services and resources. The rehabilitation nurse should be aware of the client's access needs and educate both the client and family members to empower them to obtain access to health care services and resources. Many nursing interventions to increase client access to services and resources will be done in conjunction with other members of the interdisciplinary rehabilitation team. The nurse needs to monitor and co-ordinate efforts of social services, rehabilitation counselors, and community agencies. The rehabilitation nurse should be aware of the client's access needs and educate both the client and family members to empower them to obtain access to health care services and resources.

References

American Hospital Association. (1992). *A healthier America: Reforming our health care system.* Chicago: Author.

Colter, M. (Ed.). (1996). Perspectives on chronic illness: Treating patients and delivering care. *American Behavioral Scientist, 39*(6). Thousand Oaks: Sage.

Congressional Budget Office. (1992). *Projections of national health expenditures.* Washington, DC: Author.

Congressional Budget Office. (1993). *Trends in health spending: An update.* Washington, DC: Author.

DeJong, G., & Sutton, J. P. (1995). Rehab 2000: The evolution of medical rehabilitation in American health care. In P. K. Landrum, N. D. Schmidt, & A. McLean (Eds.), *Outcome-oriented rehabilitation: Principles, strategies, and tools for effective program management.* Baltimore, MD: Aspen.

Farley, A. M. (1992). *Nursing and the disabled across the life span.* Boston: Jones and Bartlett Publishers.

Granger, C., & Hamilton, B. (1994). The uniform data system for medical rehabilitation reports of first admission for 1992. *American Journal of Physical Medical Rehabilitation, 73*(1), 51–55.

Jehle, F. F. (1992). *The complete and easy guide to Social Security and Medicare* (9th ed.). Charlotte, VT: Williamson.

Letsch, S. (1993). National health care spending 1991. *Health Affairs, 21*(1), 94–110.

Lubkin, I. M. (1995). *Chronic illness impact and interventions* (3rd ed.). Boston: Jones and Bartlett Publishers.

Melvin, J., & Zollar, C. (Eds.). (1993). *A focus for the health care reform debate.* Washington, DC: National Association of Rehabilitation Facilities.

Meili, P. (1993). The rehabilitation market. *Rehabilitation Management,* April/May, 96–102.

U.S. Department of Health and Human Services, (1991). *Healthy People 2000: National promotion and disease prevention objectives.* Washington, DC: Author.

Wieseke, A., & Bantz, D. (1992). Economic awareness of registered nurses employed in hospitals. *Nursing Economics, 10*(6), 406–412.

Suggested Readings

American Hospital Association. (1987). *Directory of national self-help and mutual aid resources.* Evanston, IL: Self-Help Center.

Enders, A. (1990). Funding for assistive technology and related services: An annotated bibliography. *Physical and Occupational Therapy in Pediatrics, 10*(2), 147–173.

Folland, S., Goodman, A., & Stano, M. (1993). *The economics of health and health care.* New York: Macmillan.

Ginzberg, E. (1990). High-tech medicine and rising health care costs. *Journal of the American Medical Association, 263*(13), 1820–1822.

Groch, S. A. (1991). Public services available to persons with disabilities in major U.S. cities. *Journal of Rehabilitation, 57*(3), 23–26.

Henry, W. (1991). Managing chronic health conditions is a critical need ignored by many. *Trustee, 46*(30), 20–21.

Landay, E. (Ed.). (1990). *The complete Medicare handbook*. Rocklin, CA: Prima.

Pell, A. E. (1990). *Making the most of Medicare: A guide through the Medicare maze*. Minneapolis, MN: DCI Publishing.

Pope, A., & Taylor, A. R. (Eds.). (1991). *Disability in America*. Washington, DC: National Academy Press.

Resources for Rehabilitation. (1991). *Resources for people with disabilities and chronic conditions*. Lexington, MA: Author.

Index

Page numbers in **boldface** are pages on which a figure appears; page numbers in *italic* are pages on which a table appears.

3

ISBN 0-07-105482-0

90000